Non-Flavivirus Encephalitis

Non-Flavivirus Encephalitis

Edited by **Roy McClen**

hayle medical

New York

Published by Hayle Medical,
30 West, 37th Street, Suite 612,
New York, NY 10018, USA
www.haylemedical.com

Non-Flavivirus Encephalitis
Edited by Roy McClen

International Standard Book Number: 978-1-63241-300-0 (Hardback)

Printed in China.

Contents

	Preface	**VII**
Part 1	**General Problems of Epidemiology**	**1**
Chapter 1	**Zoonotic and Animal Vector Mediated Encephalitides** Colleen Mikelson and Sean Richards	**3**
Chapter 2	**Zoonoses Surveillance in Italy (2000-2009): Investigation on Animals with Neurological Symptoms** Cristina Casalone, Barbara Iulini, Maria Domenica Pintore, Cristiana Maurella, Elena Bozzetta, Carlo Cantile, Gualtiero Gandini, Maria Teresa Capucchio, Arianna Calistri, Antonio D'angelo and Maria Caramelli	**29**
Part 2	**Viral Pathogens**	**59**
Chapter 3	**Virus-Induced Encephalitis and Innate Immune Responses – A Focus on Emerging or Re-Emerging Viruses** Melanie Denizot, Vincent G. Thon-Hon, Shiril Kumar, Jim W. Neal and Philippe Gasque	**61**
Chapter 4	**Herpes Simplex Type 1 Encephalitis** Feyzi Birol Sarica	**87**
Chapter 5	**Virology and Pathology of Encephalitis in Alien Hosts by Neurotropic Equine Herpesvirus 9** Hideto Fukushi and Tokuma Yanai	**111**
Chapter 6	**Blood-Brain Barrier Disruption and Encephalitis in Animal Models of AIDS** Nicole A. Renner, Andrew A. Lackner and Andrew G. MacLean	**131**
Chapter 7	**Equine Herpesvirus 9 (EHV-9) Induced Encephalitis in Nonhuman Primates** Tokuma Yanai, Atsushi Kodama, Hiroki Sakai, Hideto Fukushi, Takeshi Kuraishi, Seisaku Hattori and Chieko Kai	**147**

Chapter 8	**Coronaviruses as Encephalitis - Inducing Infectious Agents** Pierre J. Talbot, Marc Desforges, Elodie Brison and Hélène Jacomy	157
Chapter 9	**Subacute Sclerosing Panencephalitis and Other Lethal Encephalitis Caused by Measles Virus Infection: Pathogenesis and New Approaches to Treatment** Fernandez-Muñoz R., Carabaña J. Caballero M., Ortego J., Liton P.B., Duque B.M, Martin-Cortes A., Serrano-Pardo A., Muñoz-Alia M.A., Porras-Mansilla R., Alvarez-Cermeño J.C. and Celma M.L.	175
Chapter 10	**Encephalitic Development in Alphaviral Infection** Slobodan Paessler and Katherine Taylor	203
Chapter 11	**Human Rabies Epidemiology and Diagnosis** Brett W. Petersen and Charles E. Rupprecht	247
Part 3	**Protozoan Pathogens**	279
Chapter 12	**Toxoplasmic Encephalitis** Yaowalark Sukthana	281
Chapter 13	**Encephalitis Due to Free Living Amoebae: An Emerging Issue in Human Health** Jacob Lorenzo-Morales, Carmen Mª Martín-Navarro, Enrique Martínez-Carretero, José E. Piñero and Basilio Valladares	307
Chapter 14	**Autoimmunity in the Mediation of Granulomatous Amoebic Encephalitis: Implications for Therapy** Chandirasegaran Massilamany and Jay Reddy	317
Part 4	**Multicellular Pathogens**	339
Chapter 15	**Encephalitis Due to *Loa loa*** Jean Paul Akue	341
	Permissions	
	List of Contributors	

Preface

Non-flavivirus encephalitis is a group of disorders involving chronic inflammation of the brain other than the ones caused by the flavivirus genes. This is a comprehensive book which encompasses the various aspects of non-flavivirus encephalitises of distinct etiology and discusses the basic problems of epidemiology like the analysis of zoonotic and animal vectors of encephalitis causative agents and methodologies as well as approaches for encephalitis zoonoses investigations. The members of various virus species are considered as the causative agents of this disorder, and these viral pathogens, their pathology, epidemiology, diagnostics and molecular mechanisms of encephalitis development by such viruses as SIV/HIV, measles virus, alphaviruses, herpes simplex virus type 1 and equine herpesvirus 9, coronaviruses and rhabdovirus have been discussed in this insightful book. The book also presents the analysis of protozoan pathogens like amoebae and toxoplasma and multicellular pathogens like human Filaria Loa Loa - a filarial worm restricted to the West Africa.

This book is a result of research of several months to collate the most relevant data in the field.

When I was approached with the idea of this book and the proposal to edit it, I was overwhelmed. It gave me an opportunity to reach out to all those who share a common interest with me in this field. I had 3 main parameters for editing this text:

1. Accuracy - The data and information provided in this book should be up-to-date and valuable to the readers.
2. Structure - The data must be presented in a structured format for easy understanding and better grasping of the readers.
3. Universal Approach - This book not only targets students but also experts and innovators in the field, thus my aim was to present topics which are of use to all.

Thus, it took me a couple of months to finish the editing of this book.

I would like to make a special mention of my publisher who considered me worthy of this opportunity and also supported me throughout the editing process. I would also like to thank the editing team at the back-end who extended their help whenever required.

Editor

Part 1

General Problems of Epidemiology

1

Zoonotic and Animal Vector Mediated Encephalitides

Colleen Mikelson and Sean Richards
University of Tennessee Chattanooga
United States of America

1. Introduction

When discussing human diseases in general, the majority (61%) of them are zoonotic, or are able to be transferred between animals and humans (Taylor et al., 2001), either through the bite of an arthropod, exposure to the pathogen through direction contact with animal products (urine, feces, milk, afterbirth) or when humans are a part of the pathogen's life cycle directly. In regard to diseases that are considered emerging, 75% of them are zoonotic (Taylor et al., 2001), which places more weight on the study of these pathogens and their evolution in order to better understand the risk of infection to a new host (Alexander and Day, 2010). This chapter is designed to give the reader an overview of the wide array of pathogenic etiologies, whether viral, bacterial or parasitic, that have the potential to develop into encephalitis, though in some cases, this is a rare side effect, or limited to specific groups (i.e., immunecompromised individuals). Of these diseases, all have a life cycle intimately connected with an animal vector or host in some way. Some disorders are very well known and studied as a means of vector transmitted encephalitis (e.g., Eastern Equine Encephalitis), while others are just emerging as serious health risks associated with encephalitic symptoms (e.g., Chandipura Virus Encephalitis, Nipah and Henipa virus).

2. Viral related diseases

Viral infections are important in the induction of encephalitis. Arboviruses are transmitted by arthropods (e.g., mosquitoes, ticks, sand flies) and are maintained through biological transmission between a vertebrate host (Kuno & Chang, 2005). Biological transmission of such a pathogen involves several factors (Reviewed by Scott, 1988). The virus must be able to reproduce in both the arthropod and vertebrate host, then be able to produce a high enough viral titer in the blood of the vertebrate to be passed back to the vector Reviewed by Scott, 1988). It is well known that RNA viruses tend to have a high mutation rate because of unfaithful replication in host cells, among other things (Domingo, 1997). However, to maintain a relationship with both vertebrate and arthropod vectors, observed mutation rates are reduced, as is with New World Alpha viruses (Weaver et al., 1991). When selective pressures are applied to the virus between two alternating hosts, the virus population responds with adaptations fit for both environments in order to optimize suitability in a dual host system (Weaver et al., 1999; Cooper & Scott, 2001).

These viruses can be maintained in either a zoonotic or an epizootic cycle; the former involving endemic birds, rodents or non-human primates as reservoir hosts (Weaver et al., 1999), the latter is involved in epidemics or outbreaks of the disease in livestock or humans. Reservoir hosts are abundant and readily available in the vector habitat, are attractive to the vector as a potential host, and allow for viral replication sufficient to infect previously uninfected vectors, but low enough to prevent a fatal infection (Scott, 1988). Epidemics of these diseases arise when efficient bridge vectors are able to pass on the virus to new, and potentially dead-ended, hosts (e.g. humans) (Weaver et al., 1999; Armstrong & Theodore, 2010). Also critical to the success of viral transmission is the vector competence, or the ability of the vector to successfully infect a new host with the virus; moreover the vector is able to become infected with the pathogen from wild caught samples, able to efficiently bite the host, and the presence of the virus detectable in wild-caught vertebrate samples (Sudia et al., 1969). But these viruses are not limited to arthropod transfer. Other viruses are linked to bats and other wild animals to ensure their survival. The viral families included in this review are Arenaviridae, Bunyaviridae, Flaviviridae, Paramyxoviridae, Rhabdoviridae and Togaviridae.

2.1 Family Arenaviridae: Lymphocytic Choriomeningitis (LCM) Virus

The Arenaviridae are a family of viruses whose members are generally associated with rodent-transmitted disease in humans. The Lymphocytic Choriomeningitis (LCM) Virus is released in mouse urine and feces, as well as nasal secretions, saliva, milk and semen. The infectious route can be through direct contact with infected items or inhalation of aerosolized virus particles. Hamsters and guinea pigs are other rodent that can be infected (Barton & Mets, 2001). Meningoencephalitis was reported by Barton and Hyndman (2000) after infection with Lymphocytic Choriomeningitis Virus. Maternal infection has been shown to produce teratogenic effects (Larsen et al., 1993; Barton et al., 1995; Bonthius & Perlman, 2007).

2.2 Bunyaviridae Family: Californian Serogroup, Toscana Virus and Rift Valley Fever Virus

2.2.1 Californian Serogroup: Jamestown Canyon and La Cross Virus

The Jamestown Canyon Virus is endemic to Michigan and is primarily transmitted by *Aedes stimulans* (Woodland mosquito) with the white tail deer as its preferred host, and is able to pass the virus transovarially (Boromisa & Grimstad, 1986; Zamparo et al., 1997). In one study, 27% of the population showed specific neutralizing antibody to the virus (Grimstad et al., 1986), however this virus has been detected along the east coast of the U.S. as well (Zamparo et al., 1997). Fatal cases of encephalitis have been reported (Grimstad et al., 1982). The La Cross virus is transmitted through *Ochlerotatus triseriatus* (Eastern treehole mosquito) as well as *Ae. albopictus* (Tiger mosquito) in Tennessee (Erwin et al., 2002) with small rodent hosts primarily in the Midwest and southern Appalachian region (Georgiev, 2009). Numerous outbreaks of the virus have been reported (Rust et al., 1999; McJunkin et al., 2001).

2.2.2 Toscana Virus

The Toscana virus (TOSV) (genus *Phlebovirus*), is located primarily in the Mediterranean. It was first isolated in Italy, with subsequent cases in Spain, Portugal, France, Greece, Portugal and Germany and Cyprus (Charrel et al., 2005). The sandfly, *Phlebotomus perniciosus* is the primary vector and reservoir, with no connection yet as to a specific mammalian or avian host (Charrel et al., 2005). Occupational exposure to sandfly habitat correlated with seroprevalence of the virus, with up to 77.2% of the forestry workers testing positive for the antibody (Valassina et al., 2003). This virus is responsible for encephalitis complications, without accompanying meningitis (Dionisio et al., 2001; Valassina et al., 2003).

2.2.3 Rift Valley Fever Virus

Rift Valley Fever Virus (RVFV) is named from the region of Kenya from which it was first isolated (Daubney et al., 1931). A wide range of mosquito genera have been shown to maintain the enzoonic cycle (e.g., *Aedes, Ochlerotatus, Stegomyia, Anopheles, Culex, Neomelaniconion, Eretmapodites)*, with *Aedes vexans* and *Culex erraticus* showing successful transmission to other animals to serve as bridge vectors (as reviewed by Pfeffer and Dobler (2010)). Infection in pregnant ruminants induces abortion at all stages of pregnancy to the magnitude that this event is referred to as an "abortion storm" (Kasari et al., 2008). Aborted fetuses, birthing material and body fluids of infected animals carry high viral loads and contact with these materials is a possible pathway for human infection (Pepin et al., 2010). Encephalitis was reported in outbreaks in Egypt and Saudi Arabia (Laughlin et al., 1979; Madani et al., 2003).

2.3 Flaviviridae Family: Japanese Encephalitis Virus Serogroup, Tick Borne Encephalitis and Dengue Fever Encephalitis

2.3.1 Japanese Encephalitis Virus Serogroup: Japanese, St. Louis, and Australian Encephalitis Virus and West Nile Virus

With over 50,000 cases occurring each year, the Japanese Encephalitis Virus (JEV) is responsible for the most cases of epidemic encephalitis worldwide (Weaver & Barrett, 2004). Pigs are suspected to be the main amplification host for the virus involving human infection due to their proximity to human habitation. Ardeid birds (e.g., herons and egrets) serve as the natural hosts. The mosquito vector, *Culex tritaeniorhynchus,* feeds on all hosts (birds, pigs and humans) and finds suitable habitat in the flooded rice paddies of Southeast Asia. Humans and horses are susceptible, but are considered dead end hosts (reviewed by Pfeffer and Dobler (2010)).

The primary vectors for the St. Louis Encephalitis Virus (SLEV) are *Cx. Pipiens* and *Cx. Quinquefasciatus,* in the western U.S., *Cx. Tarsalis,* and *Cx. Nigripalpus* in Florida. Various birds serve as reservoirs (McLean et al., 1993; Georgiev, 2009). Outbreaks have been reported in almost every American state, along with Canada, and Central and South America (Calisher, 1994). Evidence suggests that SLEV was introduced into North America from South America and is locally circulated. Sequence comparisons from various strains show that the overall genome sequence is more conserved than other members of the Japanese serogroup (May et al., 2008). Basal diversification northward is estimated to have initiated around 177-247 years ago (Baillie et al., 2008). Vertical transmission of the St. Louis virus was studied by Flores et al. (2010). Vertical transmission is used as an overwinter mechanism for *Culex quinquefasciatus* in the temperate areas of Argentina, where St. Louis encephalitis is endemic. Lab studies confirmed that larva and adults both are capable of acquiring the virus.

Australian Encephalitis can be caused by two viral agents, the Murray Valley Encephalitis Virus or Kunjin Virus, which are distributed in both Australia and Papua New Guinea. In Western Australia, the virus is monitored through the testing of serum from sentinel chickens (Hall et al., 1995). The virus is focused in the western part of the country, linked to the growth of the primary mosquito vector, *Culex annulirostris.* This habitat also supports important reservoir species, wading birds, of which, the rufous night heron (*Nycticorax caledonicus*) is of particular importance (as reviewed by Russell et al. (2000)). The last outbreak of the disease was in 1974; 22 patients were admitted, with four deaths reported, but eleven recovered without lasting effects (Bennett, 1976). In 2000, the wet season brought record breaking rainfall, increasing the breeding ground for the vector which resulted in nine cases of encephalitis in Western Australia. A survey of sentinel chickens showed that the virus was moving southward and human infections were outside a previously determined enzootic area. New monitoring boundaries were established for the disease after this outbreak occurred (Broom et al., 2002).

West Nile Virus (WNV) was first isolated from the West Nile region of Uganda, with a relatively recent emergence of the virus in the U.S., first infecting several birds in a New York City zoo, which displayed meningoencephalitis and myocarditis. From these samples, nationwide awareness of the virus was sparked and linked to extensive bird mortality in the U.S. (Briese et al., 1999; Hayes, 2001; McLean et al., 2001). Further investigation using antigenic mapping and phylogenetic analysis linked the origin of the virus to Israel, isolated from a deceased goose (Lanciotti et al., 1999). The cycle is maintained between birds, mainly passerine, and *Culex sp.*, which serves as the predominate vector (as reviewed by Pfeffer and Dobler (2010)). Central nervous system infection can result in encephalitic onset in approximately 1% of the patients (Solomon et al., 2003).

2.3.2 Tick Borne Encephalitis and Powassan virus

There are three main groups of Tick Borne Encephalitis Virus (TBEV): Western (Central, eastern and northern Europe), Siberian (Russia, eastern Europe), Far-Eastern (Eurasia, Asia and Japan) and one main group of Powassan virus (North America, Far eastern Russia), all of which have been reported to be the causative agent in meningoencephalitis (reviewed by Günther & Haglund (2005)). The virus is transmitted by Ixodes ticks (*Ix. Ricinus* and *Ix. Persulcatu*) and small rodents (*Myodes* and *Apodemus*) (Pfeffer & Dobler, 2010). Because of a tick's extended feeding time on a host, high viral titers in the parasite's saliva glands are not necessary for successful pathogen transmission and enable another means of infecting ticks attached in the same area. Saliva-assisted transmission (SAT) occurs between ticks of close proximity by pharmacological active molecules released into the wound site, which facilitates co-feeding, allowing for passage of the virus from tick to tick in close proximity to each other (Kaufman, 2010). Human and domesticated animals are not considered to be reservoirs, so passage from tick to tick is an important part of the pathogenic cycle (Pfeffer & Dobler, 2010). The Powassan Virus, originally known as Deer Tick Virus, has had several outbreaks, mainly in North America (New York, Ontario and Quebec) that have lead to encephalitic onset of those infected (Gholam et al., 1999). This virus has three distinct enzootic cycles: *Ix. cookei* and woodchucks and mustelids, *Ix. marxi* and squirrels, and *Ix. Scapularis* and white-footed mice (Ebel, 2009).

2.3.3 Dengue Fever Encephalitis

There are four serotypes of the Dengue Fever Virus (DEN-1-4). In this lifecycle, humans serve as the amplifying host and are able to re-infect new female mosquitoes (*Ae. aegypti* in urban areas, *Ae. Albopictus* in suburban/rural areas) (Becker et al., 2010). Central nervous system involvement is suspected to be responsible for potential encephalitic onset (Lum et al., 1996; Muzaffar et al., 2006). The wide geographical breath of this disease puts approximately 2.5 billion people as risk of disease contraction (WHO, 2009).

2.4 Paramyxoviridae Family: Hendra and Nipah Viruses

Both Hendra (formerly equine morbillivirus) and Nipah are emerging encephalitic viruses. Though first associated with equine infection in 1994, other human fatal human cases followed in Australia (O'Sullivan et al., 1997). Flying foxes or fruit bats (genus *Pteropus*) serve as the virus reservoir (Halpin et al., 2000), while transmission to domestic animals (horses, pigs, cows) allows for virus amplification and a pathway for human infection. Domesticated animals are suspected to become infected with the virus after contact with bat urine, discarded fruit or birthing material (as reviewed by Wang et al. (2008)). Bats themselves transfer the virus both horizontally through feces, urine or saliva (Plowright et al., 2008) and can be passed through the placenta (Williamson et al., 2000).

Nipah virus is another highly fatal paramyxovirus transmitted by bats with a domesticated livestock amplification host (Harcourt et al., 2000; Epstein et al., 2006). The first outbreak was among pig farmers in Malaysia (Mohd Nor et al., 2000), and further south into Singapore (Paton et al., 1999), in 1998-1999. The Malaysia outbreak showed no spill over from its pig farming source, with a morality rate of 40% of infected people. The second, more severe outbreak was in Bandladesh, with a mortality rate of 75%. This strain of Nipah was shown to be different than the Malaysian strain, and characterized by its lack of amplifying host (Epstein et al., 2006) and ability to be transferred from human to human, supported by in increased risk of infection when cohabitating with an infected individual (Vincent P. Hsu, 2004). Pig to pig transmission is through inhalation of aerosolized virus particles and is highly infectious (Mohd Nor et al., 2000). Similar to Hendra, partially eaten fruit from an infected bat is a possible mechanism to initial infection in pigs, due to significant viral presence in bat saliva, or through contact with bat urine (Chua et al., 2002). The farm where the first outbreak occurred had numerous fruit trees, a major attractant for the bats (Chua et al., 2002). More recent studies looked at date palm sap, commonly consumed by humans and bats. Harvesting season coincided with the Banglash outbreak, so Salah et al. (2011) experiment with physical barriers to restrict bat consumption and help curb the spillover into humans facilitated by consumption of contaminated date palm sap.

2.5 Rhabdoviridae Family: Rabies and Chandipura virus and Australian bat lyssavirus (ABLV)

The rabies virus (genus *Lyssavirus*) is still an important cause of fatal cases of encephalitis (Mallewa et al., 2007). The most likely route for human infection is through bite wound, where the virus contaminated saliva enters into the bloodstream of the new host. The virus can also be obtained through mucous membrane passage or virus inhalation from bat-infested caves. The only documented human-human transfer was via corneal transplant (as reviewed by Krebs et al. (1995)). Rabies infections have largely been brought under control in developing countries through the vaccination of domestic dogs, though dogs bites in developing countries is the main pathway of human infection. Raccoons (Smith et al., 1995), as well as bats (silver-haired and eastern pipistrelle) are the most common animals to be infected in the U.S., with bats presenting more cryptic cases of rabies infections due to a lack of obvious bite wounds (Messenger et al., 2002). Mutations of the virus through serial passes through hosts can create quasispecies, suggesting a mechanism to the accommodation to a novel hosts (Morimoto et al., 1998; Kissi et al., 1999). Bourhy et al. (1999) showed, through an analysis of European strains of the virus, local genetic differentiation is taking place, facilitated by physical barriers. Evidence suggests substitution rates in the nucleoprotein gene is related to its infection adaption in bats (Hughes et al., 2005).

One of the lesser known viral encephalides is the Chandipura virus (genus *Vesiculovirus*). Even though it is not well reported in the literature (Van Ranst, 2004), it was responsible for considerable encephalitic outbreaks in India in the last decade, in 2003 and again in 2007 (Rao et al., 2004; Narasimha Rao et al., 2008; Gurav et al., 2010). Viral transmission is through Phlebotomid sandflies (genus *Sergentomyia)* (Mavale et al., 2005) and is mainly found in India, but has also been isolated from sand flies in West Africa (Fontenille et al., 1994). The potential and need for further research in this emerging human pathogen is great (Potharaju & Potharaju, 2006).

Australian bat lyssavirus (ABLV) is another encephalitic virus found in Pteropid bats, and as the name implies, this rabies-like virus is found in Australia (Warrilow et al., 2002). Two fatal encephalitis cases were confirmed to be caused by ABLV. The first in 1996 from an animal handler (Allworth et al., 1996); the second had been bitten by a flying fox (Hanna et al., 2000). Serologic testing done in the Philippines suggest that this virus is also present there, though no active infections were found in the bats sampled (Arguin et al., 2007).

2.6 Togaviridae Family: Old and New World Alpha Viruses

Alpha viruses have been delineated as either New or Old World, depending on their geographical distribution; New World being primarily in the Americas, while Old World is in the Africa, Europe, Asia and Australia (Paredes et al., 2005). Besides their spatial differences, these viruses typically manifest different disease characteristics. Old World infections usually are more benign, with rash and arthritic symptoms, while the New World alpha virus infections can result in febrile disease with possible encephalitis onset (Paredes et al., 2005). However, several Old World viruses have showed to develop into encephalitis, with Chikungunya virus (CHIKV) and a variant of Semliki Forest virus (SFV) as such examples.

2.6.1 Old World: Chikungunya, Me Tri and Ross River Virus

Chikungunya Virus (CHIKV) was first isolated in Africa, with outbreaks reported in the Congo and Senegal (Diallo et al., 1999; Pastorino et al., 2004). CHIKV is transmitted by gallery forest mosquitoes, from wild forest primates and rodents (genus *Aedes*) (Diallo et al., 1999). Outbreaks of the virus in La Réunion, an island in the south Pacific followed by wide spread infection in India, Sri Lanka and Indonesia, resulted in considerable central nervous system involvement, including encephalitis (Rampal et al., 2007; Robin et al., 2008; Rajapakse et al., 2010), with human-human transmission facilitated mainly by *Aedes aegypti* in urban areas (Lahariya & Pradhan, 2006). A similar Old World Virus that has shown encephalitis onset is Me Tri virus, first isolated from *Culex tritaeniorhynchus* mosquitoes in the Me Tri Village of North Vietnam (Ha et al., 1995), though later it was classified as a Semliki Forest Virus (SFV) variant that had undergone homologous recombination, though this is the first variant of SFV outside of Africa (Tan et al., 2008). Ross River Virus is also an Old World alpha virus, suspect of encephalitic onset, though causation is lacking as to whether or not those isolated incidents were truly caused by Ross River virus (Harley et al., 2001).

2.6.2 New World Alpha Viruses: Eastern, Western and Venezuelan Equine Encephalitis Virus

Eastern Equine Encephalitis Virus (EEEV) is primarily found the Atlantic and Gulf Coast states, but cases have been reported further north into Canada, and into South America (Argentina and Peru) (Hansen & Docherty, 1999). Passerine birds serve as the amplification host for the virus (Chamberlain et al., 1954; Komar et al., 1999) and *Culiseta melanura*, a mainly ornithophic mosquito, maintains the lifecycle in endemic areas between bird hosts, though other genera have be able to become infected (Armstrong & Theodore, 2010). The virus starts its replication in the mid-gut epithelial cells and maintains a persistent infection in the mosquito, eventually reaching the salivary glands to ensure viral transfer (Georgiev, 2009). Mosquito with a wider range of hosts (*Coquillettidia, Culex, Ochlerotatus, Aedes, spp.*) serve to infect dead-end hosts (humans and horses) (Pfeffer & Dobler, 2010), with often fatal consequences for both (Pfeffer & Dobler, 2010).

Western Equine Encephalitis virus undergoes a similar endemic cycle in birds as EEEV does, with *Culex tarsalis* as the maintaining mosquito vector, although there is a cycle between rodents and *Ochlerotatus melanimon* in South America (Pfeffer & Dobler, 2010). WEEV can be found in North, South and Central America (Weaver et al., 1997), though *C. tarsalis* is well sustained in the Western U.S. in areas of agriculture and stream drainages (Zacks & Paessler, 2010).

Unlike the previous alpha viruses, the Venezuelan Equine Encephalitis Virus (VEEV) is maintained mainly in a mosquito/rodent cycle and amplification and further amplification is seen in horses and humans (Pfeffer & Dobler, 2010). *C. Melanoconion* serves as the enzootic strain vector among rodent hosts. The key to epidemic/epizootic transmission is through a the selection of the E2 envelope protein mutation of ID or IE subtypes (Pfeffer & Dobler, 2010), from which the IAB and IC subtypes emerge, and go on to infect equines and humans through *Ochlerotatus taeniorhynchus* (Georgiev, 2009). For additional details of the VEEV virus, mosquito vectors (both enzoonic and epizoonic), as well as the transmission cycle, please see the review by Weaver et al. (2004).

3. Bacterial Encephalitides

3.1 Brucellosis: *Brucella*

There are six 'classical' strains of *Brucella* genus, found in specific animals, *Brucella ovis, Brucella canis, Brucella neotomae, Brucella abortus, Brucella melitensis, and Brucella suis* (Moreno et al., 2002), with the latter three strains capable of infecting humans and human producing brucellosis (de Jong et al., 2010). These three strains are also able to infect reticuloendothelial tissues as well as reproductive tract cells, which results in abortions or sterility (de Jong et al., 2010). Neurological affects can manifest into Neurobrucellosis, with meningoencephalitis as a potential complication, though a rare occurrence among those affected (Shakir et al., 1987; Al Deeb et al., 1989). *Brucella* has also been detected in terrestrial wildlife populations (Godfroid, 2002), as well as marine mammals (Foster et al., 2002) and has been shown to jump from wildlife reservoirs to domestic herds in close proximity to each other. The study done by Beja-Pereira et al. (2009) showed that elk were the origin species for the *Brucella* outbreak in cattle herds in the greater Yellowstone area. For the greater population, human infection is usually caused by consumption of dairy products contaminated with the bacterium (De Massis et al., 2005). The risk of infection increases with animal contact, especially around periods of perturbation, which puts farm workers/ranchers, veterinarians and meat-packing employers at greater risk of infection (Seleem, Boyle et al. 2010).

3.2 Leptospirosis: *Leptospira*

Leptospirosis is caused by two species of *Leptospira; L. interrogans* and *L. borgpetersenii. L. interrogans* is effective in surviving in the environment, while *L. borgpetersenii* is host dependent. Genome analysis between these two pathogenic strains showed that the host dependent strain had approximately 700 bp smaller genome and overall lower gene density than *L. interrogans*, and an obligate host to host transmission cycle (Bulach et al., 2006). Leptospires reproduce in the kidneys are shed through the urine of infected animals. Disease contraction occurs with exposure to urine and pathways to the body include skin abrasions, passage of the mucous membranes or consumption of contaminated water. Rodents are asymptomatic and are reservoirs for the bacterium, which facilitates and maintains infection in domesticated animals, as well as from passage to animal to animal in herds (Antony, 1996; Ko et al., 2009). A review of global occurrences of leptospirosis was done by Pappas et al. (2008), which showed the endemic areas of the world were mainly located in the Caribbean and Central and South America, as well as in Southeast Asia and Oceania, though the authors reported that it is probably an incomplete list due to lack of data from developing countries and unreliable reports from other parts of the world. The human leucocyte- like antigen DQ-6 (HLA-DQ6) polymorphism in has showed an increased risk of leptospirosis via consumption of contaminated water (Lingappa et al., 2004). Encephalitis onset has been reported (Dimopoulou et al., 2002).

3.3 Listeriosis: Listeria monocytogenes

Human *Listeria* infections most often occur because of consumption of contaminated food products, but *Listeria* is also shed in the feces of infected livestock. When the manure is spread on crop fields, food, soil and water contamination becomes an issue (Swaminathan & Gerner-Smidt, 2007). This pathogen is capable of living in a wide range conditions, tolerating in both an extensive temperature and pH range (0.5-45C, pH 4.3-9.8) (Gandhi & Chikindas, 2007). *L. monocytogenes* is capable of infecting a variety of hosts (Roberts & Wiedmann, 2003), but mainly reported in livestock (Low & Donachie, 1997). Human encephalitic cases have been reported (Johnson & Colley, 1969; Armstrong & Fung, 1993). The genetic changes seen in two lineages of *L. monocytogenes*, lineage II, the more environmentally resistant strain, and lineage I, the more host adapted lineage, was found to be in the cell wall and membrane biogenesis and motility-related genes (Orsi et al., 2008).

3.4 Lyme's Disease: Borrelia *burgdorferi*

The Lyme's disease (Lyme borreliosis) spirochete (*Borrelia burgdorferi*) is spread through ixodid ticks. Humans make up a small portion of bloodmeals, but can become infected through bites of *Ixodes dammini/scapularis* in the eastern U.S., *Ixodes pacificus* in the western United States and *Ixodes ricinus* in Europe. *Ixodes dammini*'s primary host is the white-footed mouse, *Peromyscus eucopus*, and the white-tailed deer, *Odocoileus virginianus*. In the western US, fence lizards (*Sceloporus occidentalis*) and Columbian black-tailed deer are reservoirs (as reviewed by Lane et al. (1991)). A study done in California found that woodrats serve as the reservoir hosts while *Ixodes neotomae* maintains the spirochete, though it does not facilitate human transfer (Brown & Lane, 1992). After the spirochete is ingested in the initial bloodmeal, protective outer surface proteins are produced as a buffer from digestion mechanisms in the tick's midgut. There it will stay until the tick molts and engages in its second bloodmeal. Feeding triggers spirochete reproduction, followed by migration to the salivary glands, allowing for host transfer (Spielman et al., 1987). The bacterium enter the host's skin and migrate out from the bite site and create the characteristic bull's eye mark of infection (Steere, 2001). A small portion of patients suffer from neurological complications (similar to neuroborreliosis in animal models (Steere, 2001)), which can result in meningoencephalitis (Broderick et al., 1987; Oschmann et al., 1998).

3.5 *Rickettsiaceae*: Scrub Typhus, Q Fever, Human Monocytic Ehrlichiosis, Rocky Mountain Spotted Fever and Colorado Tick Fever, and Epidemic Typhus

Scrub Typhus, or tsutsugamushi disease, is caused by *Orientia tsutsugamushi*, grouped into a separate genus in the Rickettsiaceae family (Tamura et al., 1995; Perlman et al., 2006). The trombiculid mite vectors (*Leptotrombidium deliense*) feed on mice and humans in their chigger stage, or parasitic larval stage, which is responsible for the transmission of the bacterium. Vertical transmission is also possible (Traub & Wisseman, 1974). The disease is endemic in a region, known as the 'tsutsugamushi triangle', ranging from Afghanistan, China, Korea, the islands of the southwestern Pacific, and northern Australia (Kelly et al., 2009) and encephalomyelitis was observed (Kim et al., 2000; Seong et al., 2001)

Query fever (commonly referred to as Q Fever) is a worldwide zoonosis caused by *Coxiella burnetii*, an obligatory intracellular organism which is a member of the family Rickettsiaceae, though genetic comparison revealed it is closer homology to *Legionella pneumophila* (Vogel, 2004; Parker et al., 2006). It enters the phagolysosome and later develops into the parasitophorous vacuole (PV), characterized by low pH, acid hydrolases and cationic peptides (Voth & Heinzen, 2007). These strange optimal conditions for growth make the culturing of this bacterium difficult (Omsland et al., 2009). Meningoencephalitis, though rare, is a potential complication of infection (Sawyer et al., 1987; Raoult et al., 2000). The bacterium is shed in large volumes during the birthing process (Welsh et al., 1958) and through milk production (Fishbein & Raoult, 1992). Domesticated ruminants (cattle, sheep, goats) are the predominate bridge to human infection, making slaughterhouses workers, farmers and livestock researchers at the greatest risk for direct infection (McQuiston & Childs, 2002), though it has been detected in other domestic and wild animals (Marrie et al., 1988; Buhariwalla et al., 1996; Stein & Raoult, 1999). The bacterium can also be isolated from environmental samples where livestock reside (DeLay et al., 1950). Ticks are considered a reservoir, though not a disease vector (Mediannikov et al., 2010). There is also evidance of wind-blown induced infections of cites downwind of sheep farms (Tissot-Dupont et al., 1999).

Ehrlichia chaffeensis (Family Anaplasmataceae) is the causative agent for human monocytic ehrlichiosis (HME) (Dumler, Madigan et al. 2007). White tail deer (*Odocoileus virginianus*), rodents and other wildlife have been shown to harbor *E. chaffeensis*, which is transmitted to humans via *Ixodes* ticks (*Amblyomma americanum*) (Telford et al., 1996; Lockhart et al., 1997; Walls et al., 1998; A. A. Kocan, 2000; Varela-Stokes, 2007). Genera *Ehrlichia* does not undergo transovarial transmission, so the perpetuation of infected ticks is through horizontal transfer from mammals to ticks (Rikihisa, 2003). Encephalitis is a reported complication of the disease (Ratnasamy et al., 1996; Paddock & Childs, 2003; Stone et al., 2004), which is found in the Atlantic, southeastern, and south central states (Paddock & Childs, 2003).

Despite the name, Rocky Mountain Spotted Fever (RMSF) has been reported in at least 42 states and the District of Columbia (Treadwell et al., 2000). The lifecycle and transmission of *R.* rickettsii is primarily through transoverial. Infected female ticks give rise to infected eggs, which develop into infected larva/nymphs, which feed on small rodents and adults infect humans, an incidental host. Uninfected ticks can also feed on infected rodents to acquire the bacterium. Close contact during mating is also able to pass the virus (Walker, 1996). The main vectors for RMSF are the *Dermacentor variabilis* (American dog tick); in the northwestern US and Canada, and *D. andersoni* (Rocky Mountain Wood Tick) and the Lone Star Tick,

Amblyomma americanum. In Latin America, *Amblyomma cajennense* (Cayenne Tick) is a human vector (Alderdice & Burgess, 1998; Thorner et al., 1998; Treadwell et al., 2000; Dumler & Walker, 2005). Meningoencephalitis can be a side effect of this disease (Horney & Walker, 1988; Sexton & Corey, 1992). To a smaller extent, Colorado Tick fever (CTF), transmitted by *D. andersoni,* manifested as meningoencephalitis in the past (Draughn et al., 1965).
Similar to RMSF and CTF, *Rickettsia prowazekii* is the causative agent of epidemic typhus, transmitted by the body louse (*Pediculus humanus corporis*). *R prowazekii* is not carried in the saliva, rather excreted in the feces and present in ruptured lice remains, so open bite wounds, conjunctivae, and mucous membranes are pathways into the body (Andersson & Andersson, 2000). Infection can still occur without a lice infestation through aerosols of fecal dust, which can maintain viable pathogens for several months (Raoult & Roux, 1999). The lice themselves also succumb to the *R. prowazekii* infection, suffering from rupture of the infected epithelial cells and subsequent loss of blood, which is witnessed by the red color shift of the infected louse, and death within a week of infection (Houhamdi et al., 2002).

4. Parasitic Encephalitis: Human African Trypanosomiasis, Schistosomiasis and Toxoplasmosis

4.1 Human African Trypanosomiasis: *Trypanosoma brucei*

In humans, a *Trypanosoma brucei infection results in* Human African Trypanosomiasis, or sleeping sickness, of which the central nervous system becomes involved later in the disease onset (Kennedy, 2004; Bentivoglio et al., 2011). The blood-sucking tsetse fly (genus *Glossina*) is insect vector of *Trypanosoma brucei gambiense,* of which, humans are the parasitic reservoir. *T.b. rhodesiense* is a subspecies, and whose main reservoir is game animals and cattle, and results in an acute form of the disease (Bentivoglio et al., 2011). A bloodmeal from an infected animal starts the lifecycle of the trypanosomes. Procyclic trypomastigotes are ingested and multiply via binary fission in the fly's midgut cells. From there they travel through to the salivary glands and transform into epimastigotes then metacyclic trypomastigotes, which are capable of being transferred to a human host. The metacyclic trypomastigotes transform into trypomastigotes, are carried throughout the body and allowed to multiply in blood, lymph and spinal fluid (reviewed by Kennedy (2004)). Infection is usually fatal, but rare cases of recovery have been documented without chemotherapy treatment (Deborggraeve et al., 2008). A study done by Courtin et al. (2006) suggests that host genetics, specifically, single nucleotide polymorphisms in the *IL10*$_{-592\,\mathrm{A}}$ allele is associated with a lower risk of disease. A review done by Solano et al. (2010) of both tsetse fly genetics and genetic susceptibility of the host highlights the complexity of this disease.

4.2 Schistosomiasis: *Schistosoma*

Schistosomiasis (also called bilharzias) is caused by schistosomes, blood-dwelling fluke worms of the genus *Schistosoma.* Encephalitic onset is observed as Neuroschistosomiasis (Devine et al., 2008; Carod-Artal, 2010). Infection is worldwide, but is limited to areas conducive to maintaining the complex life cycle of the fluke, which involves a snail and human host and an aquatic environment to as passage between hosts. Eggs are released into waterway and hatch to form miracidia. These then penetrate the snail intermediate host. Sporocysts are formed, followed by cercariae, which can penetrate the human host, turning into schistosomulae. Adult worms reside in mesenteric venules. Once reproduction occurs, eggs move to either the intestine or ureters and are then released in the feces or urine respectively, completing the cycle and the means of egg release is species dependent (Cox, 2002). The main schistosomes infecting human are *S. mansoni*, *S. haematobium*, and *S. japonicum* and their respective snail hosts, *Biomphalaria*, *Bulinus* and *Oncomelania*. *S. mansoni* is found in Africa, the Arabian peninsula, and South America, with humans as its main host, but can also infect rodents and primates (as reviewed by (Gryseels et al., 2006; Brooker, 2010). The biodiversity of an area, as can the genetic diversity of a population, can play a role in the risk of human *S. mansoni* infection. Johnson et al. (2009) found when *Biomphalaria glabrata* was raised along with non-host snails, 60–80 per cent fewer cercariae were produced, resulting in a decreased risk of human infection.

4.3 Toxoplasmosis: Toxoplasma gondii

Toxoplasma gondii is responsible for toxoplasmosis, and cases of severe encephalitis have been reported, especially in immnocompromised individuals (i.e., transplant, AIDS and lymphatic cancer patients) (Frenhel et al., 1975; Araujo & Remington, 1987; Luft & Remington, 1992; Touahri et al., 2002; Derouin et al., 2008). As an obligate intracellular parasite, producing many asymptomatic infections, this parasite has balanced host immune detection and successful infection and reproduction and passage through blood-brain, placenta and intestinal barriers (Lambert & Barragan, 2010). This phylum is named for the apical complex that assistants host cell infection (Lim & McFadden, 2010). Although Family Felidae are the sole definitive host (allowing for sexual reproduction) (Hutchison, 1965), wide range of warm-blooded animals (including livestock) and birds can act as a intermediate host (Jacobs et al., 1960; Work, 1967; Tenter et al., 2000; Innes, 2010). Initial infection is through ingestion of raw or undercooked meat containing oocysts or live organisms (Jacobs et al., 1960) or through fecal matter contact (Dubey et al., 1970). Cysts are also persistent in the environment through a wide range of conditions (Frenkel et al., 1975), and after exposure to sodium hypochlorite or ozone (Wainwright et al., 2007). Infection can occur in three forms of the parasite: tachyzoites, bradyzoites found in cysts of infected tissue or the oocysts that are released in feces. Ingestion of cysts leads to rapid infection through the release of the bradyzoite in the digestive tract followed by integration into epithelial cells of the small intestine (Dubey, 1996). There are three strains of *T. gondii*. Type I is virulent with low genetic diversity, while Type II and III are distinct lineages and are non-virulent (Sibley & Boothroyd, 1992; Howe & Sibley, 1995; Ajzenberg et al., 2004). The epigenetic mechanisms of these parasites have been investigated as a means of parasite physiology and potential therapeutics (Dixon et al., 2010).

5. Conclusion

The variety of encephalitic diseases mediated by arthropod and mammalian vectors, and requiring humans as a host in a parasitic lifestyle, is vast. With the advent of more sophisticated molecular technologies and a greater understanding of these diseases and their genetic codes, novel vaccines could be developed to help curb or prevent future infections (Seshadri et al., 2003; Diamond & Mehlhop, 2008; Ertl, 2009). As genomes become available, a further characterization of phylogenetic relationships can be made (Mavarez et al., 2002; Bourhy et al., 2005; Jackson et al., 2010). PCR applications, including multiplex PCR (Paris et al., 2008), nested PCR (James et al., 2011), heteroduplex PCR (Lee et al., 2002), reverse transcriptase PCR and direct sequencing (Telford et al., 1997), restriction fragment length polymorphic analysis (Freylikhman et al., 2008), DNA microsatellite markers (Shrivastava et al., 2005) and microarray technology (Gobert et al., 2009; Omsland et al., 2009) will aid in the detection of the pathogens to a greater level of sensitivity and specificity than previously achieved. Aside from genetic advances, immunological based assays utilize antibody/antigen specificity to detection many pathogens (Enyaru et al., 2010). On the landscape scale, geospatial analysis of vector or reservoir migration may help understand the spread of these diseases (Eisen & Eisen, 2011), as well as continued vigilance as cities and residential areas continue to sprawl further in the vector habitat (Alig et al., 2004; Estep et al., 2010; Matthews, 2011; Plowright et al., 2011). Research concerning vector control should also be expanded as a means of infection control (Solano et al., 2010). Climate change also has the potential to change the vector dynamics and should be considered when developing strategies to combat encephalitic diseases mediated by arthropod and mammalian vectors (Gubler et al., 2001; Lindgren & Gustafson, 2001; Bi et al., 2003).

6. References

A. A. Kocan, G. C. L., L. C. Whitworth, G. L. Murphy, S. A. Ewing, and R. W. Barker (2000). Naturally occurring Ehrlichia chaffeensis infection in coyotes from Oklahoma. *Emerging Infectious Diseases*, Vol. 6, No. (5), pp. 477-480, 1080-6040

Ajzenberg, D., A. L. Bañuls, et al. (2004). Genetic diversity, clonality and sexuality in *Toxoplasma gondii. International Journal for Parasitology*, Vol. 34, No. (10), pp. 1185-1196, 0020-7519

Al Deeb, S. M., B. A. Yaqub, et al. (1989). Neurobrucellosis. *Neurology*, Vol. 39, No. (4), pp. 498-498, 0028-3878

Alderdice, J. M. and I. F. Burgess (1998). The travels of a lone star tick. *Journal of Clinical Pathology*, Vol. 51, No. (5), May, pp. 403-403, 0021-9746

Alexander H. K. and T. Day (2010). Risk factors for the evolutionary emergence of pathogens. *J. R. Soc. Interface*, Vol. 7, No. (51), pp. 1455–1474, 1742-5662

Alig, R. J., J. D. Kline, et al. (2004). Urbanization on the US landscape: looking ahead in the 21st century. *Landscape and Urban Planning*, Vol. 69, No. (2-3), pp. 219-234, 0169-2046

Allworth, A., K. Murray, et al. (1996). A case of encephalitis due to a lyssavirus recently identified in fruit bats. *Commun Dis Intell*, Vol. 20, No. (504), pp.,

Andersson, J. O. and S. G. E. Andersson (2000). A century of typhus, lice and Rickettsia. *Research in Microbiology*, Vol. 151, No. (2), pp. 143-150, 0923-2508

Antony, S. J. (1996). Leptospirosis – An Emerging Pathogen in Travel Medicine: A Review of its Clinical Manifestations and Management. *Journal of Travel Medicine*, Vol. 3, No. (2), pp. 113-118, 1708-8305

Araujo, F. G. and J. S. Remington (1987). Toxoplasmosis in immunocompromised patients. *European Journal of Clinical Microbiology & Infectious Diseases*, Vol. 6, No. (1), pp. 1-2-2, 0934-9723

Arguin, P. M., K. Murray-Lillibridge, et al. (2007). Serologic Evidence of Lyssavirus Infections among Bats, the Philippines. *Emerging Infectious Diseases*, Vol. 8, No. (3), pp. 258-262, 1080-6040

Armstrong, P. M. and G. A. Theodore (2010). Eastern Equine Encephalitis Virus in Mosquitoes and Their Role as Bridge Vectors. *Emerging Infectious Diseases*, Vol. 16, No. (12), pp. 1869-1874, 1080-6059

Armstrong, R. W. and P. C. Fung (1993). Brainstem Encephalitis (Rhombencephalitis) Due to *Listeria monocytogenes*: Case Report and Review. *Clinical Infectious Diseases*, Vol. 16, No. (5), pp. 689-702, 1058-4838

Baillie, G. J., S. O. Kolokotronis, et al. (2008). Phylogenetic and evolutionary analyses of St. Louis encephalitis virus genomes. *Molecular Phylogenetics and Evolution*, Vol. 47, No. (2), pp. 717-728, 1055-7903

Barton, L. L. and N. J. Hyndman (2000). Lymphocytic Choriomeningitis Virus: Reemerging Central Nervous System Pathogen. *Pediatrics*, Vol. 105, No. (3), pp. e35-e35, 0031-4005

Barton, L. L. and M. B. Mets (2001). Congenital Lymphocytic Choriomeningitis Virus Infection: Decade of Rediscovery. *Clinical infectious diseases*, Vol. 33, No. (3), pp. 370-374, 1058-4838

Barton, L. L., C. J. Peters, et al. (1995). Lymphocytic choriomeningitis virus: an unrecognized teratogenic pathogen. *Emerging Infectious Diseases*, Vol. 1, No. (4), pp. 152-153, 1080-6059

Becker, N., D. Petrić, et al. (2010). Medical Importance of Mosquitoes. Heidelberg, Springer.

Beja-Pereira, A., B. Bricker, et al. (2009). DNA Genotyping Suggests that Recent Brucellosis Outbreaks in the Greater Yellowstone Area Originated from Elk. *Journal of Wildlife Diseases*, Vol. 45, No. (4), October 1, 2009, pp. 1174-1177, 1943-3700

Bennett, N. (1976). Murray Valley encephalitis, 1974: clinical features. *The Medical Journal of Australia*, Vol. 2, No. (12), pp. 446-450, 0025-729X

Bentivoglio, M., R. Mariotti, et al. (2011). Neuroinflammation and brain infections: Historical context and current perspectives. *Brain Research Reviews*, Vol. 66, No. (1-2), pp. 152-173, 0165-0173

Bi, P., S. Tong, et al. (2003). Climate Variability and Transmission of Japanese Encephalitis in Eastern China. *Vector-Borne and Zoonotic Diseases*, Vol. 3, No. (3), pp. 111-115, 1530-3667

Bonthius, D. J. and S. Perlman (2007). Congenital Viral Infections of the Brain: Lessons Learned from Lymphocytic Choriomeningitis Virus in the Neonatal Rat. *PLoS Pathogens*, Vol. 3, No. (11), pp. e149, 2157-3999

Boromisa, R. D. and P. R. Grimstad (1986). Virus-Vector-Host Relationships of Aedes stimulans and Jamestown Canyon Virus in a Northern Indiana Enzootic Focus. *American Journal of Tropical Medicine and Hygiene*, Vol. 35, No. (6), pp. 1285-1295, 1476-1645

Bourhy, H., J. A. Cowley, et al. (2005). Phylogenetic relationships among rhabdoviruses inferred using the L polymerase gene. *Journal of General Virology*, Vol. 86, No. (10), October 1, 2005, pp. 2849-2858, 1465-2099

Bourhy, H., B. Kissi, et al. (1999). Ecology and evolution of rabies virus in Europe. *Journal of General Virology*, Vol. 80, No. (10), October 1, 1999, pp. 2545-2557, 1465-2099

Briese, T., X.-Y. Jia, et al. (1999). Identification of a Kunjin/West Nile-like flavivirus in brains of patients with New York encephalitis. *The Lancet*, Vol. 354, No. (9186), pp. 1261-1262, 0140-6736

Broderick, J., B. Sandok, et al. (1987). Focal encephalitis in a young woman 6 years after the onset of Lyme disease: tertiary Lyme disease? *Mayo Clinic Proceedings*, Vol. 62, No. (4), pp. 313-316, 0025-6196

Brooker, S. (2010). Estimating the global distribution and disease burden of intestinal nematode infections: Adding up the numbers - A review. *International Journal for Parasitology*, Vol. 40, No. (10), pp. 1137-1144, 0020-7519

Broom, A. K., M. D. A. Lindsay, et al. (2002). Investigation of the Southern Limits of Murray Valley Encephalitis Activity in Western Australia During the 2000 Wet Season. *Vector-Borne and Zoonotic Diseases*, Vol. 2, No. (2), 2002/06/01, pp. 87-95, 1530-3667

Brown, R. N. and R. S. Lane (1992). Lyme disease in California: a novel enzootic transmission cycle of *Borrelia burgdorferi*. *Science*, Vol. 256, No. (5062), pp. 1439-1442, 0036-8075

Buhariwalla, F., B. Cann, et al. (1996). A Dog-Related Outbreak of Q Fever. *Clinical Infectious Diseases*, Vol. 23, No. (4), pp. 753-755, 1058-4838

Bulach, D. M., R. L. Zuerner, et al. (2006). Genome reduction in *Leptospira borgpetersenii* reflects limited transmission potential. *Proceedings of the National Academy of Sciences*, Vol. 103, No. (39), pp. 14560-14565, 1091-6490

Calisher, C. H. (1994). Medically important arboviruses of the United States and Canada. *Clinical microbiology reviews*, Vol. 7, No. (1), pp. 89-116, 0893-8512

Carod-Artal, F. J. (2010). Neuroschistosomiasis. *Expert Review of Anti-Infective Therapy*, Vol. 8, No. (11), pp. 1307-1318, 1478-7210

Chamberlain, R. W., R. K. Bikes, et al. (1954). Studies on the North American Arthropod-Borne Encephalities. *American Journal of Epidemiology*, Vol. 60, No. (3), pp. 278-285, 1476-6256

Charrel, R., P. Gallian, et al. (2005). Emergence of Toscana virus in Europe. *Emerging Infectious Diseases*, Vol. 11, No. (11), pp. 1657-1663, 1080-6040

Chua, K., B. Chua, et al. (2002). Anthropogenic deforestation, El Niño and the emergence of Nipah virus in Malaysia. *Malaysian Journal of Pathology*, Vol. 24, No. (1), pp. 15-21, 0126-8635

Chua, K. B., C. Lek Koh, et al. (2002). Isolation of Nipah virus from Malaysian Island flying-foxes. *Microbes and Infection*, Vol. 4, No. (2), pp. 145-151, 1286-4579

Cooper, L. A. and T. W. Scott (2001). Differential Evolution of Eastern Equine Encephalitis Virus Populations in Response to Host Cell Type. *Genetics*, Vol. 157, No. (4), pp. 1403-1412, 1943-2631

Courtin, D., L. Argiro, et al. (2006). Interest of tumor necrosis factor-alpha -308 G/A and interleukin-10 -592 C/A polymorphisms in human African trypanosomiasis. *Infection, Genetics and Evolution*, Vol. 6, No. (2), pp. 123-129, 1567-1348

Cox, F. E. G. (2002). History of human parasitology. *Clinical microbiology reviews*, Vol. 15, No. (4), Oct, pp. 595-612, 0893-8512

Daubney, R., J. R. Hudson, et al. (1931). Enzootic hepatitis or rift valley fever. An undescribed virus disease of sheep cattle and man from east africa. *The Journal of Pathology and Bacteriology*, Vol. 34, No. (4), pp. 545-579, 1555-2039

de Jong, M. F., H. G. Rolan, et al. (2010). Innate immune encounters of the (Type) 4th kind: Brucella. *Cellular Microbiology*, Vol. 12, No. (9), Sep, pp. 1195-1202, 1462-5814

De Massis, F., A. Di Girolamo, et al. (2005). Correlation between animal and human brucellosis in Italy during the period 1997–2002. *Clinical Microbiology and Infection*, Vol. 11, No. (8), pp. 632-636, 1469-0691

Deborggraeve, S., M. Koffi, et al. (2008). Molecular analysis of archived blood slides reveals an atypical human Trypanosoma infection. *Diagnostic Microbiology and Infectious Disease*, Vol. 61, No. (4), pp. 428-433, 0732-8893

DeLay, P., E. Lennette, et al. (1950). Q fever in California; recovery of *Coxiella burnetii* from naturally-infected air-borne dust. *Journal of Immunological*, Vol. 65, No. (2), pp. 211-220, 1550-6606

Derouin, F., H. Pelloux, et al. (2008). Prevention of toxoplasmosis in transplant patients. *Clinical Microbiology and Infection*, Vol. 14, No. (12), pp. 1089-1101, 1469-0691

Devine, M. J., P. A. Wilkinson, et al. (2008). Neuroschistosomiasis presenting as brainstem encephalitis. *Neurology*, Vol. 70, No. (23), Jun, pp. 2262-2264, 0028-3878

Diallo, M., J. Thonnon, et al. (1999). Vectors of Chikungunya virus in Senegal: current data and transmission cycles. *American Journal of Tropical Medicine and Hygiene*, Vol. 60, No. (2), pp. 281-286, 1476-1645

Diamond, M. S. and E. Mehlhop. (2008). The Molecular Basis of Antibody Protection Against West Nile Virus, In: *Human Antibody Therapeutics for Viral Disease*, S. K. Dessain, pp. (125-153), Springer Berlin Heidelberg, Retrieved from <http://dx.doi.org/10.1007/978-3-540-72146-8_5>

Dimopoulou, I., P. Politis, et al. (2002). Leptospirosis presenting with encephalitis-induced coma. *Intensive Care Medicine*, Vol. 28, No. (11), pp. 1682-1682-1682, 0342-4642

Dionisio, D., M. Valassina, et al. (2001). Encephalitis without Meningitis Due to Sandfly Fever Virus Serotype Toscana. *Clinical Infectious Diseases*, Vol. 32, No. (8), pp. 1241-1243, 1058-4838

Dixon, S. E., K. L. Stilger, et al. (2010). A decade of epigenetic research in *Toxoplasma gondii*. *Molecular and Biochemical Parasitology*, Vol. 173, No. (1), pp. 1-9, 0166-6851

Domingo, E. (1997). Rapid Evolution of Viral RNA Genomes. *Journal of Nutrition*, Vol. 127, No. (5), pp. 958S-961S, 1541-6100

Draughn, D. E., O. F. Sieber, et al. (1965). Colorado Tick Fever Encephalitis. *Clinical Pediatrics*, Vol. 4, No. (10), pp. 626-628, 0009-9228

Dubey, J. (1996). *Toxoplasma Gondii*, In: *Medical Microbiology*, S. Baron, The University of Texas Medical Branch at Galveston, Retrieved from http://www.ncbi.nlm.nih.gov/books/NBK7752/

Dubey, J. P., N. L. Miller, et al. (1970). The *Toxoplasma gondii* Oocyst from cat feces. *The Journal of Experimental Medicine*, Vol. 132, No. (4), pp. 636-662, 1540-9538

Dumler, J. S. and D. H. Walker (2005). Rocky Mountain Spotted Fever — Changing Ecology and Persisting Virulence. *New England Journal of Medicine*, Vol. 353, No. (6), pp. 551-553, 1533-4406

Ebel, G. D. (2009). Update on Powassan Virus: Emergence of a North American Tick-Borne Flavivirus. *Annual Review of Entomology*, Vol. 55, No. (1), 2010/01/01, pp. 95-110, 1545-4487

Eisen, L. and R. J. Eisen. (2011). Using Geographic Information Systems and Decision Support Systems for the Prediction, Prevention, and Control of Vector-Borne Diseases, In: *Annual Review of Entomology*, pp. (41-61), Annual Reviews, Retrieved from <<Go to ISI>://000286841900003>

Enyaru, J. C., J. O. Ouma, et al. (2010). Landmarks in the evolution of technologies for identifying trypanosomes in tsetse flies. *Trends in Parasitology*, Vol. 26, No. (8), pp. 388-394, 1471-4922

Epstein, J., H. Field, et al. (2006). Nipah virus: Impact, origins, and causes of emergence. *Current Infectious Disease Reports*, Vol. 8, No. (1), pp. 59-65, 1523-3847

Ertl, H. C. J. (2009). Novel Vaccines to Human Rabies. *Plos Neglected Tropical Diseases*, Vol. 3, No. (9), Sep, pp., 1935-2735

Erwin, P. C., T. F. Jones, et al. (2002). La Crosse Encephalitis in Eastern Tennessee: Clinical, Environmental, and Entomological Characteristics from a Blinded Cohort Study. *American Journal of Epidemiology*, Vol. 155, No. (11), pp. 1060-1065, 1476-6256

Estep, L. K., N. D. Burkett-Cadena, et al. (2010). Estimation of Dispersal Distances of *Culex erraticus* in a Focus of Eastern Equine Encephalitis Virus in the Southeastern United States. *Journal of Medical Entomology*, Vol. 47, No. (6), Nov, pp. 977-986, 0022-2585

Fishbein, D. B. and D. Raoult (1992). A Cluster of *Coxiella Burnetii* Infections Associated with Exposure to Vaccinated Goats and their Unpasteurized Dairy Products. *American Journal of Tropical Medicine and Hygiene*, Vol. 47, No. (1), July 1, 1992, pp. 35-40, 1476-1645

Flores, F. S., L. A. Diaz, et al. (2010). Vertical Transmission of St. Louis Encephalitis Virus in *Culex quinquefasciatus* (Diptera: Culicidae) in Córdoba, Argentina. *Vector-Borne and Zoonotic Diseases*, Vol. 10, No. (10), pp. 999-1002, 1530-3667

Fontenille, D., M. Traore-Lamizana, et al. (1994). First Isolations of Arboviruses from Phlebotomine Sand Flies in West Africa. *American Journal of Tropical Medicine and Hygiene*, Vol. 50, No. (5), pp. 570-574, 1476-1645

Foster, G., A. P. MacMillan, et al. (2002). A review of *Brucella sp.* infection of sea mammals with particular emphasis on isolates from Scotland. *Veterinary Microbiology*, Vol. 90, No. (1-4), pp. 563-580, 0378-1135

Frenhel, J. K., B. M. Nelson, et al. (1975). Immunosuppression and toxoplasmic encephalitis: Clinical and experimental aspects. *Human Pathology*, Vol. 6, No. (1), pp. 97-111, 0046-8177

Frenkel, J. K., A. Ruiz, et al. (1975). Soil Survival of Toxoplasma Oocysts in Kansas and Costa Rica. *American Journal of Tropical Medicine and Hygiene*, Vol. 24, No. (3), pp. 439-443, 1476-1645

Freylikhman, O. A., Y. A. Panfyorova, et al. (2008). Study of Heterogeneity of *Coxiella burnettii* Strains by Analysis of groEL Gene Restriction Fragment Length Polymorphism. *Bulletin of Experimental Biology and Medicine*, Vol. 146, No. (3), Sep, pp. 338-340, 0007-4888

Gandhi, M. and M. L. Chikindas (2007). Listeria: A foodborne pathogen that knows how to survive. *International Journal of Food Microbiology,* Vol. 113, No. (1), Jan, pp. 1-15, 0168-1605

Georgiev, V. S. (2009). Arthropod-Borne Viral Encephalitis, In: *National Institute of Allergy and Infectious Diseases, NIH,* V. S. Georgiev, pp. (151-162), Humana Press, Retrieved from <http://dx.doi.org/10.1007/978-1-60327-297-1_19>

Gholam, B. I. A., S. Puksa, et al. (1999). Powassan encephalitis: a case report with neuropathology and literature review. *Canadian Medical Association Journal,* Vol. 161, No. (11), pp. 1419-1422, 1488-2329

Gobert, G., L. Moertel, et al. (2009). Developmental gene expression profiles of the human pathogen *Schistosoma japonicum. BMC Genomics,* Vol. 10, No. (1), pp. 128, 1471-2164

Godfroid, J. (2002). Brucellosis in wildlife. *Rev Sci Tech,* Vol. 21, No. (2), pp. 277-286, 0253-1933

Grimstad, P. R., C. H. Calisher, et al. (1986). Jamestown Canyon Virus (California Serogroup) is the Etiologic Agent of Widespread Infection in Michigan Humans. *American Journal of Tropical Medicine and Hygiene,* Vol. 35, No. (2), pp. 376-386, 1476-1645

Grimstad, P. R., C. L. Shabino, et al. (1982). A Case of Encephalitis in a Human Associated with a Serologic Rise to Jamestown Canyon Virus. *American Journal of Tropical Medicine and Hygiene,* Vol. 31, No. (6), pp. 1238-1244, 1476-1645

Gryseels, B., K. Polman, et al. (2006). Human schistosomiasis. *The Lancet,* Vol. 368, No. (9541), pp. 1106-1118, 0140-6736

Gubler, D. J., P. Reiter, et al. (2001). Climate Variability and Change in the United States: Potential Impacts on Vector- and Rodent-Borne Diseases. *Environmental Health Perspectives,* Vol. 109, No., pp. 223-233, 0091-6765

Günther, G. and M. Haglund (2005). Tick-Borne Encephalopathies: Epidemiology, Diagnosis, Treatment and Prevention. *Cns Drugs,* Vol. 19, No. (12), pp. 1009-1032, 11727047

Gurav, Y. K., B. V. Tandale, et al. (2010). Chandipura virus encephalitis outbreak among children in Nagpur division, Maharashtra, 2007. *Indian Journal of Medical Research,* Vol. 132, No., pp. 395-399, 0971-5916

Ha, D. Q., C. H. Calisher, et al. (1995). Isolation of a Newly Recognized Alphavirus from Mosquitoes in Vietnam and Evidence for Human Infection and Disease. *American Journal of Tropical Medicine and Hygiene,* Vol. 53, No. (1), pp. 100-104, 1476-1645

Hall, R. A., A. K. Broom, et al. (1995). Immunodominant epitopes on the NS1 protein of MVE and KUN viruses serve as targets for a blocking ELISA to detect virus-specific antibodies in sentinel animal serum. *Journal of Virological Methods,* Vol. 51, No. (2-3), pp. 201-210, 0166-0934

Halpin, K., P. L. Young, et al. (2000). Isolation of Hendra virus from pteropid bats: a natural reservoir of Hendra virus. *Journal of General Virology,* Vol. 81, No. (8), pp. 1927-1932, 1465-2099

Hanna, J., I. Carney, et al. (2000). Australian bat lyssavirus infection: a second human case, with a long incubation period. *Med J Aust.,* Vol. 172, No. (12), pp. 597-599,

Hansen, W. and D. E. Docherty. (1999). Eastern Equine Encephalitis In: *Field Manual of Wildlife Diseases: General Field Procedures and Diseases of Birds*, M. Friend and J. C. Franson, pp. (171-174), US Department of the Interior, US Geological Survey, Retrieved from

Harcourt, B. H., A. Tamin, et al. (2000). Molecular Characterization of Nipah Virus, a Newly Emergent Paramyxovirus. *Virology*, Vol. 271, No. (2), pp. 334-349, 0042-6822

Harley, D., A. Sleigh, et al. (2001). Ross River Virus Transmission, Infection, and Disease: a Cross-Disciplinary Review. *Clinical microbiology reviews*, Vol. 14, No. (4), pp. 909-932, 0893-8512

Hayes, C. G. (2001). West Nile Virus: Uganda, 1937, to New York City, 1999. *Annals of the New York Academy of Sciences*, Vol. 951, No. (1), pp. 25-37, 1749-6632

Horney, L. and D. Walker (1988). Meningoencephalitis as a Major Manifestation of Rocky Mountain Spotted Fever. *Southern Medical Journal*, Vol. 81, No. (7), pp. 915-918, 0038-4348

Houhamdi, L., P.-E. Fournier, et al. (2002). An Experimental Model of Human Body Louse Infection with *Rickettsia prowazekii*. *Journal of Infectious Diseases*, Vol. 186, No. (11), December 1, 2002, pp. 1639-1646, 1537-6613

Howe, D. K. and L. D. Sibley (1995). *Toxoplasma gondii* Comprises Three Clonal Lineages: Correlation of Parasite Genotype with Human Disease. *Journal of Infectious Diseases*, Vol. 172, No. (6), pp. 1561-1566, 1537-6613

Hughes, G. J., L. A. Orciari, et al. (2005). Evolutionary timescale of rabies virus adaptation to North American bats inferred from the substitution rate of the nucleoprotein gene. *Journal of General Virology*, Vol. 86, No. (5), May 1, 2005, pp. 1467-1474, 1465-2099

Hutchison, W. M. (1965). Experimental Transmission of *Toxoplasma gondii*. *Nature*, Vol. 206, No. (4987), pp. 961-962, 0028-0836

Innes, E. A. (2010). A Brief History and Overview of *Toxoplasma gondii*. *Zoonoses and Public Health*, Vol. 57, No. (1), Feb, pp. 1-7, 1863-1959

Jackson, A. P., M. Sanders, et al. (2010). The Genome Sequence of *Trypanosoma brucei gambiense*, Causative Agent of Chronic Human African Trypanosomiasis. *Plos Neglected Tropical Diseases*, Vol. 4, No. (4), pp. e658, 1935-2735

Jacobs, L., J. S. Remington, et al. (1960). A Survey of Meat Samples from Swine, Cattle, and Sheep for the Presence of Encysted Toxoplasma. *The Journal of Parasitology*, Vol. 46, No. (1), pp. 23-28, 0022-3395

James, M. C., R. W. Furness, et al. (2011). The importance of passerine birds as tick hosts and in the transmission of *Borrelia burgdorferi*, the agent of Lyme disease: a case study from Scotland. *Ibis*, Vol. 153, No. (2), Apr, pp. 293-302, 0019-1019

Johnson, M. and E. Colley (1969). *Listeria monocytogenes* encephalitis associated with corticosteroid therapy. *Journal of Clinical Pathology*, Vol. 22, No. (4), pp. 465-469, 1472-4146

Johnson, P. T. J., P. J. Lund, et al. (2009). Community diversity reduces *Schistosoma mansoni* transmission, host pathology and human infection risk. *Proceedings of the Royal Society B: Biological Sciences*, Vol. 276, No. (1662), pp. 1657-1663, 1471-2954

Kasari, T. R., D. A. Carr, et al. (2008). Evaluation of pathways for release of Rift Valley fever virus into domestic ruminant livestock, ruminant wildlife, and human populations in the continental United States. *Javma-Journal of the American Veterinary Medical Association*, Vol. 232, No. (4), Feb, pp. 514-529, 0003-1488

Kaufman, W. (2010). Ticks: Physiological aspects with implications for pathogen transmission. *Ticks and Tick-borne Diseases*, Vol. 1, No. (1), pp. 11-22, 1877-959X

Kelly, D. J., P. A. Fuerst, et al. (2009). Scrub Typhus: The Geographic Distribution of Phenotypic and Genotypic Variants of Orientia tsutsugamushi. *Clinical Infectious Diseases*, Vol. 48, No. (Supplement 3), pp. S203-S230, 1058-4838

Kennedy, P. G. E. (2004). Human African trypanosomiasis of the CNS: current issues and challenges. *The Journal of Clinical Investigation*, Vol. 113, No. (4), pp. 496-504, 0021-9738

Kim, D.-E., S.-H. Lee, et al. (2000). Scrub Typhus Encephalomyelitis With Prominent Focal Neurologic Signs. *Archives of Neurology*, Vol. 57, No. (12), pp. 1770-1772, 0375-8540

Kissi, B., H. Badrane, et al. (1999). Dynamics of rabies virus quasispecies during serial passages in heterologous hosts. *Journal of General Virology*, Vol. 80, No. (8), August 1, 1999, pp. 2041-2050, 1465-2099

Ko, A. I., C. Goarant, et al. (2009). Leptospira: the dawn of the molecular genetics era for an emerging zoonotic pathogen. *Nature Reviews Microbiology*, Vol. 7, No. (10), Oct, pp. 736-747, 1740-1526

Komar, N., D. J. Dohm, et al. (1999). Eastern equine encephalitis virus in birds: relative competence of European starlings (*Sturnus vulgaris*). *American Journal of Tropical Medicine and Hygiene*, Vol. 60, No. (3), pp. 387-391, 1476-1645

Krebs, J. W., M. L. Wilson, et al. (1995). Rabies: Epidemiology, Prevention, and Future Research. *Journal of Mammalogy*, Vol. 76, No. (3), pp. 681-694, 0022-2372

Kuno, G. and G. J. Chang (2005). Biological transmission of arboviruses: reexamination of and new insights into components, mechanisms, and unique traits as well as their evolutionary trends. *Clinical microbiology reviews*, Vol. 18, No. (4), pp. 608-637, 0893-8512

Lahariya, C. and S. Pradhan (2006). Emergence of chikungunya virus in Indian subcontinent after 32 years: a review. *Journal of vector borne diseases*, Vol. 43, No., pp. 151-160, 1537-6591

Lambert, H. and A. Barragan (2010). Modelling parasite dissemination: host cell subversion and immune evasion by *Toxoplasma gondii*. *Cellular Microbiology*, Vol. 12, No. (3), Mar, pp. 292-300, 1462-5814

Lanciotti, R. S., J. T. Roehrig, et al. (1999). Origin of the West Nile Virus Responsible for an Outbreak of Encephalitis in the Northeastern United States. *Science*, Vol. 286, No. (5448), pp. 2333-2337, 0036-8075

Lane, R., J. Piesman, et al. (1991). Lyme borreliosis: relation of its causative agent to its vectors and hosts in North America and Europe. *Annual Review of Entomology*, Vol. 36, No., pp. 587, 1545-4487

Larsen, P., S. Chartrand, et al. (1993). Hydrocephalus complicating lymphocytic choriomeningitis virus infection. *The Pediatric Infectious Disease Journal*, Vol. 12, No. (6), pp. 528-531, 0891-3668

Laughlin, L. W., J. M. Meegan, et al. (1979). Epidemic Rift Valley fever in Egypt: observations of the spectrum of human illness. *Transactions of the Royal Society of Tropical Medicine and Hygiene*, Vol. 73, No. (6), pp. 630-633, 0035-9203

Lee, J. H., H. Hassan, et al. (2002). Identification of mosquito avian-derived blood meals by polymerase chain reaction-heteroduplex analysis. *American Journal of Tropical Medicine and Hygiene*, Vol. 66, No. (5), pp. 599-604, 1476-1645

Lim, L. and G. I. McFadden (2010). The evolution, metabolism and functions of the apicoplast. *Philosophical Transactions of the Royal Society B-Biological Sciences*, Vol. 365, No. (1541), Mar, pp. 749-763, 0962-8436

Lindgren, E. and R. Gustafson (2001). Tick-borne encephalitis in Sweden and climate change. *The Lancet*, Vol. 358, No. (9275), pp. 16-18, 0140-6736

Lingappa, J., T. Kuffner, et al. (2004). HLA-DQ6 and ingestion of contaminated water: possible gene-environment interaction in an outbreak of Leptospirosis. *Genes and Immunity*, Vol. 5, No. (3), pp. 197-202, 1466-4879

Lockhart, J. M., W. R. Davidson, et al. (1997). Isolation of *Ehrlichia chaffeensis* from wild white-tailed deer (*Odocoileus virginianus*) confirms their role as natural reservoir hosts. *Journal of Clinical Microbiology*, Vol. 35, No. (7), pp. 1681-1686, 1098-660X

Low, J. C. and W. Donachie (1997). A review of *Listeria monocytogenes* and listeriosis. *Veterinary Journal*, Vol. 153, No. (1), pp. 9-29, 1090-0233

Luft, B. J. and J. S. Remington (1992). Toxoplasmic Encephalitis in AIDS. *Clinical Infectious Diseases*, Vol. 15, No. (2), pp. 211-222, 1058-4838

Lum, L. C. S., S. K. Lam, et al. (1996). Dengue Encephalitis: A True Entity? *American Journal of Tropical Medicine and Hygiene*, Vol. 54, No. (3), pp. 256-259, 1476-1645

Madani, T. A., Y. Y. Al-Mazrou, et al. (2003). Rift Valley Fever Epidemic in Saudi Arabia: Epidemiological, Clinical, and Laboratory Characteristics. *Clinical Infectious Diseases*, Vol. 37, No. (8), pp. 1084-1092, 1058-4838

Mallewa, M., A. R. Fooks, et al. (2007). Rabies Encephalitis in Malaria-Endemic Area, Malawi, Africa. *Emerging Infectious Diseases*, Vol. 13, No. (1), pp. 136-139, 1080-6040

Marrie, T. J., H. Durant, et al. (1988). Exposure to Parturient Cats: A Risk Factor for Acquisition of Q Fever in Maritime Canada. *Journal of Infectious Diseases*, Vol. 158, No. (1), pp. 101-108, 1537-6613

Matthews, K. R. (2011). Controlling and Coordinating Development in Vector-Transmitted Parasites. *Science*, Vol. 331, No. (6021), Mar, pp. 1149-1153, 0036-8075

Mavale, M. S., G. Geevarghese, et al. (2005). Vertical and Venereal transmission of Chandipura Virus (Rhabdoviridae) by *Aedes aegypti* (Diptera: Culicidae). *Journal of Medical Entomology*, Vol. 42, No. (5), 2005/09/01, pp. 909-911, 0022-2585

Mavarez, J., C. Steiner, et al. (2002). Evolutionary history and phylogeography of the schistosome-vector freshwater snail *Biomphalaria glabrata* based on nuclear and mitochondrial DNA sequences. *Heredity*, Vol. 89, No. (4), pp. 266-272, 1365-2540

May, F. J., L. Li, et al. (2008). Genetic variation of St. Louis encephalitis virus. *Journal of General Virology*, Vol. 89, No. 8, pp. 1901-1910, 1465-2099

McJunkin, J. E., E. C. de los Reyes, et al. (2001). La Crosse Encephalitis in Children. *New England Journal of Medicine*, Vol. 344, No. (11), pp. 801-807, 1533-4406

McLean, R. G., L. J. Kirk, et al. (1993). Avian Hosts of St. Louis Encephalitis Virus in Pine Bluff, Arkansas, 1991. *American Journal of Tropical Medicine and Hygiene*, Vol. 49, No. (1), pp. 46-52, 1476-1645

McLean, R. G., S. R. Ubico, et al. (2001). West Nile Virus Transmission and Ecology in Birds. *Annals of the New York Academy of Sciences*, Vol. 951, No. (1), pp. 54-57, 1749-6632

McQuiston, J. H. and J. E. Childs (2002). Q Fever in Humans and Animals in the United States. *Vector-Borne and Zoonotic Diseases*, Vol. 2, No. (3), pp. 179-191, 1530-3667

Mediannikov, O., F. Fenollar, et al. (2010). *Coxiella burnetii* in Humans and Ticks in Rural Senegal. *Plos Neglected Tropical Diseases*, Vol. 4, No. (4), pp. e654, 1935-2735

Messenger, S. L., J. S. Smith, et al. (2002). Emerging Epidemiology of Bat-Associated Cryptic Cases of Rabies in Humans in the United States. *Clinical Infectious Diseases*, Vol. 35, No. (6), September 15, 2002, pp. 738-747, 1058-4838

Mohd Nor, M. N., C. H. Gan, et al. (2000). Nipah virus infection of pigs in peninsular Malaysia. *Revue scientifique et technique (International Office of Epizootics)*, Vol. 19, No. (1), pp. 160-165, 0253-1933

Moreno, E., A. Cloeckaert, et al. (2002). Brucella evolution and taxonomy. *Veterinary Microbiology*, Vol. 90, No. (1-4), pp. 209-227, 0378-1135

Morimoto, K., D. C. Hooper, et al. (1998). Rabies virus quasispecies: Implications for pathogenesis. *Proceedings of the National Academy of Sciences*, Vol. 95, No. (6), March 17, 1998, pp. 3152-3156, 1091-6490

Muzaffar, J., P. Venkata Krishnan, et al. (2006). Dengue encephalitis: why we need to identify this entity in a dengue-prone region. *Singapore Med Journal*, Vol. 47, No. (11), pp. 975-957, 0037-5675

Narasimha Rao, S., N. S. Wairagkar, et al. (2008). Brain Stem Encephalitis Associated with Chandipura in Andhra Pradesh Outbreak. *Journal of Tropical Pediatrics*, Vol. 54, No. (1), February 1, 2008, pp. 25-30, 0142-6338

O'Sullivan, J. D., A. M. Allworth, et al. (1997). Fatal encephalitis due to novel paramyxovirus transmitted from horses. *The Lancet*, Vol. 349, No. (9045), pp. 93-95, 0140-6736

Omsland, A., D. C. Cockrell, et al. (2009). Host cell-free growth of the Q fever bacterium *Coxiella burnetii*. *Proceedings of the National Academy of Sciences*, Vol. 106, No. (11), pp. 4430-4434, 1091-6490

Orsi, R., Q. Sun, et al. (2008). Genome-wide analyses reveal lineage specific contributions of positive selection and recombination to the evolution of *Listeria monocytogenes*. *BMC Evol Biol*, Vol. 8, No., pp. 233, 1471-2148

Oschmann, P., W. Dorndorf, et al. (1998). Stages and syndromes of neuroborreliosis. *Journal of Neurology*, Vol. 245, No. (5), pp. 262-272, 0340-5354

Paddock, C. D. and J. E. Childs (2003). *Ehrlichia chaffeensis*: a Prototypical Emerging Pathogen. *Clinical microbiology reviews*, Vol. 16, No. (1), pp. 37-64, 0893-8512

Pappas, G., P. Papadimitriou, et al. (2008). The globalization of leptospirosis: worldwide incidence trends. *International Journal of Infectious Diseases*, Vol. 12, No. (4), Jul, pp. 351-357, 1201-9712

Paredes, A., S. Weaver, et al. (2005). Structural biology of old world and new world alphaviruses, In: *Infectious Diseases from Nature: Mechanisms of Viral Emergence and*

Persistence, C. J. Peters and C. H. Calisher, pp. (179-185), Springer Vienna, Retrieved from <http://dx.doi.org/10.1007/3-211-29981-5_14>

Paris, D. H., S. D. Blacksell, et al. (2008). Real-time multiplex PCR assay for detection and differentiation of rickettsiae and orientiae. *Transactions of the Royal Society of Tropical Medicine and Hygiene*, Vol. 102, No. (2), pp. 186-193, 0035-9203

Parker, N. R., J. H. Barralet, et al. (2006). Q fever. *The Lancet*, Vol. 367, No. (9511), pp. 679-688, 0140-6736

Pastorino, B., J. J. Muyembe-Tamfum, et al. (2004). Epidemic resurgence of Chikungunya virus in democratic Republic of the Congo: Identification of a new central African strain. *Journal of Medical Virology*, Vol. 74, No. (2), pp. 277-282, 1096-9071

Paton, N. I., Y. S. Leo, et al. (1999). Outbreak of Nipah-virus infection among abattoir workers in Singapore. *The Lancet*, Vol. 354, No. (9186), pp. 1253-1256, 0140-6736

Pepin, M., M. Bouloy, et al. (2010). Rift Valley fever virus (*Bunyaviridae: Phlebovirus*): an update on pathogenesis, molecular epidemiology, vectors, diagnostics and prevention. *Veterinary Research*, Vol. 41, No. (6), pp., 1297-9716

Perlman, S. J., M. S. Hunter, et al. (2006). The emerging diversity of Rickettsia. *Proceedings of the Royal Society B: Biological Sciences*, Vol. 273, No. (1598), pp. 2097-2106, 1471-2954

Pfeffer, M. and G. Dobler (2010). Emergence of zoonotic arboviruses by animal trade and migration. *Parasites & Vectors*, Vol. 3, No. (1), pp. 1-15, 1756-3305

Pfeffer, M. and G. Dobler (2010). Emergence of zoonotic arboviruses by animal trade and migration. *Parasites & Vectors*, Vol. 3, No. (35), pp., 1756-3305

Plowright, R., P. Foley, et al. (2011). Urban Habituation, Connectivity, and Stress Synchrony: Hendra Virus Emergence from Flying Foxes (*Pteropus spp.*). *EcoHealth*, Vol. 7, No., pp. S36-S37 1612-9202

Plowright, R. K., H. E. Field, et al. (2008). Reproduction and nutritional stress are risk factors for Hendra virus infection in little red flying foxes (*Pteropus scapulatus*). *Proceedings of the Royal Society B: Biological Sciences*, Vol. 275, No. (1636), pp. 861-869, 1091-6490

Potharaju, N. R. and A. K. Potharaju (2006). Is Chandipura virus an emerging human pathogen? *Archives of Disease in Childhood*, Vol. 91, No. (3), pp. 279-280, 1468-2044

Rajapakse, S., C. Rodrigo, et al. (2010). Atypical manifestations of chikungunya infection. *Transactions of the Royal Society of Tropical Medicine and Hygiene*, Vol. 104, No. (2), pp. 89-96, 0035-9203

Rampal, M. Sharda, et al. (2007). Neurological complications in Chikungunya fever. *Journal of Association of Physicians of India*, Vol. 55, No., pp. 765-769, 0004-5772

Rao, B. L., A. Basu, et al. (2004). A large outbreak of acute encephalitis with high fatality rate in children in Andhra Pradesh, India, in 2003, associated with Chandipura virus. *The Lancet*, Vol. 364, No. (9437), pp. 869-874, 0140-6736

Raoult, D. and V. Roux (1999). The body louse as a vector of reemerging human diseases. *Clinical Infectious Diseases*, Vol. 29, No. (4), pp. 888-911, 1058-4838

Raoult, D., H. Tissot-Dupont, et al. (2000). Q Fever 1985-1998: Clinical and Epidemiologic Features of 1,383 Infections. *Medicine*, Vol. 79, No. (2), pp. 109-123, 0025-7974

Ratnasamy, N., E. D. Everett, et al. (1996). Central Nervous System Manifestations of Human Ehrlichiosis. *Clinical Infectious Diseases*, Vol. 23, No. (2), pp. 314-319, 1058-4838

Rikihisa, Y. (2003). Mechanisms to Create a Safe Haven by Members of the Family Anaplasmataceae. *Annals of the New York Academy of Sciences*, Vol. 990, No. (1), pp. 548-555, 1749-6632

Roberts, A. J. and M. Wiedmann (2003). Pathogen, host and environmental factors contributing to the pathogenesis of listeriosis. *Cellular and Molecular Life Sciences*, Vol. 60, No. (5), May, pp. 904-918, 1420-682X

Robin, S., D. Ramful, et al. (2008). Neurologic Manifestations of Pediatric Chikungunya Infection. *Journal of Child Neurology*, Vol. 23, No. (9), pp. 1028-1035, 1708-8828

Russell, R. C. and D. E. Dwyer (2000). Arboviruses associated with human disease in Australia. *Microbes and Infection*, Vol. 2, No. (14), pp. 1693-1704, 1286-4579

Rust, R. S., W. H. Thompson, et al. (1999). Topical Review: La Crosse and Other Forms of California Encephalitis. *Journal of Child Neurology*, Vol. 14, No. (1), pp. 1-14, 1708-8828

Salah, U., J. Hossain, et al. (2011). Use of Infrared Camera to Understand Bats' Access to Date Palm Sap: Implications for Preventing Nipah Virus Transmission. *EcoHealth*, Vol., No., pp. 1-9, 1612-9202

Sawyer, L. A., D. B. Fishbein, et al. (1987). Q Fever: Current Concepts. *Reviews of Infectious Diseases*, Vol. 9, No. (5), pp. 935-946, 0162-0886

Scott, T. W. (1988). Vertebrate host ecology, In: *The arboviruses: epidemiology and ecology*, T. P. Monath, pp. (257-280), CRC Press,

Seong, S., M.-S. Choi, et al. (2001). *Orientia tsutsugamushi* infection:overview and immune responses. *Microbes and Infection*, Vol. 3, No. (1), pp. 11-21, 1286-4579

Seshadri, R., I. T. Paulsen, et al. (2003). Complete genome sequence of the Q-fever pathogen *Coxiella burnetii*. *Proceedings of the National Academy of Sciences*, Vol. 100, No. (9), pp. 5455-5460, 1091-6490

Sexton, D. J. and G. R. Corey (1992). Rocky Mountain "Spotless" and "Almost Spotless" Fever: A Wolf in Sheep's Clothing. *Clinical Infectious Diseases*, Vol. 15, No. (3), pp. 439-448, 1058-4838

Shakir, R. A., A. S. N. Al-Din, et al. (1987). Clinical categories of neurobrucellosis. A report on 19 cases. *Brain*, Vol. 110, No. (1), pp. 213-223, 1460-2156

Shrivastava, J., B. Z. Qian, et al. (2005). An insight into the genetic variation of *Schistosoma japonicum* in mainland China using DNA microsatellite markers. *Molecular Ecology*, Vol. 14, No. (3), pp. 839-849, 1365-294X

Sibley, L. D. and J. C. Boothroyd (1992). Virulent strains of *Toxoplasma gondii* comprise a single clonal lineage. *Nature*, Vol. 359, No. (6390), pp. 82-85, 0028-0836

Smith, J. S., L. A. Orciari, et al. (1995). Molecular epidemiology of rabies in the United States. *Seminars in Virology*, Vol. 6, No. (6), pp. 387-400, 1044-5773

Solano, P., S. Ravel, et al. (2010). How can tsetse population genetics contribute to African trypanosomiasis control? *Trends in Parasitology*, Vol. 26, No. (5), pp. 255-263, 1471-4922

Solomon, T., M. H. Ooi, et al. (2003). West Nile encephalitis. *BMJ*, Vol. 326, No. (7394), pp. 865-869, 1756-1833

Spielman, A., J. M. C. Ribeiro, et al. (1987). Dissemination and salivary delivery of Lyme disease spirochetes in vector ticks (Acari: Ixodidae). *Journal of Medical Entomology*, Vol. 24, No., pp. 201-205, 0022-2585

Steere, A. C. (2001). Lyme Disease. *New England Journal of Medicine*, Vol. 345, No. (2), pp. 115-125, 1533-4406

Stein, A. and D. Raoult (1999). Pigeon Pneumonia in Provence: A Bird-Borne Q Fever Outbreak. *Clinical Infectious Diseases*, Vol. 29, No. (3), pp. 617-620, 1058-4838

Stone, J. H., K. Dierberg, et al. (2004). Human Monocytic Ehrlichiosis. *JAMA: The Journal of the American Medical Association*, Vol. 292, No. (18), pp. 2263-2270, 0098-7484

Sudia, W. D., V. Newhouse, et al. (1969). Venezuelan equine encephalitis virus-vector studies following a human case in Dade County, Florida. *Mosquito News* Vol. 29, No., pp. 596-600, 0027-142X

Swaminathan, B. and P. Gerner-Smidt (2007). The epidemiology of human listeriosis. *Microbes and Infection*, Vol. 9, No. (10), pp. 1236-1243, 1286-4579

Tamura, A., N. Ohashi, et al. (1995). Classification of *Rickettsia tsutsugamushi* in a New Genus, *Orientia* gen. nov., as *Orientia tsutsugamushi* comb. nov. *International Journal of Systematic Bacteriology*, Vol. 45, No. (3), pp. 589-591, 0020-7713

Tan, L. V., D. Q. Ha, et al. (2008). Me Tri virus: a Semliki Forest virus strain from Vietnam? *Journal of General Virology*, Vol. 89, No. (9), pp. 2132-2135, 1465-2099

Taylor, L. H., S. M. Latham, et al. (2001). Risk factors for human disease emergence. *Philosophical Transactions of the Royal Society of London. Series B: Biological Sciences*, Vol. 356, No. (1411), pp. 983-989, 0962-8436

Telford, S. R., P. M. Armstrong, et al. (1997). A new tick-borne encephalitis-like virus infecting New England deer ticks, Ixodes dammini. *Emerging Infectious Diseases*, Vol. 3, No. (2), pp. 165-170, 1080-6059

Telford, S. R., J. E. Dawson, et al. (1996). Perpetuation of the agent of human granulocytic ehrlichiosis in a deer tick-rodent cycle. *Proceedings of the National Academy of Sciences*, Vol. 93, No. (12), pp. 6209-6214, 1091-6490

Tenter, A. M., A. R. Heckeroth, et al. (2000). *Toxoplasma gondii*: from animals to humans. *International Journal for Parasitology*, Vol. 30, No. (12-13), pp. 1217-1258, 0020-7519

Thorner, A. R., D. H. Walker, et al. (1998). Rocky Mountain Spotted Fever. *Clinical Infectious Diseases*, Vol. 27, No. (6), pp. 1353-1360, 1058-4838

Tissot-Dupont, H., S. Torres, et al. (1999). Hyperendemic focus of Q fever related to sheep and wind. *American Journal of Epidemiology*, Vol. 150, No. (1), pp. 67-74, 1476-6256

Touahri, T., M. Pulik, et al. (2002). Toxoplasmic Encephalitis in a Non-HIV Patient With Follicular Lymphoma. *International Journal of Hematology*, Vol. 75, No. (1), pp. 111-112-112, 0925-5710

Traub, R. and C. L. Wisseman (1974). The Ecology of Chigger-Borne Rickettsiosis (Scrub Typhus). *Journal of Medical Entomology*, Vol. 11, No., pp. 237-303, 0022-2585

Treadwell, T. A., R. C. Holman, et al. (2000). Rocky Mountain spotted fever in the United States, 1993-1996. *American Journal of Tropical Medicine and Hygiene*, Vol. 63, No. (1), pp. 21-26, 1476-1645

Valassina, M., M. Cusi, et al. (2003). A Mediterranean arbovirus: The Toscana virus. *Journal of NeuroVirology*, Vol. 9, No., pp. 577-583, 1538-2443

Valassina, M., M. Valentini, et al. (2003). Serological Survey of Toscana Virus Infections in a High-Risk Population in Italy. *Clinical and Vaccine Immunology*, Vol. 10, No. (3), pp. 483-484, 1556-679X

Van Ranst, M. (2004). Chandipura virus: an emerging human pathogen? *The Lancet*, Vol. 364, No. (9437), pp. 821-822, 0140-6736

Varela-Stokes, A. S. (2007). Transmission of Ehrlichia chaffeensis from lone star ticks (*Amblyomma americanum*) to white-tailed deer (*Odocoileus virginianus*). *Journal of Wildlife Diseases*, Vol. 43, No. (3), July 1, 2007, pp. 376-381, 1943-3700

Vincent P. Hsu, M. J. H., † Umesh D. Parashar,* Mohammed Monsur Ali,‡ Thomas G. Ksiazek,* Ivan Kuzmin,* Michael Niezgoda,* Charles Rupprecht,* Joseph Bresee,* and Robert F. Breiman† (2004). Nipah virus encephalitis reemergence, Bangladesh. *Emerging Infectious Diseases*, Vol. 10, No. (12), pp., 1080-6040

Vogel, J. P. (2004). Turning a tiger into a house cat: using *Legionella pneumophila* to study *Coxiella burnetii*. *Trends in Microbiology*, Vol. 12, No. (3), pp. 103-105, 0966-842X

Voth, D. E. and R. A. Heinzen (2007). Lounging in a lysosome: the intracellular lifestyle of *Coxiella burnetii*. *Cellular Microbiology*, Vol. 9, No. (4), pp. 829-840, 1462-5822

Wainwright, K. E., M. A. Miller, et al. (2007). Chemical Inactivation of *Toxoplasma gondii* Oocysts in Water. *The Journal of Parasitology*, Vol. 93, No. (4), pp. 925-931, 0022-3395

Walker, D. (1996). Rickettsiae, In: *Medical Microbiology*, B. Baron, pp. University of Texas Medical Branch at Galveston, Retrieved from

Walls, J. J., K. M. Asanovich, et al. (1998). Serologic Evidence of a Natural Infection of White-Tailed Deer with the Agent of Human Granulocytic Ehrlichiosis in Wisconsin and Maryland. *Clinical and Vaccine Immunology*, Vol. 5, No. (6), pp. 762-765, 1556-679X

Wang, L.-F., J. S. Mackenzie, et al. (2008). Disease Outbreaks Caused by Emerging Paramyxoviruses of Bat Origin, In: *Emerging Infections in Asia*, Y. Lu, M. Essex and B. Roberts, pp. (193-208), Springer US, Retrieved from <http://dx.doi.org/10.1007/978-0-387-75722-3_12>

Warrilow, D., I. L. Smith, et al. (2002). Sequence Analysis of an Isolate from a Fatal Human Infection of Australian Bat Lyssavirus. *Virology*, Vol. 297, No. (1), pp. 109-119, 0042-6822

Weaver, S. C. and A. D. T. Barrett (2004). Transmission cycles, host range, evolution and emergence of arboviral disease. *Nature Reviews Microbiology*, Vol. 2, No. (10), pp. 789-801, 1740-1526

Weaver, S. C., A. C. Brault, et al. (1999). Genetic and Fitness Changes Accompanying Adaptation of an Arbovirus to Vertebrate and Invertebrate Cells. *The Journal of Virology*, Vol. 73, No. (5), pp. 4316-4326, 1465-2099

Weaver, S. C., C. Ferro, et al. (2004). Venezuelan Equine Encephalitis. *Annual Review of Entomology*, Vol. 49, No. (141-174), pp., 1545-4487

Weaver, S. C., W. Kang, et al. (1997). Recombinational history and molecular evolution of western equine encephalomyelitis complex alphaviruses. *The Journal of Virology*, Vol. 71, No. (1), pp. 613-623, 1465-2099

Weaver, S. C., T. W. Scott, et al. (1991). Molecular evolution of eastern equine encephalomyelitis virus in North America. *Virology*, Vol. 182, No. (2), pp. 774-784, 0042-6822

Welsh, H. H., E. H. Lennette, et al. (1958). Air-borne transmission of Q fever: the role of parturition in the generation of infective aerosols. *Annals of the New York Academy of Sciences*, Vol. 70, No. (3), pp. 528-540, 1749-6632

WHO. Dengue and dengue haemorrhagic fever, In: *Media centre* Available from: <http://www.who.int/mediacentre/factsheets/fs117/en/>

Williamson, M. M., P. T. Hooper, et al. (2000). Experimental Hendra Virus Infectionin Pregnant Guinea-pigs and Fruit Bats (*Pteropus poliocephalus*). *Journal of Comparative Pathology*, Vol. 122, No. (2-3), pp. 201-207, 0021-9975

Work, K. (1967). Isolation of *Toxoplasma Gondii* from the flesh of sheep, swine and cattle. *Acta Pathologica Microbiologica Scandinavica*, Vol. 71, No. (2), pp. 296-306, 1600-0463

Zacks, M. A. and S. Paessler (2010). Encephalitic alphaviruses. *Veterinary Microbiology*, Vol. 140, No. (3-4), pp. 281-286, 0378-1135

Zamparo, J. M., T. G. Andreadis, et al. (1997). Serologic evidence of Jamestown Canyon virus infection in white-tailed deer populations from Connecticut. *Journal of Wildlife Diseases*, Vol. 33, No. (3), pp. 623-627, 1943-3700

2

Zoonoses Surveillance in Italy (2000-2009): Investigation on Animals with Neurological Symptoms

Cristina Casalone[1], Barbara Iulini[1] et al.*
[1]*Istituto Zooprofilattico Sperimentale of Piemonte, Liguria and Valle D'Aosta*
Italy

1. Introduction

Zoonoses are defined by the World Health Organization (WHO) as "Those diseases and infections naturally transmitted between vertebrae animals and man" (WHO 1959) (Palmer et al., 1998). They may be caused by viruses, bacteria, including chlamidiae and rickettsiae, fungi, protozoa, helminths and arthropods (Krauss et al., 2003), and transmitted directly (through contact with skin, hair, eggs, blood or secretions) or indirectly (by insect vectors and ingestion of contaminated food). Currently, 1415 pathogens for humans have been identified and of these approximately 61% (868) are agents of zoonoses, some of which manifest with neurological signs; 132 agents are also associated with emerging zoonoses (Asjo et al., 2007; Matassa, 2007; Taylor et al. , 2001). Neurological zoonoses are widespread, especially in the developing countries where they are not even diagnosed in most cases.

Emerging zoonoses of recently identified pathogens are Lyme disease, cryptosporidiosis, West Nile disease, transmissible spongiform encephalopathy, and possible variants of the avian influenza virus, which have found new favourable conditions for spreading. In contrast, re-emerging zoonoses are well-known diseases considered as eradicated in a given country but recur with an exponentially increasing incidence, such as tuberculosis, leptospirosis, rabies (Matassa, 2007).

Pathogens are constantly evolving and spreading in different countries through animals that act as an asymptomatic reservoir and release pathogens into the environment (Krauss et al., 2003). Among these, wild animals, both mammals and migratory birds, play an important role.

* Maria Domenica Pintore[1], Cristiana Maurella[1], Elena Bozzetta[1], Carlo Cantile[2], Gualtiero Gandini[3], Maria Teresa Capucchio[4], Arianna Calistri[5], Antonio D'angelo[4], Maria Caramelli[1]
[2] *Department of Animal Pathology, University of Pisa, Italy*
[3]*Department of Veterinary Medical Sciences of the University of Bologna, Italy*
[4]*Department of Animal Pathology, University of Turin, Italy*
[5]*Department of Histology, Microbiology and Medical Biotechnologies University of Padova, Italy*

Neurological diseases include those caused by highly pathogenic neurotropic agents such as rabies viruses and opportunistic agents that may develop disease in the immunocompromised. These agents belong to the genus Rhabdovirus, Herpesvirus, Flavivirus, Alphavirus, Bornavirus and Circovirus; others are bacteria such as *Listeria monocytogenes, Borrelia garinii* and *Borrelia afzelii, Chlamydophila psittaci, Campylobacter jejuni,* or parasites such as *Toxoplasma gondii, Encephalitozoon cuniculi,* and *Halicephalobus gingivalis.* Recognized neurozoonotic agents among the fungi are *Aspergillus* spp., *Mucor* spp., *Candida* spp. and *Cryptococcus neoformans.*
Within the group of food-borne zoonoses, *E. coli* O157: H7 is a particularly relevant syndrome because ruminants, especially cattle, are the main reservoir of the bacterium, while milk and dairy products and meat are the vehicle of infection.
At a 2004 meeting on emerging zoonoses jointly organized by the WHO, FAO and OIE, the factors that contribute to the emergence of zoonoses were carefully analyzed: greater pathogen adaptation and resistance (new strains); increased drug resistance; increased susceptibility of humans and animals; climate change and so on.
Currently, there are about 60 (DPR 320/54 and European Directive 2003/99/EC), notifiable animal diseases in Italy, many of which are zoonoses, but this list is always likely to change. It is also worth pointing out that the existence of animal reservoirs (domestic and wild) and complex transmission mechanisms, by vector and food, make collaboration between human and veterinary medicine essential for ensuring public health safety.
The objective of this study was to investigate the presence of neurological zoonoses or zoonotic agents in Italy, and to estimate the epidemiological impact of neurological diseases potentially transmissible to humans. It is important to assess which species are at risk of disease and which are the best reservoirs for pathogens in order to understand the cause of their onset and which measures could be taken against their spread.

2. Materials and methods

From 01 January 2008 to 31 December 2009, 990 animals of different species presenting with neurological signs were investigated in the different participating study centres.
All subjects underwent clinical examination and only cases with central nervous system (CNS) involvement were analyzed further. Serum or whole blood and cerebrospinal fluid of some animals (CSF) were collected and examined. When the animals died or were slaughtered, necropsy was performed and samples were collected from the various organs and the CNS. Depending on the symptoms reported, samples from the spinal cord, muscles and nerves were also taken. The tissues were frozen for cultural and/or molecular investigations and fixed in 10% buffered formalin for histological and immunohistochemical (IHC) analysis.
Moreover, a retrospective investigation of cases recorded in the database of the participating study centres from 01/01/2000 to 31/12/2007 was performed. The case history of 570 animals dead or slaughtered, presenting with neurological signs and inflammatory lesions was examined. Among these, all the cases had already been diagnosed as affected by a zoonotic disease and those with lesions related to inflammatory diseases potentially transmissible to humans were selected.
In order to identify the pathogenic agent, suspected cases were submitted to cultural, biomolecular and IHC investigation using frozen or formalin-fixed tissue and/or previously stored CSF.

A total of 1560 cases were studied in the period from 2000 to 2009 (Graph. 1).

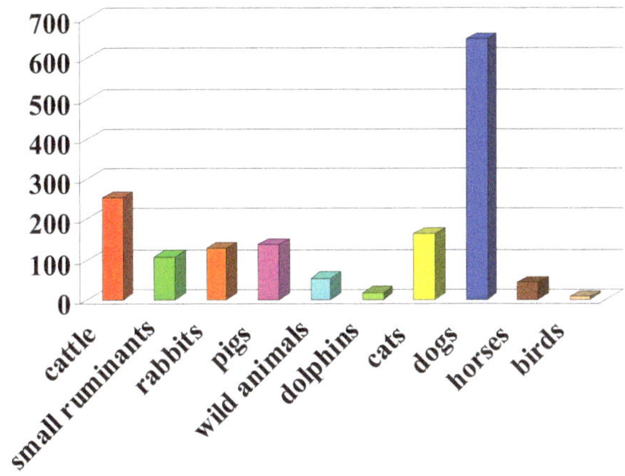

Graph. 1. Graphic representation of different species of animals studied in the period from 2000 to 2009

Cerebrospinal fluid examination: CSF samples were collected from the cisterna magna or lumbar level. Quantitative determination of total protein was carried out by photometric colorimetric testing, using as a normal range for total protein 0-30 mg/dl for fluid from the cisterna magna and 0-45 mg/dl from the lumbar region. Cell count was performed by blood cell count using a Fuchs-Rosenthal chamber, taking 0-5 cells/ mcl as the normal range, while the sediment obtained by cytocentrifugation (600 rpm for 10 min) was read by light microscopy after Romanonsky-type staining (Diff Quick Stain).

Neuropathological examination: the CNS was divided by a paramedian cut in two parts including the cerebral hemisphere, cerebellum and medulla oblongata. Coronal sections of formalin-fixed brain were made at the level of the brain stem, cerebellum, thalamus, hippocampus, and basal ganglia, including the cerebral cortex and any other areas presenting with gross lesions.

To evaluate the histological lesions, each sample was processed, embedded in paraffin, and microtome sections of about 4-5 μm were prepared; the sections were stained with haematoxylin-eosin. When necessary, specific histologic stains were also carried out, e.g., Masson's trichrome, Weigert van Gieson, Congo red, Luxol fast blue-cresyl violet (for evaluation of myelin), Bielschowsky silver-impregnation (for evaluation of axons), Gram staining, Grocott, Giemsa and Good-Pasture, periodic acid-Schiff's reagent (PAS) and Gomori trichrome, methenamine silver (for the recognition of fungal elements), mucicarmine (for recognition of *Cryptococcus neoformans*) and Ziehl Neelsen (for recognition of protozoan elements), as described in standard protocols (S. Daniel and T. Zanin, 1997).

When the histological investigation did not allow a definite diagnosis, samples were subjected to IHC, cultural and molecular (PCR) examination.

Immunohistochemical (IHC) examination: on histological sections with suspected lesions, specific antigens for *Listeria* spp. *Encephalitozoon cuniculi, Streptococcus suis, Neospora caninum*, and *Toxoplasma gondii* were investigated. Antibodies from commercially available kits were used according to the methods specific for the antigen. Deparaffinized and rehydrated sections were subjected to different types of unmasking according to the protocols: microwave (750 W), trypsin (0.1% with 0.1% Ca carbonate) or in a bain-marie (citrate buffer pH 6.1 to variable temperature). After rinsing, the sections were incubated for 4-12 h at 37°C or overnight at 4°C with specific monoclonal antibodies diluted (1:50; 1:500; 1:1000) in PBS. Subsequent antibody detection was carried out using biotinylated goat anti-mouse or anti horse secondary antibody diluted (1:200-1:1000) in PBS, for 20 min at room temperature, followed by the avidina-biotin-peroxidase complex. (Vectastain ABC kit, Vector Laboratories). Immunoreactivity was visualized using 3,3'-diaminobenzidine as chromogen; the sections were counterstained with Mayer's haematoxylin counterstain.
Cultural examination: bacteria isolation provides a first incubation at 35-37° C for 24-48 h on selective (Demi-Fraser; Oxford agar; Mac Conkey) and non-selective culture medium (blood agar with 5% sheep blood). Biochemical identification of the isolated strain was carried out on pure culture with an API Rapid system.
Biomolecular examination: frozen brain biopsies were individually macerated in a laminar flow bench and total nucleic acids were purified using a NucliSENS® easyMAG® system (bioMérieux, Inc., Durham, NC, USA) according to the manufacturer's instructions. Formalin-fixed paraffin-embedded samples were initially deparaffinizated using a xylene-based technique prior to nucleic acid extraction. All samples were tested for cellular adequacy and absence of PCR inhibitors by PCR amplification of the b-actin gene DNA (for DNA extraction) or cDNA (for RNA extraction) as previously described (Salata et al., 2009).
The samples were tested by real-time RT-PCR for West Nile Virus (WNV) and enterovirus-RNA detection using the oligonucleotide primers and TaqMan probe targeting the WNV E gene (Lanciotti et al. , 000) or the enteroviral genome 5' untranscribed region (Donaldson et al., 2002). In the procedure used, the nucleic acid (about 60 ng) was combined with Superscript® One Step RT-PCR System reagents (Invitrogen Ltd, Paisley, UK), primers and probe, reaching a total reaction volume of 20 µl, and amplified in a LightCycler® 2.0 real-time PCR System (Roche Diagnostics S.p.A., Monza, Italy).
Real-time PCR assays were used to test for the presence of *Toxoplasma gondii* (Lin et al. , 2000), *Borrelia burgdorferi* (Exner et al., 2003), *Listeria* spp. and *L. monocytogenes* (Rodríguez-Lázaro et al. ,2004), and *Chlamydia* spp. (Yang et al., 2006) with some modifications. Briefly, the extracted nucleic acid (about 60 ng) was assayed with an ABI PRISM 7700 sequence detector system (Applied Biosystems, Foster City, CA, USA) in 25 µl of a PCR mixture containing 12.5 µl TaqMan universal master mix, 15 pmol of each primer, and 10 pmol of the probe under standard amplification conditions.
End-point PCR assays were used to assay all samples for Borna virus (Cotto et al., 2003), tick-borne encephalitis virus (Puchhammer-Stoeckl et al., 1995), herpesvirus (Rose et al. , 1997) and fungi (Sutar et al., 2004). Reverse transcription, if necessary, was performed as described by Bergonzini et al., 2009. Thermal cycling conditions were: one cycle at 95°C for 10min and 40 cycles at 95°C for 30 s; 50-60°C for 45 s; 72°C for 1 min; and an additional cycle at 72°C for 10 min.
To detect herpesvirus, a set of degenerate PCR primers targeting the highly conserved DNA polymerase genes of the Herpesvirus family was used, while in the case of fungi the rDNA internal transcribed spacer sequences were targeted by primers. Subsequently, herpesvirus

or fungi typing was carried out by bi-directional sequencing of amplicons using the BigDye1 Terminator v3.1 Cycle Sequencing Kit on a 3100 Genetic Analyzer (Applied Biosystems). After alignment with the SeqScape v2.5 software (Applied Biosystems), the sequences were compared with the ones available in GenBank by using the NCBI BLAST tool.
Electron-microscopy: in suspected cases of Leishmaniasis, Protothecosis and Neosporosis, electron microscopical investigations were carried out for the morphological identification of the aetiological agents. Selected tissues were cut into small pieces of about 3 mm3 which were post-fixed with osmium tetroxide, dehydrated with ethanol and embedded in epoxy resin. Sections of 1 micron thick were cut by ultramicrotome, stained with toluidine blue and observed by light microscopy. Selected blocks were then sectioned in ultra-thin sections, stained with uranyl acetate and lead citrate and observed by electron microscopy.
Muscle biopsy: muscle biopsies were received fresh and wrapped in gauze moistened with saline solution and then were snap frozen by immersion in isopentane precooled in liquid nitrogen and stored at -80 °C. Eight μm-thick sections were stained and reacted with a standard panel of histochemical stains and enzyme reactions (H&E, PAS, ORO, Gomori trichrome, ATPase pH 4.3 and 9.8, NADH-TR, SDH, COX, non specific esterase).
Nerve biopsy: nerve samples of 1 to 2 cm in length, depending on the nerve tested, were fixed in 2.5% glutaraldehyde solution in slight tension on a rigid support, to avoid artifacts of the nerve fibers. After washing in phosphate buffer, the samples were post-fixed in osmium tetroxide, dehydrated with ethanol of increasing concentration and embedded in epoxy resin. Sections of 1 micron thick were cut by ultramicrotome, stained with toluidine blue and observed by light microscopy.

3. Results

In 660 animals (42%), traumatic, vascular, congenital, muscular and articular diseases were diagnosed by clinical examination; no CNS involvement was found. In 353 subjects (23%), probable zoonoses were identified; 82 of these (73 dogs and 9 cats) showed neuropathological lesions associated with viral infections of unknown origin and therefore considered as "potential zoonoses" in the literature (Graph. 2). In 337 (22%) cases, pathologies not transmissible to humans were present: neoplasia, toxic-degenerative and bacterial diseases, distemper, FIV, FELV, FIP, IBR, CAEV Visna, border disease, etc., and therefore were not considered in this study. In 194 cases (12%), no diagnosis was established because the case history was incomplete and/or tissues were unsuitable for biomolecular investigations. Sixteen animals (1%) showed no lesions (Graph. 3). Overall, 16 zoonoses were detected in 271 animals of different species (Table 1).
Encephalitozoonosis - In 110 (31.5%) rabbits, *Encephalitozoon cuniculi* was isolated. The clinical signs were variable, reflecting the site of lesions in the brain: convulsions, discoordination, paresis or paralysis and stiff neck were reported. The thalamus and hippocampus presented with more severe damage. In all animals there was a granulomatous meningo-encephalitis characterized by perivascular cuffs and focal granulomas composed of epithelioid histiocytes and lymphocytes, some of which showed a centre composed of amorphous eosinophilic material (Fig. 1). In all, 78% of these subjects were serologically positive for *Encephalitozoon cuniculi*; and in some cases IHC and Ziehl-Neelsen stain highlighted individual or aggregates of parasites within the granulomas, thus confirming the diagnosis (Figs. 2 and 3).
Listeriosis - In 47 (13.5%) cases (33 cattle and 14 sheep) *Listeria* spp. was isolated. Clinically, the animals showed depression, fever, paralysis, twisted neck, tremors, ataxia, motion

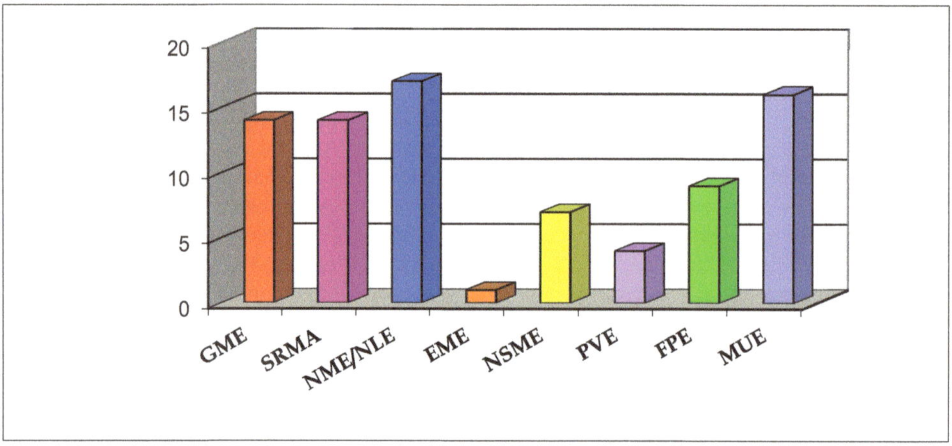

* GME: Granulomatous Meningoencephalitis; SRMA: Steroid-responsive meningitis-arteritis; NEM/NLE: Encephalo-mielitis/Leuco-encephalitis necrotizing; EME: Eosinophilic maningo-encephalitis; NSME: Non suppurative meningo-encephalitis; PVE: Periventricular encephalitis ; FPE: Feline polio-encephalomielitis ; MUE: Meningoencephalomyelitis of undetermined etiology

Graph. 2. Graphic representation of diseases of "**unknown aetiology**".

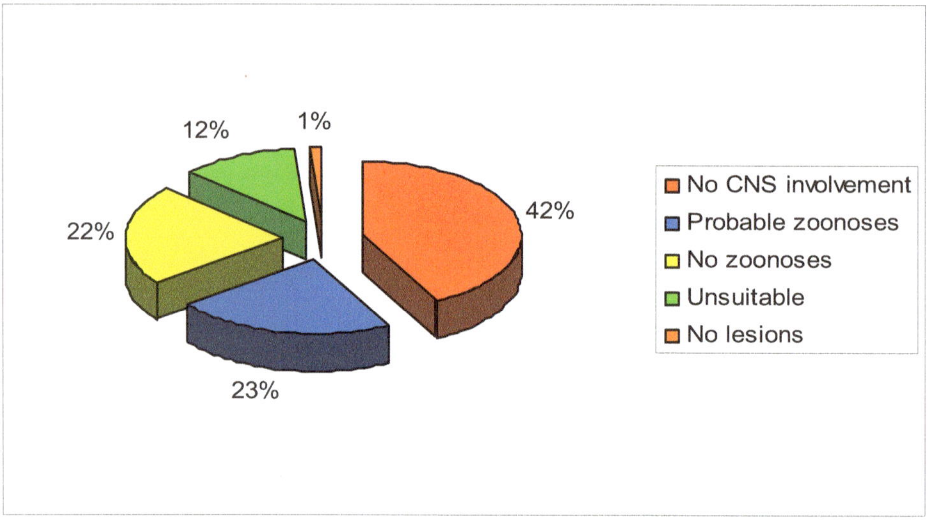

Graph. 3. Graphic representation of results obtained in this study

ZOONOSES	CATTLE	SMALL RUMINANTS	DOGS	CATS	HORSES	PIGS	DOLPHINS	RABBITS	BIRDS	WILD ANIMALS
Halicephalobiasis					2					
Neosporosis	4		11							
Borna disease		2								
Toxoplasmosis			2	1		2	2			
Rickettsiosis			1							
Nocardiosis			1							
Cryptococcosis			3	1						
Protothecosis			1							
Leishmania disease			1							
West Nile disease					15					
Unknown aetiology			73	9						
Listeriosis	33	14								
Colibacillosis	15	1				5				
Encephalitozoonosis								110		
Coenurosis	1	16								
Streptococcosis						26				
Chlamydiosis	1									

Table 1. Zoonoses diagnosed in the period of study

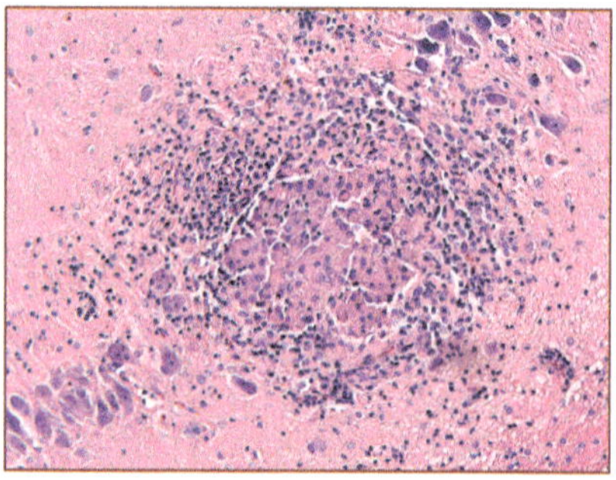

Fig. 1. Rabbit. *Encephalitozoon cuniculi*: parassitic granuloma in the hippocampus (HE, 20x).

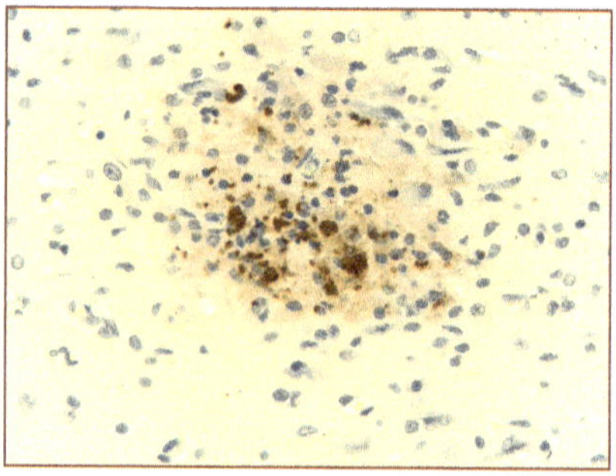

Fig. 2. Rabbit. *Encephalitozoon* cuniculi: parassitic antigen within a granuloma reaction (IHC, 40x).

handling, dysphagia, recumbency and death. The histological lesions showed a nonsuppurative meningo-encephalitis characterized by microabscesses (Fig. 4) and perivascular cuffings of lymphocytes and monocytes, distributed from the obex to the thalamus. The most severely affected areas were the pons and the midbrain, where often variable degree of haemorrhage was often observed. When fresh or frozen tissue (26 cases) was available, *Listeria monocytogenes* was isolated by cultural examination; moreover, IHC analysis showed the bacterial antigen predominantly in the microabscesses, less frequently in the perivascular cuffs (Fig. 5).

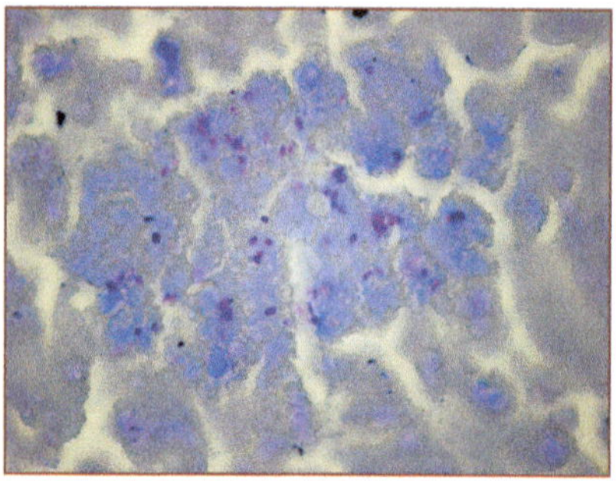

Fig. 3. Rabbit. *Encephalitozoon* cuniculi: parasites within a cerebral granuloma (ZN, 40x).

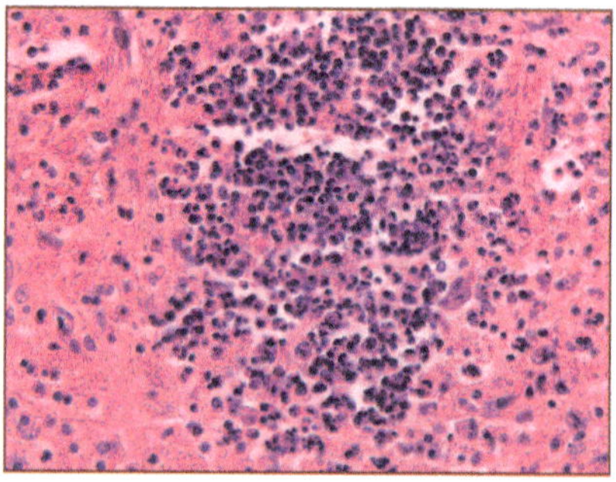

Fig. 4. Cow. *Listeria monocytogenes*: microabscess in the brain stem (HE, 40x).

Streptococcosis - In 26 (7.5%) pigs, a bacterial meningo-encephalitis was caused by *Streptococcus suis*. All our cases involved fattening piglets, 2 to 6 months of age, presenting with depression, anorexia, weight loss, ataxic gait, opisthotonus, and pedalling. The histopathological lesions showed a suppurative meningitis or mild to severe meningo-encephalitis (Fig. 6), diffuse lympho-histiocytic perivascular cuffing with some neutrophils, vasculitis, neuronal degeneration and haemorrhage; sometimes the lesions extended to the choroid plexus. In 14 cases, the bacterium was isolated directly from the CNS, and in 6 of these, also from other organs such as spleen, kidney, liver, lungs and trachea. Moreover, in

12 cases *S. suis* was found only at the level of the trachea and lungs, but only 6 of these had neuropathological lesions. IHC confirmed *S. suis* serotype 2 infection in 10 cases (Fig. 7).

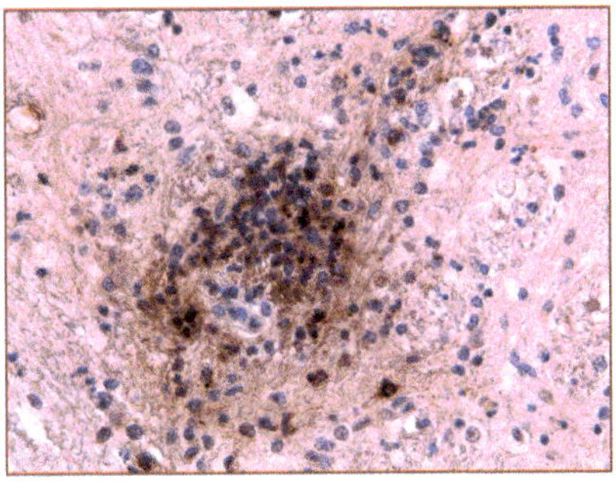

Fig. 5. Cow. *Listeria monocytogenes*: bacterial antigen within a microabscess (IHC, 40x).

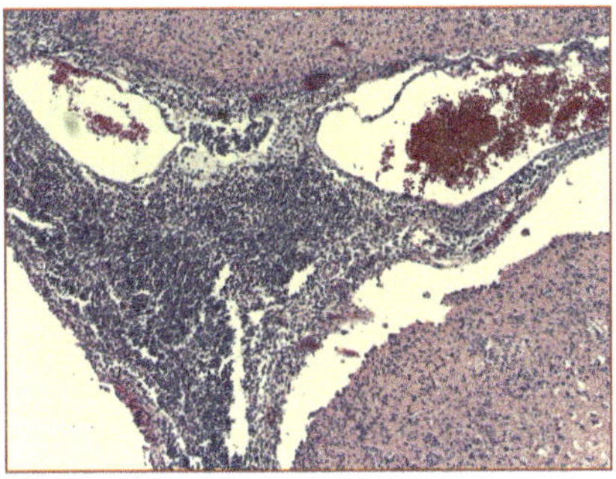

Fig. 6. Pig. *Streptococcus suis:* suppurative meningo-encephalitis (HE, 10x).

Colibacillosis - In 21 (6%) cases, involving 15 calves, 1 lamb and 5 piglets, *E. coli* was isolated. All presented with hyperacute or acute septicaemia, depression, ataxic gait, opisthotonus and sudden death. The neuropathological lesions were similar in all cases and showed a massive suppurative meningo-encephalitis characterized by mononuclear cells and a high amount of neutrophils. There was also marked vasculitis throughout the brain; in some cases, abscess-like lesions were visible, predominantly in the brainstem. The diagnosis was confirmed by bacterial culture.

Coenurosis - In 17 (5 %) cases (1 cattle and 16 sheep) larvae of the *Taenia multiceps* tapeworm were identified. Clinical signs and severity of the acute phase depended on the number of eggs ingested, the extent of inflammatory response, and the location of the parasite in the CNS. The clinical records reported weight loss, apathy, adynamia, tendency to isolation, depression, blindness, head tilt and ataxia. Histologically, focal haemorrhage or malacia caused by the migratory phase of the larval stage (acute stage), were observed at the level of the cerebral hemispheres or in the caudal brainstem. In the chronic phase, the visible cysts were surrounded by atrophic tissue. The diameter of the cysts, single or multiple, varied from 1 to 4.5 cm and appeared as an empty space surrounded by a granulomatous reaction composed of macrophages, giant cells, lymphocytes and plasma cells, and a few granulocytes. Outwardly, many macrophages, more or less extensive haemorrhage, fibrin or fibrin-purulent leptomeningitis and mononuclear perivascular cuffs were sometimes observed. In many cases it was possible to extract the parasitic cysts in which the cephalic protoscolices were visible.

West Nile encephalitis - West Nile virus was isolated in 15 (4%) horses. The horses were 9 females and 6 males, 2 to 19 years of age, mostly trotters from the provinces of Ferrara and Bologna. The horses underwent detailed neurological examination, blood-biochemical and serological tests. The blood-biochemical tests showed no significant changes, except in 5 horses in which there were slight alterations of inflammatory proteins in the acute phase. Three horses were asymptomatic, 12 had clinical signs attributable to acute forms such as dysorexia and depression, weakness, low-grade fever, hypersensitivity to touch and sound, ataxia of all four limbs (4 cases) or the hind limbs (4 cases), paraparesis (6 cases) or tetraparesis (3 cases), and three subjects presented with neurological signs indicative of intracranial involvement. In most cases (10 animals) these signs were mild to moderate and quickly improved with recovery in all subjects. Only two horses were euthanatized because of severe disease progression; sampling of CSF, necropsy and histological examination of the CNS were performed. The first test showed moderate, predominantly mononuclear pleocytosis, and the histopathological examination revealed lesions distributed mainly at the caudal brainstem and the thoracic and lumbar spinal cord. In detail, a mild to moderate nonsuppurative encephalomyelitis characterized by perivascular cuffs of mononuclear inflammatory cells, glial nodules and focal gliosis in the gray matter were observed. In the spinal cord the lesions were bilateral and symmetrical, involving the gray matter, particularly the lateral and ventral horns (Fig. 8). At this level, a nonsuppurative inflammation was identified sometimes associated with neuronal degeneration, gliosis, neuronophagia and occasionally neutrophils. Small glial foci involved the white matter in both the spinal cord and brainstem; oedema and mild inflammatory infiltrate characterized by mononuclear cells were observed in the meninges.

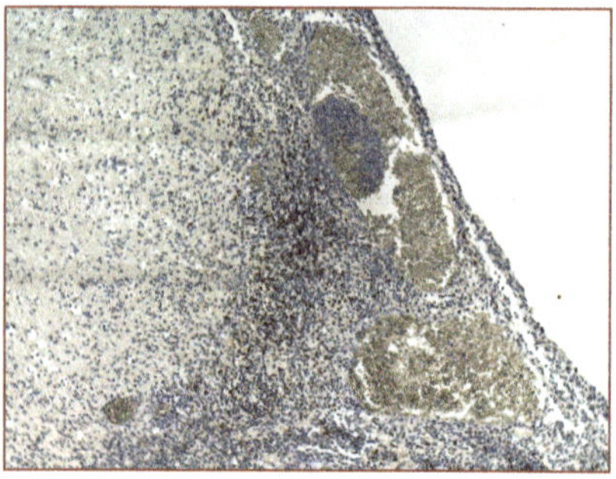

Fig. 7. Pig. *Streptococcus suis:* bacterial antigen within macrophages and neutrophils cytoplasm (IHC, 10x).

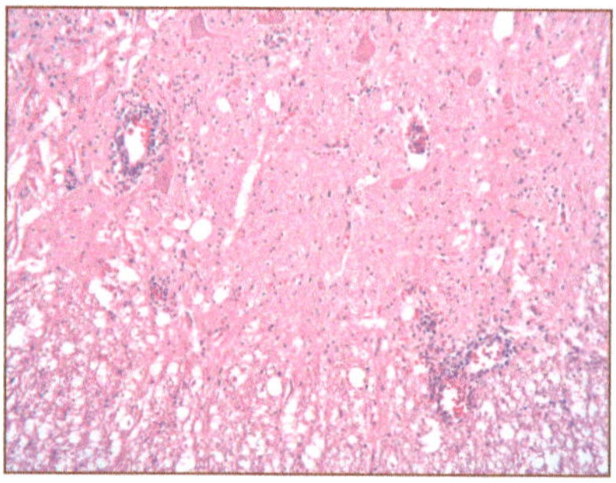

Fig. 8. Horse. *West Nile virus:* inflammatory infiltrate of mononuclear cells in the ventral horn of spinal cord (HE, 10x).

Neosporosis - In 4 calves and 11 dogs (4%) the protozoan *Neospora caninum* was found. The calves were a few days old and showed ataxia and limb paralysis. Histology showed similar nonsuppurative lesions in both the peripheral and the CNS. In detail, there were nonsuppurative meningomyelitis (meningo-encephalomyelitis in one case), polyradiculoneuritis, fibrosis of the peripheral nerves and neurogenic muscle atrophy. A large infiltration of lymphocytes and plasma cells was detected in the spinal meninges and nerve emergence of all spinal cord segments, especially at the level of cervico-thoracic and lombo-sacral intumescence. The inflammatory infiltrate appeared most abundant in the ventral roots along the perivascular spaces. In the most affected areas there was multifocal leucomyelitis and protozoan aggregates morphologically attributable to tachyzoites of the genus *Neospora*. In the spinal gray matter, a diffuse gliosis and chromatolysis of motor neurons were observed. The peripheral nerves showed Wallerian degeneration and marked fibrosis. The diagnosis was confirmed by PCR.

The dogs had paralysis, muscle weakness, ataxia, opisthotonus, head tilt and dysphagia. In 9 dogs the CNS was affected with meningo-encephalitis and myelitis; the other 2 dogs presented with polymyositis and chronic axonal neuropathy. An adult dog showed a severe cerebellar necrotizing inflammation with lymphoplasmacytic leptomeningitis, oedema of the white matter, incomplete atrophy and necrosis of the folia, with extensive loss of Purkinje and granular layer cells, often replaced by reactive astrocytes. In some areas, the lesions were more severe, with necrosis, cavitation and the presence of gitter cells and haemosiderin pigment within macrophages. This nonsuppurative inflammation also extended to the subpial neuroparenchyma of the medulla oblongata and pons. The other brain areas were affected less frequently. Clusters of tachyzoites or protozoal cysts were found scattered within the lesions and sometimes in normal nervous tissue. The diagnosis was confirmed by electron microscopy and IHC (Figs. 9-10).

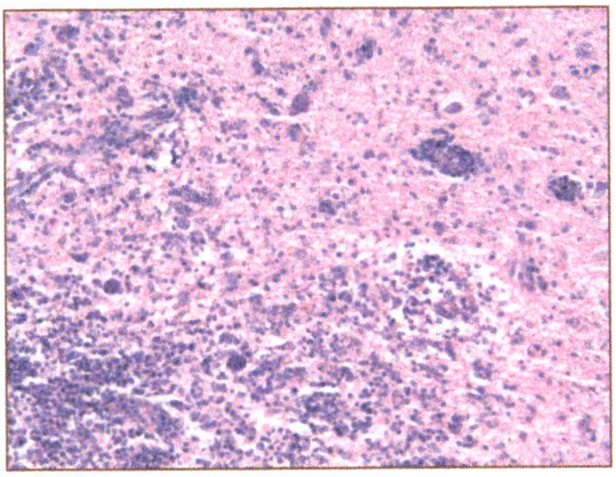

Fig. 9. Dog. *Neospora caninum*: granulomatous inflammation and protozoan cysts in cerebellum (HE, 0x).

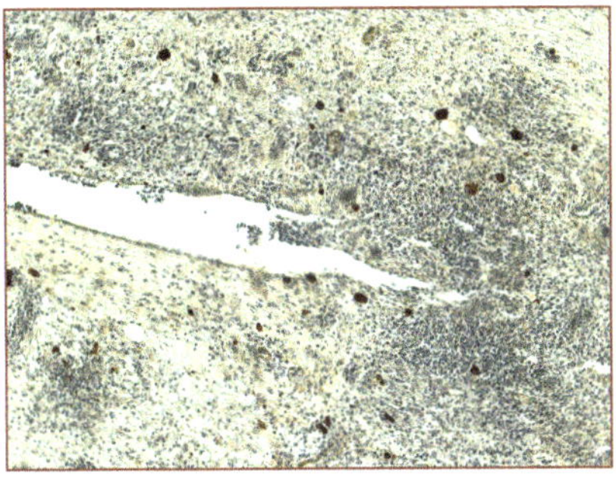

Fig. 10. Dog. *Neospora caninum:* protozoan cysts react with specific antigen in cerebellum (IHC, 40x).

Toxoplasmosis - In 7 animals (2 dogs, 1 cat, 2 pigs and 2 dolphins) (2%) *Toxoplasma gondii* was isolated in the CNS. In the dogs, reported signs were fever, paralysis, vomiting and diarrhoea; the cat had nonspecific signs such as depression, anorexia and fever, vomiting, diarrhoea, prostration, swollen lymph nodes, ataxia, behavioural changes, and circling; the pigs showed ataxia, vomiting and diarrhoea. The histological lesions were typical of a subacute or chronic nonsuppurative meningo-encephalitis characterized by prominent perivascular cuffing of mononuclear cells and multifocal microglial nodules scattered in the surrounding neuropil. In the gray matter there were astrogliosis and mild to moderate neuronal necrosis characterized by vacuolation and chromatolysis. In the most affected areas (pons), lymphocytic vasculitis associated with haemorrhage, oedema and plasmorrhagia was predominant. Single or multiple roundish, basophilic toxoplasma cysts were found scattered in the tissue . The diagnosis was confirmed by IHC and RT-PCR. (Figs. 11-12).

Cryptococcosis - In 4 subjects (2 dogs and 2 cats) (1%) *Cryptococcus neoformans* was isolated. The cats presented with cutaneous nodules, nystagmus, mydriasis, seizures, and also nasal ulcers and sneezing in one case; the dogs showed only neurological symptoms, with seizures, ataxia and abnormal behaviour. The histopathological findings differed between the two species. In the dogs there was a granulomatous meningo-encephalomyelitis, the leptomeninges, brain and spinal cord showed marked multifocal granulomatous inflammatory lesions, with large numbers of macrophages, lymphocytes and plasma cells; in the cats, the inflammatory response was mild. In all cases there were numerous clusters of fungal bodies spread throughout the parenchyma, consisting of circular structures with a slightly eosinophilic core surrounded by a clear halo (capsule) lending it a typical soap bubble appearance, and some were in gemmating phase. The capsule was strongly mucicarmine and PAS positive. The gray matter showed a moderate gliosis. The diagnosis was confirmed by staining of histological sections with mucicarmine. (Fig.13).

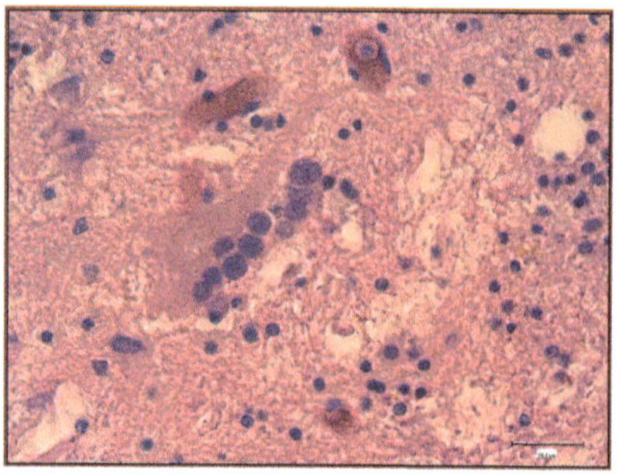

Fig. 11. Dolphin. *Toxoplasma gondii:* protozoan cysts in brain (HE,40x).

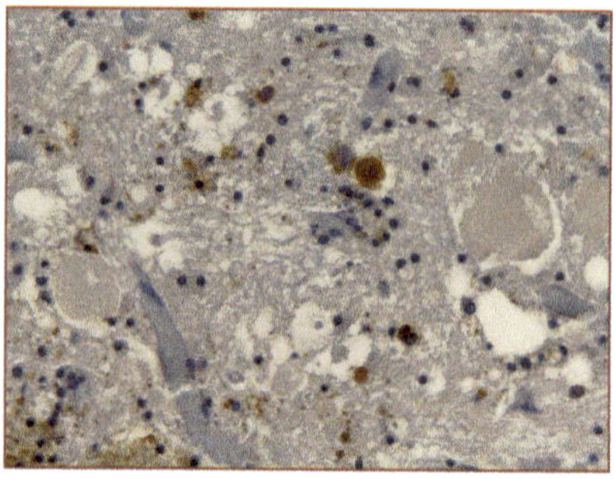

Fig. 12. Dolphin. *Toxoplasma gondii:* protozoan cysts react with specific antigen in brain (IHC, 40x).

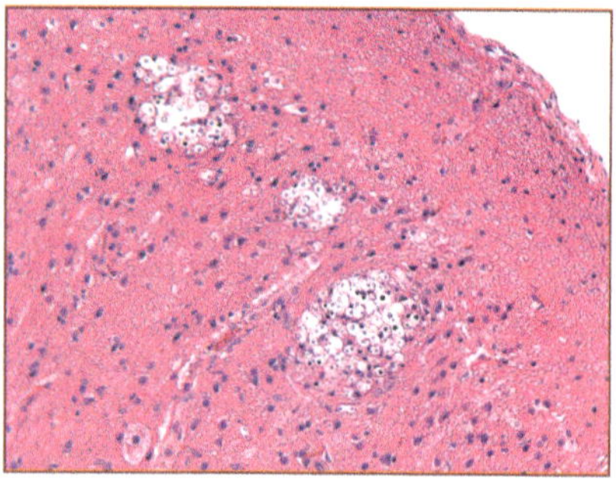

Fig. 13. Cat. *Criptococcus neoformans:* packed yeast bodies with soap bubble appearance in the cerebral cortex (HE,10x).

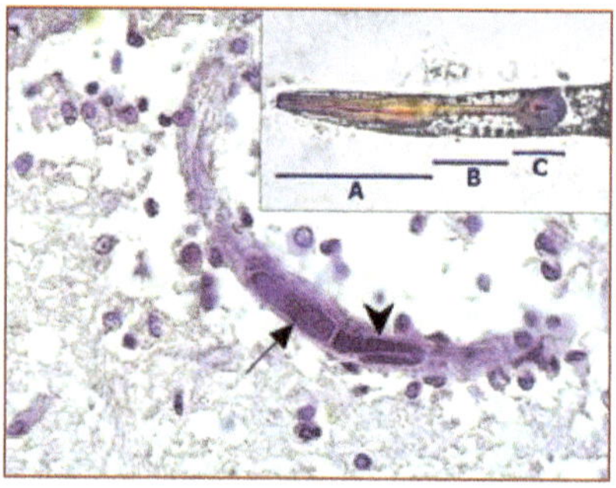

Fig. 14. Horse. *Halicephalobus gingivalis*: tangential section of a mature female in a necrotic area. Morphology of the rhabditiform oesophagus: A: body; B: isthmus; C: bulb (HE, 100x). From Mandara et al. Neuropatologia e neuroimmaging, Poletto ed., 2011.

Halicephalobiasis - In 2 (0.5%) horses, *Halicephalobus gingivalis* was isolated and showed a multifocal neurological syndrome characterized by ataxia, circling, hyperexcitability alternating with depression and blindness in the left eye in one of two subjects. There was also stiffness, recurrent epistaxis and profuse sweating. Rectal temperature and clinical-biochemistry tests were normal. The neuroanatomical site of the lesion was diagnosed at the intracranial level. Neuropathological lesions were very similar. A granulomatous meningo-encephalitis extended predominantly in the cerebellum, brainstem and diencephalon and appeared to be characterized by perivascular infiltrates consisting of lymphocytes, plasma cells, numerous macrophages, multinucleated giant cells and scattered eosinophils. Parasitic elements, 10 to 15 μm in diameter, often oriented around the blood vessels, were present within the inflammatory lesions in the neuroparenchyma, meninges and subarachnoid space (Figs. 14 and 15).

Borna disease - In two sheep (0.5%) bornavirus meningo-encephalitis was diagnosed. The animals showed anorexia, ataxia, abnormal behaviour. The neuropathological examination showed a severe nonsuppurative polioencephalomyelitis with perivascular cuffs of lymphocytes particularly around small-calibre veins of the frontal and temporal cortex, hippocampus, amygdala, and midbrain. At the hippocampal level there were also widespread gliosis with fibrillary astrocytes and neuronal necrosis (Fig. 16). The diagnosis was confirmed by real-time PCR and nested PCR.

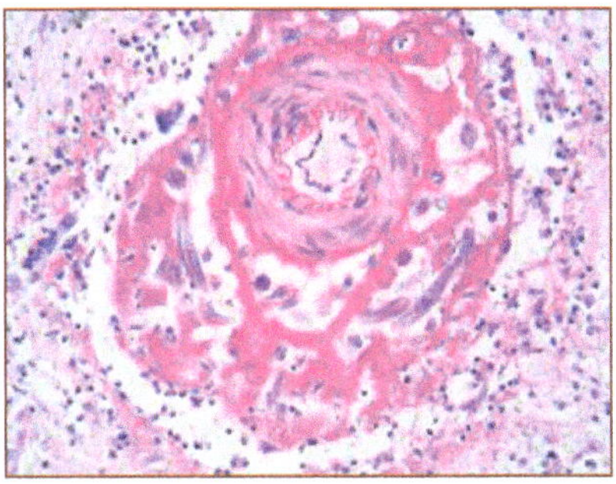

Fig. 15. Horse. *Halicephalobus gingivalis*: perivascular granulomatous infiltrate with presence of nematode around an arteriola (arrows) (HE, 40x)
From Mandara et al. Neuropatologia e neuroimmaging , Poletto ed., 2011.

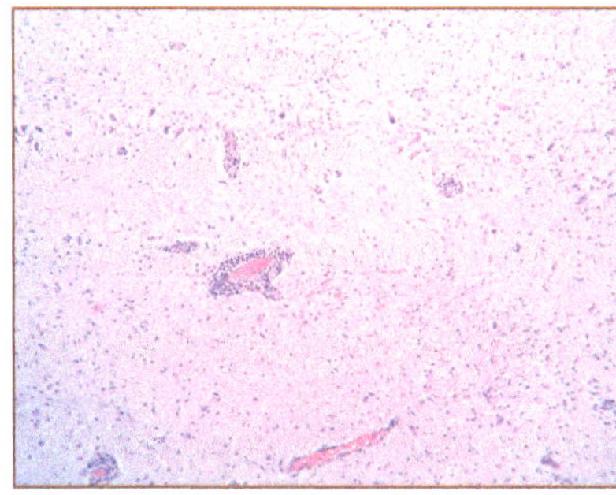

Fig. 16. Sheep. *Bornavirus*: perivascular cuffs and inflammatory infiltrate of mononuclear cells in hippocampus associated with pyramidal cells necrosis (HE, 4x)

Chlamydiosis - In a 6-year-old cattle (0.2%) bacterium of the genus *Chlamydi*a spp. was isolated. The animal presented with abnormal behaviour, muscular tremors which increased when stressed, paralysis, weight loss, decreased milk production and corneal clouding. Histology showed a diffuse inflammation characterized by prominent lymphoplasmacellular and histiocytic perivascular cuffs, associated with vasculitis with few granulocytes. In the cortex there were neuronal necrosis, neuronophagia and marked gliosis (Fig. 17). The lesions were more pronounced at the level of the pons. The diagnosis was confirmed by real-time PCR.

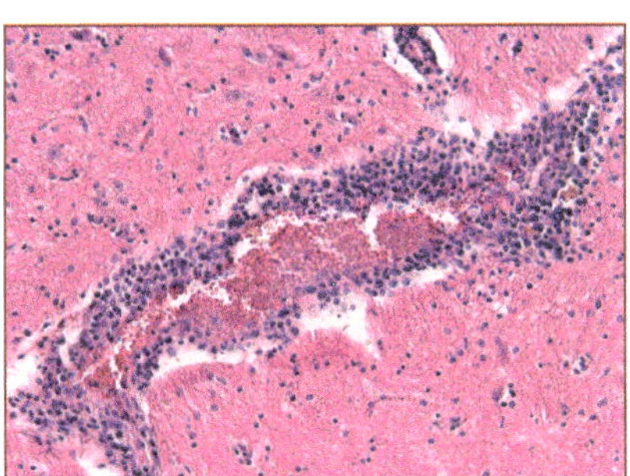

Fig. 17. Cow. *Clamydia spp.*: perivascular cuffs of mononuclear cells (HE, 20x)

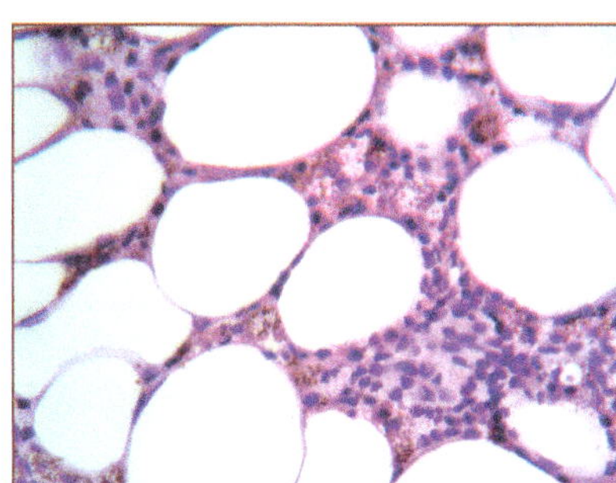

Fig. 18. Dog. *Leishmania infantum*: inflammatory infiltrate and numerous amastigotes in the epidural adipose tissue (HE, 40x)

Leishmaniasis - In one dog (0.2%) adult parasites of the genus *Leishmania* were isolated from a spinal granuloma in an extra-dural site compressing the spinal cord. The animal presented with lymphadenopathy and paraparesis. The lesion consisted of epidural adipose tissue infiltrated by inflammatory cells, primarily composed of macrophages, granulocytes, plasma cells and lymphocytes. In the cytoplasm of the macrophages, there was a large number of small spherical structures due to uniform amastigote forms of *Leishmania* spp. The diagnosis was confirmed by IHC (Fig. 18).

Nocardiosis - In one dog (0.2%) *Nocardia asteroides* was isolated. Macroscopically, there was an abscess-like lesion in the brain stem (Fig. 19). The dog showed fever, depression, difficulty walking and cranial nerve deficits. Histology revealed a piogranulomatous infiltrate consisting of neutrophils, macrophages and lymphocytes. Moreover, aggregates of club-shaped eosinophilic bacteria were found. The diagnosis was confirmed by bacterial culture.

Protothecosis - In one dog (0.2%) achlorophilic algae were isolated. The reported signs were gastrointestinal bleeding with chronic diarrhoea, depression, anorexia, and difficulty walking. Histology showed granulomatous lesions in the neuroparenchyma and meninges consisting of numerous macrophages, lymphocytes, plasma cells and some eosinophils. In the granulomatous foci there were numerous round bodies of variable size surrounded by a PAS positive capsule (Fig. 20), which were identified as achlorophilic algae of the genus *Prototheca*. The diagnosis was confirmed by electron microscopy.

Rickettsiosis - In one dog (0.2%) a microorganism of the genus *Rickettsia* spp. was isolated The reported signs were fever, depression, lethargy, tetraparesis, ataxia, hyperesthesia, vestibular syndrome, seizures, and petechiae in the mucous membranes. Microscopically, there were a nonsuppurative meningo-encephalitis and vasculitis characterized by lymphohistiocytic-type cells and plasma cells infiltrating the nervous tissue and meninges; necrotic areas were also observed (Fig. 21). In this case the diagnosis was confirmed by PCR.

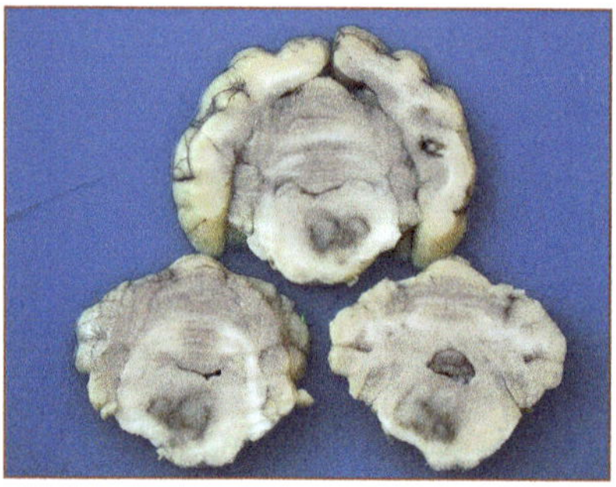

Fig. 19. Dog. *Nocardia asteroides:* abscessual lesion in the brain stem.

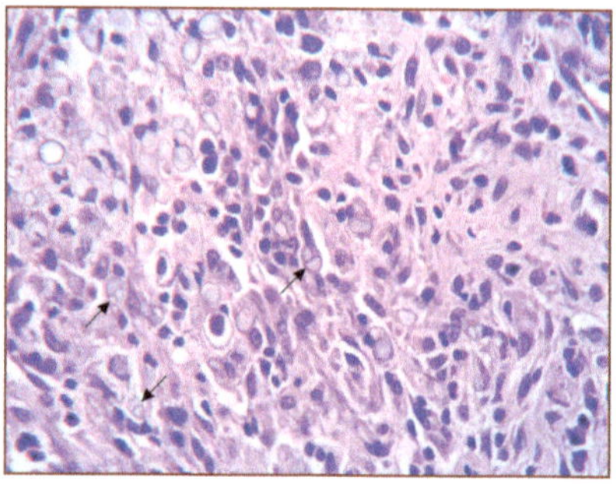

Fig. 20. Dog. *Prototheca:* numerous algae with a periodic acid-Schiff (PAS) -positive (arrows) (PAS, 40x)

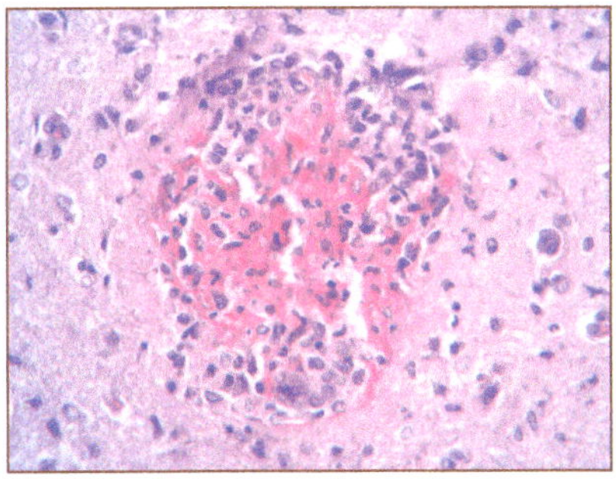

Fig. 21. Dog. *Rickettsia:* mononuclear vasculitis and fribrinoid necrosis of cerebrale arteriola (HE, 40x)

4. Discussion

In this study we investigated and analyzed the prevalence of neurological zoonoses in Italy in the decade between January 2000 and December 2009.A total of 16 different zoonotic diseases were diagnosed in 271 subjects of different animal species: 7 diseases were caused by parasites, 6 by bacteria, 2 by viruses and one case was due to achlorophilic algae. Farm animals were the species most affected; no diseases were found in birds or wild animals.

In 82 (23%) cases involving dogs and cats, the disease was of **"unknown aetiology"**. Such inflammatory diseases are prevalent in the dog, with a clear preference for breed and sometimes with family involvement. In our study, the species most affected was the dog (Graph.2). These disorders may, in fact, be triggered by an as yet unidentified pathogen and are therefore to be considered "potential zoonoses" (Schwab et al., 2007). The histological lesions were often suggestive of viral infections, but no causative agent has ever been isolated so far. Both rabies and canine distemper have been suggested as possible causes, presumably as expressions of atypical infection with these viruses (Summers et al., 1995). New diagnostic techniques may be useful to identify the pathogens responsible for these diseases and assess their possible zoonotic risk.

In the group of defined zoonoses, **Encephalitozoonosis**, a parasitic disease, was found in 86% of the rabbits investigated (110 out of 128) coming from different provinces in Piedmont. *Encephalitozoon cuniculi,* an obligate intracellular parasite of microsporidia, can affect a wide range of mammals: rabbit, dog, cat, horse, fox, and humans as well. In the rabbit it usually presents as a chronic asymptomatic disease; in other species, especially in immunocompromised humans, more severe infections can lead to death (Mertens et al., 1997). The transmission route is probably by ingestion of food or water contaminated by spores shed with the urine of infected rabbits. Some authors suggest a vertical transmission in lagomorphs (Giordano et al., 2005). The disease is more common in pet rabbits (37-68%) than in the wild (Kunzel et al., 2010). In our study, 104 affected rabbits belonged to the group of meat animals, and only 6 were pets. Cases of human infection by microsporidia have been reported worldwide, but the natural reservoirs and modes of transmission remain to be elucidated (Furuya, 2009). *E. cuniculi* ranks third among the microsporidia that affect humans, after *E. bieneusi* and *E. bowel,* and it is also the cause of rare disseminated microsporidiosis forms, as described in a recent case of a woman with AIDS in Italy (Tasone et al. , 2002). Many authors believe that the reported data are underestimated. Infection control in rabbit-breeding is very important and should not underestimate the risks to food-industry workers. While the disease in rabbits is potentially transmissible to humans, it represents a significant risk only for individuals with severe immune system impairment. Didier et al. have identified three *E. cuniculi* strains (I rabbit, II mouse, III dog) based on the number of repeated sequences in the ribosomal internal transcribed region. All confirmed cases in humans since 1994, related to immunocompromised patients, mainly HIV-seropositive, were due exclusively to the dog and rabbit strain (Weber et al. , 1997; Kunzel et al. , 2010). It would therefore be interesting to analyse the cases described in this study with accurate biomolecular investigation in order to determine which strain they belong to.

Listeriosis, an infectious bacterial disease caused by *Listeria monocytogenes*, accounted for 13.5% of the zoonoses reported here. The infection is transmitted mainly through the consumption of contaminated food, but also by direct contact with infected animals. Compared to other food-borne diseases, it has a low incidence and high mortality rate in invasive neurological forms (20-30%) (Matassa, 2007). *L. monocytogenes* is a neurotropic bacterium and is more efficient than other neuroinvasive Gram-positive bacteria, including those of the Streptococcus genus, and it is one of the most common causes of bacterial meningitis in North America and Western Europe (Drevets et al., 2008).

Immunocompromised individuals, diabetics, alcoholics, the elderly and children can develop an invasive, often fatal form that is characterised by meningitis, septicaemia, endocarditis, pneumonia, arthritis, osteomyelitis and hepatitis; in pregnant women its can cause abortion (Matassa, 2007; Ramaswamy et al., 2007). In our study, as reported by other authors, we found a higher prevalence of the disease in ruminants as compared with other domestic mammals, suggesting that these species may constitute an important source of human infection, given the variety of foods derived from them (Oevermann et al., 2008). An epidemiological human study detected the presence of the bacterium in the stool of asymptomatic healthy subjects, but further studies are needed to understand the impact of these subjects on transmission (Drevets et al., 2008). Listeriosis is now considered an endemic infection in France and northern Europe (with peaks during the summer), unlike in Italy where it occurs sporadically (Bianchi et al., 1995). Recently reported humans cases in Italy are: Genoa (n=1) (Viscoli et al., 1991); Monza (n=2) (Bianchi et al., 1995); Milan (n=1) (Ponticelli et al., 2005); and Naples (n=1) (Reynaud et al. , 2007).

Among the pigs investigated in this study, **Streptococcosis** was diagnosed in 26 (7.5%) cases, all involving very young animals from fattening farms. The disease is caused by *Streptococcus suis*, a Gram positive bacterium, facultative anaerobic, which persists in the tonsils, sinuses, reproductive and digestive systems and can cause severe forms of meningitis, endocarditis and septicaemia. Piglets become infected after contact with colonized sows, which are healthy carriers; the infection can be transmitted to humans through direct contact with symptomatic animals or carriers or through ingestion of contaminated meat (Wertheim et al. , 2009).

Higher rates of infection are attributed to stressing factors, poor hygiene and/or concurrent disease. *S. suis* has been isolated from other animals such as ruminants, dogs, cats, horses and wild animals, and it is believed to be a commensal in the intestinal flora (Staats et al. , 1997). According to the polysaccharide capsule, 35 serotypes have been identified, including serotype 2 which is the main cause of infections in humans. The first human case was reported in 1968 in Denmark (Arends et al., 1988); since then, hundreds of cases have been reported around the world, many of which fatal (Lun et al., 2007; Wertheim et al., 2009). These multiple and severe outbreaks of *S. suis* in humans have raised public concern about its role as a zoonotic agent. Human infection manifests as a purulent meningitis, fever,

vomiting, dizziness, ataxia, petechiae, muscle pain, paralysis and hearing loss; sometimes toxic forms may develop, with septic shock leading to death (Lun et al., 2007). The histological lesions in humans resemble those found in pigs. The infection typically affects men between 47 and 55 years of age and is considered an occupational condition or it may be linked to particular dietary habits of a population. Previous studies using serological tests and nasopharyngeal swabs have found low positivity to serotype 2 *S. suis* in high-risk individuals such as veterinarians and pig farmers, confirming the role of humans as healthy carriers. Its prevalence, duration and importance in the spread of the disease remains to be investigated (Elbers et al., 1999; Wertheim et al., 2009). In this population subset, it probably behaves as an opportunistic pathogen that causes symptomatic lesions in special circumstances such as stress, AIDS and cancer. In Western countries the disease occurs only sporadically; in Italy three cases have been reported to date: one in a subject with neoplasia (Manzin et al., 2007), the other two were due to occupational exposure in a farmer and a butcher (Perseghin et al., 1995; Camporese et al., 2007). Most likely, prevalence data are underestimated because in its early stages of infection the disease is very often mistaken for a simple flu that resolves with generic antibiotic therapy in immunocompetent individuals. The difficulty of determining the true incidence of infection on farms makes real risk assessment problematic. For this reason it is important to maintain biosafety standards on farms and to consider potential *S. suis* infection in cases presenting with neurological signs.
In 17 (5%) ruminants we diagnosed **Coenurosis,** an infection caused by the larval stage of *Taenia multiceps,* a flatworm that develops in the intestine of canids (definitive hosts) which release hundreds of eggs with the faeces. Ruminants are the intermediate hosts, and the oncospheres often spread via the bloodstream in the body with possible CNS involvement. Normally, it is a solitary lesion involving one hemisphere and clinical signs vary depending on the location (Scott, 2000); during their migration the larvae may carry bacteria causing bacterial meningoencephalitis (Christodoulopoulos, 2007).
Only very rarely are humans affected; most cases have been reported in the developing countries (Africa and Asia) with a high mortality rate (Crusz , 1948; Fain, 1956; Raper and Edockeray, 1956; Hermos et al., 1970). In Europe coenurosis in sheep has been reported in England, Ireland and France; in Italy it is mainly present in Sardinia, Latium, Puglia and Sicily. Man is considered an accidental dead-end host, where the infection most often develops in nervous, muscular and subcutaneous tissues. The first case of human coenurosis dates to 1913 (Brumpt, 1913); to date only a few hundred human cases have been described (Ing et al., 1998; Scala et al., 2006), some of which occurred in Italy (Sabbatani et al., 2004), at least five of which in Sardinia (Turtas et al., 1989).
In the CNS the parasite is localized predominantly in the submeningeal cortex, creating cysts that grow and compress the surrounding tissue, but it has also been found within the cerebral parenchyma and the spinal cord (Ing et al., 1998; Beniflá et al., 2007). In the Italian cases the cysts were generally located in the cerebral hemispheres in an eccentric position, and more rarely in the cerebellum. Several factors may increase the spread of the disease in sheep: illegal slaughtering, high number of dogs on the farm, and inappropriate use of antihelminthics (Scala et al. , 2006).
Colibacillosis was confirmed in 15 calves, 1 sheep and 5 pigs (6% of total), all under 2 months of age. *E. coli* is a bacterium that usually lives in symbiosis with animals and humans, colonizing the gut, but some strains have developed virulence through the production of toxins or attachment factors. In particular, *E. coli* O157: H7 causes severe haemorrhagic enteritis and the haemolytic uremic syndrome (HUS), a disease that has

recently raised concern for the health of infants. HUS affects mostly very young children and the elderly and is characterized by acute renal failure and haemolytic anaemia; the mortality rate is 5%.

A serious complication, more common in adults, is thrombotic thrombocytopenic purpura which produces neurological signs. The syndromes caused by *E. coli* O157: H7 verocytotoxin belong to both the food-borne diseases and zoonoses because ruminants, particularly cattle, are the main reservoir of the bacterium. Milk, dairy products and undercooked meat carry the infection; human transmission is also very common (Matassa, 2007).

In adult cattle the course of infection is asymptomatic, except for cases of necrotizing mastitis in dairy cows. In calves, as occurred in the cases we report here, very serious septicaemic forms may appear starting from the earliest days of life, whereas lambs and piglets are less likely to be affected. In Italy the first case of *E. coli* O157 infection was reported in 1988. Since notification of the disease is not required and all reports are made on a voluntary basis, the final data are certainly underestimated. The most affected regions are Lombardy, Piedmont, Latium and Puglia. As of 2004 there were 439 reported cases of HUS, the majority of which occurred in children between 0 and 6 years of age (80%) (Matassa , 2007).

West Nile Disease (WNV), a zoonoses caused by a flavivirus (RNAvirus), is transmitted by mosquitoes of the genus *Culex*. In this series it was found in 15 horses (4%) and probably it is understimated. Host amplifiers of the virus are migratory wild birds. The disease has seasonal trends and is more common in wetlands and marshy areas or near rivers, along the route of migratory birds (Castillo-Olivares et al. , 2004).

The virus can infect several species of vertebrates (mammals, birds and reptiles); humans and the horse are accidental dead-end hosts because viraemia is short and does not favour the spread. In the horse, the course of the disease is often asymptomatic or mildly symptomatic, rarely is it fatal. In our series, 10 horses had mild clinical signs and recovered, three were asymptomatic but sero-positive, and only two showed severe signs and were slaughtered. In humans, it appears as a influenza-like syndrome, and only 1% of cases are fatal.

WNV in Italy was first reported in Tuscany in 1998 (Cantile et al., 2000); it then reappeared 10 years later around the Po Delta in 2008, where the virus resulted phylogenetically very close to that found in Tuscany where the disease is now endemic. In July 2009, the infection recurred as in 2008 but then spread to other regions. Since 2002, the Ministry of Health has established a national surveillance plan, both active and passive, to control the introduction and circulation of the virus and insect vectors in areas considered at risk.

The viral agent may induce a variety of clinical signs depending on the subtype and its geographic distribution (Gubler, 2007; Zeller et al., 2004). In our cases, the course of disease was short, evolving toward rapid improvement; neurological symptoms may sometimes go unrecognized and show only nonspecific signs. Therefore, the presence of asymptomatic or mildly symptomatic horses could lead to underestimation of the spread of disease. The WNV is a notifiable zoonosis, potentially fatal for humans, especially in the elderly, children and immunocompromised; therefore, monitoring of virus circulation in the country and wetland reclamation are important for reducing insect vectors.

During our investigations, **Neosporosis** due to *Neospora caninum* was found in 15 (4%) subjects (4 cattle and 11 dogs). It is a protozoan of the family *Sarcocystidae*, whose life cycle is not yet clear; tachyzoites and cysts are the only stages of the cycle identified to date. The presence of cysts has been described only in nervous tissue (brain, spinal cord, nerves and retina), except for a solitary cyst in the eye muscle. The oocysts of the parasite have been isolated only from the faeces of dogs, which is considered to be both a definitive and intermediate host (Dubey et al., 1996; Cantile et al. , 2002).

It can be transmitted both orally and vertically; in cattle the infection is feared especially because of severe economic losses due to its effects on reproduction, such as embryo absorption, abortion, return to heat, infertility and increased neonatal mortality with severe CNS infection in the calf (Dubey et al., 2003). In this study we observed lesions compatible with congenital or neonatal infection in calves, prevalently CNS lesions in adult dogs, and peripheral nervous system lesions (poliradiculoneuritis) in young subjects, as reported elsewhere (De Meerschman et al., 2005; Cantile et al., 2002). Although some authors have claimed no zoonotic role for *Neospora caninum* (Dubey , 2003), there is recent evidence that the protozoan may be responsible for neurological syndromes in immunocompromised HIV-seropositive individuals, causing opportunistic infections with *Toxoplasma gondii* (Lobato et al., 2006).

In 2% of cases **toxoplasmosis** was diagnosed, a parasitic infection caused by *Toxoplasma gondii*, an intracellular protozoa of the genus *Toxoplasma*, which affects several species of birds and mammals, including humans. The cat is the definitive host that spreads the oocysts into the environment through faeces, and other animals become infected through contaminated food and water. Toxoplasma can cause subclinical or clinical infection.

In our study all cases presented with neurological signs, one of the dogs also showed a concomitant infection with *Neospora caninum*. In domestic animals the disease generally has a very low prevalence, but it can represent a real risk of transmission to humans directly or through food. In pigs the reproductive (still-born and premature births) and respiratory (pneumonia) systems are most often affected, only rarely have myocarditis and encephalitis been reported, with a mortality rate of over 50% (Dubey et al., 2008). Among poultry, toxoplasmosis is very rare, mainly occurring in family-owned farms (Goodwin et al., 1994), while symptomatic toxoplasmosis in the horse has not yet been reported to date, although the infection is possible.

Sheep and goats have a high rate of abortion and still births, but there have been reports of lambs seven months of age with numerous cysts distributed throughout the carcass after slaughter (Dubey et al., 1989). In cats, as in humans, most infections are asymptomatic and rarely involve other organs or the CNS, as in kittens with congenital infection or immunodeficiency (FIV-FeLV) (Davidson et al., 1993). In dogs the disease is more severe in pups; the most frequent signs are pneumonia, hepatitis and encephalitis. The two dolphins analyzed in this study were from strandings that occurred between 2007 and 2009 along the coast of Liguria (Italy).

This fact is of considerable importance for studying the pathogen's epidemiology and for the safety of public health and cetaceans. Many authors believe that toxoplasma may have infected the sea through the discharge of sewage along the coastline or ship ballast waters contaminated by onboard rodents, cats, or contaminated soil.

In this way, the dolphins may have been infected following ingestion of contaminated water and fish. The prevalence of this disease in animals is probably underestimated: the data are few and often not comparable because of differences in methods and the types of samples analyzed. One third of the human population is seropositive against *T. gondii* and this seroprevalence makes it an important agent of zoonosis. EC Directive 99/2003 provides that Member States report, depending its epidemiological status, all cases of disease and seropositivity detected, until a common control and surveillance system has been adopted.

Cryptococcosis is an occasional systemic infection caused by *Cryptococcus neoformans*, an opportunistic yeast-like fungus of the genus *Cryptococcus*. This disease is rare among domestic animals except dogs and cats; in fact, these two species were the only ones involved in our study. The most frequently isolated species are *C. neoformans* (serotype AD) and *C. gattii* (serotype BC). The latter are considered the most aggressive serotype (Lacaze et al., 2002). Pigeons are considered the main vector because their high body temperature protects them from disease. In immunocompetent birds cryptococcosis remains confined to the upper airways and sinuses because it prefers temperatures below 40 °C. The cat is the species most often affected and the most common route of infection is through the respiratory system; often, as in dogs, it also involves the eye and the CNS (15% of cases) (Berthelin et al., 1994). In natural conditions the immune response in humans provides resistance to infection, but in 85% of cases cryptococcosis affects the lungs and the CNS in debilitated patients within settings such as AIDS, tuberculosis, leukaemia and lymphoma (Summers et al., 1995; Kerl, 2003; Chuck et al., 1989; Nagrajan et al., 2000; Fernandes et al., 2000). *C. gattii* has also been reported in association with skin lesions in patients undergoing prolonged corticosteroid therapy (Bellissimo-Rodrigues et al., 2010). Even in the cat prolonged corticosteroid use may aggravate the infection, but there are no data demonstrating whether immunosuppressive diseases such as FIV and FeLV may predispose individuals to cryptococcosis (Gerds-Grogan et al., 1997; Kerl, 2003). In our cases, histopathological lesions were similar to those described previously (Summers et al., 1995). The cats showed low to moderate nonsuppurative inflammatory response, despite wide dissemination of the cyst both in the meninges and the neuroparenchyma; the response in the dogs was much more cellular, with granulomatous lesions and epithelioid macrophages, lymphocytes and plasma cells in the brain and meninges.

Halicephalobus gingivalis, a nematode which lives in soil and decaying plant material, was identified in two case of equine meningo-encephalitis. The parasite is pathogenic in the horse and man and infection occurs through skin injuries with spreading of the worm to other organs, including the CNS. In our cases *H. gingivalis* was found in two horses, one from Tuscany and the other from Veneto. In the horse the pathology is characterized by disseminated granulomas in the skin and other organs; granulomatous encephalomyelitis is often reported. In humans the infection is always fatal and affects the CNS (Gardiner et al., 1981). In our series only the CNS was involved and the histological lesions were similar to those described elsewhere (Mandrioli et al., 2002). The parasite was first fully described by Stefanski in 1954, from a gingival granuloma in a horse in Poland (Anderson et al., 1982). Four cases in horses have been reported so far in Italy, all native animals which apparently had never left the country, confirming the presence of the parasite in Italy (Cantile et al., 1997; Mandrioli et al., 2002). Worldwide, only three humans cases with fatal outcome have been reported, in all of which the CNS was involved (Akagami et al., 2007; Gardiner et al., 1981; Shadduck et al., 1979), but no human case has been reported in Italy so far.

Borna disease was diagnosed in 2 sheep. This infectious disease caused by an RNA virus of the Bornaviridae family affects domestic and wild animals, mainly horses and sheeps. In these species Borna virus has a low morbidity, but subclinical persistent infection is probably common (Summer 1995). The virus is transmitted through salivary, nasal and conjunctival secretions, water and contaminated food. Il virus is highly neurotropic, with constant replication in the CNS and spinal cord; however, it can spread throughout the body in infants or the immunocompromised. The disease is characterized, as in our cases, by a nonsuppurative meningo-encephalomyelitis, with infiltration of mononuclear cells that affects the gray matter of the CNS. The wide spectrum of susceptible species also includes human beings in which it is still uncertain whether the virus is responsible for the development of some forms of nervous disorders. Recent studies have shown a high prevalence of specific antibodies in the serum and/or CSF of patients with neuropsychiatric disorders (Ludwig et al., 1997; Richt et al., 2001).

Chlamydiosis is caused by an obligate intracellular organism of the genus *Chlamydia* that can infect many birds and mammals, including humans. Transmission can occur by digestive, respiratory, venereal and congenital routes, whereas aborted foetuses from infected animals and animals with subclinical infections cause the pathogen to spread into the environment (Nietfeld, 2001; McCafferty, 1990). *Chlamydiae* are primary causes of pneumonia, polyarthritis, conjunctivitis and encephalitis, and sheep is the species most affected. In the cow the infection usually manifests in a generalized form affecting mainly foetuses (vertical transmission) and calves under 6 months of age (Storz et al., 1971). In bibliography have been described cases of sporadic encephalitis in adult cattle with aetiology unclear ; often Chlamydia infection and viruses has been reported as cause of this disease. (Theil et al.., 1998). In our series a chlamydial infection was detected in only one case, a 7-year-old cow with less severe neuropathological lesions than those described previously (Piercy et al., 1999; Storz et al., 1971); probably this animal could have been at an early stage of disease.

Some authors have reported marked seropositivity in people in close contact with animals infected by Chlamydia, confirming the hypothesis that animals can be a source of infection for humans (Schachter et al., 1973; Storz et al., 1971). In humans the disease can appear with unapparent forms or with pneumonia, septicaemia and death; sometimes therapy-resistant conjunctivitis can occur. Because of the pathogen's wide diffusion and the few cases reported in humans, many others may not have been recognized (Shewen, 1980). However, cases have been reported of human chlamydiosis transmitted from sheep (Roberts et al., 1967), cattle (Sarateanu et al., 1961) and cats (Schachter et al., 1969; Ostler et al., 1969), or due to laboratory accidents while handling infected samples (Barwell, 1955; Vulgar et al. , 1974).

Leishmaniasis is a parasitic disease caused in the Mediterranean by *L. infantum*, a protozoan of the genus *Leishmania*, an obligate intracellular parasite of macrophages and dendritic cells of the skin. It is transmitted by the bite of bloodsucking vectors of the genus *Phlebotomus*; it affects several species, particularly dogs and humans. The disease can be subacute and follow a chronic course with variable symptoms; in more severe cases the animal often dies from renal failure. Other affected organs are those of the reticuloendothelial system (lymph nodes, spleen, liver and bone marrow) and sometimes associated with polymyositis and arthrosynovitis (Matassa, 2007). The CNS is a rather unusual target of the parasite, but some cases have been reported in both dogs and humans (Vinuelas et al., 2001; Melo et al., 2009).

In humans the disease is always severe, especially in the immunocompromised, such as HIV-seropitive individuals or transplant recipients. Sometimes, the symptoms are very severe with loss of sensation in the lower limbs, deafness, multiple paralysis of cranial nerve and axonal demyelination and degeneration (Hashim et al., 1995). In recent decades, various climatic factors have changed the normal areal of carriers and new leishmaniasis outbreaks have occurred in areas that were previously considered free, like the foothills of the Alps. Since 1995, outbreaks have been reported in Liguria, Tuscany, Lombardy, Piedmont and Valle D'Aosta, and rarely also in Veneto, Trentino and Friuli (Matassa, 2007).

Nocardiosis is a bacterial disease caused by the Gram-positive bacterium *Nocardia asteroides*. Usually, the infection arises in the lung following inhalation of spores; CNS involvement occurs in 13% of cases (Bosnic et al. , 2010; Cianfoni et al., 2010). As highlighted in our case, *Nocardia* generally causes solitary brain lesions, but cases have also been reported of multiple abscesses, which are very rare in dogs (Smith et al., 2007; Munana, 1996; Kaplan, 1985). The disease has been reported in the brain of immunocompromised dogs and humans due to concomitant diseases (systemic lupus erythematosus or AIDS) or immunosuppressive therapy (cyclosporine, chemotherapy) (Smith et al., 2007). Brain infections can occur after penetrating trauma, due to extension of infection to adjacent structures (internal ear and dental root) or via the bloodstream (Dow et al. , 1988; Munana, 1996). Drug therapy is not always effective.

Protothecosis is caused by achlorophil algae of the genus *Prototheca*, including five species widely distributed in the environment, especially in organic matter. It is considered an emerging disease in humans and animals. Infection occurs primarily through skin lesions in contact with contaminated water, but the algae can colonize the skin, even the nails, the respiratory and digestive systems. In cattle the algae cause clinical and subclinical mastitis refractory to treatment, with high economic losses and potential risk to public health; systemic forms are rare (Marques et al., 2006). In dogs and cats it can present both as localized cutaneous and systemic forms (Ginel et al., 1997; Dillberger et al., 1988; Krohne, 2000); respiratory and cutaneous forms have also been reported in the goat (Macedo et al., 2008).

Systemic protothecosis involving the eye and the CNS have been reported in dogs (Stenner et al., 2007); in our case only cerebral lesions were found. In humans the disease has low pathogenicity in immunocompetent subjects, with local indolent skin lesions, whereas in the immunocompromised it may occur as a scattered form and not infrequently associated with such other pathogens as *Candida*, *Staphylococcus aureus*, herpes simplex, and *Cryptococcus* spp. (Lass-Florl et al. , 2007).

Rickettsiosis was diagnosed in only one subject in this series; the disease is caused by an obligate intracellular organism considered to be an intermediate form between a virus and a bacterium of the genus *Rickettsiae*. The disease is a tick-borne zoonosis. Many *Rickettsiae* cause diseases involving the CNS in animals and humans (Parola et al., 2005), one of the most important is *R. conorii* transmitted by the dog tick (*Rhipicephalus sanguineus*) that causes Mediterranean spotted fever in humans. In recent years, the number of cases of rickettsiosis in dogs and humans has increased significantly in Italy, in conjunction with climate change (temperature and rainfall) and environmental (human-dog contact) factors that allow for prolonged survival of the carrier. The most affected regions are Sicily, Sardinia, Latium, Liguria and Piedmont (Garavelli et al., 1990; Cocco et al., 2003; Cascio et al., 2006; Beninati et al., 2002).

Given the wide diffusion of the vector and the pathogen in Italy, the incidence of rickettsiosis was surprisingly low in this series, which may have been due to the fact that many cases go undiagnosed or are asymptomatic without showing neurological signs and are not recognized. Vector control is an indispensable means to prevent diseases transmitted by ticks; rickettsioses should therefore always be included in the differential diagnosis of cases with neurological signs, especially following an arthropod bite.

5. Conclusions

In our investigation, among the many neurological cases potentially attributable to infectious agents, about 27% were confirmed as a zoonosis, but there remain many cases of inflammation not classified and potentially constituting a health risk. The results of this research show that animals can be an important reservoir for agents of neurozoonoses; therefore, monitoring of neurological diseases of animals should be designed to reduce the number of infections in humans and may be a good model for the study of therapeutic strategies in cases of infection. Neurozoonosis monitoring in animals may also allow for the surveillance of possible emerging or re-emerging infectious agents.

From available literature data it is clear that the population segments most affected by zoonoses are children, the elderly and the immunocompromised, particularly those with AIDS and chemotherapy or transplant recipients. The best way to protect these at-risk groups is through prevention, which can only be done through a national surveillance network. Further studies should also aim to identify the pathogenesis and the possible etiologic agents of idiopathic inflammatory disease or those of "unknown aetiology" to exclude the likelihood of potentially zoonotic agents.

6. Acknowledgment

We thank Debora Corbellini, Caterina Lucia Florio, Paola Gazzuola, Tiziana Avanzato and Saverio Bessone for their technical assistance.

The authors declare that this study was carried out under the following Research Projects: IZSPLV 14/06; IZSPLV 13/08 ; Monitoring Project "A new strategy to deal with the TSE in Italy" funded by the Ministry of Health; Research Project "Monitoring of Streptococcus suis infections in pigs fattening farm " funded by Cassa di Risparmio di Cuneo.

7. References

Akagami, M.; Shibahara, T.; Yoshiga, T. et al. (2007). Granulomatous nephritis and meningoencephalitis caused by Halicephalobus gingivalis in a pony gelding. *J Med Vet Sci*, 69, 1187-1190

Anderson, R.C.; Bain, O. (1982). Keys to genera of the superfamilies Rhabditoidea, Dioctophymatoidea, Trichinelloidea and Muspiceoidea p 1-8 in: CIH Keys to the Nematode *Parasites of Vertebrates*, Commonwealth Agricultural Bureaux

Arends, JP.; Zanen, H.C. (1988). Meningitis caused by Streptococcus suis in humans. *Rev. Infect Dis*, 10: 131-137

Asjo, B.; Kruse, H. (2007). Zoonoses in the Emergence of Human viral diseases. *Emerging Viruses in Human Population*, 15-41

Barwell, C.F. (1955). Laboratory infection in man with virus of enzootic abortion of ewes. *Lacent* 2, 1369-1370

Bellissimo-Rodrigues, F.; Baciotti, M.; Zanatto, M.P.; Silva, J.O.; Martins, M.A.; Martinez, R. (2010). Cutaneus cryptococcosis due to Cryptococcus gattii in a patient on chronic corticotherapy. *Revista da Sociedade Brasileira de Medicina Tropical*, 43(2): 211-212

Benifla, M.; Barrelly, R.; Shelef, I.; El-On, J.; Cohen, A.; Cagnano, E. (2007). Huge hemispheric intraparenchymal cyst caused by Taenia multiceps in a child. *J. Neurosurg*. (6 suppl. Pediatrics), 107: 511-514

Beninati, T.; Lo, N.; Noda, H.; Esposito, F.; Rizzoli, A.; Favia, G..; Genchi, C. (2002). First detection of Spotted Fever Group Rickettsiae in Ixodes ricinus from Italy. *Emerging Infection Diseases*, 8: 983-986

Bergonzini, V.; Calistri, A.; Salata, C.; Del Vecchio, C.; Sartori, E.; Parolin, C.; Palù, G. (2009). Nef and cell signaling transduction: a possible involvement in the pathogenesis of human immunodeficiency virus-associated dementia. *J Neurovirol.*15:238-248

Berthelin, C.F.; Legendre, A.M.; Bailey, C.S.; Kass, P.H.; Wolf, A.M. (1994). Cryptococcosis of the nervous system in dogs, 2. Diagnosis, treatment, monitoring and prognosis. *Progress in Vet. Neurology,* 5 (4): 136-146

Bianchi, G.; Appollonio, I.; Piolti, R.; Pozzi, C.; Frattola, L. (1995). Listeria rhombencephalitis: report of two cases with early diagnosis and favourable out come. *Clinical Neurology and Neurosurgery,* 97: 344-348

Bosnic, D.; Baresic, M.; Anic, B.; Sentic, M.; Cerovec, M.; Mayer, M.; Cikes, N.(2010). Rare zoonosis (Hemotrophic mycoplasma anfection) in a newly diagnoded systemic lupus erythematosus patient followed by a Nocardia asteroides pneumonia. *Braz. J. Infect Dis,* 14 (1): 92-95

Brumpt, E. (1913). Precis de parasitologie. 2nd ed. Paris: Masson and Co., 1913: 281

Camporese, A.; Tizianel, G..; Bruschetta, G..; Cruciatti, B. (2007). Pomes A. Human meningitis caused by Streptococcus suis: the first case report from north-eastern Italy. *Le Infezioni in Medicina,* 2: 111-114

Cantile, C.; Rossi, G,; Braca, G. et al. (1997). A horse with Halicephalobus deletrix encephalitis in Italy. *Eur J Vet Pathol,* 3, 29-33

Cantile, C.; Di Guardo, G.; Eleni, C.; Arispici, M. (2000). Clinical and neuropathological features of West Nile virus equine encephalomyelitis in Italy . *Equine Vet J. ,* Jan;32(1)

Cantile, C.& Arispici M. (2002). Necrotizing cerebellitis due to Neospora caninum infection in an old dog. *J. Vet. Med,* 2002; 49: 47-50

Cascio, A.; Iaria, C.; (2006). Epidemiology and clinical features of Mediterranean Spotted Fever in Italy. *Parassitologia,* 48: 131-133

Castillo-Olivares, J.; Wood, J. (2007). West Nile virus infection of horses. *Vet. Res,* 35: 467–483

Christodoulopoulos, G. (2007).Two rare clinical manifestations of coenurosis in sheep. *Vet. Parasitology,* 143: 368-370

Chuck, S.L.; Sande, M.A. (1989). Infections with Cryptococcus neoformans in the acquired immunodeficiency syndrome. *N. Engl. J. Med,* 321 (12): 794-799

Cianfoni, A.; Calandrelli, R.; De Bonis, P.; Pompucci, A; Lauriola, L.; Colosimo, C. (2010). Nocardia brain abscess mimicking high-grade necrotic tumor on perfusion MRI. *Jour. of Clinical Neuroscience*1-3

Cocco, R.; Sanna, G.; Cillara, M.G.; Tola, S.; Ximenes, L.; Pinnaparpaglia, M.L.; Masala, G. (2003). Ehrlichiosis and Rickettsiosis in a canine population of Northern Sardinia. *Ann. N.Y. Acad. Sci,* 126-130

Cotto, E.; Neau, D.; Cransac-Neau, M.; Auriacombe, M.; Pellegrin, J.L.; Ragnaud, J.M.; Fillet, A.M.; Belnard, M.; Fleury, H.; Lafon, M.E. (2003). Borna disease virus RNA in immunocompromised patients in southwestern France. *J Clin Microbiol.* 41:5577-5581

Crusz, H. (1948).On an English case of an intramedullary spinal coenurus in man, with some remarks on the identity of Coenurus spp. *Infesting man. J Helminthol,* 22(2):73-6

Daniel, S. & Zanin, T. (1997). Manuale di Tecnica Cito-Istologica. Documentazione Scientifica Editrice Bologna

Davidson, M.G.; Rottman, J.B.; English, R.V.; Lappin, M.R.; Tompkins, M.B. (1993). Feline immunodeficiency virus predisposes cats to acute generalized toxoplasmosis. *Anim. J. Path*, 1486-1497

De Meerschman, F.; Focant, C.; Detry, J.; Rettigner, C.; Cassart, D.; Losson, B. (2005). Clinical, pathological and diagnostic aspects of congenital neosporosis in a series of naturally infected calves. *Vet Rec*, 157 (4): 115-118

Didier, E.S.; Vossbrinck, C.R.; Baker, M.D.; Rogers, L.B.; Bertucci, D.C.; Shadduck, J.A. (1995). Identification and characterization of three Encephalitozoon cuniculi strains. *Parasitology*, 111 (pt 4): 411-421

Dillberger, J.E.; Homer, B.; Daubert, D.; Altman, N.H. (1988). Protothecosis in two cats. *J Am Vet Med Assoc.*, Jun 1;192(11):1557-9

Donaldson, K.A.; Griffin, D.W.; Paul, J.H. (2002). Detection, quantitation and identification of enteroviruses from surface waters and sponge tissue from the Florida Keys using real-time RT-PCR. *Water Res*. 36(10):2505-14

Dow, S.W. ; LeCouteur, R.A. ; Henik, R.A. ; Jones, R.L. ; Poss, M.L. (1988). Central nervous system infection associated with anaerobic bacteria in two dogs and two cats. *Journal of Vet. Inter. Med*, 2: 171-176

Drevets, D.A.; Bronze, M.(2008). Listeria monocitogenes: epidemiology, human disease, and mechanisms of brain anvasion. *FEMS Immunol Med. Microbiol* , 53: 151-165

Dubey, J.P. & Jones, J.L.(2008). Toxoplasma gondii infection in humans and animals in the United States. *Intern .J. for Parasitology* , 38: 1257-1278

Dubey, J.P. & Kirkbride, C.A. (1989). Enzootic toxoplasmosis in sheep in North-Central United-States. *J. Parasitology*, 673-676

Dubey, J.P.(2003). Review of Neospora caninum and neosporosis in animals. *The Korean Journal of Parasitology*, 41: 1-16

Dudey, J.P. & Lindsay, D.S. (1996). A Review of Neospora caninum and neosporosis. *Veterinary Parasitology*, 67: 1-59

Elbers, A.R.; Vecht, U.; Osterhaus, A.D. et al. (1999). Low prevalence of antibodies against the zoonotic agents Brucella abortus, Leptospira spp., Streptococcus suis sierotype II, hantavirus and lymphocytic choriomeningitis virus among veterinarians and pig farmers in the southern part of The Netherlands. *Vet. Q*, 21: 50-54

Exner, M.M.; Lewinski, M.A. (2003). Isolation and detection of Borrelia burgdorferi DNA from cerebral spinal fluid, synovial fluid, blood, urine, and ticks using the Roche MagNA Pure system and real-time PCR. *Diagn Microbiol Infect Dis*. 46:235-240

Fain, A. (1956). Coenurus of Taenia brauni Setti parasitic in man and animals from the Belgian Congo and Ruanda-Urundi. *Nature*, Dec 15;178(4546):1353

Fernandes, O.; de FL, Costa, T.R.; Costa, M.R.; Soares, A.J.; Pereira, AJSC ;Silva, M.; do RR. (2000).Cryptococcus neoformans isolados de pacientes com AIDS. *Revista da Sociedade Brasileira de Medicina Tropical*, 33(1): 75-78

Furuya, K.; Spore-Forming. (2009). Microsporidian Encephalitozoon: current understanding of infection and prevention in Japan. *Jpn. J. Infect. Dis*, 62: 513-422

Garavelli, P.L.; Orsi, P.G.; Azzini, M. (1990) . Febbre Bottonosa mediterranea. Analisi di 48 casi nell'alessandrino. *Minerva Medica*, 81: 49-57

Gardiner, C.H,; Koh, D.S; Cardella, T.A. (1981). Micronema in man: Third fatal infection. *Am J Trop Med Hyg*, 30, 586-589

Gerds-Grogan, S.; Dayrell-Hart, B. (1997). Feline Cryptococcosis: a retrospective evaluation. *J. Am. Anim. Hosp. Assoc*, 33 (2): 118-122

Ginel, P.J.; Pérez, J.; Molleda, J.M.; Lucena, R.; Mozos, E. (1997). Cutaneous protothecosis in a dog. *Vet Rec.* , Jun 21;140(25):651-3

Giordano, C.; Weigt, A.; Vercelli, A.; Rondena, M.; Grilli, G.; Giudices, C. (2005). Immunohistochemical identification of Encephalitozoon cunicoli in phacoclastic uveitis in four rabbits. *Vet. Ophthalmology* , 8: 271-275

Goodwing, M.A.; Dubey, J.P.; Hatkin, J. (1994). Toxoplasma gondii peripheral neuritis in chickens. *J. Vet. Diagn. Invest*, 382-385

Gubler, D.J. (2007). The Continuing Spread of West Nile Virus in the Western Hemisphere. *Clinical Infectious Diseases*, 45:1039–46.

Hashim, F.A.; Ahmed, A.E.; el Hassan, M.; el Mubarak, M.H.; Yagi, H.; Ibrahim, E.N.; Ali, M.S.(1995). Neurologic changes in visceral leishmaniosis. *Am. J. Trop. Med. Hyg.*, 52: 149-154

Hermos, J.A.; Healy, G.R.; Schultz, M.G.; Barlow, J.; Church, W.G. (1970). Fatal human cerebral coenurosis. *JAMA*, 213: 1461-1464

Ing, M.B.; Schantz, P.M.; Turner, J.A. (1998). Human Coenurosis in North America: Case report and Review. *Cli. Inf. Diseases*, 27: 519-523

Kaplan, K. (1985).Brain abscess. *Med. Clin. of North Amecica*, 69: 345-360

Kerl, M.E. (2003). Update on canine and feline fungal diseases. *Vet. Clin. Small. Anim*, 33: 721-747

Krauss, H.; Weber, A.; Appel, M.; Enders, B.; Isenberg, H.D.; Schiefer, H.G.; Slenczka, W.; Von Graevenitz, A.; Zahner, H. (2003). Zoonoses, Infectious Diseases Transmissible from Animals to Humans. *ASM Press* 3rd ed. pp. xiii-xiv

Krohne, S.G.. (2000). Canine systemic fungal infections. *Vet Clin North Am Small Anim Pract.* Sep;30(5):1063-90.

Kunzel, F. & Joachim, A.(2010). Encephalitozoonosis in rabbits. *Parasitol. Res.*, 106: 299-309

Lacaz, C.S.; Heins-Vaccari, E.M.; Hernandez-Arriagada, G.L.; Martins, L.R.; Preparo, CAL.; Corim, S.M.; Martins, M.A. (2002). Primary cutaneus cryptococcosis due to cryptococcus neoformans var. gattii serotype B, in an immunocompetent patient. *Rev. Inst. Med. Trop. S. Paulo*, 44 (4): 225-228

Lanciotti, R.S.; Kerst, A.J.; Nasci, R.S.; Godsey, M.S.; Mitchell, C.J. (2000). Savage HM, et al. Rapid detection of west nile virus from human clinical specimens, field-collected mosquitoes, and avian samples by a TaqMan reverse transcriptase-PCR assay. *J Clin Microbiol.* 38:4066-71

Lass-Florl, C. & Mayr, A. (2007). Human Protothecosis. *Clinical Microbiology Reviews*, 230-242.

Lin, Mei-Hui; Tse-Ching, Chen; Tseng-tong, Kuo; Ching-Chung Tseng; and Ching-Ping Tseng. (2000). Real-Time PCR for Quantitative Detection of Toxoplasma gondii. *J Clin Microbiol.*38:4121-4125

Lobato, J.; Silva, D.A.; Mineo, T.W.; Amaral, J.D.; Segundo, G.R.; Costa-Cruz, J.M.; Ferreira, M.S.; Borges, A.S.; Mineo, J.R. (2006). Detection of immunoglobulin G antibodies to Neospora caninum in humans: high seropositivity rates in patients who are infected by human immunodeficiency virus or have neurological disorders.*Clin Vaccine Immunol.* Jan;13(1):84-9

Lun, Z.R.; Wang, Q.P.; Chen, X.G.; Li, A.X.; Zhu, X.Q. (2007). Streptococcus suis: an emerging zoonotic pathogen. *Lancet Infect Dis.* 7: 201-209

Macedo, JTSA.; Riet-Correra, F.; Dantas, AFM. & Simoes, SVD. (2008). Cutaneous and nasal Protothecosis in a goat. *Vet. Pathol,* 45: 352-354

Mandrioli, L. (2002). Encefalite granulomatosa da Halicephalobus gingivalis in un cavallo. *Ippologia,* 1, 27-38

Matassa, E. (2007). Zoonosi e sanità pubblica. Un approccio interdisciplinare per un problema emergente. Libro della Sprinter

McCafferty, M.C. (1990). Immunity to Chlamydia psittaci with particular reference to sheep. *Vet. Microbiology* , 25: 87-99

Melo, G.D., Marcondes, M., Vasconcelos, Machado GF. (2009). Leukocyte entry into the CNS of Leishmania chagasi naturally infected dogs. *Vet. Parasitology* , 162: 248-256

Mertens, R.B.; Didier, E.S. ; Fishbein, M.C. ; Bertucci, D.C. ; Rogers, L.B. ; Orenstein, J.M.(1997). Encephalitozoon cuniculi Microsporidiosis: Infection of the brain, heart,kidney, trachea, adrenal gland and urinary bladder in a patient with AIDS. *Mod. Pathology,* 10: 68-77

Munana, K.R. (1996). Encephalitis and meningitis. *Vet. Clin. of North America: Small Animal Practice.* 1996; 26: 857-874

Manzin, A.; Palmieri, C.; Serra, C., Saddi, B.; Princivalli, M.S.; Loi, G..; Angioni, G.; Tiddia, F.; Varaldo, P.E.; Facinelli, B. (2008). Streptococcus suis meningitis without history of animal contact, Italy. *Emerging Infectious Diseases,* 14: 1946-1947

Nagrajan, S.; Gugnani, H.C.; Kowshik, T. (2000). Case Report: Meningitis due to Cryptococcus neoformans var. neoformans serotype AD associated with pulmonary tuberculosis. *Mycoses* 43: 67-69

Nietfeld, J.C. (2001). Chlamydial infections in small ruminants. *Update on Small Ruminant Medicine,* 17: 301-314

Oevermann, A.; Botteron, C.; Seuberlich, T.; Nicolier, A.; Friess, M.; Doherr, M.G.; Heim, D.; Hilbe, M.; Zimmer, K.; Zurbriggen, A.; Vandevelde, M. (2008). Neuropathological survey of fallen stock: Active surveillance reveals high prevalence of encephalitic listeriosis in small ruminants. *Vet. Microbiology* 130 , 320-329.

Ostler, N.B.; Schachter, J., Dawson, C.R. (1969). Acute follicular congiuntivitis of epizootic origin. Feline pneumonitis. *Archs. Ophthal,* 82: 587-591

Palmer, S.R.; Soulsby, L.; Simpson, DIH. (1998). Zoonoses, biology, Clinical Practice and Public Health Control 3-5. Oxfod University Press

Parola, P.; Paddock, C.D.; Raoult, D. (2005). Tick-Borne Rickettsioses around the World: emerging diseases challenging old concepts. *Clinical Microbiology Reviews,* 18: 719-756

Perseghin, P.; Bezzi, G.; Troupioti, P.; Gallina, M. (1995). Streptococcus suis meningitis in an Italian blood donor. *The Lancet,* 346: 1305-1306

Piercy, D.W.T.; Griffiths P.C.; Teale, C.J. (1999). Encephalitis related to Chlamydia psittaci infection in a 14-week-old calf. *Vet. Rec.* 144: 126-128.

Porticelli, C.; Campise, MR. (2005). Neurological complications in kidney transplant recipients. J. Nephrol, 18: 521-528

Puchhammer-StoecklE., C.; Kunz, C.W.; Mandl and F.X. Heinz, (1995). Identification of tick-borne encephalitis virus ribonucleic acid in tick suspensions and in clinical specimens by a reverse transcription-nested polymerase chain reaction assay, Clin Diagn Virol.4:321–326

Ramaswamy, V.; Cresence, V.M.; ReJitha, J.S.; Lekshmi, M.U.; Dharsana, K.S.; Prasad, S.P.; ViJila, H.M. (2007). Listeria-review of epidemiology and pathogenesis. *J. Microbiol. Immunol. Infect*, 40: 4-13

Rajeshwari, Sutar; Joseph, K.; David, K.; Ganesan; Anup, K.; Ghosh, Sunit Singhi; ; Chakrabarti and Anand K. Bachhawat. (2004).Comparison of ITS and IGS1 regions for strain typing of clinical and non-clinical isolates of Pichia anomala. *J Med Microbiol.* 53:119-123

Raper, A.B.; Dockeray, G.C. (1956). Coenurus cysts in man: five cases from East Africa. *Ann Trop Med Parasitol*, Jun;50(2):121-8

Reynaud, L.; Graf, M.; Gentile, I.; Cerini, R.; Ciampi, R.; Noce, S.; Borrelli, F.; Viola, C.; Gentile, F.; Briganti, F.; Borgia, G. (2007). A rare case of brainstem encephalitis by Listeria monocitogenes with isolated mesencephalic localization. Case raport and review. *Diagnostic Microbiology and Infection Disease*,58: 121-123

Richt, J.A.; Pfeuffer, I.; Christ, M.; Frese, K.; Bechter, K. & Herzog, S. (1997). Borna disease virus infection in animals and humans. *Emerging Infectious Diseases*, 3: 343-352

Richt, J.A.& Rott, R. (2001). Borna disease virus: a mystery as an emerging zoonotic pathogen. *Vet J.*, Jan;161(1):24-40

Roberts, W.; Grist, N.E.; Giroud, P. (1967). Human abortion associated with infection by ovine abortion agent. *Br. Med. J.* 4: 37-39

Rodríguez-Lázaro, D.; Hernández, M.; Pla M. (2004). Simultaneous quantitative detection of Listeria spp. and Listeria monocytogenes using a duplex real-time PCR-based assay. *FEMS Microbiol Lett.* 233:257-267

Rose, T.M.; Strand, K.B.; Schultz, ER.; Schaefer, G.; Rankin, G.W.; Jr, Thouless M.E.; Tsai, C.C.; Bosch, ML. (1997). Identification of two homologs of the Kaposi's sarcoma-associated herpesvirus (human herpesvirus 8) in retroperitoneal fibromatosis of different macaque species. *J Virol.* 71(5):4138-4144

Sabbatani, S.; Zucchelli, M.; Calducci, F.; Roncaroli, F.; Chiodo, F. (2004).A case of cerebral cenurosis . *Infez. Med*, 12: 205-210

Salata, C.; Curtarello, M.; Calistri, A.; Sartori, E.; Sette, P.; de Bernard, M.; Parolin, C.; Palù, G. (2009). vOX2 glycoprotein of human herpesvirus 8 modulates human primary macrophages activity. *J Cell Physiol.* 219(3):698-706.

Sarateanu, D.; Sorodoc, G.; Surdan, C.; Fuhrer Anagnoste, B. (1961). Pneumonia in calves due to pararickettsia and the possibility of human contamination. *Studii Cerc. Inframicrobiol*, 12: 353-362

Scala, A.; Varcasia, A. (2006). Updates on morphobiology, epidemiology and molecular characterization of coenurosis in sheep. *Parassitologia.*, 48(1-2):61-63

Schachter, J.; Ostler, H.B.; Meyer, K.F. (1969). Human infection with the agent of felin pneumonitis. *Lancet 1*, 1063-1065

Schachter, J.; Storz, J.; Tarizzo, M.L.; Bogel, K. (1973). Chlamydiae as agents of human and animal disease. *Bull Wld. Hlth. Org*, 49: 443-449

Schwab, S.; Herden, C.; Seeliger, F.; Papaioannou, N.; Psalla, D.; Polizopulou, Z.; Baumgärtner, W. (2007). Non-suppurative meningoencephalitis of unknown origin in cats and dogs: an immunohistochemical study. *J Comp Patho*l., Feb-Apr;136(2-3):96-110

Shadduck, I.A.; Ubelaker, J.; Telford, V.Q.; (1979). Micronema deletrix meningoencephalitis in an adult man. *Am J Clin Pathol*, 72, 640-643

Shewen, P.E. (1980). Chlamydial Infection in Animals: A Review. *Can. Vet. J.* ,21: 2-11

Smith, P.M.; Haughland, S.P.; Jeffery, N.D. (2007).Brain abscess in a dog immunosuppressed using cyclosporine. *The Vet. Journal* , 173: 675-678

Staats, J.J.; Feder, J.; Okwumabua, O.; Chengappa, MM. (1997). Streptococcus suis: past and present. *Vet. Res. Commun.*, 21: 381-407

Stenner, V.J.; Mackay, B.; King, T.; Barrs, V.R.; Irwin, P.; Abraham, L.; Swift, N.; Langer, N.; Bernays, M.; Hampson, E.; Martin, P.; Krockenberger, M.B.; Bosward, K.; Latter, M.; Malik, R. (2007). Protothecosis in 17 Australian dogs and a review of the canine literature. *Med Mycol.*, May;45(3):249-66

Storz, J.; Eugster, A.K.; Altera, K.P.; Olander, H.J. (1971). Behavior of different bovine chlamydial agents in newborn calves. *J. Comp. Pathol.* ,A; 81: 299-307

Summers, B.A.; Cummings, J.F. & De Lahunta, A. (1995) Veterinary Neuropathology

Taylor, L.H.; Latham, S.M.; Woolhouse, M.E. (2001). Risk factors for human disease emergence *Philos Trans R Soc Lond B Biol Sci* , 356-983

Tosoni, A.; Nebuloni, M.; Ferri, A.; Bonetto, S.; Antinori, S.; Scaglia, M.; Xiao, L.; Moura, H.; Visvesvara, G.S.; Vago, L.; Costanzi. (2002). Disseminated Microsporidiosis caused by Encephalitozoon cuniculi III (Dog Type) in an Italian AIDS patient: a retrospective study. *Modern Pathology*, 15: 577-583

Turtas, S.; Perria, C.; Brambilla, M.; Pau, A. (1989). Follow up of 5 cases of cerebral coenurosis.XXXVIII *Congr. Soc. It. Neurochirurgia.*, 735-740

Vinuelas, J.; Garcia-Alonso, M.; Ferrando, L.; Navarrete, I.; Molano, I.; Miron, C.; Carcelen, J.; Alonso, C,; Nieto, C.G. (2001). Meningeal leishmaniosis induced by Leishmania infantum in naturally infected dogs. *Vet. Parasitology*, 101: 23-27

Viscoli, C.; Garaventa, A.; Ferrea, G..; Manno, G..; Taccone, A.; Terragna, A. (1991). Listeria monocitogenes brain abscesses in a girl with acute lymphoblastic leukaemia after late central nervous system relapse. *Eur. J. Cancer*, 27: 435-437

Weber, R.; Deplazes, P.; Flepp, M.; Mathis, A.; Baumann, R.; Sauer, B.; Kuster, H.; & Luthy, R.(1973). Cerebral Microsporidiosis due to Encephalitozoon cuniculi in a patient with human immunodeficiency virus infection. *The New England Journal of Medicine*,13: 474-478.

Wertheim, H.F.L.; Nghia, Ho, D.N.; Taylor, W.; Schultsz, C. (2009). Streptococcus suis: an Emerging Human Pathogen. *Emerging Infections.*, 48: 617-625

Yang, J.M.; Liu, H.X.; Hao, Y.X.; He, C.; Zhao, D.M. (2006). Development of a rapid real-time PCR assay for detection and quantification of four familiar species of Chlamydiaceae. *J Clin Virol.* 36:79-81.

Zeller, H.G.. & Schuffenecker, I. (2004). West Nile virus: an overview of its spread in Europe and the Mediterranean basin in contrast to its spread in the Americas. *Eur J Clin Microbiol Infect Dis.* , Mar;23(3).

Part 2

Viral Pathogens

3

Virus-Induced Encephalitis and Innate Immune Responses – A Focus on Emerging or Re-Emerging Viruses

Melanie Denizot[1], Vincent G. Thon-Hon[1],
Shiril Kumar[1], Jim W. Neal[2] and Philippe Gasque[1]
[1]*GRI/IRG, Immunopathology and Infectious Disease Research Grouping (IRG, GRI), EA4517, University, CHR Felix Guyon and CYROI of La Reunion*
[2]*Neuropathology Laboratory, Dept of Histopathology, Cardiff University Medical School., CF14 4XN*
[1]*France*
[2]*UK*

1. Introduction

A wide variety of emerging and re-emerging viruses (e.g. arboviruses, 'arthropod-borne viruses') contributes to neurological diseases. Infections can be associated with new viral variants that are more efficiently transmitted and lead to massive outbreak and increased reports of complicated cases involving the CNS (Tsetsarkin et al., 2007; Vazeille et al., 2007). It is also possible that viruses may have acquired increased neurovirulence by a previously non-neurotropic virus. Viruses that appear to have recently become more neurovirulent include for example the West Nile flavivirus (WNV), Chikungunya alphavirus (CHIKV) and the enterovirus 71 (ENV71) (Griffin, 2010). In addition to these newer challenges, Japanese encephalitis flavivirus (JEV), rabies, polio, measles virus (MV), human immunodeficiency virus (HIV) and human herpes virus (HHV) remain important causes of neurologic diseases. Focusing on CHIKV, this is an alphavirus of the *Togaviridae* family transmitted by mosquitoes of the Aedes (*Ae*) genus. The alphavirus group comprises 29 viruses, six of which of the 'Old World, ie Africa' can cause human joint disorders (arthralgia evolving to arthritis), namely CHIKV, O'nyong-nyong virus (ONNV), Semliki forest virus (SFV), Ross River (RRV), Sindbis virus (SINV), Mayaro virus (MAYV) while the so-called 'New World' such as Eastern equine encephalitis virus (EEEV) and Venezuelan equine encephalitis virus (VEEV) can cause severe brain damage (Das et al., 2010; Jaffar-Bandjee et al., 2009). Interestingly, CHIKV-associated neuropathology was first described in the 1960s but it is the unprecedented incidence rate in the Indian Ocean with efficient clinical facilities that allowed a better description of cases with severe encephalitis, meningoencephalitis, peripheral neuropathies and deaths among newborns (mother-to-child infection), infants and elderly patients (Das et al., 2010; Jaffar-Bandjee et al., 2009). The follow-up of the neonates contaminated by CHIKV clearly indicates poor outcomes and neurodevelopment defects (Jaffar-Bandjee et al., 2011). Neurological manifestations described in adults requiring hospitalization involved cases of encephalopathy frequently associated with the presence of IgM anti-CHIKV in the CSF, encephalitis, Guillain-Barre, encephalomyeloradiculitis and rare deaths (Economopoulou et al., 2009; Lemant et al., 2008). In recent histopathological studies, CHIKV infection in adults was associated with bilateral frontoparietal white matter lesions with restricted diffusion, which is described as an early sign of viral encephalitis (Ganesan et al., 2008). Focal perivascular lymphocytic infiltrates were also present in area of active demyelination and some degree of microglial activation was also noted in the gray matter which may contribute to bystander neuronal loss (Ganesan et al., 2008). Although data are still scarce, the number of cases with CNS involvement appears to support the neurotropic/neuroinfectious activity of CHIKV. This unique CNS infection illustrated by subventricular white matter lesions and intraparenchymal haemorrhages have been confirmed experimentally. CHIKV diseases can be reproduced in several animal models and the virus was shown to infect mouse/macaque brains and to replicate in cultures of glial and neuronal cells (Gardner et al., 2010; Labadie et al., 2010; Solignat et al., 2009; Wang et al., 2008; Ziegler et al., 2008). The incidence of neuroinfection is dramatically increased following either the injection of high viral titers, the route of injection (intranasal > intraperitoneal), in young animals (less than two week-old) or in mice failing to mount a robust interferon response (i.e. IFNAR knockout animals). Thus, experimental infections where mice were inoculated subcutaneously showed rapid and robust replication (10^6-10^7 PFU/ml) of CHIKV in the brain particularly of newborn mice. Interestingly, infected mice showed signs of illness suggestive of human clinical pathology such as loss of balance, difficulty of walking, dragging of the hind limbs, skin lesions but with rare mortality. CHIKV neuroinfection is particularly severe in IFNAR -/- mice and targets the leptomeninges, the choroid plexus and ependymal cells lining the subventricular zone (SVZ) also known as one of the neural stem cell niche in adult brains. The nature of the receptor(s) mediating cell attachment and infection remains to be characterized but the role of apoptotic blebs carrying the virus from cell to cell has recently been established as in a Trojan-horse paradigm (see below). On the one hand, the local innate immune response is the key to the control of viral infection but could also, on the other, contribute to neuronal loss through the uncontrolled release of cytotoxic inflammatory cytokines, complement proteins or proapoptotic molecules (TNF-α, FasL, granzymes) (Hauwel et al., 2005). We will review herein the pathological mechanisms as well as the innate immune mechanisms engaged during encephalitis and with special emphasis on chikungunya.

2. Encephalitis and clinical manifestations

The clinical hallmark of acute viral encephalitis includes classically fever, headache, and altered level of consciousness. Other associated clinical observations are disorientation, behavioral and speech disturbances and seizures. These clinical signs distinguish a patient with encephalitis from one with viral meningitis, who can have headache, nuchal rigidity, and fever (Whitley and Gnann, 2002). Clinical findings reflect disease progression and the specific areas of CNS involvement, which is determined by the tropism of different viruses for different cell types expressing different viral receptors. Neurons are most likely to be targeted by several viruses such as polioviruses which preferentially infect motor neurons and rabies which selectively infects neurons of the limbic system (Griffin, 2010). Oligodendrocytes, the myelin-forming cells can also be infected (e.g. HHV6, SFV) and leading to direct or indirect demyelination (Fazakerley et al., 2006; Mock et al., 1999). Other cells within the CNS can also be the site of viral replication and for instance with mumps virus which can infect epithelial cells of the choroid plexus. The involvement of ependymal cells of the SVZ can result in hydranencephaly following infection for instance by adenoviruses or coxsackie viruses.

Viruses vary greatly in their capacity to induce encephalitis. For some viruses (e.g. mumps), neuroinfection is a common but a relatively benign part of the syndrome.

For others (flaviviruses such as JEV or WNV), although the infection is highly asymptomatic, CNS infection when it occurs is the most prominent clinical feature. A third group of viruses are those which commonly cause infection, but only rarely cause encephalitis (herpes simplex virus, HSV or CHIKV). In this group, newborns and elderly patients are at risk because they either have a poor or inappropriate immune response against the infectious challenge (Hoarau et al., 2010).

A paramyxovirus isolated from a Malaysian patient with encephalitis showed *in vitro* characteristics similar to Hendra virus (HeV), a new morbillivirus previously isolated from horses and human in 1995. Subsequent virological studies have shown that the Malaysian pathogen, now named Nipah virus (NiV), is closely related to, but distinct from HeV and that the two belong to a new genus within the family paramyxoviridae capable of causing major outbreaks of encephalitis. Patients present with fever, headache, dizziness, vomiting, and altered mental state.

Finally, there are viruses for which human infection inevitably and exclusively results in CNS disease (e.g. rabies). In addition to acute pathology, other viruses (e.g. measles) can cause syndromes of post-infectious encephalopathy with the capacity of the virus to hide into tissue sanctuaries. The capacity of these viruses to reactivate the viral cycle is poorly understood and may be the results of immune escape mechanisms.

3. Molecular and cellular mechanisms for virus entry into the CNS

The clinical manifestations of many virus infections are dependent on whether or not virus gains access to susceptible cells within the CNS. Therefore, the mechanisms by which viruses penetrate the CNS are of prime importance in understanding the pathogenesis of the disease. To understand the invasion process it is necessary to describe one of the defensive structures that prevent microbial invasion. The CNS is enclosed completely by three different but connected blood-brain interfaces (Abbott et al., 2010).

A blood -brain barrier (BBB) composed of brain micro-vascular endothelial cells (BMEC) with intercellular tight junctions and supported by astrocytes, pericytes and the basement membrane. The second is highly vascularized and fenestrated barrier localized at the choroid plexus between blood and cerebrospinal fluid (CSF), which also allows passage of some blood components and, thirdly, an interface provided by avascular arachnoid epithelium, underlying the dura, and completely enclosing the CNS (Abbott et al., 2010; Weiss et al., 2009).

There are at least four different mechanisms by which viruses can gain access into the CNS. First, viruses may gain access by infecting the BMEC or may be transported across the BMEC (Jarvis and Nelson, 2002). Infection of the BMEC may provide a portal for viral entry into the CNS and disrupting the BBB function. A number of viruses such as cytomegalovirus (CMV) (Jarvis and Nelson, 2002), HIV (Moses et al., 1993) and arboviruses (Dropulic and Masters, 1990) are able to infect the BMEC at least *in vitro*. In acute viral encephalitis, capillary and endothelial inflammation of cortical vessels is a striking pathological finding, occurring primarily in the grey matter or grey white junction and this observation may facilitate virus entry. For example, HIV may gain access to CNS *in vivo* by this paracellular route as a result of endothelium activation by TNFα and other proinflammatory cytokines (Fiala et al., 1997).

Second, viruses may transmigrate across the BBB within virally infected leukocytes. For HIV, several studies suggest that virus shedding from infected CD4+ T cells, macrophages, and monocytes during migration through the BBB can instigate CNS replication into the parenchyma (Nottet et al., 1996; Persidsky et al., 1997; Schmidtmayerova et al., 1996). CMV can also be transferred to CNS by virus infected mononuclear phagocytes and bi-directional cell to cell transmission between infected monocytes and endothelial cells (Drevets and Leenen, 2000).

Third, viruses can also penetrate the CNS by taking advantage of incomplete closure of the BBB. Despite the intercellular tight junctions between the capillary endothelial cells in most regions of the BBB, certain areas of the CNS such as the choroid plexus, posterior pituitary, and circumventricular organs are not completely protected by the BBB due to a fenestrated endothelial cell layer and sparse basement membrane (Zhang and Tuomanen, 1999). A number of blood-borne viruses including mumps (Herndon et al., 1974), HIV (Bagasra et al., 1996) and CHIKV (Couderc et al., 2008) have been suggested to penetrate across the choroid plexus micro- vessels and infect the epithelium. In the CSF space, viruses can subsequently infect the ependymal cells and the surrounding brain tissue.

Finally, viruses can spread to the CNS through peripheral neuronal routes, like the motor neurons of the spinal cord ,olfactory neurons, retinal neurons, oculomotor neurons and trigeminal nerves , which are directly connected to the CNS, thus providing a convenient route for neurotropic viruses (Mori et al., 2005; Tirabassi et al., 1998). Viruses including HSV (Barnett et al., 1993), rabies virus (Jackson, 2003) and VEEV (Charles et al., 1995) are able to replicate within peripheral nerves and are transported into the CNS from the PNS along axons as the result of axonal transport of neurons. Certain enteroviruses can also spread to the CNS by infecting enteric neurons (Morrison and Fields, 1991). Virus spread within the CNS by retrograde, anterograde or cell to cell diffusion mechanisms.

4. Infection and replication of viruses in brain cells

4.1 Primary receptors used by viruses to infect CNS cells

The presence of cell membrane proteins that act as virus receptors determines whether a cell can be invaded by a virus or not. Dependent on the receptor(s) chosen, some viruses may infect nearly all mammalian cell types or only a small subset of cells from certain species. We herein have chosen to highlight only some of the receptors used by a few emerging or re-emerging viruses to infect specific cell types in the brain and to cause encephalitis. Several comprehensive reviews have discussed the role of different receptors for rabies (Acethylcholine nicotinic receptors, NCAM CD56 as well as the P75 neurotrophin receptor, NTR) (Lafon, 2005) and, hence, this aspect will not be discussed herein.

4.1.1 Nectin-1 and 2 are cellular receptors for HSV

Nectins are immunoglobulin (Ig)-like Cell Adhesion Molecules (CAMs) involved in the formation of various intercellular junctions and the establishment of apical-basal polarity at cell-cell adhesion sites (Takai et al., 2008). The nectin family which comprises 4 members, nectin-1 or poliovirus receptor related 1 (PRR1 also called HveC, CD111, HIgR), nectin-2 (also termed PRR2, HveB, CD112), nectin-3 and nectin-4. Each of them contains an extracellular region with three Ig-like domains, a single transmembrane region, and a cytoplasmic tail region. Nectin-1, -2 and -3 are expressed ubiquitously in multiple cell types such as epithelia, fibroblasts and neurons, whereas nectin-4 is mainly expressed in the human placenta. Nectin-1 and -2 have been identified as HSV entry mediators (Hve) **(see Table 1)**. Nectin-1 can serve as entry receptors for both HSV-1 and HSV-2 (Geraghty et al., 1998). In contrast, nectin-2 has more limited entry activity. Indeed, human nectin-2 is only a weak entry receptor for HSV-2 and certain strains of HSV-1 carrying out mutations in the glycoprotein D (Lopez et al., 2000). A more recent study also assessed the roles of the two known entry receptors, HVEM and nectin-1, in neuronal infection in the CNS and the development of encephalitis in a mouse model (Kopp et al., 2009). Intracranial injection of HSV was performed directly into the hippocampus of Wild-type (WT), HVEM KO, nectin-1

Name	HSV	Rabies	HIV	Polio	WNV	CHIKV
Virus family	Alpha herpesvirus	Rhabdovirus	Retrovirus	Picorna virus	Flavivirus	Alphavirus
Genome	(+)DNA double stranded linear	(-)RNA single stranded linear	(+)RNA single stranded linear	(+)RNA single stranded linear	(+)RNA single stranded linear	(+)RNA Single stranded linear
Envelope	yes	yes	yes	No	yes	yes
Route of brain entry	Trigeminal Nerve Olfactory nerve	Retrograde axonal	Cell mediated BBB crossing	Retrograde Axonal + BBB crossing	Direct BBB crossing	Blood- CSF crossing
Receptors	Nectin-1, Nectin-2, HSPG	NCAM (CD56) AChR P75 NTR	CD4, CCR5, CXCR4	Nectin-1(PRR1), Nectin-2(PRR2)	DC-SIGN (myeloid cells)	Apoptotic bleb-mediated cell entry
Targets (CNS)	Neurons	Neurons	Myeloid cells microglia	Neurons	Myeloid cells Microglia	Epithelial cells Ependymal cells Neurons Glia
Clinics	Encephalitis Herpetic neuralgia Meningitis Myelitis	Guillain Barre like syndrome Progressive encephalitis paralysis	Dementia Encephalitis Myelitis Neuropathy	Paralysis Respiratory arrest	Encephalitis Meningitis Myopathy	Encephalopathy Encephalitis Guillain Barre
Geographic distribution	Worldwide	Europe Asia Africa Americas	Worldwide	India Africa	Europe Americas Africa	Africa Asia India (Europe) (Reunion)

(See text for abbreviation)

Table 1. Encephalitis due to emerging and re-emerging viruses

KO and double KO mice. The results indicated that nectin-1 deficient mice showed no signs of disease after intracranial inoculation, and no HSV antigens were detectable in the brain parenchyma. However, HSV antigens were detected in non-parenchymal cells lining the ventricules. In the double KO mice, the results showed an absence of disease and no detectable expression of viral antigens even in non-parenchymal cells, indicating that infection of these cells in the nectin-1 KO mice was dependent on the expression of HveM.

4.1.2 CD46 is a cellular receptor for HHV6 and measles

CD46 also designated as membrane cofactor protein (MCP) is a member of a family of glycoproteins acting as regulators of complement activation, but has subsequently been shown to link innate immunity to adaptative immunity (Seya et al., 1986). CD46 mediates the inactivation of its natural complement ligands C3b and C4b and acts as a cofactor for serine protease factor I (Lublin et al., 1988). CD46 thus protect host cells from homologous complement attack which could result in extensive cytolysis and widespread tissue damage. Another function of CD46 is to promote T cell differentiation from a helper Th1 to a regulatory Tr1 phenotype, depending on IL-2 concentrations (Cardone et al., 2010). Human CD46 is alternatively spliced into several isoforms, resulting in a varying number of extracellular domains and two different cytoplasmic tails, Cyt1 and Cyt2 (Seya et al., 1999). CD46 seems to be constitutively recycled from the cell surface via clathrin-coated pits and transported to perinuclear multivesicular bodies (Crimeen-Irwin et al., 2003). The importance of CD46 in the homeostasis of the organism is highlighted by its ubiquitous expression on the surface of all nucleated human cells (Liszewski et al., 1991).
Human CD46 is a cellular receptor for Human Herpesvirus 6 (HHV-6) (Santoro et al., 1999) and MV (Dorig et al., 1993). The authors demonstrated that both acute infection and cell to cell fusion mediated by HHV-6 were specifically inhibited by a monoclonal antibody to CD46; fusion was also blocked by soluble CD46. Interestingly, they showed that nonhuman cells resistant to HHV-6 fusion and entry became susceptible upon expression of recombinant human CD46. Concerning the study of MV infection in the CNS, a murine model of MV-induced pathology was developed from several lines of transgenic mice expressing human CD46 molecule with Cyt1 or Cyt2 (Evlashev et al., 2000). The results of their experiments showed that all transgenic mice expressing CD46 protein in the brain were highly sensitive to intracerebral infection by the MV Edmonston strain, in comparison to nontransgenic controls. In addition, the two isoforms of CD46, Cyt1 and 2, are functionally similar in mediating MV entry into the brain.

4.1.3 Ephrins are cellular receptors for Hendra virus (HeV) and Nipah virus (Niv)

The Eph (erythropoietin-producing hepatocellular) receptors are the largest family of tyrosine kinase receptors (TRKs). They interact with cell surface bound ligands, the ephrins (Eph receptor interacting proteins) that are a highly conserved class of proteins with many homologous members. Based on structural differences, two classes of ephrins can be classified: ephrins-A (A1 to A6) are attached to the plasma membrane via glycophosphatidyl inositol (GPI) moiety and ephrins B (B1 to B3) crossing the plasma membrane and possessing a short cytoplasmic tail. Eph receptors have diverse functions, such as widespread effects on the actin cytoskeleton, cell-substrate adhesion, intercellular junctions, cell shape, and cell movement (Egea and Klein, 2007; Himanen et al., 2007; Pasquale, 2005; Pasquale, 2008).

Two independent studies identified Ephrin B2 (EFNB2) as the receptor for HeV and NiV, which are emergent paramyxovirus. Of the ten potential receptor-encoding plasmids they used to transfect non-permissive HeLa cells, only the human EFNB2 plasmid confers HeV fusion permissiveness. They further demonstrated that soluble EFNB2 blocks both viruses fusion in human EFNB2-transfected HeLa cells. They also showed that both HeV and NiV glycoprotein G and EFNB2 soluble protein could be specifically and reciprocally captured by ELISA. In addition, both viruses glycoprotein G were efficiently coprecipitated by EFNB2/Fc. Another study identified EFNB2 as an entry receptor for NiV (Negrete et al., 2005). The authors also reported that EFNB2 binds to the NiV glycoprotein G. They observed that soluble Fc-fusion proteins of EFNB2 effectively blocked NiV fusion and entry into permissive cell types. Moreover, transfection of EFNB2 into non-permissive cells renders them permissive for NiV fusion and entry. Interestingly they found that soluble EFNB2 inhibited NiV-envelope-mediated infection of microvascular endothelial cells and primary cortical rat neurons. EFNB3 was later discovered as an additional receptor for NiV using the Chinese hamster ovary cell line (CHO-pgsA745) that does not express ephrins endogenously (Negrete et al., 2006). Interestingly, the authors characterized the important conserved Leu-Trp residues in the G-H loop of EFNB2 and B3 that are critical for their binding with NiV glycoprotein G.

4.1.4 Scavenger receptor class B member 2 (SCARB2) and EV71

The concept of scavenger receptors (SCAR) was first described by their ability to bind modified low-density lipoproteins (Goldstein et al., 1979). SCAR can bind a variety of natural/endogenous, modified host, microbial (bacterial, viral, fungal, and parasitic), environmental, soluble or particulates ligands by endocytosis and phagocytosis (reviewed in (Mukhopadhyay and Gordon, 2004)). SCARB2 (also known as lysosomal integral membrane protein II or CD36b like-2) belongs to the scavenger receptor class B subfamily, which also includes SCARB1 and CD36 (Calvo et al., 1995; Eskelinen et al., 2003). SCARB2 is a type III double-transmembrane protein with N- as well as C-terminal cytoplasmic tails and is located primarily in lysosomes and endosomes. SCARB2 participates in membrane transportation and the reorganization of the endosomal-lysosomal compartment (Kuronita et al., 2002). Deficiency of SCARB2 in mice causes ureteric pelvic junction obstruction, deafness and peripheral neuropathy (Gamp et al., 2003). SCARB2 is widely expressed in lysosomes and late endosomes (reviewed in (Eskelinen et al., 2003).

Since its identification in California in 1969 (Schmidt et al., 1974), enterovirus 71 (EV71) has been recognized as a frequent cause of epidemics of hand-foot-and-mouth disease (HFMD) associated with severe neurological sequelae in some cases (Blomberg et al., 1974). EV71 infections can progress to aseptic meningitis, acute flaccid paralysis and fatal encephalitis (McMinn, 2002). A recent paper demonstrated that SCARB2 is a receptor for EV71 (Yamayoshi et al., 2009). The authors showed that EV71 binds soluble SCARB2 or cells expressing SCARB2, and the binding is inhibited by an antibody to SCARB2. Furthermore, expression of human SCARB2 enables normally unsusceptible cell lines to support EV71 propagation and develop cytopathic effects. Yet, the detail of the interaction between EV71 and SCARB2 at the cellular level, resulting in CNS infection has not been identified.

4.1.5 CD4 as the primary receptor for HIV

Human CD4 exhibits a poly-Ig-like domain structure which is homologous to an increasingly large number of recognition molecules, and consists in four tandem variable-joining (VJ)-like domains (Maddon et al., 1987). The Ig-like domains of CD4 are anchored to the membrane by a hydrophobic segment, and followed by a short cytoplasmic region. CD4 is expressed on the surface of T lymphocytes, monocytes, macrophages, and brain microglia (resident macrophages) (Wyatt and Sodroski, 1998).

HIV invades the CNS early following viral infection but provokes brain disease only years later. During the periods of progressive immunosuppression, neurological disease occurs in 15 to 20% of infected individuals which develop cognitive and motor impairments referred to as the HIV type 1 (HIV-1)-associated dementia complex also termed as HIV-associated dementia or HIV encephalopathy (Janssen et al., 1991; Price et al., 1988). Neurological disease is often associated with a marked depletion of CD4+ T lymphocytes (Navia et al., 1986). It is now know that HIV encephalitis is a common pathological manifestation characterized by monocyte infiltration into the brain, the formation of macrophage-derived multinucleated giant cells, microglial nodules, and demyelination (Sharer et al., 1985).

Considerable amount of data identified CD4 as the main entry receptor for HIV. Previous studies on the two AIDS retroviruses, human T-lymphotropic virus type III (HTLV-III) and lymphadenopathy-associated virus (LAV) helped to characterize the primary cellular receptor involved in HIV infection (Dalgleish et al., 1984; Klatzmann et al., 1984). Dalgleish and colleagues identified receptor-positive cells by assessing induction of multinucleated syncytia and by testing the susceptibility of various cell types to pseudotypes of vesicular stomatitis virus (VSV) carrying envelope antigens of HTLV strains. Their results showed that both VSV (HTLV-I) and VSV (HTLV-II) pseudotypes plated on a variety of cell types whereas the VSV (HTLV-III) was more specific to the two human T-cell lines (JM and CEM) tested. In addition, only cells expressing the CD4 antigen were sensitive to syncytium induction by HTLV-III and infection by VSV (HTLV-III) pseudotypes. After the screening of 155 monoclonal antibodies to T-cell surface antigens for their ability to inhibit the syncytia formation induced by HTLV-III, they demonstrated that pre-incubation of cells with all anti-CD4 antibodies blocked the cell fusion induced by HTLV-III. In another paper published the same year, Klatzman *et al.* (Klatzmann et al., 1984) investigated the relationship between the CD4+ tropism of LAV and the presence of CD4 on T lymphocytes. Similarly to the previous paper on HTLV-III, they reported that pre-incubation of CD4+ T lymphocytes with three monoclonal antibodies directed against the CD4 glycoprotein specifically blocked cell infection by LAV.

It is well documented that efficient entry of HIV-1 into target cells is dependent upon binding of the viral exterior envelope glycoprotein, gp120, to the CD4-amino-terminal domain (McDougal et al., 1986). After the virus binding, the HIV-1 envelope glycoproteins mediate the fusion of viral and host cell membranes to complete the fusion process. The formation of syncytia results in the membrane fusion directed by HIV-1 envelope glycoproteins expressed on the infected cell surface with uninfected CD4-positive cells. Although CD4 expression on a target cell seems to be sufficient for HIV attachment, the fusion process appeared to be more complex.

4.2 Secondary receptors of virus entry

4.2.1 Chemokine receptors CXCR4 and CCR5 as HIV infection cofactors

Chemokine receptors are part of the serpentine GTP-binding protein (G protein)-coupled receptors superfamily that include receptors for hormones, neurotransmitters, paracrine substance, inflammatory mediators, certain proteinases, taste and odorant molecules. All known human chemokines fit within four classes based on the cysteine motifs near the Nterminus. The two major classes are the CXC chemokines (CXCR1 to CXCR5) in which the first two cysteines are separated by a single residue, and the CC chemokines (CCR1 to CCR9) in which the first two cysteines are adjacent. CXCR4 (also termed fusin, HUMSTSR, LESTR, HM89, LCR1, NPYR, D2S201E) and CCR5 (also known as CKR5, CC CKR5, ChemR13, CMKBR5) are membrane-bound co-receptors for HIV entry. CXCR4 is expressed on neutrophils, myeloid cells (as well as microglia), and particularly on T lymphocytes (Loetscher et al., 1994). CCR5 mRNA expression was detected in lymphoid organs such as the thymus and spleen, and in peripheral T lymphocytes and macrophages (Raport et al., 1996). The first HIV-1 co-receptor was identified with the use of a recombinant vaccinia virus-based construct in which fusion between the HIV gp120 envelope glycoprotein (Env)-expressing cells and CD4-expressing cells would lead to the activation of a reporter gene *Escherichia coli* LacZ (Feng et al., 1996). The screening of a HeLa cDNA plasmid library and subsequent sequence analysis of the insert revealed that the protein was a member of the G protein-coupled receptor superfamily and was designated "fusin". In addition, loss-of-function experiments showed that anti-fusin antibodies blocked cell fusion and infection of primary human CD4+ T lymphocytes. Interestingly, both experiments stressed that fusin functioned preferentially for T cell line (TCL)-tropic rather than for macrophage (M)-tropic HIV-1 isolates. The discovery of fusin provided an impetus for the identification of the M-tropic HIV isolates coreceptor. Several independent reports demonstrated that CCR5 is the major coreceptor for M-tropic HIV-1 strains (Alkhatib et al., 1996; Choe et al., 1996; Deng et al., 1996; Doranz et al., 1996; Dragic et al., 1996). The evidence was based on both gain-of-function studies using recombinant CCR5, and loss-of-function studies with CCR5 chemokines ligands (MCP-1, MIP-1α, MIP-1β and RANTES) as blocking agents. After the discovery of CCR5, it was demonstrated that fusin is a chemokine receptor that specifically recognize the CXC chemokines ligands SDF-1α and SDF-1β (Bleul et al., 1996; Oberlin et al., 1996); fusin was thus renamed CXCR4.

4.2.2 Phosphatidylserine (PS), apoptotic blebs and virus spreading from cells to cells

PS is a phospholipid located on the inner leaflet of the plasma membrane (Williamson and Schlegel, 1994; Zwaal and Schroit, 1997). Its internal positioning is maintained by translocases that catalyze aminophospholipid transport from the external to the internal leaflet of the plasma membrane. The loss of PS asymmetry can occur during several cellular events including cell injury, cell activation or apoptosis (Balasubramanian and Schroit, 2003).

Two apoptotic pathways can be identified; (i) the extrinsic apoptotic pathway is initiated by members of the Tumour necrosis factor (TNF) family of death ligands that bind to TNFR death receptor family members, Tumour Necrosis Factor Receptor -related apoptosis inducing signal ligand (TRAIL) and Fas ligand (FASL). This results in the formation of the Death Inducing Signal Complex DISC at the cell membrane. DISC subsequently interacts with Fas-associated death domain protein (FADD) in caspase 8, pro caspase 3 and this activates caspase 3, resulting in host cell death (Wilson et al., 2009); (ii) The intrinsic apoptosis pathway is dependent upon the activation of host proteins such as tumour suppressor protein P53 by virus infection. This in turn activates BH-3 domain only members of the B cell lymphoma 2 (Bcl-2) family, e.g the pro-apoptotic proteins Bax and Bak. The activation of these two proteins produces pores in the outer membrane of mitochondria with the release of cytochrome C activating caspase 9 and cell death (Danial and Korsmeyer, 2004; Kroemer et al., 2007).

Apoptosis following viral infection is a robust line defence mechanism, since the cell auto destruction appears one of the best ways to limit virus production and spreading (Griffin and Hardwick, 1997). Unequivocally, the expected purpose of this cell suicide in response to infection is to short-circuit the viral expansion and to promote the clearance of dead infected cells by professional phagocytes (Fujimoto et al., 2000; Hashimoto et al., 2007). However, most viruses deal with this defensive reaction and have evolved strategies to evade or delay apoptosis (Teodoro and Branton, 1997).

Under normal cellular conditions, exposure PS serves as a recognition signal for internalization of apoptotic cells or debris. PS-mediated apoptotic clearance is a highly conserved mechanism, occurring in both professional and nonprofessional phagocytes (Henson et al., 2001). Importantly, this process does not elicit an inflammatory response (Savill et al., 2002). "Apoptotic mimicry" or the exposure of PS on the surface of a pathogen provides a signal for virus uptake and may represent a mechanism for viruses to stunt the host inflammatory response and evade immune recognition. Some viruses like CMV or HSV-1 and HSV-2, which acquire their envelopes from intracellular organelles, have externalized PS (Pryzdial and Wright, 1994; Sutherland et al., 1997). A previous study investigated the early apoptotic events in real time in intact live ND7 neuron-like cells following HSV-1 infection (Gautier et al., 2003). The authors demonstrated that infection of differentiated ND7 cells by HSV-1 triggers detectable alterations including PS exposure indicative of physiological changes associated with early stages of apoptosis.

Furthermore, control of the apoptotic process by the viruses is key, either to establish a permanent infection when they are able to block apoptosis, or to facilitate their dissemination and prevent inflammatory and immune response when they are able to control and activate the late phase of apoptosis (Chen et al., 2006). Dissemination of viral particles through the production of apoptotic blebs from host cells could confer protection from the immune system (Chen et al., 2006; Everett and McFadden, 1999). Conversely, it has been proposed that phagocytosis of these pathogen (Sindbis for example) -enriched apoptotic blebs by antigen presenting cells (e.g. dendritic cells) could contribute to a robust and uncontrolled adaptive immune response leading to autoimmunity against self-antigens contained within the blebs (Rosen et al., 1995). In the case of CHIKV, it has recently been evidenced that completion of the apoptotic process is an important element for efficient virus propagation (Krejbich-Trotot et al., 2011). Indeed, CHIKV was revealed to exploit, may be in parallel to classical ways of entry and cell exit, an ingenious way of camouflage in apoptotic blebs to enhance viral spreading to neighbouring cells while being shielded from the immune system.

4.2.3 The C-type lectin receptors and WNV cell entry

The superfamily of proteins containing lectin-like domains is a large group of extracellular metazoan proteins with diverse functions (Zelensky and Gready, 2005). The main function of the calcium-dependent 'C'-type lectins is to interact with pathogen-associated molecular patterns (PAMPs) which are well conserved and expressed by various microorganisms and to internalize these pathogens for processing and antigen presentation (Drickamer, 1995). For instance, C-type lectins contain Carbohydrate Recognition Domains (CRDs) capable of binding to conserved oligosaccharides that are commonly found on the surface glycoproteins of viruses (Cambi et al., 2005). C-type lectins are secreted as soluble proteins or produced as transmembrane proteins. The Mannan Binding Lectin (MBL), present in the plasma, is a member of the collectin family and is an example of soluble protein. MBL is

expressed by monocytes/microglia and possesses a globular carboxy terminal sequence that binds to virus proteins containing mannose molecules. The transmembrane lectins include the Mannose Membrane Receptor (MMR also known as CD206) and the Dentritic Cell-Specific ICAM-3 Grabbing Non-integrin (DC-SIGN also known as CD209) receptor that recognizes "self " intercellular adhesion molecule 2 (ICAM2) and ICAM3 (van Kooyk and Geijtenbeek, 2003). MMR contains eight CRD (Weis et al., 1998). DC-SIGN is a type II transmembrane protein which possesses a single globular-structured CRD. DC-SIGN's CRD is separated from the transmembrane region by a neck domain involved in oligomerization and which regulates carbohydrate specificity. Finally, a cytoplasmic tail is present, which includes internalization motifs and an incomplete immunoreceptor tyrosine-based activation motif (ITAM). Microglia, perivascular macrophages and dendritic cells express MMR and DC-SIGN (Burudi et al., 1999; Linehan et al., 1999; Mukhtar et al., 2002; Sallusto et al., 1995; Schwartz et al., 2002). The expression of DC-SIGN on brain microvascular endothelial cells could be advantageous for viral entry into the CNS (Mukhtar et al., 2002).
Two major lineages of WNV, L1 and L2, have been identified after the phylogenetic analyses of glycoprotein E (Lanciotti et al., 1999). L1 strains have a large distribution and have been found in Africa, Europe, the Middle-East, North and Central America whereas the L2 strain is mainly localized in Africa and Madagascar. WNV human infection is usually asymptomatic, however life-threatening neurological disease, including encephalitis or meningitis, generally occurs in older or immunocompromised individuals (Campbell et al., 2002; Granwehr et al., 2004). A recent study investigated the relative contribution of DC-SIGN in infection by glycosylated L1 and non-glycosylated L1 and L2 strains (Martina et al., 2008). The authors showed that in contrast to a non-glycosylated L1 strain, the glycosylated L1 strains use DC-SIGN as an attachment receptor on dendritic cells, leading to enhanced infection.

4.2.4 Heparan sulfate proteoglycans (HSPGs) and HSV

Heparan sulfate proteoglycans (HSPGs) are secreted and membrane associated proteins covalently attached to unbranched glycosaminoglycan heparan sulfate (HS) molecules which are composed of linear polysaccharide chains (Esko and Selleck, 2002). HS molecules are synthesized on a variety of cell surface proteins but are found consistently on members of two major families of membrane-bound proteoglycans: the transmembrane core proteins syndecans and the GPI-linked glypicans (Bernfield et al., 1999). HS can influence cell-environment interactions by binding to a heterogeneous group of growth factors, matrix ligands, and cell surface molecules. The possibility that HS could serve as an entry receptor for HSV type 1 and 2 was assessed on HEp-2 cells (WuDunn and Spear, 1989). They found that heparin blocked both virus adsorption. Different adsorption inhibitory agents including, heparin and poly-L-lysine (both bind to anions on the surface of virions and cells) and platelet factor 4 (which has a high affinity for heparin and heparan sulfate) was tested. After the incubation of these agents with HEp-2 cells either immediately before or during exposure with HSV-1 or HSV-2, an inhibition of virions adsorption by heparin was observed. Same results for poly-L-lysine and platelet factor 4 were obtained. A further study investigated the role of cell surface heparan sulfate in HSV infection using heparan sulfate-deficient mutants CHO cells (Shieh et al., 1992). They demonstrated that CHO mutants with defect in heparan sulfate biosynthesis are resistant to HSV infection and have reduced numbers of receptor for HSV.

5. Innate immune responses against viral infection in the CNS

The active and highly regulated control of immune responses in the brain is referred to as "immune privilege". The BBB, which prevents viruses, constituents of the adaptive immune system and antigen presenting cells, gaining accesses to the brain (for a review, see (Savarin and Bergmann, 2008)), is considered to be responsive for this privileged environment of the CNS. The CNS, therefore relies upon glia perivascular and meningeal cells to provide the innate immune response against virus attack (Hauwel et al., 2005). Microglia, astrocytes, ependymal cells, oligodendrocytes and neurons express Pattern Recognition Receptors (PRR)s (Suh et al., 2009) including the highly conserved Toll like receptors (TLR)s and the Retinoic inducible gene like RIG-1 receptors (RLRs) (Fujita et al., 2007) that detect the presence of "non self "as represented by viral nucleic acids.

5.1 TLRs

The TLRs are PRRs that have unique and essential function in animal immunity. TLRs comprise a family of type I transmembrane receptors, which are characterized by an extracellular leucine-rich repeat (LRR) domain and an intracellular Toll-interleukin-1 receptor (TIR) domain. LRR domains are found in a diverse set of proteins and mediate the recognition of components of foreign pathogens referred to as pathogen-associated molecular patterns (PAMPs) (for a review, see (Alexopoulou et al., 2001)). The cytoplasmic TIR domain of Toll proteins is a conserved protein-protein interaction module that is required for downstream signal transduction. So far, 10 and 12 functional TLRs have been identified in humans and mice, respectively, with TLR1-9 being conserved in both species (Takahashi et al., 2006). Microglia are the resident macrophages in the CNS and also express a wide range of TLRs (TLR1-9). Astrocytes express TLR1, 2, 3, 4, 5 and 9 whereas neurons mainly express TLR3 (Carty and Bowie, 2010). TLRs are located on the cell surface and are also distributed in the endosome so they are strategically placed to detect cytoplasmic viral RNA. TLR9 is activated by DNA rich in CpG motifs, whereas TLR7 and TLR8 recognize RNA viruses and ssRNA. TLR3 is activated by dsRNA formed during replication of viruses. TLRs signal through the adaptor molecules, myeloid differentiation primary response gene 88 (MyD88) and Trif, to initiate intracellular signaling by transcription factors such as and the IFN regulatory factors (IRFs) (Alexopoulou et al., 2001). These IRFs are translocated to the host cell nucleus where they regulate inflammatory cytokine synthesis and stimulate type I interferon synthesis (IFNα-β expression) to produce a protective response (anti-viral state) in adjacent uninfected cells (Paul et al., 2007). A further anti-viral property of the IRF is through its binding to the pro-apoptotic protein Bax and translocation to the mitochondria with activation of the mitochondrial apoptotic pathway, terminating virus replication (Chattopadhyay et al., 2010). Viruses can activate more than one TLR and it is known for example that TLR9 as well as TLR2 in dendritic cells and neuronal cells can respond to HSV to drive a protective IFN-α antiviral response (Bereczky-Veress et al., 2010; Sato et al., 2006). RNA viruses such as HIV, Rabies and WNV are more likely to be recognized by TLR3 and/or TLR7 or 8 expressed by microglia and neuronal cells (Prehaud et al., 2005; Szretter et al., 2010; Wang et al., 2004). The absence of TLR3 enhances WNV mortality in mice and increases viral burden in the brain (Daffis et al., 2008). Compared to wild-type controls, TLR3 -/- mice showed relatively little changes in peripheral viral loads. Interestingly, deficiency of TLR3 was associated with enhanced viral replication in primary cortical neuron cultures and greater WNV infection in neurons after intracranial inoculation while no significant differences where noted in viral growth kinetics or IFN-alpha/beta induction between wild-type and TLR3 KO fibroblasts, macrophages, and dendritic cells.

5.2 The RIG-I-like receptors (RLRs)

After the discovery of TLRs, several classes of PRRs, including the RLRs were identified. The RLR family consists of the three RNA helicases members: retinoic inducible gene-I (RIG-I), the melanoma differentiation-associated factor 5 (MDA5 also known as helicard or IFIH1) and the laboratory of genetics and physiology 2 (LGP2) that detect RNA viruses (Yoneyama and Fujita, 2009). RIG-I and MDA5 contain a C-terminal DExD/H box RNA helicase domain that is a characteristic amino acid signature motif of many RNA binding proteins, as well as two N-terminal caspase activation and recruitment domain (CARDs). LGP2 lacks CARD domains and has been proposed to function as a regulator of RIG-I/MDA5 signaling (Nakhaei et al., 2009). RIG-1 and MDA-5 are expressed by microglia and astrocytes, and located mainly in the cytosol and detect both short and long ds and ssRNA respectively (Furr et al., 2008; Hoarau et al., 2011). This interaction activates a series of intracellular signaling pathways using the adaptor molecules such as Interferon promoter stimulator (IPS-1) resulting in the transcription of IFNαβ interleukins and a range of anti-viral proteins. IPS-1 is key in the control of cell infection by several alphaviruses and flaviviruses including CHIKV and WNV, respectively. IPS-1-/- mice was recently shown to exhibit increased susceptibility to WNV infection marked by enhanced viral replication and dissemination with early viral entry into the CNS (Suthar et al., 2010). Moreover, infection of dendritic cells macrophages and primary cortical neurons showed that the IPS-1-dependent RLR signaling was essential for triggering IFN response (Suthar et al., 2010). Unexpectedly, infected KO mice also displayed uncontrolled inflammation that included elevated systemic type I IFN, proinflammatory cytokine and chemokine responses, increased numbers of inflammatory cells, enhanced humoral responses marked by complete loss of virus neutralization activity, and increased numbers of virus-specific CD8+ T cells and non-specific immune cell proliferation in the periphery and in the CNS. This uncontrolled inflammatory response was associated with a lack of regulatory T cell expansion that normally occurs during acute WNV infection. Thus, the enhanced inflammatory response in the absence of IPS-1 was coupled with a failure to protect against WNV infection. This is an important finding which stresses that IPS-1-dependent RLR signaling is equally important in the innate/adaptive immune responses but also in the balance of the immune response to WNV infection. With regards to CHIKV, it has recently been shown that IPS-1 is important at least in the periphery to drive a robust anti-viral response (Schilte et al., 2010).

5.3 CNS Innate immune system; Interferon type 1 and 2 responses stimulate an anti-viral response

Mice deficient for the type I IFN receptor (IFNAR) has proved the fundamental importance of the type I IFN in the control of virus replication (Couderc et al., 2008; Muller et al., 1994). Indeed, CNS virus infections are more lethal in mice deficient in IFNAR than the wild type equivalent, emphasizing the importance of IFNα/β/IFNAR pathway for anti-viral defense (Griffin, 2003; Paul et al., 2007). The type 1 interferon response is made by most CNS cells and results in a non-apoptotic anti-viral response by the host cell reducing infection by a replicating RNA virus (Katze et al., 2002). The IFN anti-viral response involves IFN binding to IFNAR on the host cell leading to the activation of Janus kinases (JAK) with phosphorylation of the activators of transcription factors (STAT1 and STAT2). These two proteins enter the nucleus to drive the expression of interferon stimulated genes (ISGs) (Goodbourn et al., 2000) . Host CNS cells in response to IFN stimulation produces a range of anti-viral ISGs, including oligoadenylate synthetase (OAS) and IFN-inducible ds RNA - dependent protein kinase (PKR) that both modulate virus replication; RNAse L and Mx that inhibit viral transcription together with the RNA deaminases (ADAR-1 and APOBEC3G) producing mutations in viral genomes (Goodbourn et al., 2000) (George et al., 2009) (Toth et al., 2009). (IRFs) IRF-7, IRF-9, and ISG54 are all increased following CNS virus infection and one IRF, ISG15, has been found to be significantly increased in astrocytes following their infection with RNA virus (Paul et al., 2007). Type 2 interferon response is due to the interferon γ again a glycoprotein expressed by activated T cells when TCR binds to their cognate antigen (Goodbourn et al., 2000). Many of the emerging viruses disable the host anti-viral response by targeting the pathways responsible for regulating IFN and anti-viral proteins.

5.4 Phagocytosis and removal of infected cells

The peculiarity of the CNS is that it is composed by a majority of cells that are non-renewable. Hence, it is fundamental to rapidly clear the infected cells and limiting bystander effects and to reduce massive neuronal loss. Apoptotic cells must be rapidly cleared from the CNS because they contain neurotoxic proteins and viruses capable of increasing host tissue infection (Griffiths et al., 2009). Apoptotic cells express a range of non-self-molecules termed Apoptotic cell- associated molecular patterns (ACAMPs) on their surface and these molecules include sugars, nucleic acids, ribonucleoproteins and oxidized low density proteins. The best characterized ACAMP is the phosphatidylserine molecule (PS) (Fadok et al., 1998) (Savill et al., 2002). Glia and macrophages express a range of receptors including the phosphatidylserine receptor (PSR), CD14 and the Scavenger receptors (SR) divided into SRA (SRA-1, SRA-II) and SR B including CD36 all expressed by microglia (Areschoug and Gordon, 2009; Husemann et al., 2002; Savill et al., 2002) which are all involved in the selective recognition and clearance of apoptotic cells. It should be stressed that these receptors may also contribute in turn to the infection of phagocytic cells.

5.5 Autophagy and control of viral infection

Autophagy is a fundamental homeostatic process that leads to the degradation and recycling of long-lived cytoplasmic proteins and organelles (Klionsky, 2007) (Yoshimori, 2004). The hallmark of autophagy is the formation of double or multiple membrane-bound vesicles called autophagosomes, which sequester a portion of the cytoplasm and fuse, after maturation, with lysosomes to digest their contents. In the same way, autophagy can also act directly, as an innate immune actor, to engulf and degrade pathogens. There is now some evidence for an antiviral role of autophagy related to viruses that specifically target neurons. The prototype virus studied was SINV, which is a positive-stranded RNA virus in the alphavirus genus. In mice, SINV produces fatal encephalitis that can be prevented by the cellular Bcl-2, an inhibitor of apoptotis (Levine et al., 1993). In a search to understand the mechanism by which Bcl-2 regulates Sindbis virus pathogenesis, a yeast two-hybrid screening was performed of a mouse brain library using Bcl-2 as bait, leading to the identification of a novel Bcl-2-interacting coiled-coil protein, Beclin 1. Beclin 1 is the mammalian homologue of yeast Atg6 and the first identified mammalian autophagy protein. Enforced neuronal expression of Beclin 1 was found to protect mice against fatal SINV encephalitis. In addition, Beclin reduces CNS SINV replication and viral-induced neuronal apoptosis (Liang et al., 1998). The ability of enforced neuronal expression of Beclin 1 to protect against lethal SINV encephalitis suggests a protective role for autophagy in host defence against an emerging neurotropic infection.

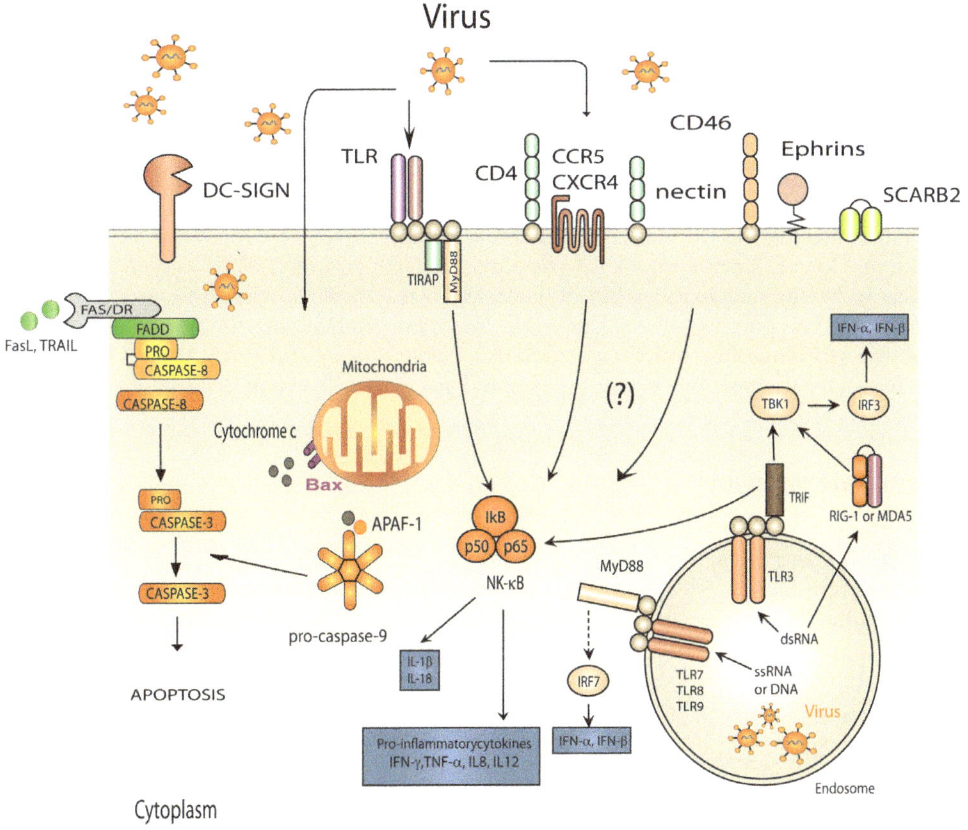

Fig. 1. **Interactions between viruses and host cell receptors**: Several receptors are known to interact with viruses and controling subsequent encephalitis. Some are receptors (e.g. CD4, CD46) involved in cell entry and signaling although the pathways which are engaged remain poorly characterized. Others are innate immune receptors such as RIG-I MDA5 and TLR which are expressed by neurons and glial cells (microglia and astrocyte) to initiate well-described signaling pathways that converge at the activation of the transcription factors (IRF3/7 and/or nuclear factor-kB (NFkB)). These key events lead to the expression of type-I interferons (IFN-α/β). The innate immune signaling pathways are intimately linked to apoptosis. The intrinsic apoptosis pathway is initiated by the release of cytochrome C from the mitochondria which promotes the formation of the apoptosome, including APAF-1 (apoptotic protease activating factor) and caspase 9 which in turn activates the effector caspase 3. The extrinsic pathway mobilized notably by TNF-α, TRAIL or FASL involves death-receptor signaling pathways linked to FADD and caspase 8. Some viruses can escape apoptosis by inducing the expression of anti-apoptotic proteins such as Bcl2.

6. Conclusion

Despite the vast genetic diversity among viruses, these pathogens face similar obstacles on the way into the CNS with the dual role of a physical and molecular barriers of the innate immune system to restrict and protect from infection. However, upon entry whether they are hidden in leukocytes or in apoptotic blebs, they will be free to interact with neurons in a rather 'immunopriviliged' environnement allowing viral persistence. However, this paradigm has been reconsidered with the observation that resident cells possess several of the key innate immune receptors involved in the recognition of the intruders and to engage a salutary antiviral response (IFN). It is now clear that other molecular interactions between the viruses and these host cells expressing primary and secondary signaling receptors will determine the outcome of the infection. Some receptors may control apoptosis or cell differentiation which in turn may have an impact on the capacity to resist viral infection and spreading. Our understanding of the molecular mechanisms of CNS diseases is still in its infancy. Increasingly, identification of virulence factors and host receptors will provide solutions for this complex puzzle. Understanding these interactions will increase our ability to control neuroinvasion and encephalitis. Moreover, it will also teach how to use these entry routes for therapeutic benefit, for example, for gene delivery of therapy of cancer and neurodegeneration.

7. Acknowledgement

The authors thanks the University of la Réunion (Felloship to GVTH), the CPER/FEDER funds (GRII Phase I-III), the ANR, INSERM (Fellowship to PG) the Regional Council of la Reunion (Fellowship to SK), the CRVOI for funds and continuous support. We express or thanks to other members of the laboratory (EA4517) for constructive criticisms and helps.

8. References

Abbott, N.J., A.A. Patabendige, D.E. Dolman, S.R. Yusof, and D.J. Begley. 2010. Structure and function of the blood-brain barrier. Neurobiol Dis. 37:13-25.

Alexopoulou, L., A.C. Holt, R. Medzhitov, and R.A. Flavell. 2001. Recognition of double-stranded RNA and activation of NF-kappaB by Toll-like receptor 3. Nature. 413:732-738.

Alkhatib, G., C. Combadiere, C.C. Broder, Y. Feng, P.E. Kennedy, P.M. Murphy, and E.A. Berger. 1996. CC CKR5: a RANTES, MIP-1alpha, MIP-1beta receptor as a fusion cofactor for macrophage-tropic HIV-1. Science. 272:1955-1958.

Areschoug, T., and S. Gordon. 2009. Scavenger receptors: role in innate immunity and microbial pathogenesis. Cell Microbiol. 11:1160-1169.

Bagasra, O., E. Lavi, L. Bobroski, K. Khalili, J.P. Pestaner, R. Tawadros, and R.J. Pomerantz. 1996. Cellular reservoirs of HIV-1 in the central nervous system of infected individuals: identification by the combination of in situ polymerase chain reaction and immunohistochemistry. AIDS. 10:573-585.

Balasubramanian, K., and A.J. Schroit. 2003. Aminophospholipid asymmetry: A matter of life and death. Annu Rev Physiol. 65:701-734.

Barnett, E.M., M.D. Cassell, and S. Perlman. 1993. Two neurotropic viruses, herpes simplex virus type 1 and mouse hepatitis virus, spread along different neural pathways from the main olfactory bulb. Neuroscience. 57:1007-1025.

Bereczky-Veress, B., N. Abdelmagid, F. Piehl, T. Bergstrom, T. Olsson, B. Skoldenberg, and M. Diez. 2010. Influence of perineurial cells and Toll-like receptors 2 and 9 on Herpes simplex type 1 entry to the central nervous system in rat encephalitis. PLoS One. 5:e12350.

Bernfield, M., M. Gotte, P.W. Park, O. Reizes, M.L. Fitzgerald, J. Lincecum, and M. Zako. 1999. Functions of cell surface heparan sulfate proteoglycans. Annu Rev Biochem. 68:729-777.

Blomberg, J., E. Lycke, K. Ahlfors, T. Johnsson, S. Wolontis, and G. von Zeipel. 1974. Letter: New enterovirus type associated with epidemic of aseptic meningitis and-or hand, foot, and mouth disease. Lancet. 2:112.

Burudi, E.M., S. Riese, P.D. Stahl, and A. Regnier-Vigouroux. 1999. Identification and functional characterization of the mannose receptor in astrocytes. Glia. 25:44-55.

Calvo, D., J. Dopazo, and M.A. Vega. 1995. The CD36, CLA-1 (CD36L1), and LIMPII (CD36L2) gene family: cellular distribution, chromosomal location, and genetic evolution. Genomics. 25:100-106.

Cambi, A., M. Koopman, and C.G. Figdor. 2005. How C-type lectins detect pathogens. Cell Microbiol. 7:481-488.

Campbell, G.L., A.A. Marfin, R.S. Lanciotti, and D.J. Gubler. 2002. West Nile virus. Lancet Infect Dis. 2:519-529.

Cardone, J., G. Le Friec, P. Vantourout, A. Roberts, A. Fuchs, I. Jackson, T. Suddason, G. Lord, J.P. Atkinson, A. Cope, A. Hayday, and C. Kemper. 2010. Complement regulator CD46 temporally regulates cytokine production by conventional and unconventional T cells. Nat Immunol. 11:862-871.

Carty, M., and A.G. Bowie. 2010. Recent insights into the role of Toll-like receptors in viral infection. Clin Exp Immunol. 161:397-406.

Catanese, M.T., H. Ansuini, R. Graziani, T. Huby, M. Moreau, J.K. Ball, G. Paonessa, C.M. Rice, R. Cortese, A. Vitelli, and A. Nicosia. 2010. Role of scavenger receptor class B type I in hepatitis C virus entry: kinetics and molecular determinants. J Virol. 84:34-43.

Charles, P.C., E. Walters, F. Margolis, and R.E. Johnston. 1995. Mechanism of neuroinvasion of Venezuelan equine encephalitis virus in the mouse. Virology. 208:662-671.

Chattopadhyay, S., J.T. Marques, M. Yamashita, K.L. Peters, K. Smith, A. Desai, B.R. Williams, and G.C. Sen. 2010. Viral apoptosis is induced by IRF-3-mediated activation of Bax. EMBO J. 29:1762-1773.

Chen, Y.B., S.Y. Seo, D.G. Kirsch, T.T. Sheu, W.C. Cheng, and J.M. Hardwick. 2006. Alternate functions of viral regulators of cell death. Cell Death Differ. 13:1318-1324.

Choe, H., M. Farzan, Y. Sun, N. Sullivan, B. Rollins, P.D. Ponath, L. Wu, C.R. Mackay, G. LaRosa, W. Newman, N. Gerard, C. Gerard, and J. Sodroski. 1996. The beta-chemokine receptors CCR3 and CCR5 facilitate infection by primary HIV-1 isolates. Cell. 85:1135-1148.

Couderc, T., F. Chretien, C. Schilte, O. Disson, M. Brigitte, F. Guivel-Benhassine, Y. Touret, G. Barau, N. Cayet, I. Schuffenecker, P. Despres, F. Arenzana-Seisdedos, A. Michault, M.L. Albert, and M. Lecuit. 2008. A mouse model for Chikungunya:

young age and inefficient type-I interferon signaling are risk factors for severe disease. PLoS Pathog. 4:e29.

Crimeen-Irwin, B., S. Ellis, D. Christiansen, M.J. Ludford-Menting, J. Milland, M. Lanteri, B.E. Loveland, D. Gerlier, and S.M. Russell. 2003. Ligand binding determines whether CD46 is internalized by clathrin-coated pits or macropinocytosis. J Biol Chem. 278:46927-46937.

Daffis, S., M.A. Samuel, M.S. Suthar, M. Gale, Jr., and M.S. Diamond. 2008. Toll-like receptor 3 has a protective role against West Nile virus infection. J Virol. 82:10349-10358.

Dalgleish, A.G., P.C. Beverley, P.R. Clapham, D.H. Crawford, M.F. Greaves, and R.A. Weiss. 1984. The CD4 (T4) antigen is an essential component of the receptor for the AIDS retrovirus. Nature. 312:763-767.

Danial, N.N., and S.J. Korsmeyer. 2004. Cell death: critical control points. Cell. 116:205-219.

Das, T., M.C. Jaffar-Bandjee, J.J. Hoarau, P. Krejbich Trotot, M. Denizot, G. Lee-Pat-Yuen, R. Sahoo, P. Guiraud, D. Ramful, S. Robin, J.L. Alessandri, B.A. Gauzere, and P. Gasque. 2010. Chikungunya fever: CNS infection and pathologies of a re-emerging arbovirus. Prog Neurobiol. 91:121-129.

Deng, H., R. Liu, W. Ellmeier, S. Choe, D. Unutmaz, M. Burkhart, P. Di Marzio, S. Marmon, R.E. Sutton, C.M. Hill, C.B. Davis, S.C. Peiper, T.J. Schall, D.R. Littman, and N.R. Landau. 1996. Identification of a major co-receptor for primary isolates of HIV-1. Nature. 381:661-666.

Doranz, B.J., J. Rucker, Y. Yi, R.J. Smyth, M. Samson, S.C. Peiper, M. Parmentier, R.G. Collman, and R.W. Doms. 1996. A dual-tropic primary HIV-1 isolate that uses fusin and the beta-chemokine receptors CKR-5, CKR-3, and CKR-2b as fusion cofactors. Cell. 85:1149-1158.

Dorig, R.E., A. Marcil, A. Chopra, and C.D. Richardson. 1993. The human CD46 molecule is a receptor for measles virus (Edmonston strain). Cell. 75:295-305.

Dragic, T., V. Litwin, G.P. Allaway, S.R. Martin, Y. Huang, K.A. Nagashima, C. Cayanan, P.J. Maddon, R.A. Koup, J.P. Moore, and W.A. Paxton. 1996. HIV-1 entry into CD4+ cells is mediated by the chemokine receptor CC-CKR-5. Nature. 381:667-673.

Drevets, D.A., and P.J. Leenen. 2000. Leukocyte-facilitated entry of intracellular pathogens into the central nervous system. Microbes Infect. 2:1609-1618.

Drickamer, K. 1995. Increasing diversity of animal lectin structures. Curr Opin Struct Biol. 5:612-616.

Dropulic, B., and C.L. Masters. 1990. Entry of neurotropic arboviruses into the central nervous system: an in vitro study using mouse brain endothelium. J Infect Dis. 161:685-691.

Economopoulou, A., M. Dominguez, B. Helynck, D. Sissoko, O. Wichmann, P. Quenel, P. Germonneau, and I. Quatresous. 2009. Atypical Chikungunya virus infections: clinical manifestations, mortality and risk factors for severe disease during the 2005-2006 outbreak on Reunion. Epidemiol Infect. 137:534-541.

Egea, J., and R. Klein. 2007. Bidirectional Eph-ephrin signaling during axon guidance. Trends Cell Biol. 17:230-238.

Eskelinen, E.L., Y. Tanaka, and P. Saftig. 2003. At the acidic edge: emerging functions for lysosomal membrane proteins. Trends Cell Biol. 13:137-145.

Esko, J.D., and S.B. Selleck. 2002. Order out of chaos: assembly of ligand binding sites in heparan sulfate. Annu Rev Biochem. 71:435-471.

Everett, H., and G. McFadden. 1999. Apoptosis: an innate immune response to virus infection. Trends Microbiol. 7:160-165.

Evlashev, A., E. Moyse, H. Valentin, O. Azocar, M.C. Trescol-Biemont, J.C. Marie, C. Rabourdin-Combe, and B. Horvat. 2000. Productive measles virus brain infection and apoptosis in CD46 transgenic mice. J Virol. 74:1373-1382.

Fadok, V.A., M.L. Warner, D.L. Bratton, and P.M. Henson. 1998. CD36 is required for phagocytosis of apoptotic cells by human macrophages that use either a phosphatidylserine receptor or the vitronectin receptor (alpha v beta 3). J Immunol. 161:6250-6257.

Fazakerley, J.K., C.L. Cotterill, G. Lee, and A. Graham. 2006. Virus tropism, distribution, persistence and pathology in the corpus callosum of the Semliki Forest virus-infected mouse brain: a novel system to study virus-oligodendrocyte interactions. Neuropathol Appl Neurobiol. 32:397-409.

Feng, Y., C.C. Broder, P.E. Kennedy, and E.A. Berger. 1996. HIV-1 entry cofactor: functional cDNA cloning of a seven-transmembrane, G protein-coupled receptor. Science. 272:872-877.

Fiala, M., D.J. Looney, M. Stins, D.D. Way, L. Zhang, X. Gan, F. Chiappelli, E.S. Schweitzer, P. Shapshak, M. Weinand, M.C. Graves, M. Witte, and K.S. Kim. 1997. TNF-alpha opens a paracellular route for HIV-1 invasion across the blood-brain barrier. Mol Med. 3:553-564.

Fujimoto, I., J. Pan, T. Takizawa, and Y. Nakanishi. 2000. Virus clearance through apoptosis-dependent phagocytosis of influenza A virus-infected cells by macrophages. J Virol. 74:3399-3403.

Fujita, T., K. Onoguchi, K. Onomoto, R. Hirai, and M. Yoneyama. 2007. Triggering antiviral response by RIG-I-related RNA helicases. Biochimie. 89:754-760.

Furr, S.R., V.S. Chauhan, D. Sterka, Jr., V. Grdzelishvili, and I. Marriott. 2008. Characterization of retinoic acid-inducible gene-I expression in primary murine glia following exposure to vesicular stomatitis virus. J Neurovirol:1-11.

Gamp, A.C., Y. Tanaka, R. Lullmann-Rauch, D. Wittke, R. D'Hooge, P.P. De Deyn, T. Moser, H. Maier, D. Hartmann, K. Reiss, A.L. Illert, K. von Figura, and P. Saftig. 2003. LIMP-2/LGP85 deficiency causes ureteric pelvic junction obstruction, deafness and peripheral neuropathy in mice. Hum Mol Genet. 12:631-646.

Ganesan, K., A. Diwan, S.K. Shankar, S.B. Desai, G.S. Sainani, and S.M. Katrak. 2008. Chikungunya encephalomyeloradiculitis: report of 2 cases with neuroimaging and 1 case with autopsy findings. AJNR Am J Neuroradiol. 29:1636-1637.

Gardner, J., I. Anraku, T.T. Le, T. Larcher, L. Major, P. Roques, W.A. Schroder, S. Higgs, and A. Suhrbier. 2010. Chikungunya virus arthritis in adult wild-type mice. J Virol. 84:8021-8032.

Gautier, I., J. Coppey, and C. Durieux. 2003. Early apoptosis-related changes triggered by HSV-1 in individual neuronlike cells. Exp Cell Res. 289:174-183.

George, C.X., Z. Li, K.M. Okonski, A.M. Toth, Y. Wang, and C.E. Samuel. 2009. Tipping the balance: antagonism of PKR kinase and ADAR1 deaminase functions by virus gene products. J Interferon Cytokine Res. 29:477-487.

Geraghty, R.J., C. Krummenacher, G.H. Cohen, R.J. Eisenberg, and P.G. Spear. 1998. Entry of alphaherpesviruses mediated by poliovirus receptor-related protein 1 and poliovirus receptor. Science. 280:1618-1620.

Goldstein, J.L., Y.K. Ho, S.K. Basu, and M.S. Brown. 1979. Binding site on macrophages that mediates uptake and degradation of acetylated low density lipoprotein, producing massive cholesterol deposition. Proc Natl Acad Sci U S A. 76:333-337.

Goodbourn, S., L. Didcock, and R.E. Randall. 2000. Interferons: cell signalling, immune modulation, antiviral response and virus countermeasures. J Gen Virol. 81:2341-2364.

Granwehr, B.P., K.M. Lillibridge, S. Higgs, P.W. Mason, J.F. Aronson, G.A. Campbell, and A.D. Barrett. 2004. West Nile virus: where are we now? Lancet Infect Dis. 4:547-556.

Griffin, D.E. 2003. Immune responses to RNA-virus infections of the CNS. Nat Rev Immunol. 3:493-502.

Griffin, D.E. 2010. Emergence and re-emergence of viral diseases of the central nervous system. Prog Neurobiol. 91:95-101.

Griffin, D.E., and J.M. Hardwick. 1997. Regulators of apoptosis on the road to persistent alphavirus infection. Annu Rev Microbiol. 51:565-592.

Griffiths, M.R., P. Gasque, and J.W. Neal. 2009. The multiple roles of the innate immune system in the regulation of apoptosis and inflammation in the brain. J Neuropathol Exp Neurol. 68:217-226.

Hashimoto, Y., T. Moki, T. Takizawa, A. Shiratsuchi, and Y. Nakanishi. 2007. Evidence for phagocytosis of influenza virus-infected, apoptotic cells by neutrophils and macrophages in mice. J Immunol. 178:2448-2457.

Hauwel, M., E. Furon, C. Canova, M. Griffiths, J. Neal, and P. Gasque. 2005. Innate (inherent) control of brain infection, brain inflammation and brain repair: the role of microglia, astrocytes, "protective" glial stem cells and stromal ependymal cells. Brain Res Brain Res Rev. 48:220-233.

Henson, P.M., D.L. Bratton, and V.A. Fadok. 2001. Apoptotic cell removal. Curr Biol. 11:R795-805.

Herndon, R.M., R.T. Johnson, L.E. Davis, and L.R. Descalzi. 1974. Ependymitis in mumps virus meningitis. Electron microscopical studies of cerebrospinal fluid. Arch Neurol. 30:475-479.

Himanen, J.P., N. Saha, and D.B. Nikolov. 2007. Cell-cell signaling via Eph receptors and ephrins. Curr Opin Cell Biol. 19:534-542.

Hoarau, J.J., M.C. Jaffar Bandjee, P. Krejbich Trotot, T. Das, G. Li-Pat-Yuen, B. Dassa, M. Denizot, E. Guichard, A. Ribera, T. Henni, F. Tallet, M.P. Moiton, B.A. Gauzere, S. Bruniquet, Z. Jaffar Bandjee, P. Morbidelli, G. Martigny, M. Jolivet, F. Gay, M. Grandadam, H. Tolou, V. Vieillard, P. Debre, B. Autran, and P. Gasque. 2010. Persistent chronic inflammation and infection by Chikungunya arthritogenic alphavirus in spite of a robust host immune response. J Immunol. 184:5914-5927.

Hoarau, J.J., P. Krejbich-Trotot, M.C. Jaffar-Bandjee, T. Das, G.V. Thon-Hon, S. Kumar, J.W. Neal, and P. Gasque. 2011. Activation and control of CNS innate immune responses in health and diseases: a balancing act finely tuned by neuroimmune regulators (NIReg). CNS Neurol Disord Drug Targets. 10:25-43.

Husemann, J., J.D. Loike, R. Anankov, M. Febbraio, and S.C. Silverstein. 2002. Scavenger receptors in neurobiology and neuropathology: their role on microglia and other cells of the nervous system. Glia. 40:195-205.

Jackson, A.C. 2003. Rabies virus infection: an update. J Neurovirol. 9:253-258.

Jaffar-Bandjee, M.C., T. Das, J.J. Hoarau, P. Krejbich Trotot, M. Denizot, A. Ribera, P. Roques, and P. Gasque. 2009. Chikungunya virus takes centre stage in virally induced arthritis: possible cellular and molecular mechanisms to pathogenesis. Microbes Infect. 11:1206-1218.

Jaffar-Bandjee, M.C., D. Ramful, B.A. Gauzere, J.J. Hoarau, P. Krejbich-Trotot, S. Robin, A. Ribera, J. Selambarom, and P. Gasque. 2011. Emergence and clinical insights into the pathology of Chikungunya virus infection. Expert Rev Anti Infect Ther. 8:987-996.

Janssen, R.S., D.R. Cornblath, L.G. Epstein, R.P. Foa, J.C. McArthur, R.W. Price, A.K.K. Asbury, A. Beckett, D.F. Benson, T.P. Bridge, C.M. Leventhal, P. Satz, A.J. Saykin, J.J. Sidtis, and S. Tross. 1991. Nomenclature and research case definitions for neurological manifestations of human immunodeficiency virus type 1 (HIV-1) infection. Neurology. 41:778-785.

Jarvis, M.A., and J.A. Nelson. 2002. Human cytomegalovirus persistence and latency in endothelial cells and macrophages. Curr Opin Microbiol. 5:403-407.

Katze, M.G., Y. He, and M. Gale, Jr. 2002. Viruses and interferon: a fight for supremacy. Nat Rev Immunol. 2:675-687.

Klatzmann, D., E. Champagne, S. Chamaret, J. Gruest, D. Guetard, T. Hercend, J.C. Gluckman, and L. Montagnier. 1984. T-lymphocyte T4 molecule behaves as the receptor for human retrovirus LAV. Nature. 312:767-768.

Klionsky, D.J. 2007. Autophagy: from phenomenology to molecular understanding in less than a decade. Nat Rev Mol Cell Biol. 8:931-937.

Kopp, S.J., G. Banisadr, K. Glajch, U.E. Maurer, K. Grunewald, R.J. Miller, P. Osten, and P.G. Spear. 2009. Infection of neurons and encephalitis after intracranial inoculation of herpes simplex virus requires the entry receptor nectin-1. Proc Natl Acad Sci U S A. 106:17916-17920.

Krejbich-Trotot, P., M. Denizot, J.J. Hoarau, M.C. Jaffar-Bandjee, T. Das, and P. Gasque. 2011. Chikungunya virus mobilizes the apoptotic machinery to invade host cell defenses. FASEB J. 25:314-325.

Kroemer, G., L. Galluzzi, and C. Brenner. 2007. Mitochondrial membrane permeabilization in cell death. Physiol Rev. 87:99-163.

Kuronita, T., E.L. Eskelinen, H. Fujita, P. Saftig, M. Himeno, and Y. Tanaka. 2002. A role for the lysosomal membrane protein LGP85 in the biogenesis and maintenance of endosomal and lysosomal morphology. J Cell Sci. 115:4117-4131.

Labadie, K., T. Larcher, C. Joubert, A. Mannioui, B. Delache, P. Brochard, L. Guigand, L. Dubreil, P. Lebon, B. Verrier, X. de Lamballerie, A. Suhrbier, Y. Cherel, R. Le Grand, and P. Roques. 2010. Chikungunya disease in nonhuman primates involves long-term viral persistence in macrophages. J Clin Invest. 120:894-906.

Lafon, M. 2005. Rabies virus receptors. J Neurovirol. 11:82-87.

Lanciotti, R.S., J.T. Roehrig, V. Deubel, J. Smith, M. Parker, K. Steele, B. Crise, K.E. Volpe, M.B. Crabtree, J.H. Scherret, R.A. Hall, J.S. MacKenzie, C.B. Cropp, B. Panigrahy, E. Ostlund, B. Schmitt, M. Malkinson, C. Banet, J. Weissman, N. Komar, H.M. Savage, W. Stone, T. McNamara, and D.J. Gubler. 1999. Origin of the West Nile virus responsible for an outbreak of encephalitis in the northeastern United States. Science. 286:2333-2337.

Lemant, J., V. Boisson, A. Winer, L. Thibault, H. Andre, F. Tixier, M. Lemercier, E. Antok, M.P. Cresta, P. Grivard, M. Besnard, O. Rollot, F. Favier, M. Huerre, J.L. Campinos, and A. Michault. 2008. Serious acute chikungunya virus infection requiring intensive care during the Reunion Island outbreak in 2005-2006. Crit Care Med. 36:2536-2541.

Levine, B., Q. Huang, J.T. Isaacs, J.C. Reed, D.E. Griffin, and J.M. Hardwick. 1993. Conversion of lytic to persistent alphavirus infection by the bcl-2 cellular oncogene. Nature. 361:739-742.

Liang, X.H., L.K. Kleeman, H.H. Jiang, G. Gordon, J.E. Goldman, G. Berry, B. Herman, and B. Levine. 1998. Protection against fatal Sindbis virus encephalitis by beclin, a novel Bcl-2-interacting protein. J Virol. 72:8586-8596.

Linehan, S.A., L. Martinez-Pomares, P.D. Stahl, and S. Gordon. 1999. Mannose receptor and its putative ligands in normal murine lymphoid and nonlymphoid organs: In situ expression of mannose receptor by selected macrophages, endothelial cells, perivascular microglia, and mesangial cells, but not dendritic cells. J Exp Med. 189:1961-1972.

Liszewski, M.K., T.W. Post, and J.P. Atkinson. 1991. Membrane cofactor protein (MCP or CD46): newest member of the regulators of complement activation gene cluster. Annu Rev Immunol. 9:431-455.

Loetscher, M., T. Geiser, T. O'Reilly, R. Zwahlen, M. Baggiolini, and B. Moser. 1994. Cloning of a human seven-transmembrane domain receptor, LESTR, that is highly expressed in leukocytes. J Biol Chem. 269:232-237.

Lopez, M., F. Cocchi, L. Menotti, E. Avitabile, P. Dubreuil, and G. Campadelli-Fiume. 2000. Nectin2alpha (PRR2alpha or HveB) and nectin2delta are low-efficiency mediators for entry of herpes simplex virus mutants carrying the Leu25Pro substitution in glycoprotein D. J Virol. 74:1267-1274.

Lublin, D.M., M.K. Liszewski, T.W. Post, M.A. Arce, M.M. Le Beau, M.B. Rebentisch, L.S. Lemons, T. Seya, and J.P. Atkinson. 1988. Molecular cloning and chromosomal localization of human membrane cofactor protein (MCP). Evidence for inclusion in the multigene family of complement-regulatory proteins. J Exp Med. 168:181-194.

Maddon, P.J., S.M. Molineaux, D.E. Maddon, K.A. Zimmerman, M. Godfrey, F.W. Alt, L. Chess, and R. Axel. 1987. Structure and expression of the human and mouse T4 genes. Proc Natl Acad Sci U S A. 84:9155-9159.

Martina, B.E., P. Koraka, P. van den Doel, G.F. Rimmelzwaan, B.L. Haagmans, and A.D. Osterhaus. 2008. DC-SIGN enhances infection of cells with glycosylated West Nile virus in vitro and virus replication in human dendritic cells induces production of IFN-alpha and TNF-alpha. Virus Res. 135:64-71.

McDougal, J.S., M.S. Kennedy, J.M. Sligh, S.P. Cort, A. Mawle, and J.K. Nicholson. 1986. Binding of HTLV-III/LAV to T4+ T cells by a complex of the 110K viral protein and the T4 molecule. Science. 231:382-385.

McMinn, P.C. 2002. An overview of the evolution of enterovirus 71 and its clinical and public health significance. FEMS Microbiol Rev. 26:91-107.

Mock, D.J., J.M. Powers, A.D. Goodman, S.R. Blumenthal, N. Ergin, J.V. Baker, D.H. Mattson, J.G. Assouline, E.J. Bergey, B. Chen, L.G. Epstein, and B.M. Blumberg. 1999. Association of human herpesvirus 6 with the demyelinative lesions of progressive multifocal leukoencephalopathy. J Neurovirol. 5:363-373.

Mori, I., Y. Nishiyama, T. Yokochi, and Y. Kimura. 2005. Olfactory transmission of neurotropic viruses. J Neurovirol. 11:129-137.

Morrison, L.A., and B.N. Fields. 1991. Parallel mechanisms in neuropathogenesis of enteric virus infections. J Virol. 65:2767-2772.

Moses, A.V., F.E. Bloom, C.D. Pauza, and J.A. Nelson. 1993. Human immunodeficiency virus infection of human brain capillary endothelial cells occurs via a CD4/galactosylceramide-independent mechanism. Proc Natl Acad Sci U S A. 90:10474-10478.

Mukhopadhyay, S., and S. Gordon. 2004. The role of scavenger receptors in pathogen recognition and innate immunity. Immunobiology. 209:39-49.

Mukhtar, M., S. Harley, P. Chen, M. BouHamdan, C. Patel, E. Acheampong, and R.J. Pomerantz. 2002. Primary isolated human brain microvascular endothelial cells express diverse HIV/SIV-associated chemokine coreceptors and DC-SIGN and L-SIGN. Virology. 297:78-88.

Muller, U., U. Steinhoff, L.F. Reis, S. Hemmi, J. Pavlovic, R.M. Zinkernagel, and M. Aguet. 1994. Functional role of type I and type II interferons in antiviral defense. Science. 264:1918-1921.

Nakhaei, P., P. Genin, A. Civas, and J. Hiscott. 2009. RIG-I-like receptors: sensing and responding to RNA virus infection. Semin Immunol. 21:215-222.

Navia, B.A., B.D. Jordan, and R.W. Price. 1986. The AIDS dementia complex: I. Clinical features. Ann Neurol. 19:517-524.

Negrete, O.A., E.L. Levroney, H.C. Aguilar, A. Bertolotti-Ciarlet, R. Nazarian, S. Tajyar, and B. Lee. 2005. EphrinB2 is the entry receptor for Nipah virus, an emergent deadly paramyxovirus. Nature. 436:401-405.

Negrete, O.A., M.C. Wolf, H.C. Aguilar, S. Enterlein, W. Wang, E. Muhlberger, S.V. Su, A. Bertolotti-Ciarlet, R. Flick, and B. Lee. 2006. Two key residues in ephrinB3 are critical for its use as an alternative receptor for Nipah virus. PLoS Pathog. 2:e7.

Nottet, H.S., Y. Persidsky, V.G. Sasseville, A.N. Nukuna, P. Bock, Q.H. Zhai, L.R. Sharer, R.D. McComb, S. Swindells, C. Soderland, and H.E. Gendelman. 1996. Mechanisms for the transendothelial migration of HIV-1-infected monocytes into brain. J Immunol. 156:1284-1295.

Pasquale, E.B. 2005. Eph receptor signalling casts a wide net on cell behaviour. Nat Rev Mol Cell Biol. 6:462-475.

Pasquale, E.B. 2008. Eph-ephrin bidirectional signaling in physiology and disease. Cell. 133:38-52.

Paul, S., C. Ricour, C. Sommereyns, F. Sorgeloos, and T. Michiels. 2007. Type I interferon response in the central nervous system. Biochimie. 89:770-778.

Persidsky, Y., M. Stins, D. Way, M.H. Witte, M. Weinand, K.S. Kim, P. Bock, H.E. Gendelman, and M. Fiala. 1997. A model for monocyte migration through the blood-brain barrier during HIV-1 encephalitis. J Immunol. 158:3499-3510.

Prehaud, C., F. Megret, M. Lafage, and M. Lafon. 2005. Virus infection switches TLR-3-positive human neurons to become strong producers of beta interferon. J Virol. 79:12893-12904.

Price, R.W., B. Brew, J. Sidtis, M. Rosenblum, A.C. Scheck, and P. Cleary. 1988. The brain in AIDS: central nervous system HIV-1 infection and AIDS dementia complex. Science. 239:586-592.

Pryzdial, E.L., and J.F. Wright. 1994. Prothrombinase assembly on an enveloped virus: evidence that the cytomegalovirus surface contains procoagulant phospholipid. Blood. 84:3749-3757.

Raport, C.J., J. Gosling, V.L. Schweickart, P.W. Gray, and I.F. Charo. 1996. Molecular cloning and functional characterization of a novel human CC chemokine receptor (CCR5) for RANTES, MIP-1beta, and MIP-1alpha. J Biol Chem. 271:17161-17166.

Rosen, A., L. Casciola-Rosen, and J. Ahearn. 1995. Novel packages of viral and self-antigens are generated during apoptosis. J Exp Med. 181:1557-1561.

Sallusto, F., M. Cella, C. Danieli, and A. Lanzavecchia. 1995. Dendritic cells use macropinocytosis and the mannose receptor to concentrate macromolecules in the major histocompatibility complex class II compartment: downregulation by cytokines and bacterial products. J Exp Med. 182:389-400.

Santoro, F., P.E. Kennedy, G. Locatelli, M.S. Malnati, E.A. Berger, and P. Lusso. 1999. CD46 is a cellular receptor for human herpesvirus 6. Cell. 99:817-827.

Sato, A., M.M. Linehan, and A. Iwasaki. 2006. Dual recognition of herpes simplex viruses by TLR2 and TLR9 in dendritic cells. Proc Natl Acad Sci U S A. 103:17343-17348.

Savarin, C., and C.C. Bergmann. 2008. Neuroimmunology of central nervous system viral infections: the cells, molecules and mechanisms involved. Curr Opin Pharmacol. 8:472-479.

Savill, J., I. Dransfield, C. Gregory, and C. Haslett. 2002. A blast from the past: clearance of apoptotic cells regulates immune responses. Nat Rev Immunol. 2:965-975.

Schilte, C., T. Couderc, F. Chretien, M. Sourisseau, N. Gangneux, F. Guivel-Benhassine, A. Kraxner, J. Tschopp, S. Higgs, A. Michault, F. Arenzana-Seisdedos, M. Colonna, L. Peduto, O. Schwartz, M. Lecuit, and M.L. Albert. 2010. Type I IFN controls chikungunya virus via its action on nonhematopoietic cells. J Exp Med. 207:429-442.

Schmidt, N.J., E.H. Lennette, and H.H. Ho. 1974. An apparently new enterovirus isolated from patients with disease of the central nervous system. J Infect Dis. 129:304-309.

Schmidtmayerova, H., H.S. Nottet, G. Nuovo, T. Raabe, C.R. Flanagan, L. Dubrovsky, H.E. Gendelman, A. Cerami, M. Bukrinsky, and B. Sherry. 1996. Human immunodeficiency virus type 1 infection alters chemokine beta peptide expression in human monocytes: implications for recruitment of leukocytes into brain and lymph nodes. Proc Natl Acad Sci U S A. 93:700-704.

Schwartz, A.J., X. Alvarez, and A.A. Lackner. 2002. Distribution and immunophenotype of DC-SIGN-expressing cells in SIV-infected and uninfected macaques. AIDS Res Hum Retroviruses. 18:1021-1029.

Seya, T., A. Hirano, M. Matsumoto, M. Nomura, and S. Ueda. 1999. Human membrane cofactor protein (MCP, CD46): multiple isoforms and functions. Int J Biochem Cell Biol. 31:1255-1260.

Seya, T., J.R. Turner, and J.P. Atkinson. 1986. Purification and characterization of a membrane protein (gp45-70) that is a cofactor for cleavage of C3b and C4b. J Exp Med. 163:837-855.

Sharer, L.R., E.S. Cho, and L.G. Epstein. 1985. Multinucleated giant cells and HTLV-III in AIDS encephalopathy. Hum Pathol. 16:760.

Shieh, M.T., D. WuDunn, R.I. Montgomery, J.D. Esko, and P.G. Spear. 1992. Cell surface receptors for herpes simplex virus are heparan sulfate proteoglycans. J Cell Biol. 116:1273-1281.

Solignat, M., B. Gay, S. Higgs, L. Briant, and C. Devaux. 2009. Replication cycle of chikungunya: a re-emerging arbovirus. Virology. 393:183-197.

Suh, H.S., C.F. Brosnan, and S.C. Lee. 2009. Toll-like receptors in CNS viral infections. Curr Top Microbiol Immunol. 336:63-81.

Suthar, M.S., D.Y. Ma, S. Thomas, J.M. Lund, N. Zhang, S. Daffis, A.Y. Rudensky, M.J. Bevan, E.A. Clark, M.K. Kaja, M.S. Diamond, and M. Gale, Jr. 2010. IPS-1 is essential for the control of West Nile virus infection and immunity. PLoS Pathog. 6:e1000757.

Sutherland, M.R., C.M. Raynor, H. Leenknegt, J.F. Wright, and E.L. Pryzdial. 1997. Coagulation initiated on herpesviruses. Proc Natl Acad Sci U S A. 94:13510-13514.

Szretter, K.J., S. Daffis, J. Patel, M.S. Suthar, R.S. Klein, M. Gale, Jr., and M.S. Diamond. 2010. The innate immune adaptor molecule MyD88 restricts West Nile virus replication and spread in neurons of the central nervous system. J Virol. 84:12125-12138.

Takahashi, K., T. Kawai, H. Kumar, S. Sato, S. Yonehara, and S. Akira. 2006. Roles of caspase-8 and caspase-10 in innate immune responses to double-stranded RNA. J Immunol. 176:4520-4524.

Takai, Y., J. Miyoshi, W. Ikeda, and H. Ogita. 2008. Nectins and nectin-like molecules: roles in contact inhibition of cell movement and proliferation. Nat Rev Mol Cell Biol. 9:603-615.

Teodoro, J.G., and P.E. Branton. 1997. Regulation of apoptosis by viral gene products. J Virol. 71:1739-1746.

Tirabassi, R.S., R.A. Townley, M.G. Eldridge, and L.W. Enquist. 1998. Molecular mechanisms of neurotropic herpesvirus invasion and spread in the CNS. Neurosci Biobehav Rev. 22:709-720.

Toth, A.M., Z. Li, R. Cattaneo, and C.E. Samuel. 2009. RNA-specific adenosine deaminase ADAR1 suppresses measles virus-induced apoptosis and activation of protein kinase PKR. J Biol Chem. 284:29350-29356.

Tsetsarkin, K.A., D.L. Vanlandingham, C.E. McGee, and S. Higgs. 2007. A single mutation in chikungunya virus affects vector specificity and epidemic potential. PLoS Pathog. 3:e201.

Van Gorp, H., P.L. Delputte, and H.J. Nauwynck. 2010. Scavenger receptor CD163, a Jack-of-all-trades and potential target for cell-directed therapy. Mol Immunol. 47:1650-1660.

van Kooyk, Y., and T.B. Geijtenbeek. 2003. DC-SIGN: escape mechanism for pathogens. Nat Rev Immunol. 3:697-709.

Vazeille, M., S. Moutailler, D. Coudrier, C. Rousseaux, H. Khun, M. Huerre, J. Thiria, J.S. Dehecq, D. Fontenille, I. Schuffenecker, P. Despres, and A.B. Failloux. 2007. Two Chikungunya isolates from the outbreak of La Reunion (Indian Ocean) exhibit different patterns of infection in the mosquito, Aedes albopictus. PLoS One. 2:e1168.

Wang, E., E. Volkova, A.P. Adams, N. Forrester, S.Y. Xiao, I. Frolov, and S.C. Weaver. 2008. Chimeric alphavirus vaccine candidates for chikungunya. Vaccine. 26:5030-5039.

Wang, T., T. Town, L. Alexopoulou, J.F. Anderson, E. Fikrig, and R.A. Flavell. 2004. Toll-like receptor 3 mediates West Nile virus entry into the brain causing lethal encephalitis. Nat Med. 10:1366-1373.

Weis, W.I., M.E. Taylor, and K. Drickamer. 1998. The C-type lectin superfamily in the immune system. Immunol Rev. 163:19-34.

Weiss, N., F. Miller, S. Cazaubon, and P.O. Couraud. 2009. The blood-brain barrier in brain homeostasis and neurological diseases. Biochim Biophys Acta. 1788:842-857.

Whitley, R.J., and J.W. Gnann. 2002. Viral encephalitis: familiar infections and emerging pathogens. Lancet. 359:507-513.

Williamson, P., and R.A. Schlegel. 1994. Back and forth: the regulation and function of transbilayer phospholipid movement in eukaryotic cells. Mol Membr Biol. 11:199-216.

Wilson, N.S., V. Dixit, and A. Ashkenazi. 2009. Death receptor signal transducers: nodes of coordination in immune signaling networks. Nat Immunol. 10:348-355.

WuDunn, D., and P.G. Spear. 1989. Initial interaction of herpes simplex virus with cells is binding to heparan sulfate. J Virol. 63:52-58.

Wyatt, R., and J. Sodroski. 1998. The HIV-1 envelope glycoproteins: fusogens, antigens, and immunogens. Science. 280:1884-1888.

Yamayoshi, S., Y. Yamashita, J. Li, N. Hanagata, T. Minowa, T. Takemura, and S. Koike. 2009. Scavenger receptor B2 is a cellular receptor for enterovirus 71. Nat Med. 15:798-801.

Yoneyama, M., and T. Fujita. 2009. RNA recognition and signal transduction by RIG-I-like receptors. Immunol Rev. 227:54-65.

Yoshimori, T. 2004. Autophagy: a regulated bulk degradation process inside cells. Biochem Biophys Res Commun. 313:453-458.

Zelensky, A.N., and J.E. Gready. 2005. The C-type lectin-like domain superfamily. FEBS J. 272:6179-6217.

Zhang, J.R., and E. Tuomanen. 1999. Molecular and cellular mechanisms for microbial entry into the CNS. J Neurovirol. 5:591-603.

Ziegler, S.A., L. Lu, A.P. da Rosa, S.Y. Xiao, and R.B. Tesh. 2008. An animal model for studying the pathogenesis of chikungunya virus infection. Am J Trop Med Hyg. 79:133-139.

Zwaal, R.F., and A.J. Schroit. 1997. Pathophysiologic implications of membrane phospholipid asymmetry in blood cells. Blood. 89:1121-1132.

4

Herpes Simplex Type 1 Encephalitis

Feyzi Birol Sarica
*Başkent University, Faculty of Medicine, Department of Neurosurgery
Turkey*

1. Introduction

Encephalitides, an acute infection of the brain parenchyma, are characterized by fever, headache and altered consciousness. Neurological deficits and focal or generalized epileptic seizures may also be seen. There are important differences in clinical presentations between encephalitides caused by viruses. While some viral encephalitides, such as Herpes simplex virus type-1 (HSV type-1) encephalitis, cause sporadic infection; others, such as Japanese B encephalitis virus and Eastern equine encephalitis virus, cause epidemic infections with specific geographic distribution. Some viruses like HSV cause fulminant encephalitis leading to death within a couple of days whereas viruses such as Measles virus can cause progressive subacute sclerosing panencephalitis lasting several months and years. HSV type-1, HSV type-2, LaCrosse encephalitis virus, St. Louis encephalitis virus usually causes encephalitis in healthy individuals, whereas HSV type-1, Cytomegalovirus, Varicella-zoster virus, Epstein-Barr virus, Human herpes virus type-6 and Enteroviruses are associated with encephalitides in immunodeficient or immunocompromised patients (Mathewson Commission, 1929; Meyer et al.,1960; Roos,1999).

Herpes simplex virus (HSV) is the most common cause of sporadic fatal encephalitis (Mathewson Commission, 1929; Meyer et al.,1960; Smith et al., 1941). Smith et al. detected inclusion bodies consistent with HSV infection from a newborn's brain with encephalitis and virus was isolated from brain tissue then (Smith et al., 1941). The first adult case of HSE was reported by Zarafonetis et al. (Zarafonetis et al., 1944). The pathological findings in this patient's brain were prominent perivascular cuffing of lymphocytes and a large number small hemorrhages in left temporal lobe. Later in several studies, this temporal lobe localization was reported to be characteristic for HSE in patients older than 3 months. In the mid 1960s, Nahmias and Dowdle found two distinct antigenic type of HSV, as HSV type-1 and HSV type-2 (Nahmias & Dowdle, 1968).

The HSE, observed in adults, is caused by HSV type-1 predominantly (Dennett et al., 1997; Whitley & Lakeman, 1995). HSV type-2 is rarely seen in healthy adults and usually causes benign CNS infection, whereas severe meningoencephalitis is seen in immunosuppressed individuals (Mommeja-Marin et al., 2003). Herpes neonatorum, transmitted from perinatal area, causes severe encephalitis in neonates (Corey et al., 1983). HSV type-1 and HSV type-2 are from Herpesviridae family. The common feature of Herpesviridae family is that they stay in life-long latent (persistent) form in the organism and they can reactivate later leading recurrent infections. Also other viruses from Herpesviridae group may lead CNS diseases (Garcia-Blanco et al., 1991).

Herpes simplex encephalitis (HSE) continues to be one of the most devastating infections of the central nervous system despite available antiviral therapy. In patients taking no treatment or receiving an ineffective anti-viral treatment such as Idoxuridine and Cytosine Arabinoside, the mortality rate is higher than 70 % (Chien et al., 1975; Longson, 1979; Whitley et al, 1977; Whitley et al, 1981). Approximately one-third of all patients diagnosed with HSE are composed of children and adolescents. In clinical diagnosis, an encephalopathic disease process with focal neurological symptoms is seen. However, these clinical findings are not pathognomonic, and many other disorders involving the central nervous system have these symptoms and these diseases can mimic HSE.
In neurodiagnostic evaluation, demonstration of temporal lobe edema and /or bleeding with magnetic resonance imaging (MRI) is supportive for diagnosis. In electroencephalogram, spike and slow wave activity is observed. HSV isolation from brain tissue with brain biopsy was a diagnostic method used in the past. Today, detection of herpes simplex virus (HSV) DNA by cerebrospinal fluid polymerase chain reaction (PCR) is the gold standard for diagnosis. PCR is an excellent test and preferred over brain biopsy. 95% of cases can be diagnosed by PCR (Chien et al., 1975; Longson, 1979; Whitley et al, 1977; Whitley et al, 1981). However in the early period after the onset of the disease, false-negative results by PCR may be seen.
Acyclovir is the preferred method of treatment and administered 10 mg / kg every 8 hours for 21 days. Even if the treatment is started early after the onset of the disease, significant neurological deficits are observed in nearly two-thirds of the surviving patients. Today in current studies, quantitative prognostic value of viral DNA by PCR both at the beginning as well as at the end of treatment and contribution of long-term anti-viral therapy for improvement in neurological outcomes are investigated (Tyler, 2004).

2.1 Etiology

HSV type-1, member of the herpes virus family, is an enveloped-virus with a large (150-250 nm in size) linear double-stranded DNA (Mathewson Commission, 1929). The viral particle is wrapped from outermost by an envelope, which is made of lipid. Viral DNA is encased within a capsid that is 85-110 nm diameter in size. The structure between the envelope and capsid is called tegument (Davison & Clements, 2005; Jerome & Ashley, 2003; Whitley, 1996). In these 3 layers, there are 25-30 structural proteins which form the structure of the virion. There are 11 glycoprotein protrusions on the surface of the envelope with antigenic properties (gB, gC,....., gM). While gB and gD glycoproteins play an important role in the attachment to and entrance of the virus into target cells, gC, gE, gG, gI, gJ and gM glycoproteins play an important role in the penetration of the virus to the cell. gG is the major protein providing antigenic specificity of the virus (Erturk, 1999; Whitley,1996; Whitley & Roizman, 2001). gC glycoprotein binds to C3b component of complement system on the surface of infected cells. gE and gI glycoproteins bind to Fc part of IgG. The antibodies against to these envelope glycoproteins neutralize the infectivity of the virus with competitive binding to receptors. The protein named as transinducing factor (Vmw65) is localized in the region of tegument and related with latent or lytic infection (Mathewson Commission, 1929). Capsid, surrounding the viral genome, and consists of 162 kapsomers and is icosahedral in shape. Icosahedral structure of capsid is supported by structural proteins VP21 and VP22a particularly (Davison & Clements, 2005; Jerome & Ashley, 2003; Whitley, 1996). Non-structural proteins, so-called Infected cell proteins (ICP), play role in

DNA replication and transcription regulation. In addition, there are some other non-structural proteins that act especially as enzymes. The most important of these enzymes are; DNA polymerase, deoxyribonuclease, ribonucleotide reductase, protein kinase and thymidine kinase. These enzymes,in similar, have also important roles in important functions such as viral DNA replication (Erturk,1999; Whitley & Roizman, 2001).
HSV is unstable in the external environment. HSV is heat-labile. Half-life of the virus is 1.5-3 hours at 37 ° C. The virus is inactivated at temperatures above 56 ° C. It can live for months at -70 ° C and protect its infectivity. It can remain alive for 48 hours at 4 ° C in humid conditions, while it is inactivated under dry conditions. It is sensitive to most proteolytic enzymes, such as trypsin, protease and aminopeptidase. Like other enveloped viruses, it is easily inactivated by ether, phenol, chloroform and formalin (Mathewson Commission, 1929; Whitley, 1996).

2.2 Epidemiogy

The most common cause of acute viral encephalitis is Varicella zoster virus and it causes a mild encephalitis course (Koskiniemi et al., 2001). Herpes simplex viruses are the agents in approximately 10% of all acute encephalitides. The most common cause of acute sporadic viral encephalitis (95% cases) is Herpes Simplex Type-1 and it causes fatal encephalitis. The incidence of HSE is reported as 2-4/1 million/year (Johnson, 1998; Koskiniemi et al., 2001; Levitz, 1998; Rantalaiho et al., 2001). All over the world, irrespective of the seasons, encephalitis occurs sporadically in all ages and does not show gender difference throughout the year (Whitley et al., 1982). Virus usually spreads via infected aerosols and through saliva (Griffin, 2000; Loon et al., 2004; Serter, 2002). Throat carriers are responsible from person to person spread of infection. The infection occurs with direct inoculation of the agent to oral, ocular, genital, anal mucosa, respiratory tract and bloodstream of susceptible people. No infection is seen through intact skin. Viral antibodies are positive in 70-90% of adults (Griffin, 2000; Roos,1999).
HSV-induced central nervous system (CNS) infections are much more severe than all other viral infections observed in the human brain. Today, the incidence of HSE is estimated to be approximately 1/250.000-500.000. Studies in United States, Britain and European countries show similar incidence rates and annual incidence has been reported as 1/300.000 (Longson, 1984; Skoldenberg et al., 1984). It was reported that medical costs for the young and adult patients hospitalized with the diagnosis of HSE in the United States in 1983 was more than $ 1 billion (Khetsuriani et al., 2002; Straus et al., 1985). HSE does not show seasonal variation throughout the year and can be seen in individuals of all ages. Approximately one-third of the cases are younger than 20 years and half of the patients are over the age of 50 (Whitley et al., 1982a, Whitley et al., 1982b).

2.3 Pathology and pathogenesis

HSV replication is a regular and a multi-step process. All herpes viruses induce long-term latent infections in the host. However, this process is not fully elucidated (Griffin, 2000). Pathological changes are characterized by ballooning degeneration of cells infected with replicated HSV and accumulation of chromatin within the cell nucleus following cellular core degeneration. Cells lost intact plasma membranes. During this process; multinucleated giant cells are formed by amitotic dividing of the nucleus. Also inside them, Cowdry type A intranuclear inclusion bodies formed by newly synthesized DNA masses are observed

(Serter, 2002). Usually, a clear area surrounded by chromatin is seen around the zone characterized by an obvious eosinophilic homogeneous appearance. These intranuclear inclusion bodies are supportive for diagnosis and usually observed in the first week of the infection, whereas they are only seen in 50% of patients. Then, migration of mononuclear cells in infected tissues, showing host immune response, can be detected. In this acute stage of HSE, congestion and / or bleeding may also be seen in the inflammatory field formed by mononuclear cells particularly in temporal lobes. This is usually asymmetrical in adults whereas a more diffuse involvement is seen in newborns (Boos & Esiri, 1986). Similar involvement can be seen in the adjacent limbic areas. After about 2 weeks, neurophagia with necrosis is observed in neurons and glial nodules occur. In addition, host immune response is also responsible for the severity of tissue damage (Serter, 2002).

Microscopic examination is usually abnormal due to enlargement of the involved areas. In the first stages, histological changes may not be dramatic and they are non-specific. Congestion of capillaries was observed in the cortex and all other changes, including petechiae, were significantly observed in subcortical white matter. Vascular changes are usually seen in the infection areas of hemorrhagic necrosis and perivascular cuffing. Perivascular cuffing becomes apparent in the second and third week of the infection. Glial nodules have been observed more frequently after the second week of the infection (Boos & Kim, 1984; Kapur et al., 1994). Microscopic appearance is characterized by inflammation dominated by necrosis, extensive perivascular mononuclear cell infiltration, gliosis and satellitosis neuronophagia (Boos & Esiri, 1986; Garcia et al., 1984). The most striking finding is observation of large areas of hemorrhagic necrosis reflecting the area of infection. In the later stages of the disease, oligodendrocytic participation and gliosis (astrocytosis as well) has been observed more often.

2.4 Pathogenesis of human disease

HSE development occurs by reaching of CNS disease causing virus to the brain. Course of illness and disease pathogenesis in humans is well known, but the arrival of virus to brain and issues related to reactivation of the virus present in the temporal lobe is still not clear. Partial understanding of the pathogenesis of HSE is a common feature for all age groups. Primary and recurrent HSV infections lead CNS disease eventually.

Primary infection in humans occurs via secretion of HSV and its spread to a seronegative sensitive person. For the occurrence of infection, contact of virus with mucosal surfaces or damaged skin is required (Cook & Stevens, 1973). As a rule, primary infection of HSV type-1 is often associated with oral mucosal disease in children or young adults. Tissue lesion, as a result of local virus replication, is usually in the form of asymptomatic gingivostomatitis (Schmutzhard, 2001). Then, viruses penetrate to mucosal receptors. As a result of viral replication in primary infection area, HSV Type-1, due to its affinity to sensitive and autonomic nerves, settles into the trigeminal nerve and olfactory tract ganglion neurons which are usually found in dorsal root ganglions.

Studies on the reactivation of the virus within the CNS have shown that certain viruses have enhanced neurotropism potential. Classical studies on animals proved that HSV reaches CNS through by both olfactory and trigeminal nerves (Johnson et al., 1968). However, especially in primary infection of humans, usage of trigeminal nerve by virus as a means of access to the CNS in a more preferred way is still a controversial issue. In HSE, settlement of the virus in temporal lobe through this route and spreading into the limbic system with replication is called as anatomical spread hypothesis. In studies conducted on patients diagnosed with HSE, herpes virus particles along the olfactory tract were shown by electron microscopic examination of tissue samples in some patients (Dinn, 1980; Ojeda et al., 1983; Twomey et al., 1979; Whitley et al., 1986).

Animal studies showed that virus transmission to CNS has occurred through a neurological pathway via olfactory tract and an infection is seen in animal brain regions similar to the medial temporal lobes in humans (Schlitt et al., 1986; Stroop & Schaefer, 1986). However, for humans, there is no evidence for such an access route. HSV reactivation is another confusing issue in the process of HSE formation. There are documentations regarding virus latency in infected brain tissue (Rock. & Frasher, 1983), but there is not enough information about the virus reactivation also taking place in this area. The disease has been suggested to occur via neuronal transmission of reactivated growing viruses to CNS right after virus reactivation in peripheral regions such as olfactory bulb or trigeminal ganglia (Davis & Mclaren, 1983; Griffith et al., 1967; Johnson et al., 1968; Stroop & Schaefer, 1986). As a result, HSV type-1 settles in its preferred remote residential areas of CNS such as the basal parts of the frontal lobes and limbic system parts of the temporal lobe via retrograde axoplasmic transport (Barnett et al., 1994; Cook & Stevens, 1973; Schmutzhard, 2000). Then type HSV-1 remains latent until another viral replication occurs. Also in animal studies, it was shown that virus can remain latent in the neuronal sub-populations of brain stem and cerebellum (Baringer & Pisani, 1994; Boggian et al., 2000; Lewandowski et al., 2002; Rock. & Frasher, 1983).

In the later stages, reactivation occurs in nuclei of these latent virus infiltrated neurons and virus proliferation is seen. Viral DNA synthesis is built together with the virus capsule and an acute infection occurs clinically (Hill, 1985). This asymptomatic acute infection, caused by reactivation of HSV type-1, is characterized with infections such as herpetic keratoconjunctivitis in residual regions (oropharyngeal, orofacial and corneal) of distribution area of trigeminal ganglia. This infection is also accompanied by typical mucocutaneous vesicular eruptions (such as herpes labialis) and mucosal ulcers. In addition, proliferating viruses of viral reactivation in this acute infection period are secreted to the external environment and constitute a source of infection for HSV type-1 (Schmutzhard, 2001).

In this infection situation, formation of infectious virus particles is accompanied by deterioration in host cells. These events are shown in various animal studies (Hill, 1985). This infection situation in latent areas can be diagnosed at this stage by demonstration of viral DNA content (20-100 copies per cell) in neural cell nuclei. Detection of viral antigenic structure is rarely possible in the latent phase. In general, synthesis of the single viral gene, called Latency Associated Transcripts (LATs), occurs in infiltrated cells. In many studies, LATs are shown to be responsible from prevention of apoptosis in infiltrated cells and that they reflect late viral reactivation (Millhouse & Wigdahl, 2000; Perng & Ciacci-Zanella, 2000).

Eosinophilic inclusion bodies containing viral antigen and herpes virus particles are found in related neurons and glial cells. Chemotherapy and UV-rays trigger immune system changes, latent virus activation leading to formation of the HSE and development of herpes labialis. HSE has been noticed to be not more frequent in immunosuppressed people. In several studies, it was observed that the disease had a more severe course in immune-competent patients. Because, the CNS disorders are estimated to occur as a result of serious contributions of immune-mediated mechanisms (Hudson et al., 1991; Levitz, 1998; Whitley & Lakeman, 1995).

Recurrent reactivation (such as herpes labialis infections) and viral replication rarely causes acute hemorrhagic necrotizing encephalitis (involving temporal cortex and the limbic system) (Barnes & Whitley, 1986; Roos,1999). Despite extensive researches in animal models, pathogenesis of HSE is not fully explained. 3 different hypotheses have been proposed in formation of the HSE via HSV type-1 (Levitz, 1998; Schmutzhard, 2001; Whitley & Lakeman, 1995). According to examinations conducted by National Institute of Allergy and Infectious Diseases (NIAID) and Common Antiviral Study Group (CASG), the primary infection has been reported to occur in about one-third of patients with HSE. After primary HSV infections, direct CNS invasion from nasal mucosa of the mouth and throat occurs through trigeminal nerve and olfactory tract. Often patients with primary infection are younger than 18 (Barnett et al., 1994; Davis & Johnson, 1979). Whereas in two-thirds of the cases, the disease occurs in the presence of existing antibodies (Nahmias et al., 1982). In 1/3 of HSE cases in this group, reactivation is seen as a result of recurrent herpes diseases in latent viruses in trigeminal ganglion and viruses multiply to cause a retrograde infection (Johnson, 1998; Schmutzhard, 2000). Endonuclease analysis of peripheral (labial) and CNS DNA isolates were compared and often the isolates were identified as similar. Only 10% of the patients had a medical history of recurrent herpes labialis (Nahmias et al., 1982). Also in 1/3 of the HSE cases, reactivation of existing latent viruses in CNS, such as brain stem and cerebellum, plays role (Levitz, 1998; Rock. & Frasher, 1983; Whitley & Lakeman, 1995). Finally, acute hemorrhagic necrotizing viral encephalitis in gray matter, particularly basal portions of the frontal lobe and limbic system of temporal lobe is seen (Barnett et al., 1994). Bilateral asymmetrical inflammation of temporal lobes is the main finding and intracerebral amygdaloid nucleus, hippocampus and insular region involvement is usually observed (Mutluer, 2002).

2.5 Clinical variability

Primary HSV infection and first viral replication usually occurs in the oropharyngeal mucosa. During this asymptomatic period, influenza infection findings, such as fatigue and general feeling of illness, are observed. Then a period of symptomatic disease which is characterized by high fever, headaches and difficulty in chewing caused by cheek and gum mucosa lesions begins and this period lasts 2-3 weeks.

High fever (89%) and headache (78%) are the most common non-specific symptoms seen in the early period of HSE. Also within this period, the basic neurological disorders are added to the course. Listed among the characteristic findings; changes in level of consciousness (confusion, hallucinations and personality changes, etc.), from sleep tendency leading to coma, were observed in 96%. Personality change was observed in 61%, whereas dysphasia was observed in 51%. Sensory aphasia (Wernicke's aphasia) due to dominant hemisphere involvement in the early period describes mild organic psycho-syndrome seen in HSE. Epileptic seizures (focal and generalized) are observed in 38% of patients and to a lesser extent, 36%, hemiparesis accompanies. Papilledema was observed in 14%, whereas ataxia is rarely observed (Bewermeyer et al., 1987; Johnson, 1998; Maihofner et al., 2002; Schmutzhard, 2000; Whitley et al., 1982). It was reported that meningeal irritation findings were not significant. Symptoms usually reach maximal level in 2-3 weeks (Loon et al., 2004; Roos,1999). Nothing is observed in herpetic skin flora (Shoji et al., 2002). In late HSE period, findings ranging from neurological residual syndrome, mild grade cognitive deficits, behavioral changes or personality changes are seen. Mostly post-infectious therapy-refractory epilepsy remains permanent (Bewermeyer et al., 1987; Schmutzhard, 2001).

However, completely atypical or chronic illness courses have also been reported (Bewermeyer et al., 1987; Panagariya et al., 2001; Whitley et al., 1989). Besides very mild courses, recurrent brain stem encephalitides were also defined (Klapper at al., 1984; Tyler et al., 1995). Because of this diversity of clinical symptoms, the diagnosis of the disease remains difficult and this causes the virostatic therapy to be applied very late.

Active mucocutaneous HSV infection accompanying immunocompromised patients is rarely observed with immunocompetent patients. Immune-suppression increases the risk of reactivation of latent HSV in cranial nerves and immune-suppressive agents in animal model studies have been shown to induce HSE. HSV type-1 was described as the main factor in brain stem and limbic system encephalitis in AIDS patients. Immune reaction that causes classical necrotizing encephalitis in advanced AIDS cases may not be seen (Roos,1999). As a result of some studies, the risk of reactivation of HSE during intracranial surgery was found and therefore pre-, peri-and post-operative application of Acyclovir treatment was proposed (Bourgeois et al., 1999). In an experimental study, induction of hypothalamic-pituitary adrenocortical axis and production of IL-1 and PG-E2 in the brain, independent of viral replication, by HSV type-1 was shown and also HSV type-1 was suggested to be a factor in the emergence of the symptoms, such as high- fever, motor hyperactivity and aggressive behavior.

2.6 Diagnosis

Clinical findings in HSE are non-specific so they cannot be used for empirical diagnosis. The presence of clinical symptoms and a localized lesion in the temporal lobe usually reflects HSE, but other diseases can also mimic this condition (Whitley et al., 1989). CSF examination is indicated for patients with mental changes even if intracranial pressure is increased. In addition, presence of a lesion in brain computed tomography (CT) or magnetic resonance imaging (MRI) was found to be related with poor neurological outcomes (Domingues et al., 1997; Domingues et al., 1998a; Domingues et al., 1998b).

In HSE cases in which viral replication cannot be blocked with early treatment, surviving patients are known to suffer heavy and large number of neurological sequelae. Therefore, early diagnosis is of great importance. Diagnosis is made with clinical symptoms, MRI, EEG and CSF examination. The sensitivity is increased with the combination of these neurodiagnostic tests, but the specificity is still insufficient (Griffin, 2000; Dupuis, 1999). In the past, the only method used to prove HSE was brain biopsy, whereas today HSV-DNA presence in CSF with PCR method is valid for the diagnosis (Lakeman & Whitley, 1995).

Specificity and sensitivity of brain CT for diagnostic aspect is less. Hemorrhagic brain lesions in temporal lobe on CT show areas of low density causing localized mass effect (Enzmann et al., 1978; Zimmerman et al., 1980). Especially bilateral involvement of temporal areas at the later stages of the disease shows that the disease is resistant to therapy. Typical changes in HSE, correlated with brain CT, show large brain damage but these changes are not compatible with the prognosis (Morawetz et al., 1983).

When HSE is suspected; cranial MRI should be applied as an emergency to prove neuropathologic changes very early. MRI suggests the findings of HSE earlier than CT (Schlesinger et al., 1995). Because MRI is a more sensitive and specific diagnostic tool, it is used instead of CT scans in majority of patients (Schlesinger et al., 1995; Sener, 2001, 2002). The characteristic MRI finding of HSE is hyperintense areas in inferior lobes including the medial part and insula and this characteristic involvement may also be observed in the frontal and parietal lobes, furthermore bilateral temporal lobe involvement has been reported to be pathognomonic as well (Aribas, 1996; Gordon, 1999; Roos,1999). This frontobasal and temporobasal hyperintense signal changes and diffusion limitation especially observed in T2-FLAIR sequences are typical (Djukic et al., 2003; Maihofner et al.,

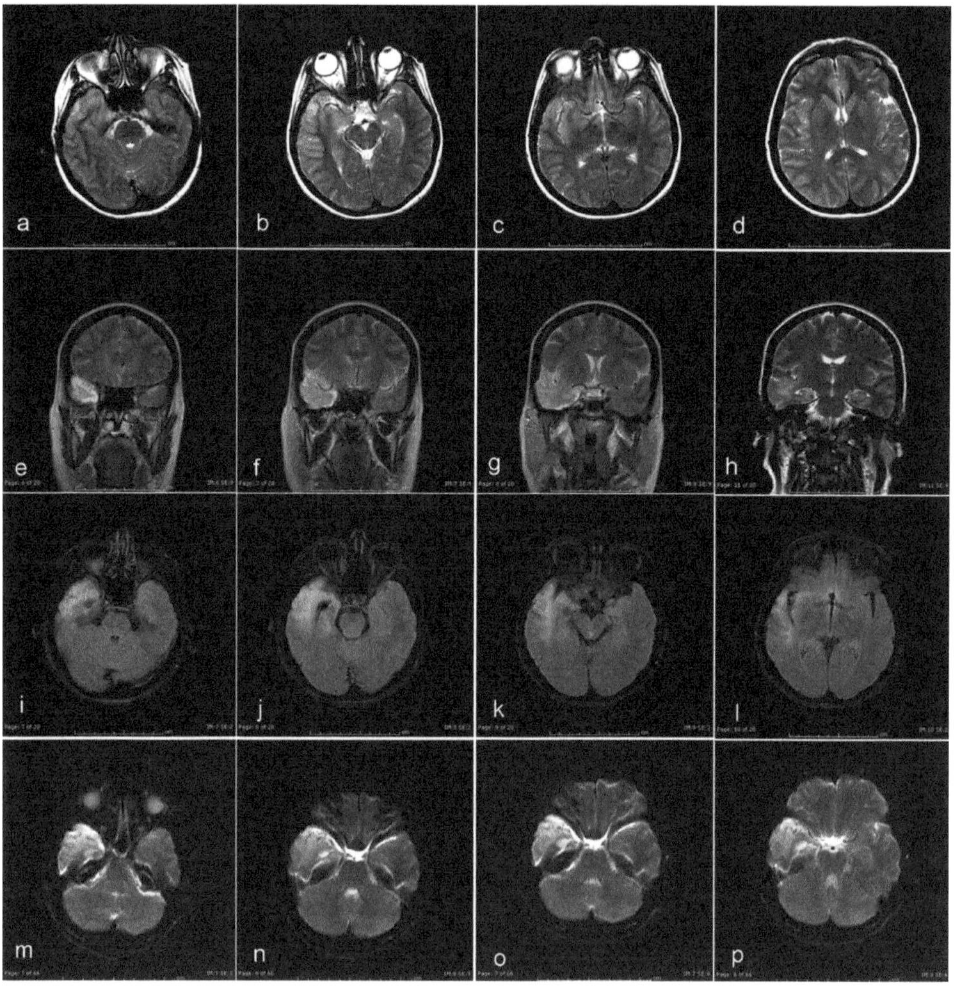

Fig. 1. T1-SE images in axial and sagittal planes, T2-TSE images in axial and coronal planes, FLAIR images in axial plane, T1-weighted SE images in axial, coronal and sagittal planes after intravenous contrast agent administration were obtained. Diffusion-weighted images of brain were obtained (b=0 b= 500, b=1000sn/mm2 and ADC mapping). Lesion consistent with herpes encephalitis was observed in examination of right supratentorial region. The lesion was in the temporal lobe, involving parahippocampal gyrus and the hippocampus, and was extending to frontobasal region. The lesion was hyperintense on T2 and FLAIR-weighted sequences, showing diffusion limitation and no contrast enhancement after intravenous injection of Gadolunium.

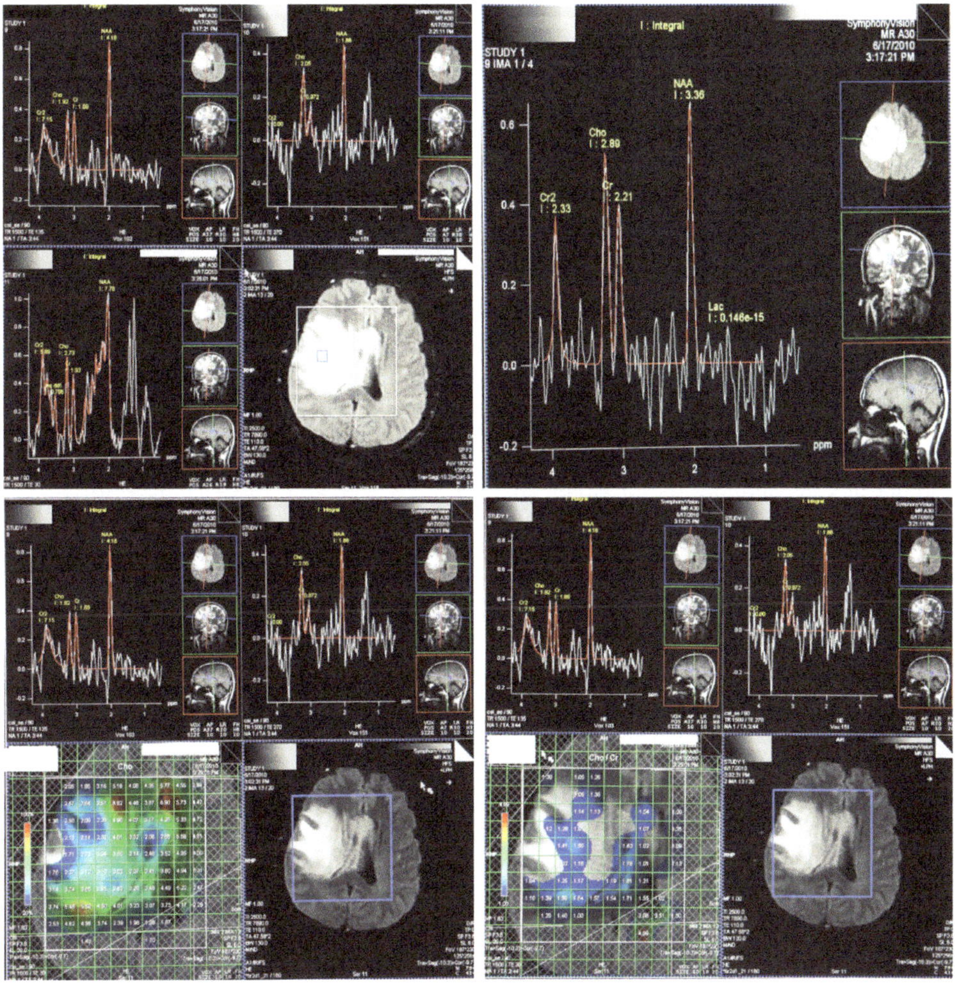

Fig. 2. Brain MR Spectroscopy evaluation of another patient was performed with CSI technique and TE of 30ms, 135ms and 270ms. Millimetric nodular lesions consistent with encephalitis were seen in right frontotemporal region, brain stem diffusely involving pons and left centrum semiovale. In spectroscopic examination, no significant choline peak was detected and a decrease was observed in NAA/Creatinine ratio.

2002; Schroth et al., 1987). In other sequences, parenchymal injury observed in the initial stage has been documented as areas of abnormal diffusion and these areas was observed to be reversible with virostatic treatment (McCabe et al., 2003). In addition, as a result of further studies, the severity of involvement observed in cranial MRI was reported to be compatible with the severity of clinical symptoms (Lamade et al., 1999).

CSF examination is another helpful method in the diagnosis of HSE and guiding in differentiation of diseases that mimic HSE. CSF examination is particularly indicated for patients with mental changes. CSF is transparent and cerebrospinal fluid pressure is usually

increased in HSE (Whitley et al., 1989). Polymorphonuclear leukocyte domination is seen in CSF in the early periods of HSE (Griffin, 2000). With disease progression, increase in WBC (lymphocytic pleocytosis) and protein level is determined. The average protein and WBC counts in CSF are approximately 100 mg / dL and 100 cells / L, respectively. The frequency of lymphocytic pleocytosis in CSF, especially when compared to patients with diseases that mimic HSE, is determined to be higher (Whitley et al., 1989). HSE leads to early hemorrhagic encephalitis so erythrocytes are often seen in CSF and this is a helpful finding for diagnosis (Mutluer, 2002). CSF glucose level is almost always within the normal range but reduction of glucose level due to consumption is typical in bacterial meningitis (Griffin, 2000; Roos,1999). In 5-10% of cases observed especially in children, the first evaluation of CSF examination can be found normal. However, CSF examination should be repeated within 24 hours, so in most cases, abnormalities can be observed (Whitley et al., 1989).
The success of CSF virus culture does not exceed 5% in encephalitis, so detection of nucleic acid by PCR in CSF at the first two weeks of infection and intrathecal antibodies at late period (after the 10th day) is recommended (Linde et al., 1997). Intrathecal specific IgG positivity begins at 10-12th day reaches its peak level at 20th day and may continue for years. Timing of CSF sampling is important for PCR. CSF sampling in early stage (first 48-72 hours) or after treatment can lead to negative results in PCR. In cases that the test is negative but there is clinical suspicion, repeated sampling of CSF for PCR and investigation of intrathecal antibodies at late stage may be diagnostic (Cinque et al., 1996; Puchhammer-Stöckl et al., 2001; Sauerbrei & Wutzler, 2002).

2.6.1 PCR detection of viral DNA

The most commonly used method for the isolation of virus is cell culture cultivation. However, CSF viral cultures of HSV type-1 are often negative (Griffin, 2000; Serter, 2002). Therefore, viral nucleic acid exploration by PCR in the CSF has become very important in patients with encephalitis. With this method, there is a possibility of detecting even small amounts of DNA and the test results within 24 hours often. Over time, CSF HSV DNA detection by PCR has become the gold standard for diagnosis (Boos & Esiri, 1986; Davis & Mclaren, 1983; Dinn, 1980; Hill, 1985; Radermecker, 1956). Different genome regions (thymidine kinase, DNA polymerase, GPB, GPC, GPG, GPD, etc.) can be used for PCR (Cinque et al., 1996; Tang et al., 1999). Studies conducted by NIAID and CASG reported that this method had a very high sensitivity (98%) and specificity (94%). In 80% of tested samples, HSV-DNA positivity still remained within 1 week or more despite anti-viral treatment in HSE patients. As a result of the studies, HSV-DNA positivity in CSF by PCR was 100% within 10 days after the onset of symptoms, 30% in 11-20th and 19% in 21-40th days (Griffin, 2000; Roos,1999; Serter, 2002). The recently developed real-time PCR method has also examined CSF samples from patients with suspected HSE. As a result of the studies, a statistical correlation between the amount of virus (viral DNA copies / mL) and decrease in level of consciousness was showed, and a direct correlation was reported between CSF viral load (HSV-DNA amount), clinical outcome and prognosis (Domingues et al., 1998a; Domingues et al., 1998b; Domingues et al., 1997). PCR negativity shows either the absence of virus in the sample or presence of inhibitory activity. False-negative results may be observed in the PCR at the beginning of HSE symptoms (the first 24-48 hours) or 10 days to 2 weeks after onset of symptoms. False-negative results may also be observed in hemorrhagic CSF samples due to inhibition of the PCR reaction by erythrocytes (Serter, 2002).

The presence of HSV-DNA in CSF shows CNS infection due to HSV. However, in immunocompromised individuals, especially low amounts of HSV-DNA may not always be the evidence of the disease. Viral DNA quantitation may be guiding in diagnosis (Aberle & Puchhammer-Stöckl, 2002). Although the clinical significance of quantification of the controversial yet, as real-time PCR quantitation can be made with precision and speed, it can provide the knowledge needed in this regard. HSV-DNA in CSF can remain positive up to 1 week after beginning of acyclovir treatment (Cinque et al., 1996). HSV-DNA positivity in spite of treatment was associated with poor prognosis (Najioullah et al., 2000).
Though difficult to perform, brain biopsy protects its value in confirmatory of diagnosis (Djukic et al., 2003; Maihofner et al., 2002; Schroth et al., 1987). Isolation of HSV from the tissue samples taken by brain biopsy is sensitive (96%) and specific (100%) method for diagnosis. However, HSV-DNA detection in CSF by PCR has replaced brain biopsy due to being a less invasive method, easy to implement and achieving faster results. Brain biopsy is preferred in cases where CSF findings are atypical, HSV-DNA detection in CSF by PCR cannot be done, antibody tests are negative and MRI and EEG findings are non-specific (Roos,1999). In patients with suspected HSE, HSE rate confirmed by brain biopsy has been reported to be 45% (Whitley, 2004). Brain biopsy procedure-related acute and chronic complications are observed in approximately 3% of patients. Brain sample collection from a diseased area with incision has the potential for acute disease and can cause epileptic seizures at chronic stage. As a result, even though in some cases it is confusing, brain biopsy is a helpful method in diagnosis.

2.6.2 Serologic evolution

Demonstration of HSV antigens via immunoperoxidase method is specific in diagnosis. Viral particles can be shown by electron microscopy in 50% of all cases (Serter, 2002). Detection of anti-HSV antibodies in CSF is another method used for the diagnosis of HSV encephalitis (Cesario et al, 1969). Detection of specific antibodies in CSF may be diagnostic when other methods are inadequate and at periods of removal of virus from CSF (usually the first 1-2 weeks after infection) (Lanciotti et al., 2000). Detection of specific IgM in CSF is diagnostic (Holzmann, 2003; Petersen & Marfin, 2002). Detection of specific IgG in CSF is also significant. However, transition of IgG from serum to CSF may be seen as a result of blood-brain barrier disruption, so demonstration of intrathecal synthesis is required. For this purpose, specific antibodies are examined quantitatively in serum and CSF samples which are taken at the same time and index obtained by proportion to each other is evaluated. If IgG in CSF is from serum origin, CSF / serum antibody ratio is 1/200-1/300 (Link & Muller, 1971). During infection of the CNS, this ratio is increases in parallel with the increase in intrathecal antibody production. This method can be used as a reliable method except conditions causing polyspecific immune activation like Multiple Sclerosis or causing severe immunosuppression. Monteyne et al. compared a variety of index calculation formulas in detection of intrathecal HSV antibody response and determined that the results are compatible except with MS patients (Blennow et al., 1994; Linde et al., 1997; Reiber & Lange, 1991).
HSV type-specific IgM and IgG antibodies can be measured via immunological methods (neutralization, complement incorporation reaction, haemagglutination, indirect immunofluorescence, "radioimmunoassay" and ELISA) (Serter, 2002; Griffin, 2000). As a rule, detection of anti-HSV antibodies in CSF at the initial phase of the disease is not possible, but after 10-14 days, intrathecal production of virus-specific antibodies becomes

provable and thus makes a retrospective diagnosis possible. Especially between 2-4th weeks of infection, an increase in antibody titers is observed. A slight increase can be seen in subsequent recurrent infections, but specific antibody levels will persist for life (Pfister & Eichenlaub, 2001). However, the sensitivity and specificity of this method is low. Because increase in antibody titers up to four times at acute and convalescent stages of primary infection has been found neither sensitive nor sufficiently useful for the diagnosis of disease in patients diagnosed with HSE via other diagnostic procedures such as biopsy. In addition, increase in antibody levels may be detected in cases of herpetic infection causing fever, such as herpes labialis (Pfister & Eichenlaub, 2001).

Increase in CSF anti-HSV antibody titers up to four-fold or greater is diagnostic. A significant increase (from 29% to 85%) is detected in 1 month till the onset. Four-fold

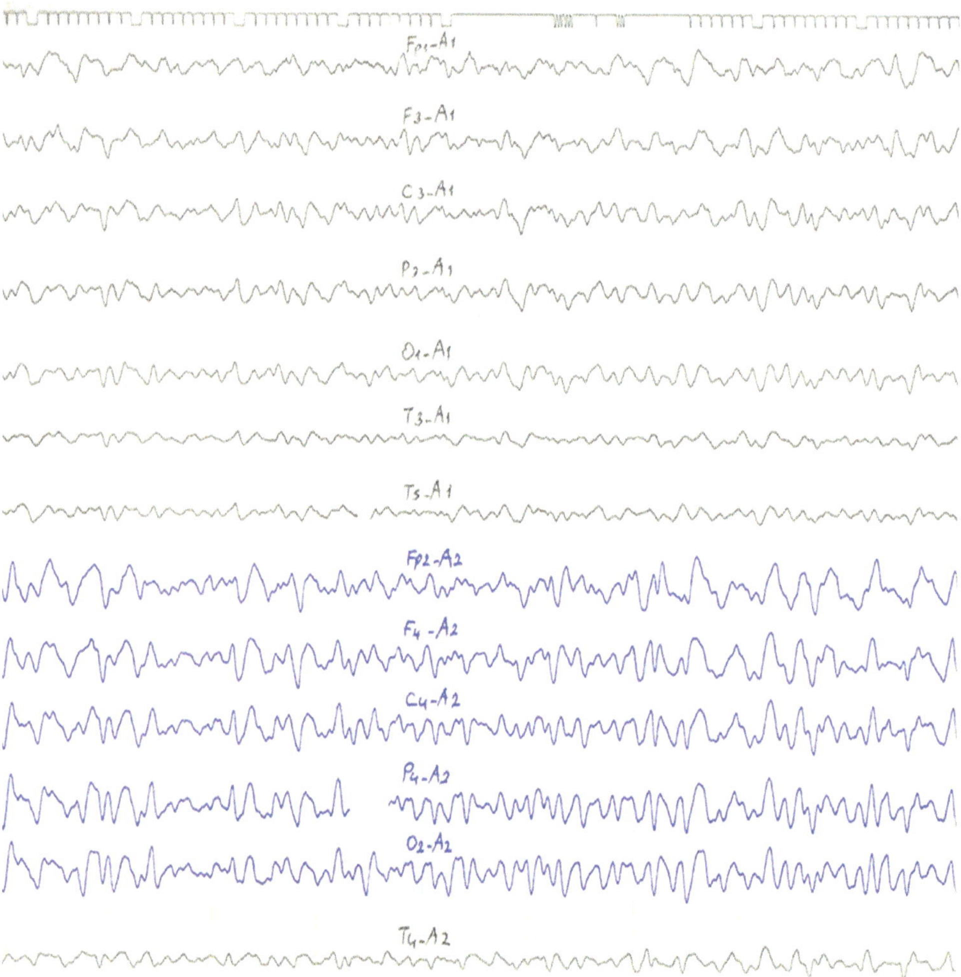

Fig. 3. PLED formation was observed in left hemisphere of the brain in EEG of the patient.

increase in CSF anti-HSV antibody titers 10 days after the start of clinical symptoms are observed in only 50% of patients diagnosed as HSE with brain biopsy. Therefore, this test is valuable only in retrospective diagnosis. In addition, a CSF / serum antibody ratio value of 20 or less has shown that there is no sensitivity during the first 10 days of the disease (Pfister & Eichenlaub, 2001).

Increased pathological levels of markers (neuron-specific enolase, NSE and S-100, etc.) showing destruction of neuronal and glial tissue in the CSF may occur in HSE. In some studies, a correlation between brain injury and these values was able to be used to estimate prognosis. However, these parameters increase in cerebral ischemia and dementia so they are not HSE specific (Studahl et al., 2000). Similarly, observation of various signal peptides, proteins, cytokines and soluble cytokine receptors (Neopterin, beta-2 microglobulin, Interleukin, interferon gamma, etc.) should be understood as an expression of strong intrathecal immune response (Griffin, 2000; Serter, 2002). In addition, a few values also increased actively in the course of HSE correlated with increases (Aurelius et al., 1993; Aurelius et al., 1994; Griffin, 2000). Serial changes observed in intrathecal cytokine and chemokine levels in patients with HSE were investigated in 4 separate clinical trials in detail. As a result of these studies; HSE identified in the acute stages of IFN-γ and IL-6 levels increased and these values, confirming the diagnosis has been reported to be helpful (Asaoka et al., 2004; Aurelius et al., 1994; Ichiyama et al., 2008; Rösler et al., 1998).

Another preferred method of early diagnosis of HSE is EEG. Frontotemporobasal dysrhythmia and a slowdown in frequency are observed in the EEG (Bewermeyer et al., 1987; Whitley et al., 1982). Periodic lateralized epileptiform discharges (PLEDs) are relative characteristic findings resulting from the temporal lobe, observed as slow and sharp wave complexes repeatedly (Chien et al., 1977; Longson, 1984; Miller & Coey, 1959; Panagariya et al., 2001; Smith et al., 1975; Upton & Grumpert, 1970). They are often observed between 2-15th days of the disease (Roos,1999). Early in the disease, abnormal electrical activity usually involves one temporal lobe, but as the disease progresses (over a period of 7-10 days), similar electrical activity may be observed in the contralateral temporal lobe. For the diagnosis of HSE, EEG sensitivity is 84% whereas specificity is only 32.5% (Enzmann et al., 1978; Zimmerman et al., 1980).

2.7 Differantial diagnosis

In a study by NIAID and CASG; brain biopsy has been performed in 432 patients with encephalopathic foci and HSE was diagnosed in 45% of these patients. Diseases mimicking HSE were found in the remaining 55% of the cases (Whitley et al., 1989; Whitley & Gnann, 2002). In this group, brain abscess, tuberculosis, cryptococcal infection and brain tumor were detected in 38 patients and other viral encephalitides caused by enterovirus and Epstein-Barr virus were detected in 38 patients. As a result, CNS HSV infection must be distinguished from these diseases mimicking HSV encephalitis (Roos,1999). Emergency medical treatment of patients with these statements is required even if PCR investigation of HSV-DNA is negative.

2.8 Treatment and prognosis

Idoxuridine is the first antiviral drug used for the treatment of HSE. However, as a result of a controlled clinical trial, this anti-viral agent was found to be ineffective and toxic (Chien et al., 1975). Later Vidarabine was defined as an effective therapeutic agent in the treatment of

HSE, but over time was replaced by Acyclovir, a more effective anti-viral agent (Whitley et al, 1977; Whitley et al, 1981).

An improvement has been achieved in the prognosis of HSE with anti-viral therapy with acyclovir. In 1984 and 1986, two studies compared the efficacy and clinical use of Acyclovir and Vidarabine (Skoldenberg et al., 1984; Whitley et al., 1986). Acyclovir (9 - [2-Hydroxymethyl] guanine) is a nucleoside analogue of deoxyguanosine. For the effectiveness of acyclovir in infected cells, phosphorylation with viral thymidine kinase is required. Acyclovir is converted to acyclovir monophosphate by viral thymidine kinase phosphorylation. The monophosphate is further converted into diphosphate and triphosphate by cellular kinases. Acyclovir-triphosphate inhibits viral DNA-polymerase selectively and competitively. In conclusion, the viral DNA chain is broken, and thus complete viral DNA synthesis is stopped. Due to lesser affinity to host cell DNA polymerases, causing a very little toxic effect in host cell is another important feature of Acyclovir-triphosphate (Dorsky & Crumpacker, 1987; Van Landingham et al., 1988).

Acyclovir prevents virus proliferation but has no protective effect on primary and secondary immune-mediated damage that developed in previously virus infected cells. Therefore, early treatment is mandatory in patients with HSE and prophylactic Acyclovir treatment should be given even if HSE is suspected (Djukic et al., 2003; Dorsky & Crumpacker, 1987; Whitley et al., 1986). When administered intravenously, Acyclovir may crystallize and cause temporary renal failure. Therefore, intravenous drug should be administered both slowly and with adequate fluid support. Similarly, especially in patients with renal failure, renal function tests should be followed closely. Acyclovir should be applied intravenously every 8 hours at 10 mg / kg dose slowly (over 1 hour). The duration of treatment should be at least 14 days, but 21 days will be better (Djukic et al., 2003; Levitz, 1998). Because worsening of the disease was defined in short-term treatment with reactivation of the virus (Baringer & Pisani, 1994; Van Landingham et al., 1988). CSF acyclovir levels are approximately 30-50% of corresponding plasma levels (Serter, 2002). HSV-DNA viral load in CSF may be used as a marker for treatment efficacy, but is independent from clinical course and cannot be correlated with it (Wildemann et al., 1997).

Factors influencing the success and long-term clinical results in a positive way are patient age <30, Glasgow coma score (GCS) >10, <4 days of disease before the treatment with Acyclovir and early start time of the therapy (Griffin, 2000). Therefore, for the effectiveness of Acyclovir, the treatment should be initiated before a significant deterioration (GCS> 10) at the level of consciousness, the symptoms of initial phase (first 4 days) and particularly before start of the dominant temporal lobe hemorrhagic necrosis. Glasgow coma scale is the preferred scale indicating the level of consciousness in literature. Regardless of the age, a patient with a GC score 6 or less was shown to have worse treatment outcomes. Children and adolescents constitute 90% of HSE diagnosed patients under the age of 30. This group of patients likely to return to normal functions with mortality rates reported to be higher than in elderly patients (Whitley et al., 1986).

The treatment of HSE is difficult and the mortality and morbidity rates still remain high despite treatment The mortality rate decreases from 70% to 20-30% with the use of acyclovir (Gnann & Salvaggio, 2004; Loon et al., 2004). In a study conducted by CASG and NIAID, 6 and 18 months of treatment with Acyclovir decreased mortality rates to 19% and 28% respectively. Regardless of their age, 38% of patients return to normal lives with normal or minor neurological sequelae. However, even with treatment, most patients have a significant permanent neurological deficit. 9% of patients with neurological deficits had moderate neurological sequelae, while 53% developed severe neurological sequelae that become permanent or fatal. Permanent neurological deficit or death occurs not by reactivation of HSV infection but as a result of the disease. The mortality rate is lower than that of children and adolescents, but studies did not show statistically significantly lower rates of mortality in elderly individuals.

In a study recurrence of HSE was reported as 26%, while other studies have reported rate as 4% and 8% (Ito et al., 2000). In a study by NIAID, no recurrences were observed after completion of treatment. As a result, even after Acyclovir treatment only a few patients had recurrence of HSE (Van Landingham et al., 1988; Wang et al., 1994). Treatment failure was attributed to post-infectious encephalomyelitis, reactivation of latent virus, inadequacy of 14-day standard treatment regimen and possible drug resistance (Griffin, 2000). In addition, despite anti-viral treatment and clinical improvement, MRI follow-ups should be done frequently for progressive changes secondary to tissue damage (Lamade et al., 1999).

As a result of a mutation in viral genes encoding thymidine kinase, resistance to acyclovir may occur in HSV. Resistant isolates of HSV had been identified in encephalitides of patients with organ transplant and HIV infection. Especially in HIV-infected patients, the prognosis is very poor if Acyclovir-resistant HSV infections were not treated (Roos,1999).

Vidarabine may be used at a dose of 15 mg / kg / day in case of acyclovir resistance. However, although in vitro effect has been shown, Vidarabine was determined to be inadequate for treatment due to failure to reach target tissues and cells adequately and its side effects. In NIAID CASG studies, new morbidity development was demonstrated in about 15-20% of patients undergoing Vidarabine treatment during long-term follow-ups. In the same study, only 13% of patients treated with Vidarabine had none or mild neurological sequelae. 22% of the patients had moderate or severe neurological sequelae and death occurred in 55% of patients during the follow-up.

Therefore, in case of intolerance to acyclovir, Foscarnet, a more effective anti-viral drug with lesser side-effects than Vidarabine, is suggested to be used (Schmutzhard, 2001). The effect of Foscarnet in the treatment of resistant HSV infections has been proven. 40 mg / kg Foscarnet administration every 8 hours for a period of 10-42 days is recommended in resistant cases. However, the recurrence rate is high after treatment with this anti-viral agent (Roos,1999; Serter, 2002).

Famcyclovir, another alternative anti-viral drug used to treat HSE, is a pro-drug. In the organism, its structure changes into Pencyclovir, having a similar effect as acyclovir. However, its affinity for the viral-DNA polymerase is less than acyclovir. Therefore, the effectiveness for the treatment of HSE is less than acyclovir (Perry & Wagstaff, 1995). Valacyclovir, developed upon mild grade modification of acyclovir, reaches a high effect level when taken orally. However, a successful HSE therapy with Valacyclovir has been defined as casuistic in the literature. Similarly, as an alternative to acyclovir in the treatment of HSE; nucleoside analogues were used (Alrabiah & Sacks, 1996; Chan et al., 2000).

Because the majority of cellular damage is immune-mediated, simultaneous use of corticosteroids in HSE treatment is controversial. However, in recent studies, combined therapies of Acyclovir and corticosteroids are mentioned (Meyding-Lamade et al., 2003; Thompson et al., 2000).

Acute treatment of HSE should be done in intensive care unit. Intracranial pressure monitoring is required in order to intervene complications more quickly and in case of increased intracerebral pressure; mild hyperventilation and administration of osmotic diuretics (Mannitol, Gycerosteril) are recommended. If sufficient effect cannot be obtained despite these treatments, craniectomy should be considered as an option to relieve intracranial pressure. Especially in cases complicated by tentorial herniation or massive brain edema, anterior temporal lobe resection and / or decompressive craniectomy is suggested to be useful (Griffin, 2000).

Epileptic seizures in the acute phase should be treated with benzodiazepines, Valproic acid or diphenylhydantoin. In the treatment of permanent symptomatic epilepsy; similarly Carbamazepine, Oxcarbazepine and Valproic acid treatment is recommended. In addition, combinations of other anti-epileptic drugs like Lamotrigine, Topiramate or Levetiracetam are often necessary (Bewermeyer et al., 1987; Djukic et al., 2003; Pfister & Eichenlaub, 2001; Schmutzhard, 2001).

3. Conclusion

Marked improvement in prognosis has been achieved with modern diagnosis and Acyclovir treatment in the last 10-15 years. However, HSE is a severe, dangerous and progressive disease. As a result of an actual multi-center study, severe permanent neurological deficits or mortalities were reported in 35% of HSE patients despite treatment with Acyclovir (Raschilas et al., 2002). As documented in past studies, late admission to hospital and administration of anti-viral therapy are the reasons for the poor prognosis (Marton et al., 1996; Raschilas et al., 2002; Schmutzhard, 2000). The prognosis is worse in older patients and those with impaired general and mental status before the onset of the therapy. Therefore, early diagnosis and anti-viral treatment should be done as quickly as possible with Acyclovir.

4. References

Aberle, S.W. & Puchhammer-Stöckl, E. (2002). Diagnosis of herpesvirus infections of the central nervous system. *J Clin Virol*, Vol.25, pp. S79-85

Alrabiah, F.A. & Sacks, S.L. (1996). New antiherpesvirus agents. Their targets and therapeutic potential. *Drugs*, Vol. 52, pp. 17–32

Aribas, E. & Turk U. (1996). Herpes simpleks virus ensefaliti: bir olgu sunumu. *Flora*, Vol.2, pp. 123-126

Asaoka, K.; Shoji, H.; Nishizaka, S.; Ayabe, M.; Abe, T. & Ohori, N. et al. (2004). Non-herpetic acute limbic encephalitis: cerebropinal fluid cytokines and magnetic resonance imaging findings. *Intern Med*, Vol.43, pp. 42-48

Aurelius, E.; Andersson, B.; Forsgren, M.; Sköldenberg, B. & Strannegard, O. (1994). Cytokines and other markers of intrathecal immune response in patients with herpes simplex encephalitis. *J Infect Dis*, Vol.170, pp. 678–681

Aurelius, E.; Forsgren, M. & Skoldenberg, B. et al. (1993). Persistent intrathecal immune activation in patients with herpes simplex encephalitis. *J Infect Dis*, Vol.168, pp. 1248–1252

Baringer, J.R. & Pisani, P. (1994). Herpes simplex virus genomes in human nervous system tissue analyzed by polymerase chain reaction. *Ann Neurol*, Vol.36, pp, 823–829

Barnes, D.W. & Whitley, R.J. (1986). CNS disease associated with varicellazoster virus and herpes simplex virus infection. *Neurol Clin*, Vol.4, pp. 265–283

Barnett, E.M.; Jacobsen, G. & Evans, G. et al. (1994). Herpes simplex encephalitis in the temporal cortex and limbic system after trigeminal nerve inoculation. *J Infect Dis,* Vol.169, pp. 782–786

Bewermeyer, H.; Huber, M. & Bamborschke, S. et al. (1987). Neue Aspekte in der Diagnsotik und Therapie der Herpes-simplex-Enzephalitis. *Internist Prax,* Vol.27, pp. 323–337

Blennow, K.; Fredman, P. & Wallin, A. et al. (1994). Formulas for the quantitation of intrathecal IgG production. Their validity in the presence of blood-brain barrier damage and their utility in multiple sclerosis. *J Neurol Sci,* Vol.121, pp. 90-96

Boggian, I.; Buzzacaro, E. & Calistri, A. et al. (2000). Asymptomatic herpes simplex type 1 virus infection of the mouse brain. *J Neurovirol,* Vol.6, pp. 303–313

Boos, J. & Esiri, M.M. (1986). *Sporadic Encephalitis I. Viral Encephalitis: Pathology, Diagnosis and Management.* Blackwell Scientific Publishers, Boston

Boos, J. & Kim, J.H. (1984). Biopsy histopathology in herpes simplex encephalitis and in encephalitis of undefined etiology. *Yale J. Biol. Med.,* Vol.57, pp. 751–755

Bourgeois, M.; Vinikoff, L.; Tubiana, A.L. & Rose, C.S. (1999). Reactivation of herpes virus after surgery for epilepsy in a pediatric patient with mesial temporal sclerosis: case report. *Neurosurgery,* Vol.44, pp. 633-635

Cesario, T.C.; Poland, J.D.; Wulff, H.; Chin, T.D. & Wenner, H.A. (1969). Six years experiences with herpes simplex virus in a children's home. *Am. J. Epidemiol.,* Vol.90, pp. 416–422

Chan, P.K.; Chow, P.C. & Peiris, J.S. et al. (2000). Use of oral valaciclovir in a 12-year-old boy with herpes simplex encephalitis. *Hong Kong Med J,* Vol.6, pp. 119–121

Chien, L.T.; Boehm, R.M.; Robinson, H.; Liu, C. & Frenkel, L.D. (1977). Characteristic early electroencephalographic changes in herpes simplex encephalitis. *Arch. Neurol,.* Vol.34, pp. 361–364

Chien, A., Whitley, et al. (1975). Boston Interhospital Virus Study Group and the NIAID Sponsored Cooperative Antiviral Clinical Study. Failure of high dose 5-deoxyuridine in the therapy of herpes simplex virus encephalitis: evidence of unacceptable toxicity. *New Engl. J. Med,* Vol.292, pp. 600–603

Cinque, P.; Cleator, G.M.; Weber, T.; Monteyne, P.; Sindic, C.J. & van Loon A.M. (1996). The role of laboratory investigation in the diagnosis and management of patients with suspected herpes simplex encephalitis: a consensus report. *J Neurol Neurosurg Psychiatry,* Vol.61, pp. 339-345

Cook, M.L. & Stevens, J.G. (1973). Pathogenesis of herpetic neuritis and ganglionitis in mice: evidence of intra-axonal transport of infection. *Infect. Immun.,* Vol.7, pp. 272–288

Corey, L.; Adams, H.G. & Brown Z.A. et al. (1983). Genital herpes simplex virus infections: clinical manifestations, course, and complications. *Ann Intern Med,* Vol.98, pp. 958–972

Davis, L.E. & Johnson, R.T. (1979). An explanation for the localization of herpes simplex encephalitis? *Ann Neurol,* Vol.5, pp.2–5

Davis, L.E. & Mclaren, L.E. (1983). Relapsing herpes simplex encephalitis following antiviral therapy. *Ann. Neurol.,* Vol.13, pp. 192–195

Davison, A.J. & Clements, J.B. Herpesviruses: general pruperties. (2005). In: *Topley and Wilson's Virology,* Mahy, B.W.J. & Ter Maulen, V., (Eds). pp. 485-505, ASM Press, Washington.

Dennett, C; Cleator, G.M. & Klapper, P.E. (1997). HSV-1 and HSV-2 in herpes simplex encephalitis: a study of sixty- four cases in the United Kingdom. *J Med Virol*, Vol.53, pp.1–3

Dinn, J.J. (1980). Transolfactory spread of virus in herpes simplex encephalitis. *Brit. Med. J.*, Vol.281, p.1392

Djukic, M.; Meyding-Lamade, U.K. & Prange, H. et al. (2003). Virale Meningoenzephalitis In: *Leitlinien für Diagnostik und Therapie in der Neurologie.* Diener, H.C., für die Kommission „Leitlinien" der Deutschen Gesellschaft für Neurologie, pp. 226-233, Thieme, Hrsg. Stuttgart

Domingues, R.B.; Fink, M.C.; Tsanaclis, S.M.; De Castro, C.C.; Cerri, G.G.; Mayo, M.S. & Lakeman, F.D. (1998a). Diagnosis of herpes simplex encephalitis by magnetic resonance imaging and polymerase chain reaction assay of cerebrospinal fluid. *J. Neurol. Sci.*, Vol.157, pp. 148–153

Domingues, R.B.; Lakeman, F.D.; Mayo, M.S. & Whitley, R.J. (1998b). Application of competitive PCR to cerebrospinal fluid samples from patients with herpes simplex encephalitis. *J. Clin. Microbiol.*, Vol.36, pp. 2229–2234

Domingues, R.B.; Lakeman, F.D.; Pannuti, C.S.; Fink, M.C. & Tsanaclis, A.M. (1997). Advantage of polymerase chain reaction in the diagnosis of herpes simplex encephalitis: presentation of 5 atypical cases. *Scand J Infect Dis*, Vol.29, pp. 229–231

Dorsky, D.I. & Crumpacker, C.S. (1987). Drugs five years later: acyclovir. *Ann Intern Med*, Vol.107, pp. 859–874

Dupuis, O.; Audibert, F.; Fernandez, F. & Frydman R. (1999). Herpes simplex virus encephalitis in pregnancy. *Obstet Gynecol*, Vol.94, pp. 810-812

Enzmann, D.R.; Ransom, B. & Norman, D. (1978). Computed tomography of herpes simplex encephalitis. *Radiology*, Vol.129, pp. 419–425

Erturk, M. Herpes simplex virusleri (1999). In: *Temel ve Klinik Mikrobiyoloji*, Ustacelebi, S., (Ed). pp. 815-827, Gunes Kitabevi, Ankara.

Garcia, J.H.; Colon, L.E.; Whitley, R.J.; Kichara, J. & Holmes, F.J. (1984). Diagnosis of viral encephalitis by brain biopsy. *Semin. Diagn. Pathol.*, Vol.1, pp. 71–80

Garcia-Blanco, M.A. & Cullen, B.R. (1991). Molecular basis of latency in pathogenic human viruses. *Science*, Vol.254, pp. 815–820

Gnann, J.W. & Salvaggio, M.R. (2004). Drugs for herpesvirus infections. In: *Infectious Diseases*, Cohen, J. & Powderly, W.G., (Eds), 2nd ed. pp. 1895-1909. Mosby, London

Gordon, K. Infection and inflammation. (1999). In: *Magnetic Resonance Imaging*, Stark, D.D. & Bradley, W.G. (Eds.), pp. 1361-1378, Mosby, St. Louis, Missouri

Griffin, D.E. (2000). Encephalitis, myelitis, and neuritis. In: *Mandell, Douglas, and Bennett's Principles and Practice of Infectious Diseases*, Mandell, G.L.; Bennett, J.E. & Dolin R, (Eds)., Fifth ed., pp. 1009-1016, Churchill Livingstone, Philadelphia

Griffith, J.R.; Kibrick, S.; Dodge, P.R. & Richardson, E.P. (1967). Experimental herpes simplex encephalitis: electroencephalographic, clinical, virologic, and pathologic observations in the rabbit. *Electroencephalogr. Clin. Neurophysiol.*, Vol.23, pp. 263–267

Hill, T.J. (1985). Herpes simplex virus latency. In: *The Herpesviruses*, Roizman, B. (Ed.), Plenum Publishing, New York

Holzmann, H. (2003). Diagnosis of tick-borne encephalitis. *Vaccine*, Vol.21, pp. S1/36-40

Hudson, S.J.; Dix, R.D. & Streilein, J.W. (1991). Induction of encephalitis in SJL mice by intranasal infection with herpes simplex virus type 1: a possible model of herpes simplex encephalitis in humans. *J Infect Dis*, Vol.163, pp. 720–727

Ichiyama, T.; Shoji, H.; Takanashi, Y.; Matsushige, T.; Kajimoto, M. & Inuzuka, T. et al. (2008). Cerebrospinal fluid levels of cytokines in non-herpetic acute limbic encephalitis: comparison with herpes simplex encephalitis. *Cytokine*, Vol.44, pp. 149-153

Ito, Y.; Kimura, H. & Yabuta, Y. et al. (2000). Exacerbation of herpes simplex encephalitis after successful treatment with acyclovir. *Clin Infect Dis*, Vol.30, pp. 185-187

Jerome, K.R. & Ashley, R.l. Herpes simplex viruses and Herpes B virus. (2003) In: *Manuel of Clinical Microbiology*, Murray, P.R., (Ed). pp. 1291-1303, ASM Press, Washington. Johnson, R.T. (1998). *Viral infections of the nervous system*, 2nd edn., Lippincott-Raven, Philadelphia-New York

Johnson, R.T.; Olson, L.C. & Buescher, E.L. (1968). Herpes simplex virus infections of the nervous system: problems in laboratory diagnosis. *Arch. Neurol.*, Vol.18, pp. 260–264

Kapur, N.; Barker, S.; Burrows, E.H.; Ellison, D.; Brice, J.; Illis, L.S.; Scholey, K.; Colbourn, C.; Wilson, B. & Locates, M. (1994). Herpes simplex encephalitis: long term magnetic resonance imaging and neuropsychological profile. *J. Neurol. Neurosurg. Psychiat*, Vol.57, pp. 1334–134

Khetsuriani, N.; Holman, R.C. & Anderson, L.J. (2002). Burden of encephalitis associated hospitalizations in the United States, 1988–1997. *Clin. Infect. Dis.*, Vol.35, pp. 175–182

Klapper, P.E.; Cleator, G.M. & Longson, M. (1984). Mild forms of herpes encephalitis. *J Neurol Neurosurg Psychiatry*, Vol.47, pp. 1247–1250

Koskiniemi, M.; Rantalaiho, T. & Piiparinen, H. et al. (2001). Infections of the central nervous system of suspected viral origin: a collaborative study from Finland. *J Neurovirol*, Vol.7, pp. 400–408

Lakeman, F.D. & Whitley, R.J. The National Institute of Allergy and Infectious Diseases Collaborative Antiviral Study Group. (1995). Diagnosis of herpes simplex encephalitis: application of polymerase chain reaction to cerebrospinal fluid from brain-biopsied patients and correlation with disease. National Institute of Allergy and Infectious Diseases Collaborative Antiviral Study Group. *J Infect Dis*, Vol.171, pp. 857–863

Lamade, U.K.M.; Lamade, W.R. & Wildemann, B.T. et al. (1999). Herpes simplex virus encephalitis: chronic progressive cerebral magnetic resonance imaging abnormalities in patients despite good clinical recovery. *Clin Infect Dis*, Vol.28, pp. 148-149

Lanciotti, R.S.; Kerst, A.J. & Nasci, R.J. et al. (2000). Rapid detection of West Nile virus from human clinical specimens, field-collected mosquitoes, and avian samples by a TaqMan reverse transcriptase-PCR assay. *J Clin Microbiol*, Vol.38, pp. 4066-4071

Levitz, R.E. (1998). Herpes simplex encephalitis: a review. *Heart Lung*, Vol.27, pp. 209–212

Lewandowski, G.; Zimmerman, M.N. & Denk LL. et al. (2002). Herpes simplex type 1 infects and establishes latency in the brain and trigeminal ganglia during primary infection of the lip in cotton rats and mice. *Arch Virol*, Vol.147, pp. 167–179

Linde, A.; Klapper, P.E. & Monteyne, P. et al. (1997). Specific diagnostic methods for herpes virus infections of the central nervous system: A consensus review by the European Union Concerted Action on Virus Meningitis and Encephalitis. *Clin Diagn Virol*, Vol.8, pp. 83-104

Link, H. & Muller, R. (1971). Immunoglobulins in multiple sclerosis and infections of the nervous system. *Arch Neurol*, Vol.25, pp. 326-344

Longson, M. (1979). Le defi des encephalitis herpetiques. *Ann. Microbiol. (Paris)*, Vol.130, pp. 5

Longson, M. (1984). The general nature of viral encephalitis in the United Kingdom. In: *Viral Diseases of the Central Nervous System*, Ellis, L.S. (Ed.), Bailliere Tindall, London.

Loon, A.M.; Cleator, G.M. & Klapper, P.E. (2004). Herpesviruses. In: *Infectious Diseases*, Cohen, J. & Powderly, W.G. (Eds). 2nd ed. pp. 2021-2039, Mosby, London

Maihofner, C.; Neundorfer, B. & Tomandl, B. et al. (2002). Herpes simplex virus encephalitis. *Med Klin*, Vol.97, pp. 493–494

Marton, R.; Gotlieb-Steimatsky, T. & Klein, C. et al. (1996). Acute herpes simplex encephalitis: clinical assessment and prognostic data. *Acta Neurol Scand*, Vol.93, pp. 149–155

Mathewson Commission. (1929). *Epidemic encephalitis: etiology, epidemiology, treatment.* Report of a Survey by the Mathewson Commission. Columbia University Press, New York

McCabe, K.; Tyler, K. & Tanabe, J. (2003). Diffusion-weighted MRI abnormalities as a clue to the diagnosis of herpes simplex encephalitis. *Neurology*, Vol.61, pp. 1015–1016

Meyding-Lamade, U.K.; Oberlinner, C. & Rau, P.R. et al. (2003). Experimental herpes simplex virus encephalitis: a combination therapy of acyclovir and glucocorticoids reduces long-term magnetic resonance imaging abnormalities. *J Neurovirol*, Vol.9, pp. 118–125

Meyer, Jr., M.H.; Johnson, R.T.; Crawford, I.P.; Dascomb, H.E. & Rogers, N.G. (1960). Central nervous system syndromes of "viral" etiology. *Am. J. Med.*, Vol.29, pp. 334–347

Miller, J.H.D. & Coey, A. (1959). The EEG in necrotizing encephalitis. *Electroencephalogr. Clin. Neurophysiol.*, Vol.2, pp. 582–585

Millhouse, S. & Wigdahl, B. (2000). Molecular circuitry regulating herpes simplex virus type 1 latency in neurons. *J Neurovirol*, Vol.6, pp. 6–24

Mommeja-Marin, H.; Lafaurie, M. & Scieux, C. et al. (2003). Herpes simplex virus type 2 as a cause of severe meningitis in immunocompromised adults. *Clin Infect Dis*, Vol.37, pp.1527-33

Morawetz, R.B.; Whitley, R.J. & Murphy, D.M. (1983). Experience with brain biopsy for suspected herpes encephalitis: a review of forty consecutive cases. *Neurosurgery*, Vol.12, pp. 654–657

Mutluer, N. (2002). Ensefalomiyelitler ve noritler. In: *Infeksiyon Hastaliklari ve Mikrobiyolojisi.* Topcu, A.W.; Soyletir, G. & Doganay, M., (Eds). pp. 1019-1023, Nobel Tip Kitabevleri, Istanbul

Nahmias, A.J. & Dowdle, W.R. (1968). Antigenic and biologic differences in herpesvirus hominis. *Prog. Med. Virol.*, Vol.10, pp. 110–159

Nahmias, A.J.; Whitley, R.J.; Visintine, A.N.; Takei, Y. & Alford Jr., C.A. The National Institute of Allergy and Infectious Diseases Collaborative Antiviral Study Group.

(1982). Herpes simplex encephalitis: laboratory evaluations and their diagnostic significance. *J. Infect. Dis.*, Vol.145, pp. 829–836

Najioullah, F.; Bosshard, S. & Thouvenot, D. et al. (2000). Diagnosis and surveillance of herpes simplex virus infection of the central nervous system. *J Med Virol,* Vol.61, pp. 468-473

Ojeda, V.J.; Archer, M.; Robertson, T.A. & Bucens, M.R. (1983). Necropsy study of olfactory portal of entry in herpes simplex encephalitis. *Med. J. Aust.*, Vol.1, pp. 79–81

Panagariya, A.A.; Jain, R.S. & Gupta, S.S. et al. (2001). Herpes simplex encephalitis in North West India. *Neurol India,* Vol.49, pp. 360–365

Perng, G.C.; Jones, C. & Ciacci-Zanella, J. et al. (2000). Virus-induced neuronal apoptosis blocked by the herpes simplex virus latency-associated transcript. *Science,* Vol.287, pp. 1500–1503

Perry, C.M. & Wagstaff, A.J. (1995). Famciclovir. A review of its pharmacological properties and therapeutic efficacy in herpesvirus infections. *Drugs,* Vol.50, pp. 396–415

Petersen, L.R. & Marfin, A.A. (2002). West Nile virus: A primer for the clinican. *Ann Intern Med,* Vol.137, pp. 173-179

Pfister, H.W. & Eichenlaub, D. (2001). Infectious inflammatory diseases of the central nervous system from the neurological and internal medicine viewpoint. *Internist (Berl),* Vol.42, pp. 991–998

Puchhammer-Stöckl, E.; Presterl, E. & Croy, C. et al.(2001). Screening for possible failure of herpes simplex virus PCR in cerebrospinal fluid for the diagnosis of herpes simplex encephalitis. *J Med Virol,* Vol.64, pp. 531-536

Radermecker, J. (1956). Systematique its electrocencephalographic des encephalitis it encephalopathies. *Electroencephalography,* Vol.Suppl. 5, pp. 1–243

Rantalaiho, T.; Farkkila, M. & Vaheri, A. et al. Acute encephalitis from 1967 to 1991. J Neurol Sci 2001; 184: 169–77.

Raschilas, F.; Wolff, M. & Delatour, F. et al. (2002). Outcome of and prognostic factors for herpes simplex encephalitis in adult patients: results of a multicenter study. *Clin Infect Dis,* Vol.35, pp. 254–260

Reiber, H. & Lange, P. (1991). Quantification of virus-specific antibodies in cerebrospinal fluid and serum: sensitive and specific detection of antibody synthesis in brain. *Clin Chem,* Vol.37, pp.1153-1160

Rock, D.L. & Frasher, N.W. (1983). Detection of HSV-1 genome in central nervous system of latently infected mice. *Nature,* Vol.302, pp. 523–531

Roos, K.L. (1999). Encephalitis. *Neurol Clin,* Vol.17, pp. 813-825

Rösler, A.; Pohl, M.; Braune, H.J.; Oertel, W.H.; Gemsa, D. & Sprenger, H. (1998). Time course of chemokines in the cerebrospinal fluid and serum during herpes simplex type 1 encephalitis. *J Neurol Sci,* Vol.157, pp. 82-89

Sauerbrei, A. & Wutzler, P. (2002). Laboratory diagnosis of central nervous system infections caused by herpesviruses. *J Clin Virol,* Vol.25, pp. S45-51

Schlesinger, Y.; Buller, R.S.; Brunstrom, J.E.; Moran, C.J. & Storch, G.A. (1995). Expanded spectrum of herpes simplex encephalitis in childhood. *J. Pediatr.* Vol.126, pp. 234–241

Schlitt, M.; Lakeman, F.D.; Wilson, E.R.; To, A.; Acoff, R.; Harsh, G.R. & Whitley, R.J. (1986). A rabbit model of focal herpes simplex encephalitis. *J. Infect. Dis.,* Vol.153, pp. 732–735

Schmutzhard, E. (2000). *Entzündliche Erkrankungen des Nervensystems*, Thieme, Stuttgart

Schmutzhard, E. (2001). Viral infections of the CNS with special emphasis on herpes simplex infections. *J Neurol,* Vol.248, pp. 469–477

Schroth, G.; Gawehn, J. & Thron, A. et al. (1987). Early diagnosis of herpes simplex encephalitis by MRI. *Neurology* Vol.37, pp. 179–183

Sener, R.N. (2001). Herpes simplex encephalitis: diffusion MR imaging findings. *Comput. Med. Imag. Graph.,* Vol.25, pp. 391–397

Sener, R.N. (2002). Diffusion MRI in Rasmussen's encephalitis, herpes simplex encephalitis, and bacterial meningoencephalitis. *Comput. Med. Imag. Graph.,* Vol.26, pp. 327–332

Serter, D. (2002). Herpes simplex viruslar. In: *Infeksiyon Hastaliklari ve Mikrobiyolojisi,* Topcu, A.W.; Söyletir, G. & Doganay, M., (Eds). pp. 1176-1186, Nobel Tip Kitabevleri, Istanbul

Shoji, H.; Wakasugi, K. & Miura, Y. et al. (2002). Herpesvirus infections of the central nervous system. *Jpn J Infect Dis,* Vol.55, pp. 6–13

Skoldenberg, B.; Forsgren, M.; Alestig, K.; Bergstrom, T.; Burman, L.; Dahlqvist, E.; Forkman, A.; Fryden, A.; Lovgren, K.; Norlin, K.; Norrby, R.; Olding-Stenkvist, E.; Stiernstedt, G.; Uhnoo, I. & Devahl, K. (1984). Acyclovir versus vidarabine in herpes simplex encephalitis: a randomized multicentre study in consecutive Swedish patients. *Lancet,* Vol. 2, pp. 707- 711

Smith, M.G.; Lennette, E.H. & Reames, H.R. (1941). Isolation of the virus of herpes simplex and the demonstration of intranuclear inclusions in a case of acute encephalitis. *Am. J. Pathol.,* Vol.17, pp. 55–68

Smith, J.B.; Westmoreland, B.F.; Reagan, T.J. & Sandok, B.A. (1975). A distinctive clinical EEG profile in herpes simplex encephalitis. *Mayo Clin. Proc.* Vol.50, pp. 469–474

Straus, S.; Rooney, J.F.; Sever, J.L. & Seilding, M.; Nusinoff-Lehrman, S. & Cremer, K. (1985). Herpes simplex virus infection: biology, treatment and prevention. *Ann. Intern. Med.,* Vol.103, pp. 404–419

Stroop, W.G. & Schaefer, D.C. (1986). Production of encephalitis restricted to the temporal lobes by experimental reactivation of herpes simplex virus. *J. Infect. Dis.,* Vol.153, pp. 721–731

Studahl, M.; Rosengren, L. & Gunther, G. et al. (2000). Difference in pathogenesis between herpes simplex virus type 1 encephalitis and tick-borne encephalitis demonstrated by means of cerebrospinal fluid markers of glial and neuronal destruction. *J Neurol ,* Vol.247, pp. 636–642

Tang, Y.; Mitchell, P.S.; Espy, M.J.; Smith, T.S. & Persing, D.H. (1999). Molecular diagnosis of herpes simplex virus infections in the central system. *J Clin Microbiol,* Vol.37, pp. 2127-2136

Thompson, K.A.; Blessing, W.W. & Wesselingh, S.L. (2000). Herpes simplex replication and dissemination is not increased by corticosteroid treatment in a rat model of focal herpes encephalitis. *J Neurovirol,* Vol.6, pp. 25–32

Twomey, J.A.; Barker, C.M.; Robinson, G. & Howell, D.A. (1979). Olfactory mucosa in herpes simplex encephalitis. *J. Neurol. Neurosurg. Psychiat.,* Vol.42, pp. 983–987

Tyler, K.L. (2004). Herpes simplex virus infections of the central nervous system encephalitis and meningitis, including Mollaret's. *Herpes,* Vol.11 (Suppl. 2), pp. 57A–64A

Tyler, K.L.; Tedder, D.G. & Yamamoto, L.J. et al. (1995). Recurrent brainstem encephalitis associated with herpes simplex virus type 1 DNA in cerebrospinal fluid. *Neurology*, Vol.45, pp. 2246-2250

Upton, A. & Grumpert, J. (1970). Electroencephalography in diagnosis of herpes simplex encephalitis. *Lancet*, Vol.1, pp. 650-652

Van Landingham, K.E.; Marsteller, H.B. & Ross, G.W. et al. (1988). Relapse of herpes simplex encephalitis after conventional acyclovir therapy. *JAMA*, Vol.259, pp.1051-1053

Wang, H.S.; Kuo, M.F.; Huang, S.C. & Chou, M.L. (1994). Choreoathetosis as an initial sign of relapsing of herpes simplex encephalitis. *Pediatr. Neurol.*, Vol.11, pp. 341-345

Whitley, R.J. Herpes simplex viruses. (1996). In: *Fields Virology*, Fields, B.N.; Knipe, D.M. & Howley, P.M., (Eds). pp. 2297-2330, Lippincott Williams & Wilkens, Philadelphia. Whitley, R.J. Viral infections of the central nervous system. (2004). In: *Infectious Diseases Cohen*, J, Powderly W.G., (Eds.), 2nd ed., pp. 267-277, Mosby, London

Whitley, R.J.; Alford Jr, C.A.; Hirsch, M.S.; Schooley, R.T.; Luby, J.P.; Aoki, F.Y.; Hanley, D.; Nahmias, A.J. ; Soong, S.J. & The National Institute of Allergy and Infectious Diseases Collaborative Antiviral Study Group. (1986). Vidarabine versus acyclovir therapy in herpes simplex encephalitis. *New Engl. J. Med.*, Vol.314, pp. 144-149

Whitley, R.J.; Cobbs, C.G.; Alford Jr., C.A.; Soong, S.J.; Morawetz, R.; Benton, J.W.; Hirsch, M.S.; Reichman, R.C.; Aoki, F.Y.; Connor, J.; Oxman, M.; Corey, L.; Hanley, D.F.; Wright, P.F.; Levin, M.; Nahmias, A. & Powell, D.A. The National Institute of Allergy and Infectious Diseases Collaborative Antiviral Study Group. (1989). Diseases that mimic herpes simplex encephalitis: diagnosis, presentation and outcome. *JAMA*, Vol.262, pp. 234-239

Whitley, R.J. & Gnann, J.W. (2002). Viral encephalitis: familiar infections and emerging pathogens. *Lancet*, Vol.359, pp. 507-513

Whitley, R.J. & Lakeman, F. (1995). Herpes simplex virus infections of the central nervous system: therapeutic and diagnostic considerations. *Clin Infect Dis*, Vol.20, pp. 414-420

Whitley, R.J.; Lakeman, A.D.; Nahmias, A.J. & Roizman, B. (1982a). DNA restriction-enzyme analysis of herpes simplex virus isolates obtained from patients with encephalitis. *New Engl. J. Med.*, Vol.307, pp. 1060-1062

Whitley, R.J. & Roizman, B. (2001). Herpes simplex virus infections. *Lancet*, Vol. 357, pp. 1513-1518.

Whitley, R.J.; Soong, S.J.; Dolin, R.; Galasso, G.J.; Chien, L.T.; Alford Jr., C.A. & The National Institute of Allergy and Infectious Diseases Collaborative Antiviral Study Group. (1977). Adenine arabinoside therapy of biopsy-proved herpes simplex encephalitis: National Institute of Allergy and Infectious Diseases Collaborative Antiviral Study. *New Engl. J. Med.*, Vol.297, pp. 289-294

Whitley, R.J.; Soong, S.J.; Hirsch, M.S.; Karchmer, A.W.; Dolin, R.; Galasso, G.; Dunnick, J.K.; Alford Jr., C.A. & The National Institute of Allergy and Infectious Diseases Collaborative Antiviral Study Group. (1981). Herpes simplex encephalitis: vidarabine therapy and diagnostic problems. *New Engl. J. Med.*, Vol.304, pp. 313-318

Whitley, R.J.; Soong, S.J.; Linneman Jr. C.; Liu, C.; Pazin, G.; Alford, C.A. & The National Institute of Allergy and Infectious Diseases Collaborative Antiviral Study Group.

(1982b). Herpes simplex encephalitis: Clinical assessment. *JAMA*, Vol.247, pp. 317–320

Wildemann, B.; Ehrhart, K. & Storch-Hagenlocher, B. et al. (1997). Quantitation of herpes simplex virus type 1 DNA in cells of cerebrospinal fluid of patients with herpes simplex virus encephalitis. *Neurology*, Vol.48, pp. 1341–1346

Zarafonetis, C.J.D.; Smodel, M.C.; Adams, J.W. & Haymaker, V. (1944). Fatal herpes simplex encephalitis in man. *Am. J. Pathol.*, Vol. 20, pp. 429–445

Zimmerman, R.D.; Russell, E.J.; Leeds, N.E. & Kaufman, D. (1980). CT in the early diagnosis of herpes simplex encephalitis. *Am. J. Roentgenol.*, Vol.134, pp. 61–66

5

Virology and Pathology of Encephalitis in Alien Hosts by Neurotropic Equine Herpesvirus 9

Hideto Fukushi and Tokuma Yanai
Gifu University
Japan

1. Introduction

Herpesviruses occasionally cause lethal infection in alien hosts by interspecies transmission such as B virus infection in humans from Macaques and pseudorabies virus infection in various animals from pigs. Most of the infection can be characterized as lethal encephalitis. One of typical examples is equine herpesvirus 9 (EHV-9), also called as gazelle herpesvirus 1 (GHV-1), which was isolated from enzootic encephalitis of Thomson's gazelles (*Gazella thomsoni*) in 1993 (Fukushi et al., 1996, Yanai et al., 1998). EHV-9 infection has been reported in non-equid species such as Thomson's gazelles, a reticulated giraffe (*Giraffa camelopardalis reticulata*) (Hoenerhoff et al., 2006), and a polar bear (*Ursus maritimus*) (Donovan et al., 2006). Experimental infections have also been investigated including domestic horses, pigs, cattle, and goats, companion animals including cats and dogs and common marmosets (*Callithrix jacchus*) (Section 3). These interspecies or cross-species infections can be characterized as viral lethal and inapparent encephalitis (Table 1).

Animals	Clinical symptoms	Lesions
Thomson's gazelles, giraffle, Polar bear, goats, cats, dogs, hamsters, mice, rats, marmosets	Lethal Infection with neurological symptoms	meningoencephalitis. Neuronal degeneration and necrosis with intranuclear inclusion bodies, gliosis, cuffing
Horse, cattle, pigs	Fever, light depression	
Onager	Abortion	

Table 1. A list of animals infected with EHV-9

1.1 Epizootiology of encephalitis in a herd of Thomson's gazelles

Epizootic encephalitis occurred in a herd of Thomson's gazelles kept in a zoo in 1993. Twelve Thomson's gazelles were first introduced into the zoo in 1992. Then eight normal newborns and one malformed newborn have been delivered. Ten gazelles died of injury by various causes. The herd consisted of ten Thomson's gazelles at the outbreak. A first occurrence was sudden death of one gazelle, and then others showed neurological symptoms in turn over 2-week period (Fig. 1). The neurological symptoms in the gazelles were depression, incoordination, nystagmus, and convulsion. Laboratory tests showed occult blood and albumin in the urine samples. Seven out of the nine gazelles died. No evidence of infection was found in this foal. The other two gazelles recovered. The remaining one was a newborn that died of malnutrition, because the sick mother gazelle refused nursing. One of the recovered gazelles delivered a healthy neonate two months later. All dead gazelles did not have apparent changes at necropsy. Microscopically, all dead gazelles except the foal of malnutrition had nonsuppurative encephalitis, which characterized by neuronal degeneration and intracellular inclusion bodies (Fukushi et al., 1996, Yanai et al., 1998).

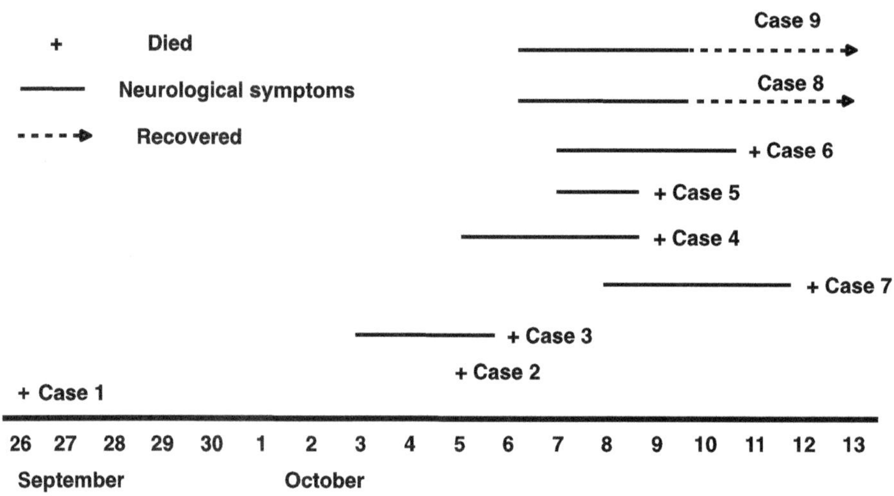

Fig. 1. Outbreak of lethal enzootic encephalitis in Thomson's gazelles

Homogenates of the brain, spinal cord, kidney, liver, lung and spleen were inoculated into Madin-Darby bovine kidney (MDBK) cells. Cells inoculated with the brain homogenate showed cytopathic effect characterized as syncitium formation accompanying nuclear inclusion bodies and detachment (Fig. 2), indicating the isolation of a virus. Physicochemical characterization of the isolate showed that the isolate was chloroform sensitive DNA virus of about 150 to 200 nm diameter. Considering the characteristics, the isolate was identified as a herpesvirus. Serum neutralization tests using antisera against pseudorabies virus, bovine herpesvirus 1, malignant catarrahl fever virus, and equine herpesvirus 1 (EHV-1) indicated that the isolated virus should be EHV-1 or EHV-1 related virus. Comparing DNA fingerprints and nucleotide sequences of a glycoprotein B gene and a glycoprotein G gene, the isolate should be regarded as a new herpesvirus, gazelles herpesvirus 1 (GHV-1) at first (Fukushi et al., 1996). DNA fingerprints of GHV-1 were different from those of EHV- 1, EHV-4, and EHV-8, although GHV-1 cross-reacted with EHV-1 and EHV-4 in neutralization tests. Southern analysis indicated that GHV-1 shared sequence homology with EHV-1.

Sequences of gB and gG homologue genes of GHV-1 are closer to EHV-1 than to other equine herpesviruses including EHV-8. Therefore GHV-1 was recognized as a new member of equine herpesvirus, equine herpesvirus 9 (EHV-9).
It should be noted that a zebra kept in the same field with the gazelles had neutralizing antibody to GHV-1 but not to EHV-1 in neutralization tests examined several months after the episode.

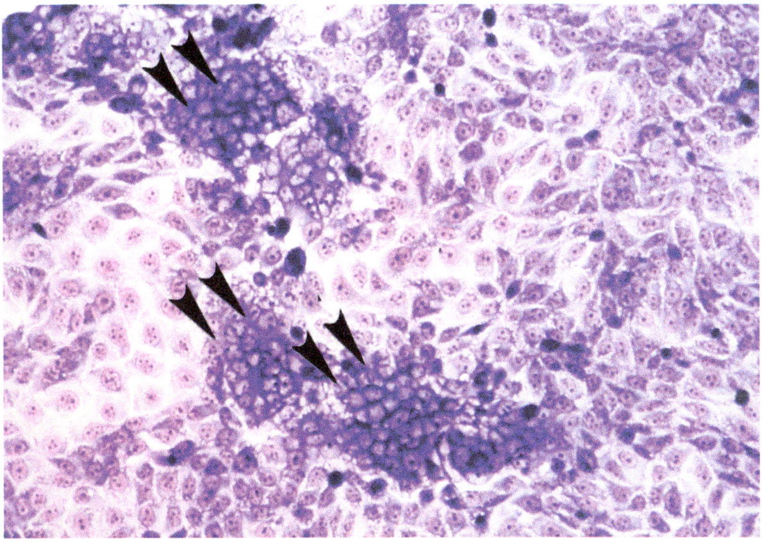

Fig. 2. CPE observed in MDBK cells inoculated with brain homogenate

1.2 A sporadic encephalitis in a giraffe

An 18-month-old male reticulated giraffe (*Giraffa camelopardalis reticulate*) housed in a zoo presented with a one and a half day history of incoordination, stumbling, and abdominal pain and died (Hoenerhoff et al., 2006). Nonsuppurative encephalitis was histopathologically found in the brain of giraffe. Several zebras (*Equus burchelli*), which were apparently healthy, were housed in a pen with the giraffe. Herpesvirus was isolated from the reticulated giraffe. The isolated virus was identified as EHV-1 by PCR and monoclonal antibody assay at first. The giraffe had been housed with a group of zebras that were serologically positive for EHV-1. Considering the situation and histopathological findings, there was a possibility that the isolate could be EHV-9. Several gene sequences of the giraffe virus were almost identical to those of EHV-9 (Samy et al., 2008). Therefore the giraffe virus was EHV-9.

1.3 Meningoencephalitis in a polar bear

A 12-year-old female polar bear (*Ursus maritimus*) developed a sudden onset of neurological symptoms in 2007 (Schrenzel et al., 2008; Donovan et al., 2009). Nonsuppurative pleocytosis of cerebrospinal fluid was observed. The bear was euthanized. Multifocal, random nonsuppurative meningoencephalitis was microscopically found involving most prominently the rostral cerebral cortex, as well as the thalamus, midbrain, and rostral medulla. Lesions consisted of inflammation, neuronal necrosis, gliosis, and both neuronal and glial basophilic intranuclear inclusion bodies. PCR for the herpesvirus DNA polymerase gene segment was positive on DNA extracted from frozen tissues and from paraffin-embedded fixed brain. The nucleotide sequence of the PCR product indicated the presence of EHV-9, which was further confirmed by following PCR for the EHV-9 gB gene segment.

Schrenzel et al. (2008) described that EHV-9 had been detected at the same zoological garden in 2 Grevy's zebras (*Equus grevysi*) from the same herd, which had been relocated near the polar bears before the polar bear case. One of the infected Grevy's zebras was 8 days old and had viral interstitial pneumonia; the other was an adult with rhinitis and intranuclear inclusion bodies. Both zebras were immunocompromised as a result of other concurrent conditions.

1.4 Abortion in an onager

Schrenzel et al. (2008) described that EHV-9 was found by a retrospective analysis of tissues from an aborted Persian onager (*Equus hemionus onager*) fetus from a zoological park in Washington, DC (Montali et al., 1985). The onager fetus was aborted after the dam came in close proximity to a Grevy's zebra. A herpesvirus was isolated from the fetus. The virus was identified as EHV-1 based on DNA fingerprinting and serological analyses (Montali et al., 1985). PCR and DNA sequencing analyses of the DNA polymerase showed that the zebras and the onager had an EHV-9 strain identical to that found in the polar bear (Schrenzel et al., 2008).

1.5 Burchell's zebras from the Serengeti ecosystem

Zebras have been suspected to be the source of EHV-9 infection. To prove the hypothesis, serological analysis was examined by using 43 sera from Burchell's zebras (*Equus burchelli*) and 21 Thomson's gazelles from the Serengeti cocsystem for neutralizaing antibodies (Borchers et al., 2008). Seven zebra sera were positive for EHV-1 and EHV-9. The trigeminal ganglia of 17 other Burchell's zebras and one Thomson's gazelles were examined by PCR for EHV-9 gB and EHV-1 ICP0 genes. One zebra ganglion was positive for EHV-9 by PCR and confirmed by sequencing. These results suggest that the Burchell's zebras were latently infected by EHV-9.

2. Virology

2.1 Virus genome

A whole genome sequence of EHV-9 has been determined as 148371 base pairs (bp) (accession number AP010838). The genome encodes at least 80 open reading frames (ORF) (Fig. 3, Table 2). There is no large deletion and insertion comparing with EHV-9 and EHV-1 genomes. All of the ORFs in EHV-1 are conserved in EHV-9 genome. The EHV-9 ORFs have been serially numbered as homologues in EHV-1 genome (Telford et al., 1992). Identities of each ORF to EHV-1 ORFs range from 86% to 99% (Table 2). ORFs showing higher identity (99 %) are glycoprotein K (ORF6), UL37 tegument protein (ORF23), VP26 capsid protein (ORF25), glycoprotein B (ORF33), thymidine kinase (ORF38), a major capside protein (ORF42), DNA packaging terminase subunit 1 (ORF44_47), a nuclear protein UL3 (ORF60) and glycoprotein E (ORF74). ORFs showing lower identity (86 %) to EHV-1 include UL45 tegument/envelope protein (ORF15) and UL4 nonstructural protein (ORF58).

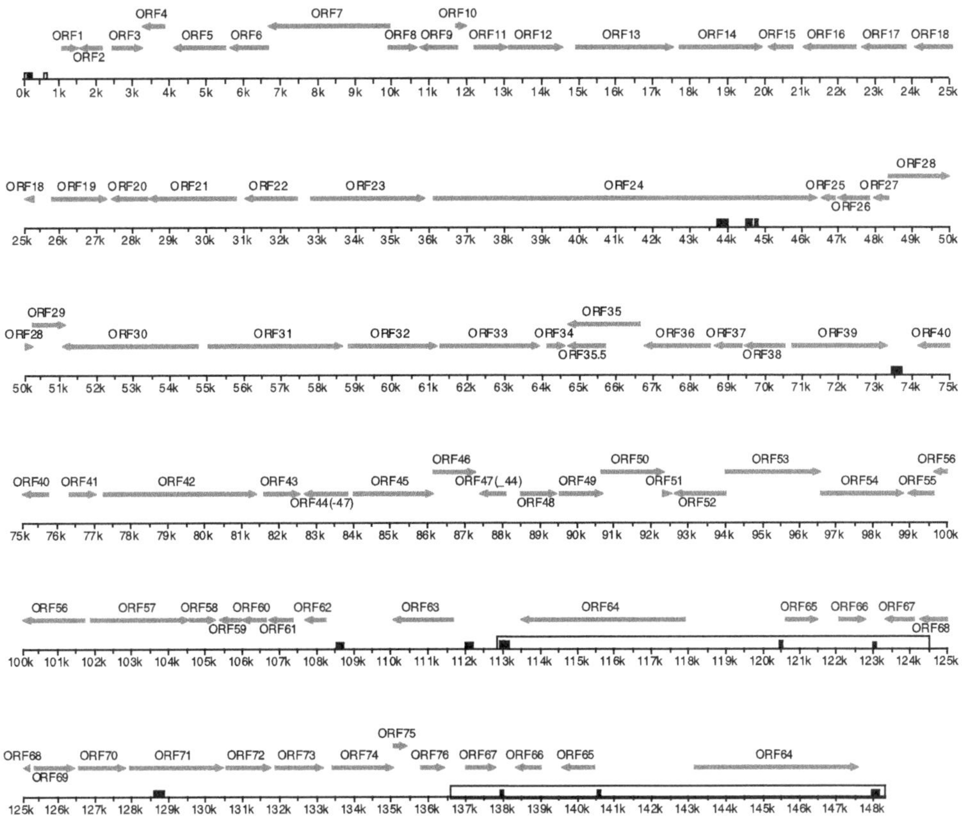

Fig. 3. Scheme of the EHV-9 genome based on the complete nucleotide sequence (AP010838)

ORF	Codons	Identity (%)	HSV-1	Predicted or confirmed functions
1	202	96	-	C-terminal hydrophobic domain
2	204	93	-	C-terminal hydrophobic domain
3	257	93	-	
4	200	93	UL55	
5	470	95	UL54	Post-translational regulator of gene expression
6	343	99	UL53	Glycoprotein (gK)
7	1079	95	UL52	Component of DNA helicase-primase complex; primase
8	245	97	UL51	Tegument protein
9	326	94	UL50	Deoxyuridine triphosphatase
10	100	95	UL49A	Envelope protein

ORF	Codons	Identity (%)	HSV-1	Predicted or confirmed functions
11	305	93	UL49	Tegument protein, VP22
12	449	97	UL48	Tegument protein; transactivator of immediate-early genes
13	868	93	UL47	Tegument protein
14	744	94	UL46	Tegument protein
15	219	86	UL45	Tegument/envelope protein
16	468	96	UL44	Envelope glycoprotein (gC); role in cell entry
17	401	96	UL43	Probable integral membrane protein
18	406	97	UL42	Processivity subunit of replicative DNA polymerase
19	497	96	UL41	Tegument protein; host shut-off factor
20	323	98	UL40	Small subunit of ribonucleotide reductase
21	790	97	UL39	Large subunit of ribonucleotide reductase
22	465	97	UL38	Capsid protein; component of intercapsomeric triplex
23	1021	99	UL37	Tegument protein
24	3439	96	UL36	Very large tegument protein
25	119	99	UL35	Capsid protein; located on tips of hexons, VP26
26	275	95	UL34	Membrane-associated phosphoprotein
27	139	95	UL33	Role in DNA packaging
28	620	93	UL32	Role in DNA packaging
29	326	98	UL31	
30	1220	97	UL30	Catalytic subunit of replicative DNA polymerase
31	1209	98	UL29	Single-stranded DNA-binding protein
32	775	98	UL28	DNA packaging terminase subunit 2
33	980	99	UL27	Envelope glycoprotein (gB); role in cell entry
34	160	93	-	Unknown
35	646	97	UL26	N-terminal protease domain acts in capsid maturation and is a capsid protein; C-teminal domain is the minor capsid scaffold protein
35.5	329	96	UL26.5	Major capsid scaffold protein
36	587	97	UL25	DNA packaging tegument protein

ORF	Codons	Identity (%)	HSV-1	Predicted or confirmed functions
37	272	96	UL24	Nuclear protein, related to neurovirulence
38	352	99	UL23	Thymidine kinase
39	850	96	UL22	Envelope glycoprotein (gH); complexes with gL; role in cell entry
40	530	97	UL21	Tegument protein
41	239	98	UL20	Integral membrane protein; role in virion egress
42	1376	99	UL19	Major capsid protein; component of hexons and pentons
43	314	98	UL18	Capsid protein; component of intercapsomeric triplex
44_47	734	99	UL15	DNA packaging terminase subunit 1
45	706	97	UL17	DNA packaging tegument protein
46	370	97	UL16	Tegument protein
48	318	93	UL14	Tegument protein
49	595	96	UL13	Tegument protein; probable serine-threonine protein kinase
50	565	96	UL12	Deoxyribonuclease; role in maturation/packaging of DNA
51	73	91	UL11	Myristylated tegument protein; role virion envelopement
52	451	98	UL10	Envelope glycoprotein (gM)
53	887	98	UL9	Replication origin-binding helicase
54	751	95	UL8	Component of DNA helicase-primase complex
55	303	96	UL7	Tegument progein
56	753	97	UL6	Minor capsid protein; role in DNA; role in DNA packaging
57	881	97	UL5	Component of DNA helicase-primase complex; helicase
58	224	86	UL4	Nuclear protein
59	182	87	-	Unknown
60	212	99	UL3	Nuclear protein
61	313	97	UL2	Uracil-DNA glycosylase
62	218	97	UL1	Envelope glycoprotein (gL); complexes with gH
63	533	90	RL2	Transcriptional regulator, ICP0

ORF	Codons	Identity (%)	HSV-1	Predicted or confirmed functions
64	1475	92	RS1	Transcriptional regulator, ICP4
65	291	94	US1	Regulatory protein ICP22
66	234	94	US10	Virion protein
67	269	94	-	Virulence determinant virion protein
68	296	93	US2	Virion protein
69	383	95	US3	Serine–threonine protein kinase
70	411	92	US4	Envelope glycoprotein (gG)
71	830	91	US5	Envelope glycoprotein (gp300)
72	402	97	US6	Envelope glycoprotein (gD); role in cell entry
73	425	94	US7	Envelope glycoprotein (gI); complexes with gE in Fc receptor
74	550	99	US8	Envelope glycoprotein (gE); complexes with gI in Fc receptor
75	130	97	US8A	Unknown
76	219	89	US9	Tegument protein

Identity was evaluated by protein-protein BLAST analysis.
-: there is no homologue in herpes simplex virus 1 (HSV-1) genome

Table 2. Characteristics of EHV-9 proteins

2.2 Host range in vitro and in nature

EHV-9 can be propagated by fetal equine kidney cells (FEK), Madine-Darby bovine kidney cells (MDBK), rabbit kidney cells (RK-13), murine fibroblast L929 cells, and human HeLa 229 cells. Cytopathic effects varied in each cell line. Lytic CPE is observed in FEK, RK-13 and HeLa 229, while syncitium formation is observed in MDBK (Fig.). EHV-9 can be also propagated in neural cells derived from a fetal equine brain as well as a fetal murine brain.
EHV-9 has been isolated from Thomson's gazelles, zebras (Borchers et al., 2008; Schrenzel et al., 2008), giraffes (Samy et al., 2009), polar bears (Schrenzel et al., 2008; Donovan et al., 2009) and onager (Schrenzel et al., 2008) as described in Section 1. Epizootiologically all of the cases in zoo animals associated with the presence of zebras. These data indicates that Burchell's zebra and other zebras might be a natural host of EHV-9 in nature.
EHV-9 can infect several animals experimentally. The experimental hosts include horse, goat, pig, cattle, hamster, mouse, rat, guineapig, dog, cat, and marmosette as described in the section 3.

2.3 Phylogenic relatedness to other related herpesviruses

The phylogenic tree constructed by using a part of glycoprotein B gene sequence indicates three groups of EHV-9, EHV-1 in horses and EHV-1 in zoo animals (Fig. 4).
EHV-1 derived from zoo animals might be considered as another type of equid herpesvirus. Unfortunately equine herpesvirus 8 glycoprotein G sequence is not available at present.

Sequences of glycoprotein G in EHV-1 derived from zoo animals would provide a clue to resolve the problem.

EHV-9 strain P19, prototype of EHV-9, is closely related to the strain 1220 which was derived from a Burcell's zebra (Borchers et al., 2008), while the isolate 4 derived from the polar bear associated with Grevy's zebra (Schrenzel et al., 2008) is distantly related to the other EHV-9s. These data suggest the EHV-9 would be strongly related to each species of zebras. Of cause, further research should be examined to prove the hypothesis.

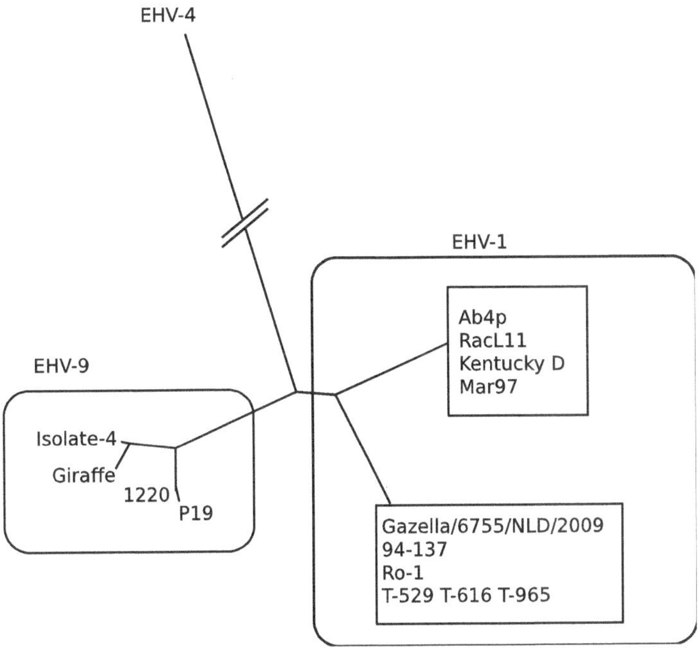

Fig. 4. A phylogenc tree of EHV-9 and other related viruses based on the glycoprotein B gene segment. The phylogenic tree was constructed by using PHYLIP package (Felsenstein, 2005). Accession numbers are as follows: EHV-9 P19 (D49800), 1220 (EU087294), Giraffe (AB439723), Isolate-4 (EU717150); EHV-1 Ab4p (AY665713), RacL11 (X95374), Kentucky D (AB279609), Mar97 (DQ095871), Gazella/6755/NLD/2009 (HM216495), 94-137 (AB280624), Ro-1 (DQ095872), T-529 (AB280630), T-616 (EU087295), T-965 (DQ095873); EHV-4 (M26171).

3. Pathology

3.1 Lethal Encephalitis in zoo, domestic and companion animals, and experimental small animals

EHV-9 caused lethal encephalitis in several animals such as Thomson's gazelles, giraffes, and polar bears naturally and goats, cats, dogs, mice, rats, hamster and marmosets experimentally. All of these infections can be regarded as encephalitis with neuronal degeneration, perivascular cuffing and gliosis. Histopathological characteristics will be described.

3.1.1 Thomson's gazelles

An outbreak of acute encephalitis occurred in a herd of Thomson's gazelle in a Japanese zoo. Seven of 9 gazelle died with or without neurological symptoms within a 3-week period as described in the section 1.1 (Fig. 5A). All animals had nonsuppurative encephalitis characterized by necrosis and degeneration of neurons (Fig. 5B), gliosis and perivascular aggregates of lymphocytes (Fig. 5C) in the cerebrum (Yanai et al., 1998). Five cases had intranuclear inclusion bodies in neurons compatible with those of herpesvirus. Immunohistochemically, a positive reaction to EHV-1 antigen was demonstrated in neurons in the necrotic areas of the cortex in all cases. The neuropathology of EHV-9 infection clearly differed from EHV-1-induced encephalitis in the horse, which is characterized by vasculitis, thrombosis, ischemia, and lack of intranuclear inclusion in neurons (Wada et al., 1991).

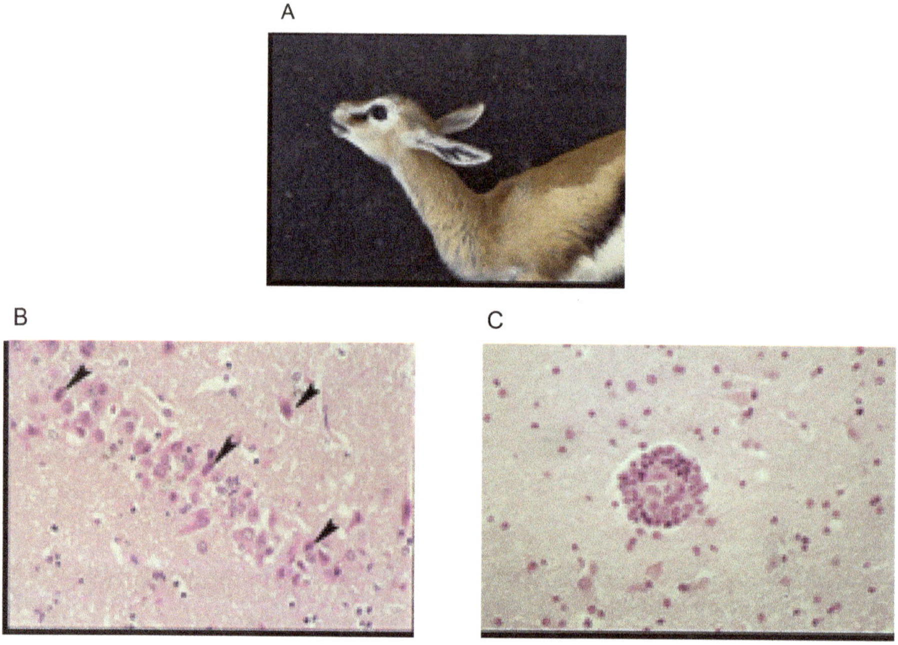

Fig. 5. A: A dead Thomson's gazelle. B: Neuronal necrosis with frequent nuclear inclusion formation. HE. C: Perivascular aggregates of lymphocytes in affected brain. HE.

3.1.2 Giraffe

Hoenerhoff et al. (2006) described as follows. The giraffe was in good body condition. There was a traumatic wound on the dorsal aspect of the tail base. There was a focal area of malacia within the cerebrum on cut section. There were no other lesions noted on gross necropsy examination.

Histopathological examination included sections of brain; cervical, thoracic, and lumbar spinal cord; heart; lungs; liver; spleen; kidneys; adrenal glands; rumen; abomasum; jejunum; ileum; and colon. There was severe multifocal nonsuppurative meningoencephalitis within the white and gray matter of the cerebral cortex, hippocampus, thalamus, midbrain, and medulla oblongata, and was most severe in the thalamus and ventrolateral portions of the cerebral cortex. Lesions were characterized by multifocal perivascular cuffs composed of moderate numbers of lymphocytes and histiocytes. The endothelium of affected blood vessels was swollen, and there were numerous microglial cell foci distributed diffusely in the gray and white matter. Multifocal neuronal necrosis was most evident in the ventral portion of the cerebral hemispheres, and areas of neuronal necrosis were occasionally associated with characteristic herpetic eosinophilic intranuclear inclusions in neurons and astrocytes.

3.1.3 Polar bear

Donovan et al. (2009) described as follows. The polar bear was in good body condition The meninges of the brain and spinal cord were diffusely congested. The caudodorsal lung lobes were edematous.

Histopathological findings were severe nonsuppurative meningoencephalitis, predominantly in the grey matter of the cerebrum. The most significantly affected region of the brain was the rostral telencephalon, particularly the rhinencephalon. Scattered regions of inflammation involved the olfactory bulbs, cerebrum, thalamus, midbrain, and rostral medulla. Inflammatory cells consisting of lymphocytes, plasma cells, macrophages, and fewer eosinophils formed perivascular cuffs within the meninges overlying the brain and Virchow-Robin spaces within the parenchyma, as well as more poorly delineated inflammatory cell infiltrates within the subjacent meninges, neuropil, and neuroparenchyma. Neuronal degeneration was characterized by peripheral localization or complete loss of Nissl substance, and neuronal necrosis consisted of cytoplasmic hyperosinophilia, loss of cytoplasmic detail, nuclear pyknosis, karyolysis, and karyorrhexis. Glial proliferation accompanied the inflammation, consisting of microgliosis and astrogliosis.

Within the nuclei of neurons and astrocytes, there were diffuse type and Cowdry type A inclusions. White matter tracts had random areas of vacuolation, axonal degeneration characterized by formation of axonal spheroids, demyelination, edema, and microg- lial and astrocytic gliosis. Additional histologic findings included mild, multifocal neutrophilic bronchiolitis, mild neutrophilic rhinitis, moderate pulmonary edema, mild lymphocytic myocarditis, and mild membranoproliferative glomerulonephritis.

3.1.4 Goats

Two young goats were inoculated intranasally with 10 ml of virus solution containing 5.25 x 10^6 PFU (Taniguchi et al., 2000a). These animals showed sudden neurological symptoms consisting of marked salivation, teeth grinding, convulsion, tremor and ataxia 8 days IP. One animal died 30 minutes after the onset of clinical signs and another was sacrificed 3 hours after the onset of teeth griding and foamy salvation. Both animals had fulminant encephalitis characterized by neuronal degeneration and necrosis with intranuclear inclusion bodies (Fig. 6).

3.1.5 Carnivors

In carnivore cats and dogs got fulminant encephalitis via nasal rout of inoculation with EHV-9, which suggested these animals to be fully susceptible to EHV-9 and that EHV-9 could cause fulminant encephalitis with high mortality in dogs and cats, as in gazelles and goats.

An acute lethal infection of EHV-9 was induced in cats by intranasal inoculation of 10^6 pfu (Yanai et al., 2003a). Four cats killed at 4, 5, 6 or 10 days after inoculation showed neurological signs consisting of hyper-excitability and aggressiveness, followed by tremors, occasional

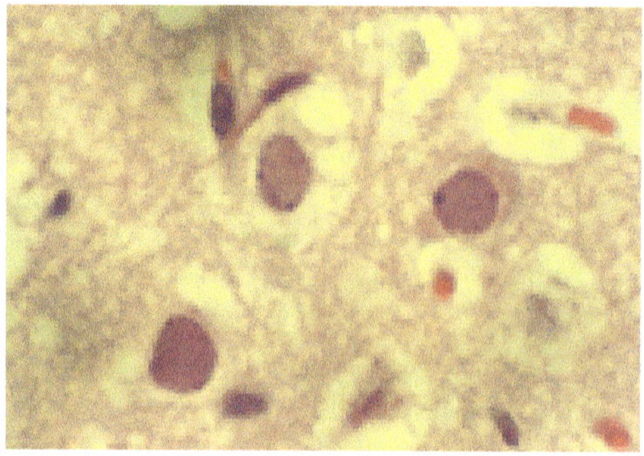

Fig. 6. Frequent intra-nuclear inclusion formation in the neuronal cells. HE stain.

convulsions, and depression. Histologically, the cats affected showed severe encephalitis characterized by neuronal degeneration and loss, intranuclear inclusions, perivascular aggregates of lymphocytes and gliosis in the cerebrum. The olfactory bulb and rhinencephalon were severely affected and collapsed, and eventually softened by complete destruction of both neuronal cells and glial cells. Using Double Label immunohistochemistry all cats showed proliferating astrocytes with double reactivities to both EHV-9 and GFAP, as well as EHV-9 antigen bearing neurons (Fig. 7A and B). These findings were most frequently observed in the intermediate stage of the infection (6th day post-inoculation by intranasal route) while in early stage of the infection (4th day post-inoculation by intranasal route), and 15th day of post-inoculation by intraperitoneal route, only small number of astrocytes showed reactivity to EHV-9. At the later stage (10th day post-ionculation), malacia was observed in the cortex together with marked decrease in the number of astrocytic cells showing GFAP reactivity as well as neuronal number decreased by collapse.

A B

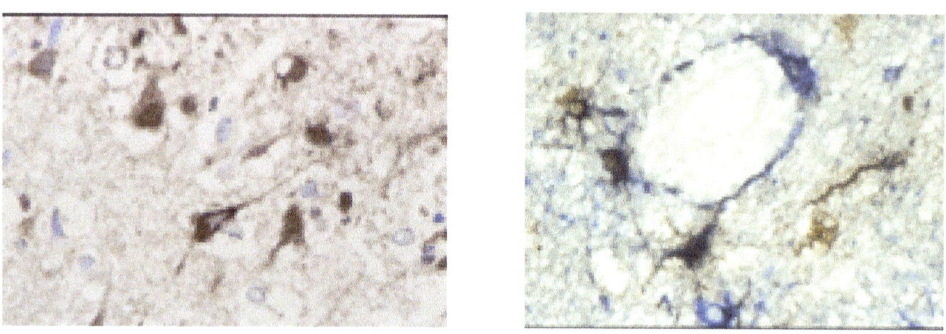

Fig. 7. A: Affected cat had encephalitis with EHV-9 antigen in the brain. IHC. ABC methods. B: Double Label immunohistochemistry showed proliferating astrocytes with double reactivities to both EHV-9 and GFAP, as well as EHV-9 antigen bearing neurons. ABC method.

EHV-9 was inoculated intranasally at 10^7 PFU in five dogs to assess its pathogenicity (Yanai et al., 2003b). Dogs affected showed weight loss, pyrexia, anorexia, and neurologic signs on the fourth day. The EHV-9 virus was recovered from the examined brain. Histologically, dogs had a fulminant encephalitis characterized by severe neuronal degeneration and loss, with intranuclear inclusions, glial reactions (Fig. 8A), perivascular aggregates of lymphocytes, and multi-focal perivascular hemorrhages (Fig. 8B). The olfactory bulb and the frontal and temporal lobes were predominantly affected. Immunohistochemistry revealed reactivity for EHV-9 antigens in neurons (Fig. 8C).

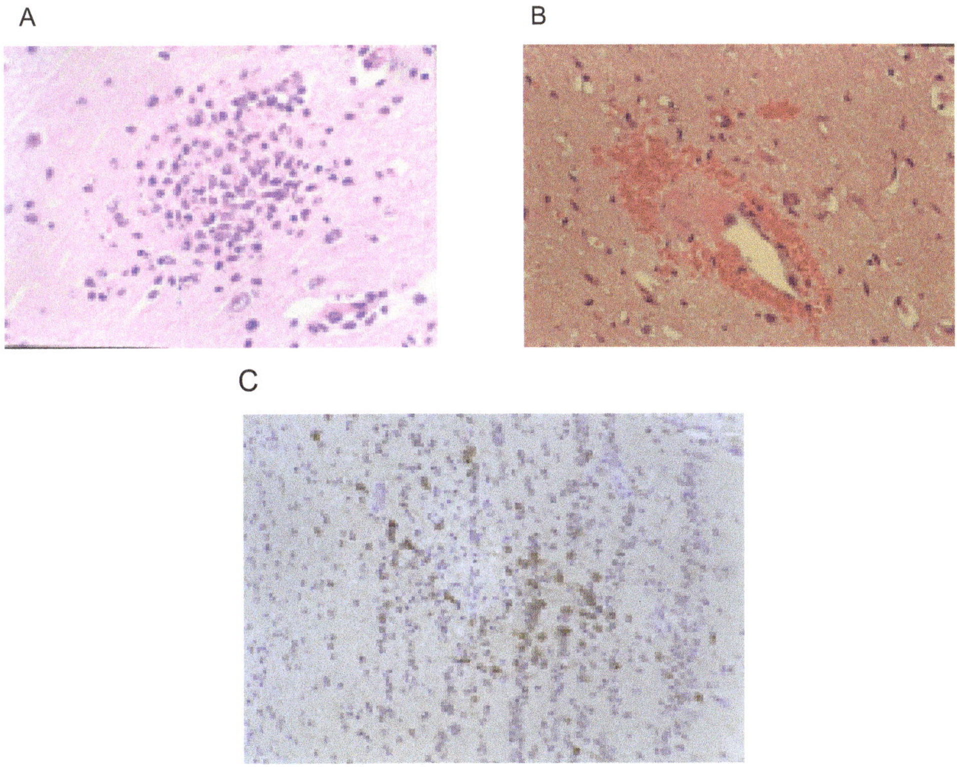

Fig. 8. A: There were frequent positive reaction to EHV-9 antigen in the neuronal cells in the olfactory bulb in a dog inoculated with EHV-9 intra-nasally. IHC. B: There were prominent glial reactions in the brain. HE stain. C: There were occasional perivascular hemorrhages in the affected brain. HE stain.

3.1.6 Rodents

In suckling mice and rats inoculated intra-cerebrally with 102 to 105 plaque-forming units (PFU) of cell-free viral suspension, growth deterioration (Fig. 9) and neurological symptoms, including depression and seizures were observed, and inoculated animals died within 8 days of inoculation (Fukushi et al., 1997). The brain of dead animal had severe neuronal degeneration and necrosis accompanied by numerous intranuclear inclusion bodies characteristic of herpesviruses.

In mice, rats and hamsters inoculated with 10^2 to 10^6 PFU via intranasal route (Fukushi et al., 1997). The animals had neurological signs, including depression or convulsion, and died of acute encephalitis characterized by neuronal degeneration and necrosis with intranuclear inclusion bodies (Fig. 10A and B). Mortality rates were 100% with 104 PFU and 33% with 10^2

PFU in young mice (Fukushi et al., 1997). Although the morphological features of E HV9-induced encephalitis was common in rodents, the hamsters were thought to more susceptible to EHV-9 via nasal route (Taniguchi et al., 2000a).

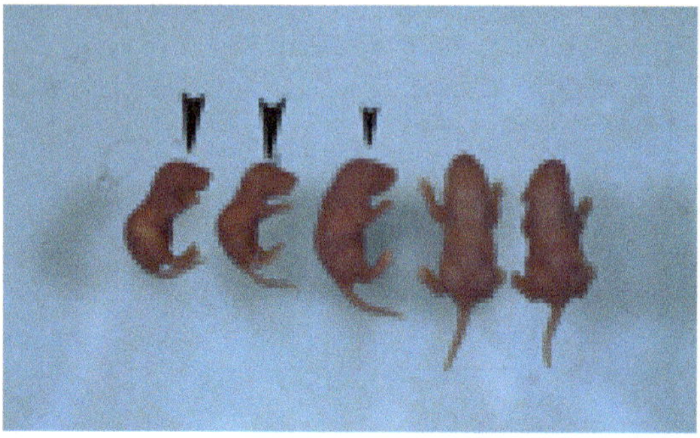

Fig. 9. A: Inoculate suckling rats (arrow heads) showed growth deterioration.

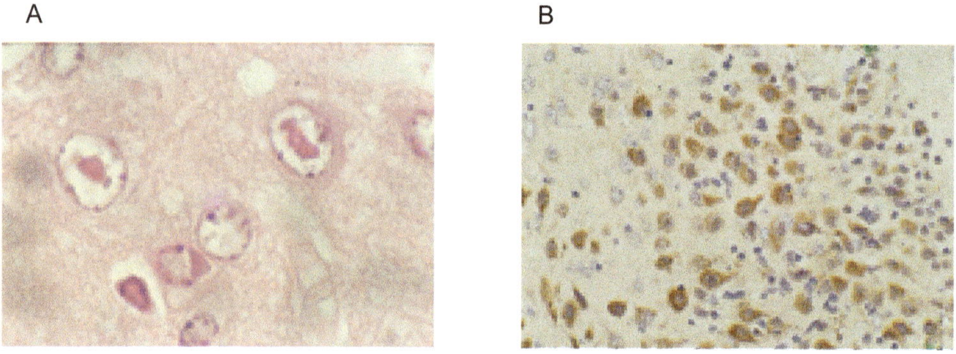

Fig. 10. A: There were frequent intranuclear inclusions in degenerating neuronal cells. A mouse inoculated with EHV-9 intra-nasally. HE stain. B: Most neuronal cells with inclusion body had positive reaction for EHV-9 antigen. A mouse inoculated with EHV-9 intra-nasally. IHC.

3.2 Inapparent encephalitis in several experimental hosts

EHV-9 also cause inapparent encephalitis in horses, cattel and pigs. Although animals inoculated with EHV-9 showed high fever and slight depression, the animals did not show neurological symptoms. These inapparent encephalitis were characterized as meningoencephalitis, gliosis and cuffing with EHV-9 antigen bearing neural cells. Histopathological characteristics will be described and discussed.

3.2.1 Horses

Two young adult horses were inoculated intranasally with 10 ml of virus solution containing 10^7 PFU and euthanized two weeks after inoculation (Taniguchi et al., 2000b). The animals showed no clinical symptom except a moderate fever (higher than 39oC). The brains showed a moderate degree of nonsuppurative encephalitis characterized by perivascular aggregates of lymphocytes (Fig. 11A) and gliosis (Fig. 11B). Neither neuronal necrosis nor intranuclear inclusions were observed in affected horses.

A B

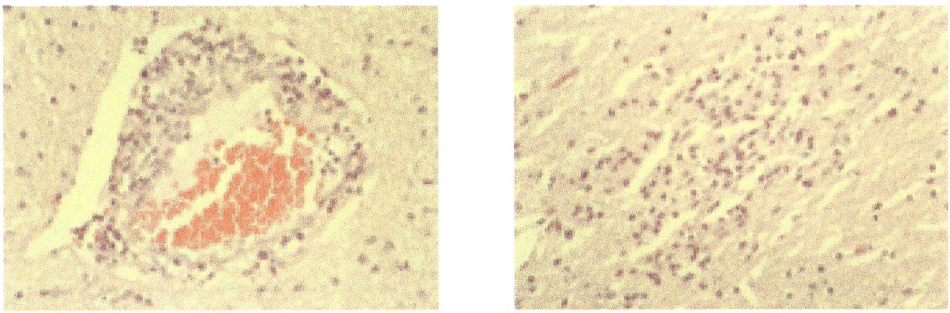

Fig. 11. A: Perivascular aggregates of lymphocytes in the affected brain. HE stain. B: Glial cells reaction was observed. HE stain.

3.2.2 Cattle

In cattle seven calves were inoculated intranasally with 10^5 and 10^7 PFU of the EHV-9 (El-Habashi et al., 2011). Three animals showed brain lesions consisting of glial reactions and perivascular aggregates of lymphocytes in the olfactory bulb and the frontal and temporal lobes. Additionally, the animal inoculated with 10^7 PFU showed neuronal degeneration and loss, as well as nuclear inclusions compatible with herpesvirus. EHV-9 was isolated from the brain of a calf and the lungs of two calves. The results suggested that cattle are susceptible to experimental infection with EHV-9 and at risk from natural infection from reservoir hosts.

3.3 Neuropathogenesis of EHV-9 by experimental infections

The infectivity and pathology of various routes including nasal, ocular, oral, intravenous (IV), or peritoneal routes of experimental infection were studied in hamsters (El-Habashi et al., 2010a). Clinically, all animals inoculated by the nasal route and ~25% inoculated by the oral and peritoneal routes showed neurological signs on days 3, 6 and 9 post-inoculation (PI), respectively. Neurological signs were not observed in animals administered EHV-9 by the IV and ocular routes. With the exception of animals administered EHV-9 by the IV route, all infected animals had lymphocytic meningoencephalitis. Although there were a number of differences in the severity and distribution of the lesions depending on the route of inoculation, the basic features of lymphocytic meningoencephalitis caused by EHV-9 were common. Lesions consisted of neuronal necrosis, perivascular aggregates of lymphocytes, plasma cells, and neutrophils, gliosis, intranuclear inclusion bodies, and diffuse lymphocytic infiltrates in the meninges. Viral antigen was detected in degenerated neurons in infected animals inoculated by the nasal, ocular, oral and peritoneal routes. The distribution of EHV-9 antigen was somewhat dependent upon inoculation route. There were no microscopic abnormalities nor viral antigen in animals treated by the IV route. This study provides new data about experimental EHV-9 infection in hamsters through routes other than the IV route. These results suggest that in the animals infected by the oral, ocular and peritoneal routes, EHV-9 might travel to the brain through nerves, other than by the olfactory route, after initial propagation at the site of viral entry.

To access transmission of EHV-9 in the nasal cavity and brain, a sagittal model using suckling hamsters was developed, and proved useful in detecting viral transmission as well as extension of pathological lesions using the sagittal section of the head (El-Habashi et al., 2010b). Suckling hamsters were inoculated intranasally with EHV-9, and were sacrificed at 6, 12, 18, 24, 36, 48 and 60 h PI. Sagittal sections of the whole heads were made to access viral kinetics and identify the progress of the neuropathological lesions. At 12-24 h PI the virus attached and propagated in the olfactory epithelium and migrated from one cell to another. At 48 h PI, the olfactory epithelium shows irregularity, necrosis, and erosion in the mucosa (Fig. 12 A), and immunohistochemistry showed encephalitis extending into the olfactory bulb, as well as virus antigen in the olfactory nerve. The trigeminal ganglion showed neuronal necrosis and neurophagia of the trigeminal ganglion cells at 48 h PI (Fig. 12B). One of the most striking findings was the presence of the viral antigen in the connection of the trigeminal sensory nerve root to the brain stem, the pons and medulla oblongata, as well as weak positive reactions in the trigeminal nerve at 60 h PI (Fig. 12C). These results suggested that the sagittal model using suckling hamsters might be useful in accessing the kinetics of neuro-virulent viruses, including EHV-9.

A B C

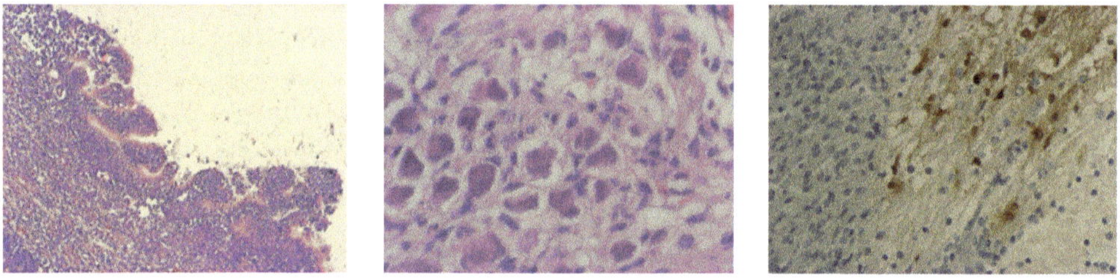

Fig. 12. A: At 48 h PI, the olfactory epithelium shows irregularity, necrosis, and erosion in the mucosa. HE stain. B: At 48 h PI, the trigeminal ganglion shows neuronal necrosis, neurophagia of the trigeminal ganglion cells. HE stain. C: Results of immunolabeling with EHV-9 antibody at 60 h PI. Presence of the viral antigen in the connection of the trigeminal sensory nerve root to the brain stem. IHC.

The kinetics and neuropathogenicity of equine herpesvirus 9 (EHV-9) were studied in hamsters by means of intraperitoneal inoculation (El-Nahass et al., 2011) (Fig. 13). Five-week-old Syrian hamsters and 5-day-old Suckling hamsters were inoculated with 50 and 15 μl of 2 x 10^6 pfu/ml of EHV-9 virus solution, respectively. After inoculation, EHV-9 antigens were detected in the peritoneal macrophages, which were possibly the primary site of virus attachment and propagation at 6 h PI (Fig. 13B). At 12 h PI, the viral antigen was observed in both the abdominal ganglions (mainly the celiac ganglions) and the peripheral nerves derived from the spinal cord. The virus antigen was seen in the dorsal root (spinal) ganglions (Fig. 13C) and in different parts of the spinal cord especially the mid-lumbar and cervical spinal cord at 24 and 36 h PI respectively. At 96 h PI, the virus antigen was detected in the most caudal part of the brain as well as the intestinal myenteric plexuses. PCR conducted on the blood, spinal cord and brain samples revealed EHV-9 DNA in both the spinal cord, at 24 h PI, and in blood, at 36 h PI. Based on these results, EHV-9 possibly traveled from the myenteric plexus or abdominal ganglions via the peripheral nerves and spinal cord, and finally reached the brain after initial propagation in the abdominal macrophages.

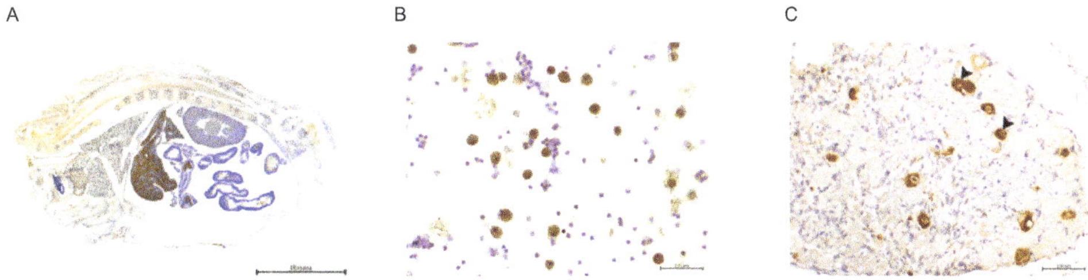

Fig. 13. A: Sagittal section of the entire body of a suckling hamster from the neck to the tail showing all internal organs. IHC. Bar, 10 nm. B: Expression of EHV-9 antigen in peritoneal macrophages at 6 h PI. Bar, 100 micrometer. C: Expression of EHV-9 antigen in the nucleus and cytoplasm of neuron in abdominal ganglion at 24 h PI. IHC. Bar, 100 micrometer.

Several routes of viral entry into the central nervous system (CNS) have been postulated in the neurotropic herpesvirus, which include the neural, olfactory, and hematogenous routes (Johnson, 1998). Other neurotropic herpes viruses, including herpes simplex virus-1 (HSV-1) and porcine herpesvirus-1, may enter the CNS via the intravenous, intramuscular, and intraperitoneal routes (Johnson, 1998). It has been previously hypothesized in hamsters and pigs that a possible route of EHV-9 infection is from the nasal mucosa along the olfactory pathway, vomeronasal organ, and/or trigeminal nerve (Fukushi et al., 2000; Narita et al., 2000) and then trans-synaptically via its connections to the hippocampus, amygdala, and cerebral cortex. Induction of encephalitis by intranasal inoculation in different animals including mice, rats (Fukushi et al., 1997), hamsters (Fukushi et al., 2000), goats (Taniguchi et al., 2000b), pigs (Narita et al., 2000), dogs and cats (Yanai et al., 2003a, b), common marmosets (Kodama et al., 2007) and cattle (El-Habashi et al., 2011) suggests that EHV-9 gains access to the brain via olfactory neurons of the olfactory mucosa specially there was inflammatory reaction in the olfactory mucosa of some of these animals and olfactory bulbs, cerebrum especially the frontal lobe, mid brain and medulla oblongata in most of these animals. Another possible route might be hematogenous dissemination from infected lungs. It is plausible to consider that EHV-9 may have entered the CNS from the nasal mucosa along the olfactory pathway to limbic structures, as was found in other virus, like Bornavirus and rabies virus infection (Gosztonyi et al., 1993).

It was proved that EHV-9 migrates from nasal cavity to the brain through the olfactory nerve after initial propagation in the olfactory receptor neurons in suckling hamster (El-Habashi et al., 2010b). At 48 h PI, EHV-9 antigen was detected in most of the olfactory receptor neurons as well as in the central processes of the olfactory epithelial neurons, olfactory nerve and olfactory bulb. The olfactory epithelium offer direct free surface on the internal lining of the nasal cavity, after propagation in olfactory receptor neurons, the virus could travel directly through olfactory nerve to the brain while the terminal nerve endings of the maxillary branch of the trigeminal nerve lie in the submucosa and could be only infected with the virus if the epithelial surface is damaged and consequently the axons are directly exposed to the virus and this suggested from suckling hamster experiment as well as common marmoset which showed necrotizing rhinitis as well as late access of the virus to the trigeminal nerve, pons and medulla oblongata (El-Habashi et al, 2010b; Kodama et al., 2007). One study compared various routes of experimental EHV-9 inoculation in Syrian hamsters (Fukushi et al., 2000), including intranasal, intravenous, intraperitoneal, intramuscular, intraocular, and subcutaneous routes, but only intranasal inoculation induced disease. However, in more recent study, possible infection by different routes of inoculation including, nasal, ocular, peritoneal and oral routes were evident. There may be discrepancies in EHV-9 infection of the brain based on the route of inoculation when animals are inoculated with the same quantity of virus (El-Habashi et al, 2010a).

4. Conclusion: EHV-9 infection as a model of cross-species viral transmissions

Based on previous experimental studies in different animals inoculated via the nasal route, the olfactory pathway (i.e. through the olfactory nerves) is the major route of transmission of EHV-9 into the CNS. However, recent study that compared different routes of inoculation clearly indicates that virus can enter the CNS after administration of EHV-9 via the oral, peritoneal, and ocular routes, and that there are differences in the distribution of antigen-positive cells and in the location and severity of the cerebral lesions. Thus, EHV-9 may gain access to the CNS through a non-olfactory route as these animals inoculated via these non-nasal routes did not exhibit EHV-9 induced rhinitis, and the olfactory bulbs showed milder lesions and fewer viral antigen-positive cells than observed in the animals infected via the nasal route.

One of the striking finding was that animals infected via the ocular route had mild and localized lesions in the rhinencephalon, which indicated that the virus had traveled to the CNS through the optic nerve. Similar to what is reported about fatal infections by Cercopithecine herpes virus 1 (B virus) in humans via ocular exposure from biological fluid from macaque monkeys (CDC, 1999).

The differences in the incubation period and paths of travel to the CNS among the various routes in resulting in a variety of clinical signs and histopathological features, suggests a dependency on the replication of the virus at the site of entry and its opportunity to access regional nerves to travel to the brain. A similar hypothesis was proposed in the case of pigs infected orally by EHV-9 (Narita et al., 2000), where the virus was thought to travel centripetally in the nerve fibers from the oral mucosa to the trigeminal ganglion, eventually entering the olfactory lobes (Chowdhury et al., 1997; Kritas, et al., 1994; Narita et al., 1976).

Previously, EHV-9 antigen was found in the neurons and neural fibers but not in the glial cells in the brain, indicating that neurons are the susceptible cells to EHV-9 in the CNS of hamsters (Fukushi et al., 2000). However, other neurotropic herpesviruses such as herpes simplex virus 1 (HSV-1) and pseudorabies virus (PRV) are known to infect glial cells as well as neurons (Johnson, 1998). Astrocytes infection of EHV-9 was described in the cases of a giraffe and a polar bear (Donovan et al., 2009; Hoenerhoff et al., 2006). Immunohistochemistry demonstrated the presence of EHV-9 antigen in the neurons and neuronal fibers including the axons and dendrites in the brain of the goat and the naturally infected bear which indicate a trans-synaptic spread of EHV-9 from neuron to neuron via the neuronal fibers (Taniguchi et al., 2000b; Donovan et al., 2009). Similar transmission has been shown in pseudorabies viral infection (Card et al, 1990). In suckling hamster study, there was necrosis of some of trigeminal ganglion cells as well as detection of the viral antigen in the same ganglion and in the connection between trigeminal sensory nerve root and the brain stem at the level of the pons and medulla oblongata. Based on previous findings, the neurotropism might be the most characteristic property of EHV-9, differentiating it from other neurotropic herpesviruses. Similar transneural passage was suggested after intranasal infection with IBR virus (Narita et al, 1979).

EHV-9 infection can be regarded as one of cross-species viral transmission. In nature, natural barriers exist to prevent the cross-species transmission as well as natural clearance such as predation by carnivors can hide the lethal cross-species transmission. An artificial situation of zoos or farms can cause cross-species transmission among carrier animals and susceptible animals. However, some species do not show clinical symptoms even though they can be infected by viruses. In EHV-9 infection, all of the animals infected by EHV-9 caused various degree of meningo-encephalitis. It is not clear what kind of factors are involved in the clinical course of EHV-9 infection.

5. References

Borchers K, Lieckfeldt D, Ludwig A, Fukushi H, Allen G, Fyumagwa R, Hoare R: Detection of equid ferpesvirus 9 DNA in the trigeminal ganglia of a Burchell's zebra from the Serengeti ecosystem. J Vet Med Sci 70: 1377–1381, 2008

Borchers K, Wiik H, Frolich K, Ludiwig H, East ML: Antibodies against equine herpesviruses and equine arteritis virus in Burchell's zebra (*Equus Burchelli*) from the Serengeti ecosystem. J Wildl Dis 41: 80-86, 2005

CDC: Hazard ID 5- Cercopithecine herpesvirus 1 (B Virus) infection resulting from ocular exposure. National Institute for Occupational Safety and Health (NIOSH). Publication 99-100, 1999

Chowdhury SI, Lee BJ, Mosier D, Sur JH, Osori FA, Kennedy G, Weiss ML: Neuropathology of bovine herpesvirus type 5 (BHV-5) meningo-encephalitis in a rabbit seizure model. J Comp Pathol 117: 295-310, 1997

Donovan TA, Schrenzel MD, Tucker T, Pessier AP, Bicknese B, Busch MD, Wise AG, Maes R, Kiupel M, McKnight C, Nordhausen RW: Meningoencephalitis in a polar bear caused by equine herpesvirus 9 (EHV-9). Vet Pathol 46:1138-43, 2009

El-Habashi N, Murakami M, EL-Nahass E, Hibi D, Sakai H, Fukushi H, Sasseville V, Yanai T: Study on the infectivity of equine herpesvirus 9 (EHV-9) by different routes of inoculation in hamsters. Vet Pathol 47: 1-7, 2010a

El-Habashi N, EL-Nahass E, Fukushi H, Hibi D,Sakai H, Sasseville V, Yanai T: Experimental intranasal infection of equine herpesvirus 9 (EHV-9) in suckling hamsters: Kinetics of viral transmission and inflammation in the nasal cavity and brain. J NeuroVirol 16: 242-248, 2010b

El-Habashi N, EL-Nahass E, Fukushi H, Namihira Y, Hagiwara H, Fukushi H, Narita M, Hirata A, Sakai H, Yanai T: Neuropathogenicity of equine herpesvirus 9 in cattle. J Eqine Vet Sci 31: 72-77, 2011

El-Nahass E, El-Habashi N, Nayel M, Kasem S, Fukushi H, Suzuki Y, Hirata A, Sakai H, Yanai T: Kinetics and pathogenicity of equine herpesvirus 9 infection following intraperitoneal inoculation in hamsters. J Comp Pathol doi:10.1016/j.jcpa.2011.01.009, 2011

Felsenstein J. PHYLIP (Phylogeny Inference Package) version 3.6. Distributed by the author. Department of Genome Sciences, University of Washington, Seattle, 2005

Fukushi H, Tomita T, Taniguchi A, Ochiai Y, Kirisawa R, Matsumura T, Yanai T, Masegi T, Yamaguchi T, Hirai K: Gazelle herpesvirus 1: A new neurotropic herpesvirus immunologically related to equine herpesvirus 1. Virology 227: 34-44,1997

Fukushi H, Taniguchi A, Yasuda K, Yanai T, Masegi T, Yamaguchi T, Hirai K: A hamster model of equine herpesvirus 9 induced encephalitis. J Neuro Virol 6: 314-319, 2000

Gosztonyi G, Dietzschold B, Kao M, Rupprecht CE, Ludwig H and Koprowski H. Rabies and Borna disease: a comparative pathogenetic study of two neurovirulent agents. Lab Invest 68: 285–95, 1993

Johnson RT: Viral infections of the nervous system, 2nd ed. Lippincott-Raven Publishers, Philadelphia. 1998

Hoenerhoff MJ, Janovitz EB, Richman LK, Murphy DA, Butler TC, Kiupel M. Fatal herpesvirus encephalitis in a reticulated giraffe (*Giraffa camelopardalis reticulata*). Vet Pathol. 43:769–772, 2006

Kodama A, Yanai T, Yomemaru K, Sakai H, Masegi T, Yamada S, Fukushi H, Kuraishi T, Hattori S, Kai C: Acute neuropathogenicity with experimental infection of equine herpesvirus 9 in common marmosets (*Callithrix jacchus*). J Med Primatol 36 : 335 - 342, 2007

Kritas SK, Pensaert MB, Mettenleiter TC: Invasion and spread of single glycoprotein deleted mutants of Aujeszky's disease virus (ADV) in the trigeminal nervous pathway of pigs after intranasal inoculation. Vet Microbiol 40: 323-334, 1994

Montali RJ, Allen GP, Bryans JT, Phillips LG, Bush M. Equine herpesvirus type 1 abortion in an onager and suspected herpesvirus myelitis in a zebra. J Am Vet Med Assoc. 187:1248–1249, 1985

Narita M, Inui S, Namba K, Shimizu Y: Trigeminal ganglionitis and encephalitis in calves intranasally inoculated with infectious bovine rhinotracheitis virus. J Comp Pathol 86: 93-100, 1976

Narita M, Ishikawa Y, Inui S. Neural changes in calves intranasally inoculated with two strains of infectious bovine rhinotracheitis virus. J Comp Pathol, 89, 489-494, 1979.

Narita M, Uchimura A, Kimura K, Tanimura N, Yanai T, Masegi T, Fukushi H, Hirai K: Brain lesions and transmission of experimental equine herpesvirus type 9 in pigs. Vet Pathol 37: 476-479, 2000

Schrenzel MD, Tucker TA, Donovan TA, Martin DM, Busch MDM, Wise AG, Maes RK, Kiupel M: New hosts for equine herpesvirus 9. Emerging Infectious Diseases 14: 1616-1619, 2008

Taniguchi A, Fukushi H, Matsumura T, Yanai T, Masegi T, Hirai K: Pathogenicity of a new neurotropic equine herpesvirus 9 (Gazelle herpesvirus 1) in horses. J Vet Med Sci 62: 215-218, 2000a

Taniguchi A, Fukushi H, Yanai T, Masegi T, Hirai K: Equine herpesvirus 9 induced lethal encephalitis in experimentally infected goats. Arch Virol 145: 2619-2627, 2000b

Telford EA, Watson MS, McBride K, Davison AJ: The DNA sequence of equine herpesvirus-1. Virology 189: 304-316, 1992

Wada R, Kanamaru T, Yokota S, Nanbu M, Matsumura T: Pathological observations on 2 horses of myeloencephalopathy associated with Equine Herpesvirus 1 (EHV-1). Bull.Equine Res.Inst.28,21-28, 1991

Yanai T, Sakai T, Fukushi H, Hirai K, Narita M, Sakai H and Masegi T: Neuro-pathological study of Gazelle Herpesvirus 1 (Equine Herpesvirus 9) infection in Thomsonis Gazelles (*Gazella thomsoni*). J Comp Pathol 119: 158-168, 1998

Yanai T, Fujishima N, Fukushi H, Hirata A, Sakai H, Masegi T: Experimental infection of equine herpesvirus 9 in dogs. Vet Pathol 40: 263-267, 2003a

Yanai T, Tsujioka S, Sakai H, Fukushi H, Hirai K, Masegi T: Experimental infection with equine herpesvirus 9 (EHV-9) in cats. J Comp Pathol 128: 113-118, 2003b

6

Blood-Brain Barrier Disruption and Encephalitis in Animal Models of AIDS

Nicole A. Renner, Andrew A. Lackner and Andrew G. MacLean
Tulane National Primate Research Center, Program in Neuroscience, Covington
USA

1. Introduction

The pathogenesis of HIV/SIV encephalitis (HIVE/SIVE) remains incompletely understood, but is associated with alterations in the blood brain barrier. In animals infected with pathogenic strains of simian immunodeficiency virus (SIV), such as SIVmac239 and SIVmac251, the virus can be consistently found in the central nervous system (CNS) within 10 to 14 days of infection: at the time of peak viremia (Lackner et al., 1994). This also appears to be true in human immunodeficiency virus (HIV)-infected humans, but the number of cases examined during peak viremia is very small (Davis et al., 1992). In SIV-infected macaques at this early time point, endothelial cells of the blood-brain barrier (BBB) are activated and integrity of the BBB is compromised (Stephens et al., 2003). As viral loads decline toward set point at roughly two months post infection the endothelial activation subsides and BBB integrity is largely restored (Sasseville et al., 1995, Lackner et al., 1994, Annunziata, 2003, Zink et al., 1998). However, in the terminal phases of disease, viral loads rise and approximately one third of animals develop SIV encephalitis (SIVE), which is associated with breakdown of the BBB.

The exact mechanisms of BBB disruption are unclear, but it is known that numerous resident and transitory cell populations in the CNS can be infected, with CD14-positive perivascular macrophages being the primary productively-infected cell type (Little et al., 1999, Gorry et al., 2003, Bissel and Wiley, 2004, Ryzhova et al., 2002, Liu et al., 2004, Brack-Werner, 1999, Trillo-Pazos et al., 2003, Williams et al., 2001, Fischer-Smith et al., 2001). Nervous system manifestations associated with HIV infection of humans or SIV infection of rhesus macaques include an encephalitis (SIV or HIV encephalitis, SIVE/HIVE) characterized by astrocytic and microglial activation and scattered perivascular aggregates of mononuclear cells and multinucleated giant cells. These perivascular lesions contain large numbers of HIV/SIV-infected cells, the majority of which are monocyte/macrophages. The presence of cells productively-infected with SIV/HIV in the parenchyma has been shown to induce a response in astrocytes (Nath, 1999, Tyor et al., 1992, Persidsky et al., 1999, Persidsky et al., 2000) which in turn may lead to decreased tight junction protein expression and a leaky BBB (Dallasta et al., 1999, Persidsky et al., 1997, Moses and Nelson, 1994, Boven et al., 2000, Luabeya et al., 2000, Andras et al., 2003, Annunziata, 2003, Kanmogne et al., 2005, Kanmogne et al., 2007, MacLean et al., 2004b, Persidsky, 1999).

Astrocytes, along with microglia, are resident cells in the brain involved in inflammation. Their role during inflammation is not well understood; it is believed that both cell types are involved in propagating and limiting inflammation (Kielian, 2004). Astrocytes and microglia are the primary cell types found in glia scar formation. They serve a vital role during injury to the brain: both astrocytes and microglia are capable of promoting an inflammatory response, but are also known to have cytoprotective and anti-inflammatory effects (Hauwel et al., 2005, Park et al., 2003). The complex nature of astrocytes' chemokine response has recently been shown to vary by pathogen (McKimmie and Graham, 2010).

2. Overview of viral encephalitides

There are numerous viruses that can cause encephalitis. For some of these viruses the encephalitis is such a prominent part of the subsequent disease that "encephalitis" is part of the name. Examples include Eastern, Western and Venezuelan encephalitis viruses and St. Louis encephalitis virus all caused by arthropod borne (arbo) viruses that belong to several different virus families (Togaviridae, Flaiviridae) (Adams 2008 and Ciota 2009). In most instances these "encephalitis viruses" cause disease by targeting neurons. In contrast lentivirurses of the family Retroviridae, such as HIV and SIV, which are the major focus of this review, cause disease by a much less direct means.

2.1 Lentiviral encephalitis

The precise mechanism of lentiviral entry to brain is still a subject of some debate. In 1982, Bill Narayan postulated the "Trojan Horse" hypothesis whereby visna virus (one of the first lentiviruses described in detail) entered brains of sheep and goats by hiding within circulating monocytes and then once in the brain, emerged to cause disease (Narayan et al., 1982). It has been proposed that circulating monocytes enter the brain during normal immune surveillance (Williams and Hickey, 1995). However, this remains an issue of debate (Fischer-Smith and Rappaport, 2005). Regardless, the predominate cell infected early in infection of the brain is the CD14+ monocyte-derived macrophage (Williams et al., 2001).

2.2 Simian immunodeficiency virus infection

The simian and human immunodeficiency viruses are closely related with HIV having originated from at least two cross species transmission events from monkeys to humans in West Africa in the mid 20th century (P Marx, personal communication and (Worobey et al., 2010). Infection of macaques (primarily rhesus macaques—*Macaca mulatta* and Pigtail macaques - *M. nemestrina*) with SIV follows a near identical course to HIV infection of humans with a peak viral load approximately two weeks following infection, subsiding to a viral set point which rises again with development of AIDS. The disease in brain also follows a similar course. SIV and HIV infection have, in addition to acute and terminal phases, a chronic, relatively asymptomatic, phase, during which very little is known about the physiology and pathology (or lack thereof) in brain. For this reason, we will focus on the acute and terminal stages of infection when encephalitis is an issue.

2.2.1 Acute infection

The precise mechanisms involved in the recruitment of the first viral-infected cell into the brain is the topic of much speculation and debate, although increased expression of VCAM-1 (CD106) by brain endothelial cells is a possibility (Sasseville et al., 1995, Sasseville et al., 1992). CD106 is one of several vascular adhesion molecules involved in directing leukocyte recruitment to tissues (Luster et al., 2005). Expression of CD106 was not limited to areas immediately adjacent to viral-infected cells, but was diffuse throughout brain, remaining elevated through at least 23 weeks post infection (well beyond peak viral load and establishment of viral set point). We have shown that CD106 expression is upregulated on endothelial cells and astrocytes following incubation with either viral-infected cells or their supernatants (MacLean et al., 2004a, MacLean et al., 2004b), and by others on astrocytes using Theiler's Murine Encephalomyelitis Virus (Rubio et al., 2010). That cell-free virus was able to stimulate endothelial cells to express CD106 may explain the diffuse staining earlier observed by Sasseville *et al.*

Both HIV and SIV use two cellular receptors in combination for infection: the CD4 molecule and a chemokine receptor, the two most common being CCR5 and CXCR4 (Moore et al., 2004). Monocyte/macrophages express these receptors and thus SIV and HIV are macrophage tropic (Salazar-Gonzalez et al., 2009). During early SIV infection, the predominate cell type productively-infected in brain is the monocyte-derived macrophage (Williams et al., 2001). Due to the many similarities between HIV infection of humans and SIV infection of macaques, SIV infection of macaques, particularly of Indian-origin rhesus macaques, has become the most widely used model for HIV pathogenesis studies.

2.2.2 Terminal disease

In humans with symptoms of AIDS dementia complex (the clinical spectrum of illness that includes individuals with HIV encephalitis), there are altered subpopulations of circulating monocytes; CD14 expression is lower, and CD16 and CD69 are both increased (Pulliam et al., 1997, Zhou et al., 2007, Munsaka et al., 2009). Similar changes in monocyte / macrophage populations are also observed throughout disease progression in macaques infected with SIV (Bissel et al., 2006b, Bissel et al., 2006a, Kuroda, 2010, Kim et al., 2005, Williams and Hickey, 2002).

While circulating monocytes are not thought to be productively-infected, the increased numbers of primed monocytes would likely lead to an increased potential for trafficking of cells capable of being infected to brain. The presence of infected monocytes is known to activate endothelial cells of the BBB to express CD106 (MacLean et al., 2004a, MacLean et al., 2004b) and leads to disruption of tight junction proteins including ZO-1 and claudin 5 (Andras et al., 2003, Ivey et al., 2009b, Kanmogne et al., 2007, Luabeya et al., 2000, Persidsky et al., 2006, Huang et al., 2009).

In contradistinction to CD106 expression, the loss of tight junction proteins is largely limited to areas close to viral infected cells (Luabeya et al., 2000, Andras et al., 2003, Kanmogne et al., 2005, Kanmogne et al., 2007, Persidsky et al., 2006), and Renner et al, in press. In those areas where encephalitis is observed, the loss of tight junction protein expression can extend over 150μm (MacLean et al., 2005). As with primary infection, productively-infected cells in brain are largely monocyte-derived macrophages, including microglia in close proximity to blood vessels (Roberts et al., 2004b, Gonzalez-Scarano and Martin-Garcia, 2005). The conceptual framework for interactions of the various cell types involved is summarized in Figure 1.

3. Blood-brain barrier disruption in HIVE/SIVE

As outlined above, lentiviruses are thought to enter the brain within circulating infected monocytes during immune surveillance. Numerous studies have been undertaken to determine the reasons underlying increased monocyte migration into brain following lentiviral infection. HIV-infected leukocytes are primed for adhesion (Hallett, 1995), having already shed L-selectin, and increased expression of CD11b/CD18 compared with monocytes from healthy controls (Elbim et al., 1999). Therefore, it is possible that even barely increased levels of chemokines expressed within the parenchyma would lead to increased migration of monocytes. Recent studies have shown that glial cells are stimulated to produce chemokines in response to inflammatory cytokines (Renner et al., 2011, Thompson and Van Eldik, 2009) known to be secreted by SIV-infected macrophages (Orandle et al., 2002). Therefore, the role played by glial cells and tight junctions requires further discussion.

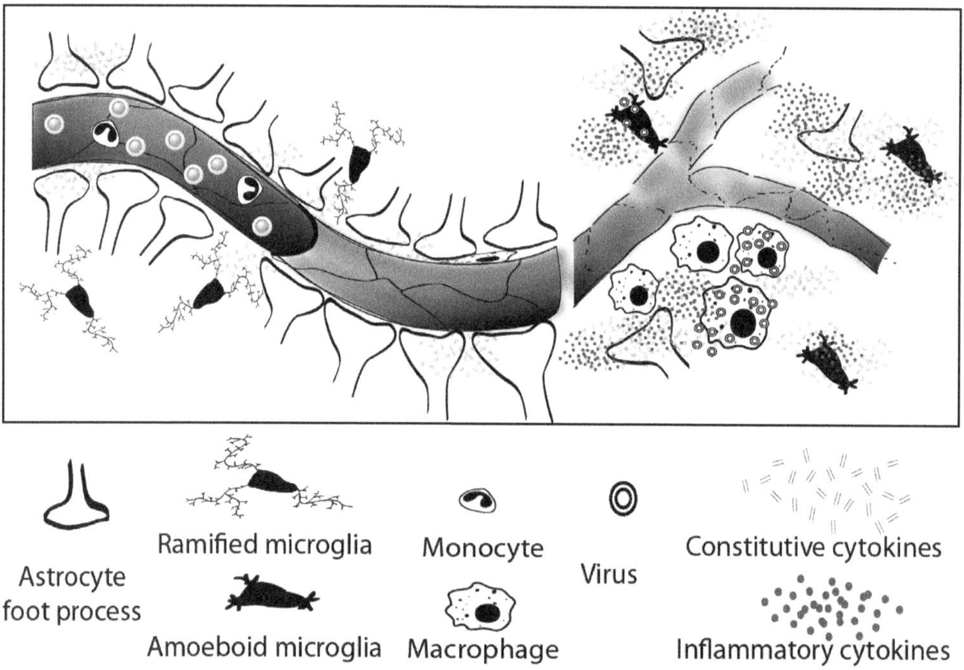

Fig. 1. Schematic of key players in the development of SIV encephalitis. At left, a cutaway section of a cerebral microvessel showing circulating blood cells. At center, normal blood vessel with tight junctions (solid lines) evident between endothelial cells. Astrocyte foot processes are highly evident with occasional microglia. Low levels of cytokines and chemokines are expressed. At right a microvessel in an encephalitic lesion, showing disrupted junctions (dashed lines), leakage of serum proteins into parenchyma, displaced astrocyte foot processes and increased cytokines/ chemokines concomitant with increased numbers of perivascular macrophages.

3.1 Tight junction proteins

The primary defining feature of the blood brain barrier (BBB) is the presence of tight junction proteins between brain microvascular endothelial cells (BMEC). Immediately subjacent to the endothelial cells, and anchoring them to the underlying tissues, is the basement membrane which is composed largely of Type IV collagen and laminin. Perivascular macrophages and the foot processes of astrocytes and microglia surround the endothelial cells (Hickey and Kimura, 1988, Graeber et al., 1992, Streit and Graeber, 1993, Lassmann et al., 1991).

Tight junctions are a fibrillary network of transmembrane proteins that can be phosphorylated to regulate physiologic processes such as replacement of perivascular macrophages by circulating monocytes. This phosphorylation can function differently depending if the stimulus is from the luminal or parenchymal side of the BBB. The presence of adhesion molecules on the luminal surface of BMEC is very important for leukocyte extravasation into the CNS (see our recent review for further details (Ivey et al., 2009a)). Tight junctions consist of at least 40 transmembrane proteins, anchorage proteins and tight junction-associated proteins in the membrane and cytosol of endothelial cells. Tight junctions are characterized as having high transendothelial electrical resistance values between 1000 and 1500 Ω/cm^2 (Butt *et al*, 1990).

A recent study by Strayer et. al. has shown that either cell-free or cell-associated gp120 (the outer envelope glycoprotein of HIV) leads to increased matrix metallopeptidase 9 (MMP9) expression which causes decreased expression of laminin and the tight junction protein claudin 5 (Louboutin et al., 2010). A possible mechanism for this could be mediated through focal adhesion kinase, which has been shown to be upregulated in areas of increased neurovascular permeability (Lee et al., 2010).

3.2 Signalling pathways in BBB disruption in HIVE/SIVE

We have recently shown that viral infected macrophages are important in disruption of the BBB *in vitro* (MacLean et al., 2004a, MacLean et al., 2004b), *ex vivo* (Ivey et al., 2009b, Renner et al., 2011) and *in vivo* (Renner *et al.*, in press). The precise mechanisms of BBB disruption are a subject of active research by numerous groups (Luabeya et al., 2000, Andras et al., 2003, Kanmogne et al., 2005, Kanmogne et al., 2007, Persidsky et al., 2006). All of these distinct signal transduction mechanisms have a common factor, however: the tight junctions are linked to the actin cytoskeleton, and the dynamics of the cytoskeleton are therefore important regulators. The importance of cytoskeleton activation will be revisited later when discussing glial cell activation.

4. Astrocytes

4.1 Summary of astrocytes in encephalitis

As illustrated in Figure 2, astrocyte foot processes are closely apposed to BMEC and ensheath more than 60% of the vessel exterior (Mathiisen et al., 2010). Through these contacts astrocytes are able to affect changes in BBB integrity during health and disease, and recruit or repel inflammatory cells through cytokines (Figure 2).

4.2 Role of astrocytes in BBB physiology

The BBB is formed during early infancy in primates (Bayer et al., 1993). The exact mechanisms underlying BBB formation are not clear, but it is known that astrocytes are critical in both maturation and maintenance of the barrier integrity (Willis et al., 2004, Al Ahmad et al., 2010). Astrocytes also act to repel circulating immune cells through secretion of eotaxin (Cardona et al., 2003), reinforcing the brain's immune-privileged status in conjunction with the selective physical properties of the BBB.

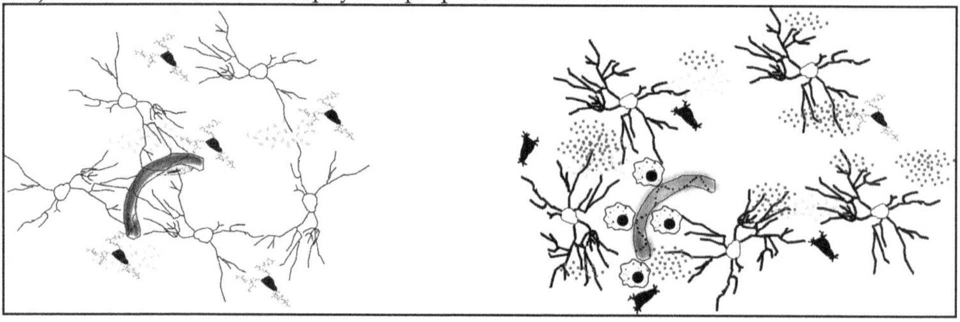

Fig. 2. Schematic of role of astrocytes in pathogenesis. Normal astrocytes (at left) have foot processes ensheathing over 60% of the endothelium and express low levels of GFAP and cytokines / chemokines. In encephalitis, there can a loss of connection to the endothelial cells, increased cytokine / chemokine secretion and altered expression of intermediate filaments, including GFAP and peripherin (right).

4.3 Astrocytes and signaling in encephalitis

Astrocytes are the primary cell type found in glia scar formation (Voskuhl et al., 2009, Kielian, 2004), and secrete cytokines and chemokines to elicit increased trafficking of leukocytes into the brain (Renner et al., 2011, Cota et al., 2000, Eugenin et al., 2006). Astrocytes also may provide a role for the resolution of inflammation by reducing the secretion of pro-inflammatory cytokines and increasing anti-inflammatory processes (Kielian, 2004, Hauwel et al., 2005, Park et al., 2003).

Decreased BBB integrity early in SIV/HIV infection allows latently-infected monocytes to enter the brain (Fischer-Smith and Rappaport, 2005). Circulating virus could induce BMEC to express CD106 diffusely (Sasseville et al., 1995, Sasseville et al., 1992) leading to increased monocyte migration into brain, where they become productively infected. Astrocytes respond to these macrophages resulting in a wide-range of cellular changes referred to as astrogliosis.

4.3.1 Astrogliosis

On activation, astrocytes undergo a morphological change: most notably an increase in ramification concomitant with upregulation of GFAP, and thickened processes. We have also observed some astrocytes in the proximity of SIV lesions to express peripherin, an alternative type III intermediate filament not normally expressed in brain (Mathew et al., 2001). Immunologically, astrocytes respond to HIV/ SIV infection through increased production of inflammatory cytokines. As outlined above, the predominate inflammatory cell type in HIVE/SIVE is the monocyte-derived macrophage. The chemokines upregulated by astrocytes in HIVE/SIVE are largely specific to monocyte/macrophages (Renner et al., 2011, Sasseville et al., 1996). This suggests the possibility of a positive feedback system being initiated: a productively-infected macrophage induces nearby astrocytes to upregulate secretion of macrophage-specific chemokines, leading to lesion formation.

The cytokine response of astrocytes includes a cornucopia of molecules including a variety of cytokines and chemokines. It is intriguing that astrocytes will secrete a different "barcode" of cytokines and chemokines in response to different classes of stimuli

(McKimmie and Graham, 2010). Below we discuss key cytokines and chemokines that are thought to play a role in SIVE/HIVE.

4.3.2 Expression and secretion of selected cytokines

Productively-infected macrophages in the encephalitic brain express Tumor Necrosis Factor alpha (TNF-α) (Orandle et al., 2002). TNF-α receptors are present in the non-encephalitic brain (Shaw and Greig, 1999), such that normal brains are primed to respond quickly to low levels of TNF-α. TNF-α induces increased chemokine production and secretion by astrocytes, and these chemokines induce monocyte migration preferentially over lymphocytes (Renner et al., 2011).

Vascular Endothelial Growth Factor (VEGF) promotes proliferation of BMEC, resulting in reorganization of the cytoskeleton and TJ proteins. This induces a decrease in BBB integrity, creating a permissive environment for monocyte migration, and also bidirectional leakage of proteins across the BBB. A possible mechanism for the VEGF pathway could be as follows: tat binds to the VEGF receptor (Nyagol et al., 2008). The VEGF receptor binds to focal adhesion kinase (Garces et al., 2006), increases of which have been implicated in BBB disruption (Ivey et al., 2009b).

Other pro-inflammatory cytokines, including interferon-γ and IL-6 are upregulated in the encephalitic brain, with far-reaching effects in neuroinflammatory events (Roberts et al., 2004a). The complement pathway is also known to be induced through interferon-γ and IL-6 signaling, propagating inflammation in the area surrounding a lesion/lesions.

4.3.3 Expression and secretion of selected chemokines

An early study of chemokine expression in brains of macaques infected with SIV showed increased CCLs 3-5 & 7, and CXCL10 (Sasseville et al., 1996), although no increase in CCLs 2 or 8 nor CXCL8 was observed in this definitive study, other later studies have "muddied the waters" somewhat: Penton-Rol used dexamethasone to stimulate cells to have increased CCL2 receptors before infecting with HIV 89.6 (Penton-Rol et al., 1999). The Clements group at Johns Hopkins has shown increased CCL2 mRNA in brain extracts using a highly accelerated encephalitis model (Witwer et al., 2009), although mRNA does not always equate with secreted protein. Additionally, the Berman group at Einstein College of Medicine has shown numerous effects of CCL2 on HIV-infected macrophages (Eugenin et al., 2003, Eugenin et al., 2006). CCL2 was among several chemokines in CSF that was not upregulated in one study using humans infected with HIV (Kolb et al., 1999), although IP-10 was upgregulated. In contrast, CCL2 was increased in pigtail macaques that develop encephalitis (Mankowski et al., 2004).

The precise cell types producing these chemokines were not identified in these studies. CCL2 mRNA was upregulated in cultured astrocytes, but remained at low levels compared to CCL7, suggesting a role for CCL7 in HIV-related encephalitis (Renner et al., 2011).

Even under noninflamed conditions CCL7 is expressed in the brain (Renner et al., 2011, Sasseville et al., 1996), which could contribute to basal levels of monocyte migration into the brain for "routine surveillance" (Williams and Hickey, 1995). That CCL7 is upregulated by astrocytes in response to cytokines present in encephalitic brains gives a potential role for controlling monocyte migration during encephalitis as well (Sasseville et al., 1996, Renner et al., 2011).

5. Microglia

Microglia are the resident macrophages in brain. These cells are believed to be derived from bone marrow, and present in brain from birth with no replenishment of these cells during the life of an individual (Williams and Hickey, 1995). In normal, healthy brain, microglia play a surveillance role. The high surface area to volume ratio is indicative of a cell "sampling" its environment (Figure 2). On activation, fine processes are no longer visible, with the microglia taking on a more amoeboid morphology. In SIV infection microglia can be recruited and productively-infected themselves (Gonzalez-Scarano and Martin-Garcia, 2005). These cells can also be induced to upregulate CD163 (Roberts et al., 2004b, Borda et al., 2008) which can be quite prominent in areas of BBB breakdown.

5.1 Summary of gliosis

The overall response to SIV or HIV infection of the CNS which primarily involves infected monocyte/macrophages is pro-inflammatory. Neuroinvasion by monocyte/macrophages initiates a positive feedback loop stimulating glial cells to respond further. Glial involvement increases not only the intensity but the area affected by inflammation, damaging local neural circuitry, and recruiting monocytes into the parenchyma. While the glial inflammatory response may seem detrimental, ablation of monocytes led to increased tissue damage in a model of retinal inflammation, implicating lesion formation as a partially neuroprotective response (London et al., 2011). Although the initial monocytes entering the brain carrying HIV/SIV may not be recruited by glial signaling, later neuroinvasion is likely driven, at least in part, by gliosis.

6. Modeling HIVE *in vitro*

6.1 Simple models – single cell type

Numerous groups have used *in vitro* models for determining the cellular and molecular events occurring during the development of HIVE. These have ranged from utilizing single cell types including astrocytes (Renner et al., 2011, Eugenin and Berman, 2007), or endothelial cells (MacLean et al., 2001, Oshima et al., 2000) to tease out initial activation steps. An *ex vivo* single cell type model has also been used recently to examine BBB disruption whereby intact microvessels are extracted and incubated with the lentiviral-infected macrophages (Ivey et al., 2009b). This method has an advantage of maintaining original tight junction orientations. However, the downside is that this technique is only suitable for assessing interactions for the first couple of hours due to viability issues with the microvessels.

6.2 2.5D model of BBB *in vitro*

More complex models involve monolayers of endothelial cells cultured above astrocytes, either on top of a collagen matrix (Biegel and Pachter, 1994, Biegel et al., 1995) or on opposite sides of a membrane (Lu et al., 2008, Persidsky et al., 1997, Eugenin et al., 2006). The coculture allows tight junction formation to occur. The endothelial cells are still a single monolayer, and for this reason, the model is referred to as 2.5D, rather than 3D. These models have been used to examine mechanisms of encephalitis.

6.3 3D model of BBB *in vitro*

A further refinement involved the growth of endothelial cells in tubes (Stanness et al., 1999), or of culturing the endothelial cells within a matrix surrounded by glial cells allowing the endothelial cells to form tubes with astrocytes extending processes to induce tight junction proteins (Al Ahmad et al., 2010). Collagen gels were used to create 3D cultures with BMEC and astrocytes. Al Ahmad et al. showed that BMEC alone were unable to localize tight junction proteins to the cell border. Coculture with astrocytes corrected this, with Claudin5 and ZO1 localized to functionally relevant positions. This clearly demonstrates the necessity for including astrocytes in BBB culture models. As of yet, these models have not been applied to encephalitis studies.

A further model that has been utilized is slice cultures (Renner et al., 2011, Noraberg, 2004). These *ex vivo* models are essentially a complex co-culture that preserves cell:cell ratios, and functional spatial relationships. This model allows one to determine precise cell types secreting chemokines in response to viral-infected cells. It will also prove useful for mechanistic studies of neuropathogenesis.

7. Summary of SIV model of encephalitis

Under normal conditions the brain allows only limited access by immune cells. Early in HIV infection the virus enters the brain through normal trafficking. This leads to a transient increase in BBB permeability, and a localized immune response. As the disease progresses to encephalitis the immune response is dramatically increased, marked by a loss of tight junction integrity, gliosis, and formation of multinucleated giant cells in the parenchyma.

The parallel between the neuropathogenesis of HIV in humans, and SIV in the rhesus macaque has led to the establishment of rhesus macaque as the predominant *in vivo* model for HIVE. The use of *in vitro* models allows for precise control for investigating pathways of lentiviral neuropathogenesis.

8. Acknowledgements

Supported by: This work was supported in part by PHS grants RR00164, MH077544 (AGM), Louisiana Board of Regents Fellowship LEQSF(2007-2012)-GF15 (NAR).

9. References

al Ahmad, A., Taboada, C. B., Gassmann, M. & Ogunshola, O. O. 2010. Astrocytes and pericytes differentially modulate blood-brain barrier characteristics during development and hypoxic insult. *J Cereb Blood Flow Metab.*

Andras, I. E., Pu, H., Deli, M. A., Nath, A., Hennig, B. & Toborek, M. 2003. HIV-1 Tat protein alters tight junction protein expression and distribution in cultured brain endothelial cells. *J Neurosci Res,* 74, 255-65.

Annunziata, P. 2003. Blood-brain barrier changes during invasion of the central nervous system by HIV-1. Old and new insights into the mechanism. *J Neurol,* 250, 901-6.

Bayer, S. A., Altman, J., Russo, R. J. & Zhang, X. 1993. Timetables of neurogenesis in the human brain based on experimentally determined patterns in the rat. *Neurotoxicology,* 14, 83-144.

Biegel, D. & Pachter, J. S. 1994. Growth of brain microvessel endothelial cells on collagen gels: applications to the study of blood-brain barrier physiology and CNS inflammation. *In Vitro Cell Dev Biol Anim,* 30A, 581-8.

Biegel, D., Spencer, D. D. & Pachter, J. S. 1995. Isolation and culture of human brain microvessel endothelial cells for the study of blood-brain barrier properties in vitro. *Brain Res*, 692, 183-9.

Bissel, S. J., Wang, G., Trichel, A. M., Murphey-Corb, M. & Wiley, C. A. 2006a. Longitudinal analysis of activation markers on monocyte subsets during the development of simian immunodeficiency virus encephalitis. *J Neuroimmunol*, 177, 85-98.

Bissel, S. J., Wang, G., Trichel, A. M., Murphey-Corb, M. & Wiley, C. A. 2006b. Longitudinal analysis of monocyte/macrophage infection in simian immunodeficiency virus-infected, CD8+ T-cell-depleted macaques that develop lentiviral encephalitis. *Am J Pathol*, 168, 1553-69.

Bissel, S. J. & Wiley, C. A. 2004. Human immunodeficiency virus infection of the brain: pitfalls in evaluating infected/affected cell populations. *Brain Pathol*, 14, 97-108.

Borda, J. T., Alvarez, X., Mohan, M., Hasegawa, A., Bernardino, A., Jean, S., AYE, P. & Lackner, A. A. 2008. CD163, a Marker of Perivascular Macrophages, Is Up-Regulated by Microglia in Simian Immunodeficiency Virus Encephalitis after Haptoglobin-Hemoglobin Complex Stimulation and Is Suggestive of Breakdown of the Blood-Brain Barrier. *Am J Pathol*, 172, 725-37.

Boven, L. A., Middel, J., Verhoef, J., De Groot, C. J. & Nottet, H. S. 2000. Monocyte infiltration is highly associated with loss of the tight junction protein zonula occludens in HIV-1-associated dementia. *Neuropathol Appl Neurobiol*, 26, 356-60.

Brack-Werner, R. 1999. Astrocytes: HIV cellular reservoirs and important participants in neuropathogenesis. *Aids*, 13, 1-22.

Cardona, A. E., Gonzalez, P. A. & Teale, J. M. 2003. CC chemokines mediate leukocyte trafficking into the central nervous system during murine neurocysticercosis: role of gamma delta T cells in amplification of the host immune response. *Infect Immun*, 71, 2634-42.

Cota, M., Kleinschmidt, A., Ceccherini-Silberstein, F., Aloisi, F., Mengozzi, M., Mantovani, A., Brack-Werner, R. & Poli, G. 2000. Upregulated expression of interleukin-8, RANTES and chemokine receptors in human astrocytic cells infected with HIV-1. *J Neurovirol*, 6, 75-83.

Dallasta, L. M., Pisarov, L. A., Esplen, J. E., Werley, J. V., Moses, A. V., Nelson, J. A. & Achim, C. L. 1999. Blood-brain barrier tight junction disruption in human immunodeficiency virus-1 encephalitis. *Am J Pathol*, 155, 1915-27.

Davis, L. E., Hjelle, B. L., Miller, V. E., Palmer, D. L., Llewellyn, A. L., Merlin, T. L., Young, S. A., Mills, R. G., Wachsman, W. & Wiley, C. A. 1992. Early viral brain invasion in iatrogenic human immunodeficiency virus infection. *Neurology*, 42, 1736-9.

Elbim, C., Pillet, S., Prevost, M. H., Preira, A., Girard, P. M., Rogine, N., Matusani, H., Hakim, J., Israel, N. & Gougerot-Pocidalo, M. A. 1999. Redox and activation status of monocytes from human immunodeficiency virus-infected patients: relationship with viral load. *J Virol*, 73, 4561-6.

Eugenin, E. A. & Berman, J. W. 2007. Gap junctions mediate human immunodeficiency virus-bystander killing in astrocytes. *J Neurosci*, 27, 12844-50.

Eugenin, E. A., D'aversa, T. G., Lopez, L., Calderon, T. M. & Berman, J. W. 2003. MCP-1 (CCL2) protects human neurons and astrocytes from NMDA or HIV-tat-induced apoptosis. *J Neurochem*, 85, 1299-311.

Eugenin, E. A., Osiecki, K., Lopez, L., Goldstein, H., Calderon, T. M. & Berman, J. W. 2006. CCL2/monocyte chemoattractant protein-1 mediates enhanced transmigration of human immunodeficiency virus (HIV)-infected leukocytes across the blood-brain barrier: a potential mechanism of HIV-CNS invasion and NeuroAIDS. *J Neurosci,* 26, 1098-106.

Fischer-Smith, T., Croul, S., Sverstiuk, A. E., Capini, C., L'heureux, D., Regulier, E. G., Richardson, M. W., Amini, S., Morgello, S., Khalili, K. & Rappaport, J. 2001. CNS invasion by CD14+/CD16+ peripheral blood-derived monocytes in HIV dementia: perivascular accumulation and reservoir of HIV infection. *J Neurovirol,* 7, 528-41.

Fischer-Smith, T. & Rappaport, J. 2005. Evolving paradigms in the pathogenesis of HIV-1-associated dementia. *Expert Rev Mol Med,* 7, 1-26.

Garces, C. A., Kurenova, E. V., Golubovskaya, V. M. & Cance, W. G. 2006. Vascular endothelial growth factor receptor-3 and focal adhesion kinase bind and suppress apoptosis in breast cancer cells. *Cancer Res,* 66, 1446-54.

Gonzalez-Scarano, F. & Martin-Garcia, J. 2005. The neuropathogenesis of AIDS. *Nat Rev Immunol,* 5, 69-81.

Gorry, P. R., Ong, C., Thorpe, J., Bannwarth, S., Thompson, K. A., Gatignol, A., Vesselingh, S. L. & Purcell, D. F. 2003. Astrocyte infection by HIV-1: mechanisms of restricted virus replication, and role in the pathogenesis of HIV-1-associated dementia. *Curr HIV Res,* 1, 463-73.

Graeber, M. B., Streit, W. J., Buringer, D., Sparks, D. L. & Kreutzberg, G. W. 1992. Ultrastructural location of major histocompatibility complex (MHC) class II positive perivascular cells in histologically normal human brain. *J Neuropathol Exp Neurol,* 51, 303-11.

Hallett, M. B. L., D. 1995. Neutrophil Priming: the Cellular Signals that say 'Amber' but not 'Green". *Immunology Today,* 16, 264-268.

Hauwel, M., Furon, E., Canova, C., Griffiths, M., Neal, J. & Gasque, P. 2005. Innate (inherent) control of brain infection, brain inflammation and brain repair: the role of microglia, astrocytes, "protective" glial stem cells and stromal ependymal cells. *Brain Res Brain Res Rev,* 48, 220-33.

Hickey, W. F. & Kimura, H. 1988. Perivascular microglial cells of the CNS are bone marrow-derived and present antigen in vivo. *Science,* 239, 290-2.

Huang, W., Eum, S. Y., Andras, I. E., Hennig, B. & Toborek, M. 2009. PPARalpha and PPARgamma attenuate HIV-induced dysregulation of tight junction proteins by modulations of matrix metalloproteinase and proteasome activities. *Faseb J,* 23, 1596-606.

Ivey, N. S., Maclean, A. G. & Lackner, A. A. 2009a. Acquired Immunodeficiency syndrome and the blood-brain barrier. *J Neurovirol,* 15, 111-22.

Ivey, N. S., Renner, N. A., Moroney-Rasmussen, T., Mohan, M., Redmann, R. K., Didier, P. J., Alvarez, X., Lackner, A. A. & Maclean, A. G. 2009b. Association of FAK activation with lentivirus-induced disruption of blood-brain barrier tight junction-associated ZO-1 protein organization. *J Neurovirol,* 1-12.

Kanmogne, G. D., Primeaux, C. & Grammas, P. 2005. HIV-1 gp120 proteins alter tight junction protein expression and brain endothelial cell permeability: implications for the pathogenesis of HIV-associated dementia. *J Neuropathol Exp Neurol,* 64, 498-505.

Kanmogne, G. D., Schall, K., Leibhart, J., Knipe, B., Gendelman, H. E. & Persidsky, Y. 2007. HIV-1 gp120 compromises blood-brain barrier integrity and enhances monocyte migration across blood-brain barrier: implication for viral neuropathogenesis. *J Cereb Blood Flow Metab*, 27, 123-34.

Kielian, T. 2004. Immunopathogenesis of brain abscess. *J Neuroinflammation*, 1, 16.

Kim, W. K., Avarez, X. & Williams, K. 2005. The role of monocytes and perivascular macrophages in HIV and SIV neuropathogenesis: information from non-human primate models. *Neurotox Res*, 8, 107-15.

Kolb, S. A., Sporer, B., Lahrtz, F., Koedel, U., Pfister, H. W. & Fontana, A. 1999. Identification of a T cell chemotactic factor in the cerebrospinal fluid of HIV-1-infected individuals as interferon-gamma inducible protein 10. *J Neuroimmunol*, 93, 172-81.

Kuroda, M. J. 2010. Macrophages: do they impact AIDS progression more than CD4 T cells? *J Leukoc Biol*, 87, 569-73.

Lackner, A. A., Vogel, P., Ramos, R. A., Kluge, J. D. & Marthas, M. 1994. Early events in tissues during infection with pathogenic (SIVmac239) and nonpathogenic (SIVmac1A11) molecular clones of simian immunodeficiency virus. *Am J Pathol*, 145, 428-39.

Lassmann, H., Zimprich, F., Vass, K. & Hickey, W. F. 1991. Microglial cells are a component of the perivascular glia limitans. *J Neurosci Res*, 28, 236-43.

Lee, J., Borboa, A. K., Chun, H. B., Baird, A. & Eliceiri, B. P. 2010. Conditional deletion of the focal adhesion kinase FAK alters remodeling of the blood-brain barrier in glioma. *Cancer Res*, 70, 10131-40.

Little, S. J., Mclean, A. R., Spina, C. A., Richman, D. D. & Havlir, D. V. 1999. Viral dynamics of acute HIV-1 infection. *J Exp Med*, 190, 841-50.

Liu, Y., Liu, H., Kim, B. O., Gattone, V. H., Li, J., Nath, A., Blum, J. & He, J. J. 2004. CD4-independent infection of astrocytes by human immunodeficiency virus type 1: requirement for the human mannose receptor. *J Virol*, 78, 4120-33.

London, A., Itskovich, E., Benhar, I., Kalchenko, V., Mack, M., Jung, S. & Schwartz, M. 2011. Neuroprotection and progenitor cell renewal in the injured adult murine retina requires healing monocyte-derived macrophages. *J Exp Med*, 208, 23-39.

Louboutin, J. P., Agrawal, L., Reyes, B. A., Van Bockstaele, E. J. & Strayer, D. S. 2010. HIV-1 gp120-induced injury to the blood-brain barrier: role of metalloproteinases 2 and 9 and relationship to oxidative stress. *J Neuropathol Exp Neurol*, 69, 801-16.

Lu, T. S., Avraham, H. K., Seng, S., Tachado, S. D., Koziel, H., Makriyannis, A. & Avraham, S. 2008. Cannabinoids inhibit HIV-1 Gp120-mediated insults in brain microvascular endothelial cells. *J Immunol*, 181, 6406-16.

Luabeya, M. K., Dallasta, L. M., Achim, C. L., Pauza, C. D. & Hamilton, R. L. 2000. Blood-brain barrier disruption in simian immunodeficiency virus encephalitis. *Neuropathol Appl Neurobiol*, 26, 454-62.

Luster, A. D., Alon, R. & Von Andrian, U. H. 2005. Immune cell migration in inflammation: present and future therapeutic targets. *Nat Immunol*, 6, 1182-90.

Maclean, A. G., Belenchia, G. E., Bieniemy, D. N., Moroney-Rasmussen, T. A. & Lackner, A. A. 2005. Simian immunodeficiency virus disrupts extended lengths of the blood--brain barrier. *J Med Primatol*, 34, 237-42.

Maclean, A. G., Orandle, M. S., Alvarez, X., Williams, K. C. & Lackner, A. A. 2001. Rhesus macaque brain microvessel endothelial cells behave in a manner phenotypically distinct from umbilical vein endothelial cells. *J Neuroimmunol,* 118, 223-32.

Maclean, A. G., Rasmussen, T. A., Bieniemy, D. & Lackner, A. A. 2004a. Activation of the blood-brain barrier by SIV (simian immunodeficiency virus) requires cell-associated virus and is not restricted to endothelial cell activation. *Biochem Soc Trans,* 32, 750-2.

Maclean, A. G., Rasmussen, T. A., Bieniemy, D. N., Alvarez, X. & Lackner, A. A. 2004b. SIV-induced activation of the blood-brain barrier requires cell-associated virus and is not restricted to endothelial cell activation. *J Med Primatol,* 33, 236-42.

Mankowski, J. L., Queen, S. E., Clements, J. E. & Zink, M. C. 2004. Cerebrospinal fluid markers that predict SIV CNS disease. *J Neuroimmunol,* 157, 66-70.

Mathew, J. S., Westmoreland, S. V., Alvarez, X., Simon, M. A., Pauley, D. R., Mackey, J. J. & Lackner, A. A. 2001. Expression of peripherin in the brain of macaques (Macaca mulatta and Macaca fascicularis) occurs in astrocytes rather than neurones and is associated with encephalitis. *Neuropathol Appl Neurobiol,* 27, 434-43.

Mathiisen, T. M., Lehre, K. P., Danbolt, N. C. & Ottersen, O. P. 2010. The perivascular astroglial sheath provides a complete covering of the brain microvessels: an electron microscopic 3D reconstruction. *Glia,* 58, 1094-103.

Mckimmie, C. S. & Graham, G. J. 2010. Astrocytes modulate the chemokine network in a pathogen-specific manner. *Biochem Biophys Res Commun,* 394, 1006-11.

Moore, J. P., Kitchen, S. G., Pugach, P. & Zack, J. A. 2004. The CCR5 and CXCR4 coreceptors--central to understanding the transmission and pathogenesis of human immunodeficiency virus type 1 infection. *AIDS Res Hum Retroviruses,* 20, 111-26.

Moses, A. V. & Nelson, J. A. 1994. HIV infection of human brain capillary endothelial cells--implications for AIDS dementia. *Adv Neuroimmunol,* 4, 239-47.

Munsaka, S. M., Agsalda, M., Troelstrup, D., Hu, N., Yu, Q. & Shiramizu, B. 2009. Characteristics of Activated Monocyte Phenotype Support R5-Tropic Human Immunodeficiency Virus. *Immunol Immunogenet Insights,* 1, 15-20.

Narayan, O., Wolinsky, J. S., Clements, J. E., Strandberg, J. D., Griffin, D. E. & Cork, L. C. 1982. Slow virus replication: the role of macrophages in the persistence and expression of visna viruses of sheep and goats. *J Gen Virol,* 59, 345-56.

Nath, A., Conant, K., Chen, P., Scott, C., Major, E.O. 1999. Transient exposure to HIV-1 tat protein results in cytokine production in macrophages and astrocytes. *Journal of biological chemistry,* 274, 17098-17102.

Noraberg, J. 2004. Organotypic brain slice cultures: an efficient and reliable method for neurotoxicological screening and mechanistic studies. *Altern Lab Anim,* 32, 329-37.

Nyagol, J., De Falco, G., Lazzi, S., Luzzi, A., Cerino, G., Shaheen, S., Palummo, N., Bellan, C., Spina, D. & Leoncini, L. 2008. HIV-1 Tat mimetic of VEGF correlates with increased microvessels density in AIDS-related diffuse large B-cell and Burkitt lymphomas. *J Hematop,* 1, 3-10.

Orandle, M. S., Maclean, A. G., Sasseville, V. G., Alvarez, X. & Lackner, A. A. 2002. Enhanced expression of proinflammatory cytokines in the central nervous system is associated with neuroinvasion by simian immunodeficiency virus and the development of encephalitis. *J Virol,* 76, 5797-802.

Oshima, T., Flores, S. C., Vaitaitis, G., Coe, L. L., Joh, T., Park, J. H., Zhu, Y., Alexander, B. & Alexander, J. S. 2000. HIV-1 Tat increases endothelial solute permeability through tyrosine kinase and mitogen-activated protein kinase-dependent pathways. *Aids,* 14, 475-82.

Park, E. J., Park, S. Y., Joe, E. H. & Jou, I. 2003. 15d-PGJ2 and rosiglitazone suppress Janus kinase-STAT inflammatory signaling through induction of suppressor of cytokine signaling 1 (SOCS1) and SOCS3 in glia. *J Biol Chem,* 278, 14747-52.

Penton-Rol, G., Cota, M., Polentarutti, N., Luini, W., Bernasconi, S., Borsatti, A., Sica, A., Larosa, G. J., Sozzani, S., Poli, G. & Mantovani, A. 1999. Up-regulation of CCR2 chemokine receptor expression and increased susceptibility to the multitropic HIV strain 89.6 in monocytes exposed to glucocorticoid hormones. *J Immunol,* 163, 3524-9.

Persidsky, Y. 1999. Model systems for studies of leukocyte migration across the blood - brain barrier. *J Neurovirol,* 5, 579-90.

Persidsky, Y., Ghorpade, A., Rasmussen, J., Limoges, J., Liu, X. J., Stins, M., Fiala, M., Way, D., Kim, K. S., Witte, M. H., Weinand, M., Carhart, L. & Gendelman, H. E. 1999. Microglial and astrocyte chemokines regulate monocyte migration through the blood-brain barrier in human immunodeficiency virus-1 encephalitis. *Am J Pathol,* 155, 1599-611.

Persidsky, Y., Heilman, D., Haorah, J., Zelivyanskaya, M., Persidsky, R., Weber, G. A., Shimokawa, H., Kaibuchi, K. & Ikezu, T. 2006. Rho-mediated regulation of tight junctions during monocyte migration across the blood-brain barrier in HIV-1 encephalitis (HIVE). *Blood,* 107, 4770-80.

Persidsky, Y., Stins, M., Way, D., Witte, M. H., Weinand, M., Kim, K. S., Bock, P., Gendelman, H. E. & Fiala, M. 1997. A model for monocyte migration through the blood-brain barrier during HIV-1 encephalitis. *J Immunol,* 158, 3499-510.

Persidsky, Y., Zheng, J., Miller, D. & Gendelman, H. E. 2000. Mononuclear phagocytes mediate blood-brain barrier compromise and neuronal injury during HIV-1-associated dementia. *J Leukoc Biol,* 68, 413-22.

Pulliam, L., Gascon, R., Stubblebine, M., Mcguire, D. & Mcgrath, M. S. 1997. Unique monocyte subset in patients with AIDS dementia. *Lancet,* 349, 692-5.

Renner, N. A., Ivey, N. S., Redmann, R. K., Lackner, A. A. & Maclean, A. G. 2011. MCP-3/CCL7 production by astrocytes: implications for SIV neuroinvasion and AIDS encephalitis. *J Neurovirol.*

Roberts, E. S., Burudi, E. M., Flynn, C., Madden, L. J., Roinick, K. L., Watry, D. D., Zandonatti, M. A., Taffe, M. A. & Fox, H. S. 2004a. Acute SIV infection of the brain leads to upregulation of IL6 and interferon-regulated genes: expression patterns throughout disease progression and impact on neuroAIDS. *J Neuroimmunol,* 157, 81-92.

Roberts, E. S., Masliah, E. & Fox, H. S. 2004b. CD163 identifies a unique population of ramified microglia in HIV encephalitis (HIVE). *J Neuropathol Exp Neurol,* 63, 1255-64.

Rubio, N., Sanz-Rodriguez, F. & Arevalo, M. A. 2010. Up-regulation of the Vascular Cell Adhesion Molecule-1 (VCAM-1) Induced By Theiler's Murine Encephalomyelitis Virus Infection of Murine Brain Astrocytes. *Cell Commun Adhes,* 17, 57-68.

Ryzhova, E. V., Crino, P., Shawver, L., Westmoreland, S. V., Lackner, A. A. & Gonzalez-Scarano, F. 2002. Simian immunodeficiency virus encephalitis: analysis of envelope sequences from individual brain multinucleated giant cells and tissue samples. *Virology,* 297, 57-67.

Salazar-Gonzalez, J. F., Salazar, M. G., Keele, B. F., Learn, G. H., Giorgi, E. E., Li, H., Decker, J. M., Wang, S., Baalwa, J., Kraus, M. H., Parrish, N. F., Shaw, K. S., Guffey, M. B., Bar, K. J., Davis, K. L., Ochsenbauer-Jambor, C., Kappes, J. C., Saag, M. S., Cohen, M. S., Mulenga, J., Derdeyn, C. A., Allen, S., Hunter, E., Markowitz, M., Hraber, P., Perelson, A. S., Bhattacharya, T., Haynes, B. F., Korber, B. T., Hahn, B. H. & Shaw, G. M. 2009. Genetic identity, biological phenotype, and evolutionary pathways of transmitted/founder viruses in acute and early HIV-1 infection. *J Exp Med,* 206, 1273-89.

Sasseville, V. G., Lane, J. H., Walsh, D., Ringler, D. J. & Lackner, A. A. 1995. VCAM-1 expression and leukocyte trafficking to the CNS occur early in infection with pathogenic isolates of SIV. *J Med Primatol,* 24, 123-131.

Sasseville, V. G., Newman, W. A., Lackner, A. A., Smith, M. O., Lausen, N. C., Beall, D. & Ringler, D. J. 1992. Elevated vascular cell adhesion molecule-1 in AIDS encephalitis induced by simian immunodeficiency virus. *Am J Pathol,* 141, 1021-30.

Sasseville, V. G., Smith, M. M., Mackay, C. R., Pauley, D. R., Mansfield, K. G., Ringler, D. J. & Lackner, A. A. 1996. Chemokine expression in simian immunodeficiency virus-induced AIDS encephalitis. *Am J Pathol,* 149, 1459-67.

Shaw, K. T. & Greig, N. H. 1999. Chemokine receptor mRNA expression at the in vitro blood-brain barrier during HIV infection. *Neuroreport,* 10, 53-6.

Stanness, K. A., Neumaier, J. F., Sexton, T. J., Grant, G. A., Emmi, A., Maris, D. O. & Janigro, D. 1999. A new model of the blood-brain barrier: co-culture of neuronal, endothelial and glial cells under dynamic conditions. *Neuroreport,* 10, 3725-31.

Stephens, E. B., Singh, D. K., Kohler, M. E., Jackson, M., Pacyniak, E. & Berman, N. E. 2003. The primary phase of infection by pathogenic simian-human immunodeficiency virus results in disruption of the blood-brain barrier. *AIDS Res Hum Retroviruses,* 19, 837-46.

Streit, W. J. & GRAEBER, M. B. 1993. Heterogeneity of microglial and perivascular cell populations: insights gained from the facial nucleus paradigm. *Glia,* 7, 68-74.

Thompson, W. L. & Van Eldik, L. J. 2009. Inflammatory cytokines stimulate the chemokines CCL2/MCP-1 and CCL7/MCP-3 through NFkB and MAPK dependent pathways in rat astrocytes [corrected]. *Brain Res,* 1287, 47-57.

Trillo-Pazos, G., Diamanturos, A., Rislove, L., Menza, T., Chao, W., Belem, P., Sadiq, S., Morgello, S., Sharer, L. & Volsky, D. J. 2003. Detection of HIV-1 DNA in microglia/macrophages, astrocytes and neurons isolated from brain tissue with HIV-1 encephalitis by laser capture microdissection. *Brain Pathol,* 13, 144-54.

Tyor, W. R., Glass, J. D., Griffin, J. W., Becker, P. S., Mcarthur, J. C., Bezman, L. & Griffin, D. E. 1992. Cytokine expression in the brain during the acquired immunodeficiency syndrome. *Ann Neurol,* 31, 349-60.

Voskuhl, R. R., Peterson, R. S., Song, B., Ao, Y., Morales, L. B., Tiwari-Woodruff, S. & Sofroniew, M. V. 2009. Reactive astrocytes form scar-like perivascular barriers to leukocytes during adaptive immune inflammation of the CNS. *J Neurosci,* 29, 11511-22.

Williams, K. C., Corey, S., Westmoreland, S. V., Pauley, D., Knight, H., Debakker, C., Alvarez, X. & Lackner, A. A. 2001. Perivascular Macrophages Are the Primary Cell Type Productively Infected by Simian Immunodeficiency Virus in the Brains of Macaques. Implications for the neuropathogenesis of aids. *J Exp Med,* 193, 905-16.

Williams, K. C. & Hickey, W. F. 1995. Traffic of hematogenous cells through the central nervous system. *Curr Top Microbiol Immunol,* 202, 221-45.

Williams, K. C. & Hickey, W. F. 2002. Central nervous system damage, monocytes and macrophages, and neurological disorders in AIDS. *Annu Rev Neurosci,* 25, 537-62.

Willis, C. L., Nolan, C. C., Reith, S. N., Lister, T., Prior, M. J., Guerin, C. J., Mavroudis, G. & Ray, D. E. 2004. Focal astrocyte loss is followed by microvascular damage, with subsequent repair of the blood-brain barrier in the apparent absence of direct astrocytic contact. *Glia,* 45, 325-37.

Witwer, K. W., Gama, L., Li, M., Bartizal, C. M., Queen, S. E., Varrone, J. J., Brice, A. K., Graham, D. R., Tarwater, P. M., Mankowski, J. L., Zink, M. C. & Clements, J. E. 2009. Coordinated regulation of SIV replication and immune responses in the CNS. *PLoS One,* 4, e8129.

Worobey, M., Telfer, P., Souquiere, S., Hunter, M., Coleman, C. A., Metzger, M. J., Reed, P., Makuwa, M., Hearn, G., Honarvar, S., Roques, P., Apetrei, C., Kazanji, M. & Marx, P. A. 2010. Island biogeography reveals the deep history of SIV. *Science,* 329, 1487.

Zhou, L. P., Shang, H., Zhang, Z. N., Wang, Y. N., Li, G. F., Shi, W. Y. & Ding, H. B. 2007. [Correlation between the function of monocytes/macrophages and disease progression in people living with HIV/AIDS in several provinces in China]. *Zhonghua Yi Xue Za Zhi,* 87, 2394-7.

Zink, M. C., Spelman, J. P., Robinson, R. B. & Clements, J. E. 1998. SIV infection of macaques--modeling the progression to AIDS dementia. *J Neurovirol,* 4, 249-59.

7

Equine Herpesvirus 9 (EHV-9) Induced Encephalitis in Nonhuman Primates

Tokuma Yanai, Atsushi Kodama, Hiroki Sakai, Hideto Fukushi,
Takeshi Kuraishi, Seisaku Hattori and Chieko Kai
The University of Tokyo, Gifu University
Japan

1. Introduction

Equine Herpesvirus 9 (EHV-9) is a new member of the equine herpesviruses which was isolated from Thomson's gazelles (*Gazella thomsoni*) that died of fulminant encephalitis in a Japanese zoo (Fukushi et al., 1997; Yanai et al., 1998). Previously, experimental infections of EHV-9 were conducted in various species of animals other than primates to clarify the infectivity and virulence of this virus and to assess the emerging aspects of EHV-9 in zoo and domestic animal populations. EHV-9 caused fatal infections with fulminant encephalitis characterized by neuronal degeneration and necrosis as well as intra-nuclear inclusion bodies in rodents (Fukushi et al., 1997; Fukushi et al., 2000), goats (Taniguchi et al., 2000), pigs (Narita et al., 2000, 2001), dogs (Yanai et al., 2003a) and cats (Yanai et al., 2003b). Based on several experimental studies of EHV-9 involving various domestic animals such as dogs and cats often found in close proximity to humans, there were grave concerns that EHV-9 could be transmitted to humans through contact with affected animals or zebras through certain routes. In order to assess the risk of EHV-9 to humans, we tried to determine the infectivity of EHV-9 in non-human primates, including common marmosets (*Callithrix jacchus*) and cynomolgus macaques (*Macaca fasciocularis*), which have strong similarities to humans, using the nasal route.

2. Marmosets

One female and four male common marmosets, aged 2 to 4 years old and weighing 285-368g, were used for this assessment (Kodama et al., 2007). Four of the marmosets were inoculated intranasally with 1ml of EHV-9 virus solution containing 10^6 plaque-forming units. The other was inoculated with 1 ml of MEM as a negative control. The inoculated animals were humanely euthanatized on Days 3, 4 and 5 following inoculation, respectively, at a point when they were in poor condition or dying from a neuronal disorder. The virus was recovered and identified by polymerase chain reaction (PCR) with the primers targeting the EHV-9 specific region of the EHV-9 gene. The PCR primers used for amplification were 5′-CTGGGTTATAGATTGTCGCCTC-3′ and 5′-CCCAGAAAGTATTACACGCGAT-3′. The neutralization test was done using the 50% plaque reduction method with the MDBK cell monolayer.

All four of the inoculated animals exhibited various neurological signs and finally collapsed. From the second day post-inoculation (dpi), all four inoculated marmosets began to exhibit signs of anorexia and depression. A decrease in body weight was noted from 3 dpi. At 3 dpi, rectal temperatures in each of the treated animals were approximately 2 to 3 degrees lower than those in the non-treated control animal, although the animals recovered from the hypothermia the following day. From 3 to 5 dpi, the inoculated animals showed varying degrees of neurological signs consisting of salivation (Fig. 1), star gazing, convulsions and finally coma. At 4 and 5 dpi the animals refused food, became severely depressed, and collapsed. One animal was euthanized based on schedule, but two animals were euthanized at 3 dpi due to poor condition, and the last one was euthanized at 5 dpi. The control animal was euthanized at 6 dpi.

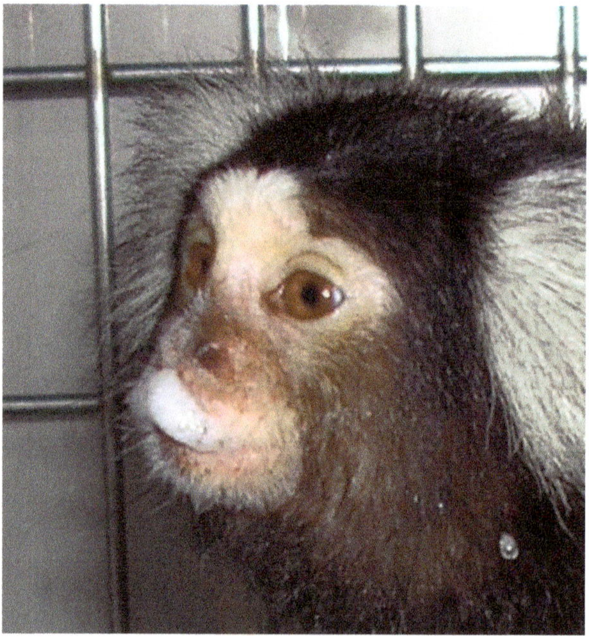

Fig. 1. Marked salivation with a large amount of foamy saliva at 4 dpi.

At necropsy, no significant abnormalities were observed in the external or visceral organs in any of the inoculated animals.

Histologically, the affected animals had severe encephalitis characterized by neuronal degeneration and necrosis with intra-nuclear inclusions, which extended from the olfactory bulb to the rhinencephalon and piriform lobe. The nuclei of affected degenerating neuronal cells exhibited severe degrees of chromatolysis or karyorrhexis, eventually resulting in neuronal loss and cellular debris (Fig. 2). The degenerating neuronal cells had frequent intra-nuclear inclusion bodies which were equivalent to herpesvirus in morphology, appearing as full-inclusion or Cowdry type A inclusions (Figs. 2 and 3). The inclusion bodies were particularly frequent in the olfactory bulb, piriform lobe and amygdaloid body in the affected animals. Cerebrum lesions were observed in all layers of the olfactory bulb, the piriform lobe (Fig. 4) and a part of the temporal lobe in an animal euthanized at 3 dpi.

The lesions then spread to the basal ganglia, except for the globus pallidus, and the limbic lobe, including the hippocampus and cingulate gyrus, basal forebrain and temporal lobe in the animals (Fig. 5). The animal euthanized at 5 dpi had widely distributed lesions in the cerebrum. No abnormalities were observed in the cerebellum or spinal cord. Immunohistochemistry to EHV-9 antibody revealed positive reactions in the nucleus, intra-nuclear inclusions and the cytoplasm in degenerating neuronal cells, and occasionally in normal-appearing neuronal cells in the marginal zone or surroundings of affected areas in the brain (Fig. 6). Prominent inclusion bodies appearing as the full-inclusion type had the most intensely positive reaction around the nuclear membrane.

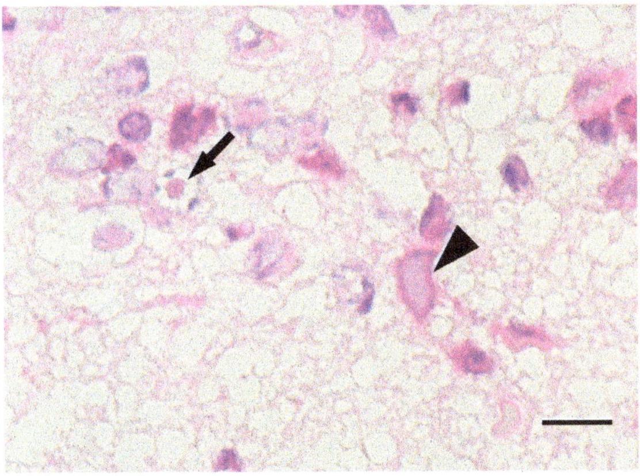

Fig. 2. Olfactory bulb; Neuronal necrosis with intra-nuclear inclusion bodies, appearing as Cowdry type A (arrow) or full-inclusion (arrow head) inclusions. HE. Bar=3.5μm.

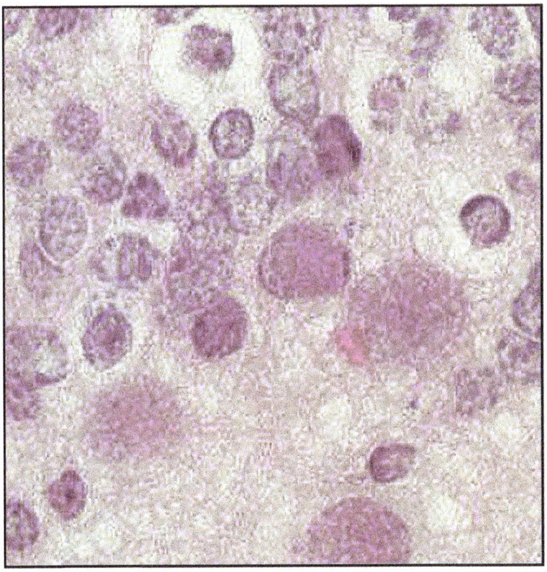

Fig. 3. Olfactory bulb; Frequent intra-nuclear inclusions. HE.

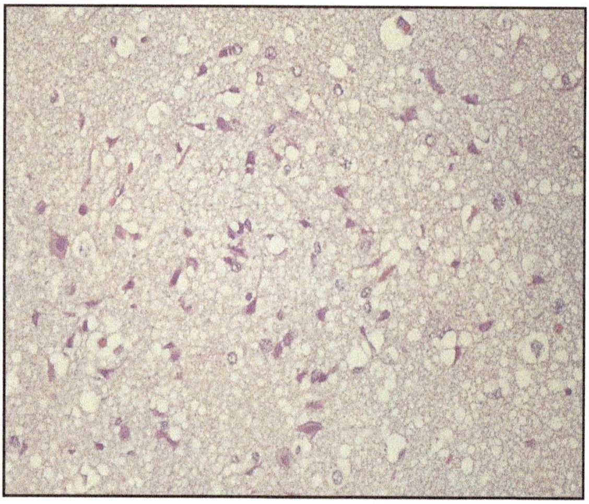

Fig. 4. Piriform lobe; Neuronal degeneration and necrosis with intra-nuclear inclusions.

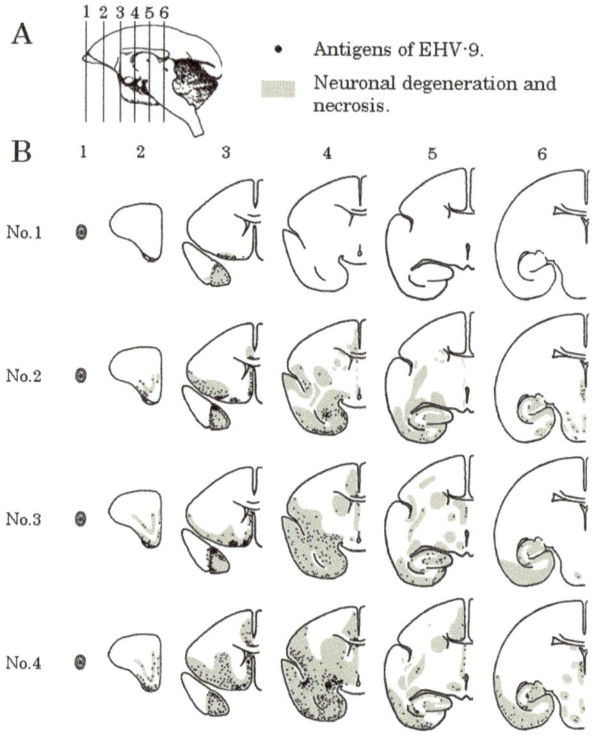

Fig. 5. Time-course extension of EHV-9 induced encephalitis in the brain.

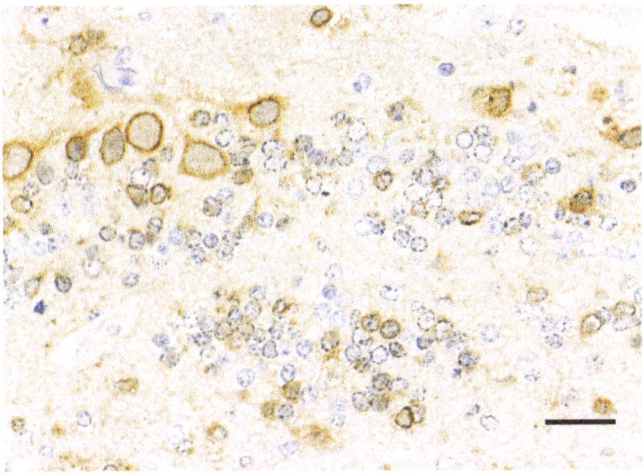

Fig. 6. Olfactory bulb. Most neuronal cells in all layers of the glomerular, mitral and granule layers are frequently positive to EHV-9 antigen. ABC method. Bar=5.7μm. Immunostaining for EHV-9 antigen. Frequent positive reactions.

In the nasal cavities of all of the animals inoculated with EHV-9, there was severe necrotizing rhinitis characterized by severe necrosis of the olfactory epithelium and olfactory glands in the olfactory area (Fig. 7). The marmosets that had been inoculated exhibited more severe desquamation of the olfactory epithelium, as well as degeneration and necrosis at 3 dpi. In addition, occasional olfactory Schwann cells were degenerative or necrotic. Frequent intra-neuronal inclusion bodies were seen in the degenerating epithelial cells in both the olfactory epithelium and olfactory glandular epithelium (Fig. 8). In the respiratory area, sight focal necrosis and ablation were occasionally observed in the mucosa. Immunohistochemically, there were frequent positive reactions in both intra-nuclear inclusion bodies and the cytoplasm of degenerating cells in the olfactory epithelium and olfactory glandular epithelium in all animals inoculated with EHV-9 (Figs. 9, 10). Occasional degenerating mucosal epithelium in the respiratory area and degenerating Schwann cells also had positive reactions.

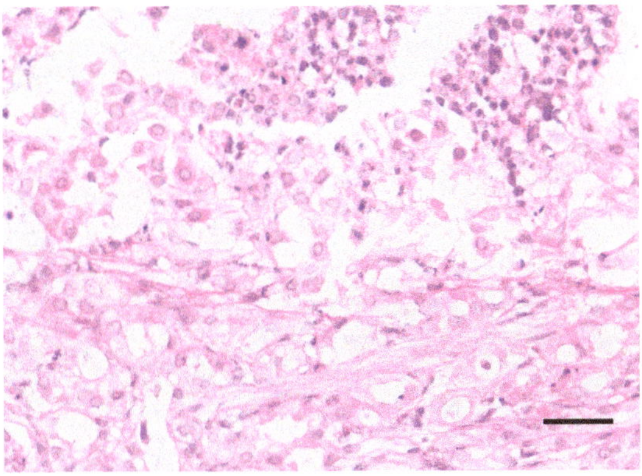

Fig. 7. Olfactory area in the nasal cavity; The degenerating epithelial epithelium and olfactory glandular epithelium with frequent intranuclear inclusions. HE. Bar = 8.6 μm

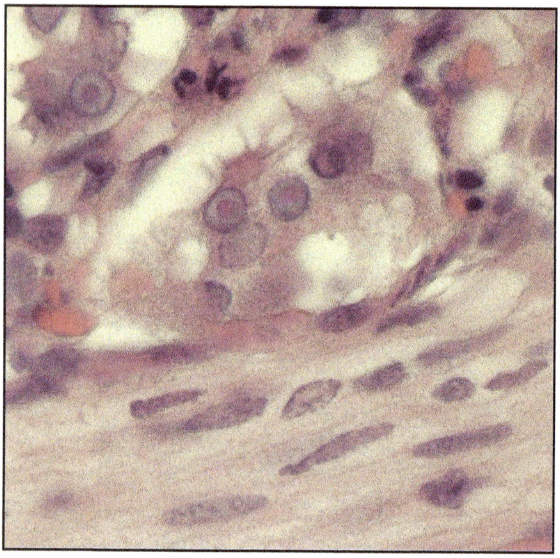

Fig. 8. Olfactory area in the nasal cavity; Frequent intra-neuronal inclusion bodies are seen epithelium and olfactory glandular epithelium. HE.

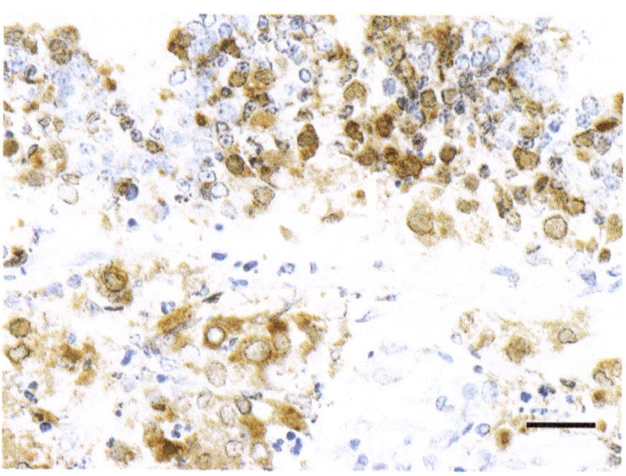

Fig. 9. Olfactory area in the nasal cavity; Positive reaction is seen in the degenerating epithelial cells in both the olfactory epithelium and olfactory glandular epithelium. Immunohistochemical stain for EHV-9. ABC method. Bar=8.6μm.

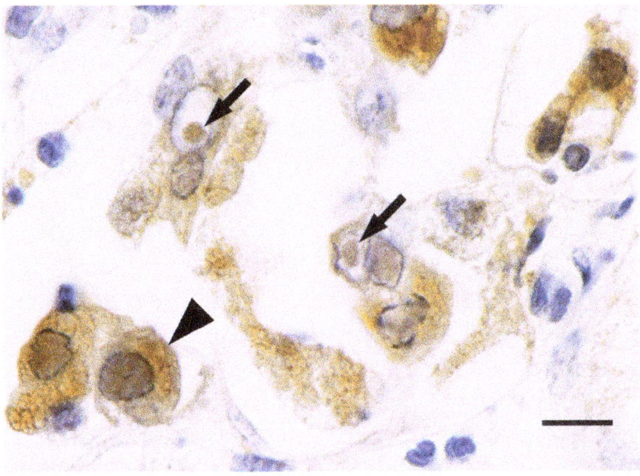

Fig. 10. Olfactory area in the nasal cavity; Positive reaction is seen at the intra-nuclear inclusion bodies (arrows), nucleus and cytoplasm (arrow head) in the degenerating olfactory glandular epihelial cells. Immunohistochemical stain for EHV-9. ABC method. Bar=3.3μm.

EHV-9 was recovered from the olfactory bulb and frontal lobe in all inoculated marmosets. In addition, EHV-9 was isolated from the lung in one marmoset and from the salivary gland and mandible lymph node in one marmoset. The recovered virus was confirmed to be EHV-9 by the PCR method. The EHV-9 virus was not neutralized by 4-times dilution serum in the neutralization test. No virus was isolated from other organs or blood.

EHV-9 demonstrated ready infectivity and rapid progression of the disease in marmosets, which indicates the possibility of EHV-9 infectivity in primates, including humans, as in other domestic animals and rodents. Nasal inoculation of EHV-9 resulted in varying degrees of encephalitis in a wide variety of animals, including rodents, domestic ruminants and companion animals. As with other novel herpesvirus infections such as pseudorabies virus infection in dogs (Yanai et al., 2003a) and B virus infection in humans (Adam and Graham, 1994), EHV-9 could possibly be more virulent in unusual hosts than in the natural host. The pathogenicity of EHV-9 to humans is currently unknown; however, we may be able to assess the virulence of EHV-9 in humans to a certain extent by using nonhuman primates as a model because nonhuman primates have many infectious diseases in common with humans. It was estimated that EHV-9 could possibly be pathogenic to humans if nonhuman primates were infected with it. We used common marmosets for the experimental infection of EHV-9 because they are commonly used for experiments and because they are known to be susceptible to some herpesviruses. Generally, nonhuman primates are highly susceptible to cross-species infectivity by human alpha-herpesvirus, including herpes simplex virus (HSV). In new world monkeys, HSV causes outbreaks characterized by severe ulcerative gingivostomatitis and encephalitis, and these outbreaks are quick to occur in zoo-housed marmosets, with marmosets being thought to be highly susceptible to HSV (Matz-Rensing et al., 2003). On the other hand, simian herpes virus, Herpesvirus B (Cercopithecine herpesvirus 1), has been implicated as the cause of approximately 40 cases of meningoencephalitis affecting persons in direct or indirect contact with laboratory macaques (Weigler, 1992).

In marmosets, as in other animals, EHV-9 shows strong neurotropism and causes selective neuronal necrosis. The distribution of lesions and the virus are most similar to those in cats

(Yanai et al., 2003b). As the most severely affected area was the olfactory bulb, the virus inoculated into the nasal cavity gained access to the olfactory bulb and then progressed along the rhinencephalon over time. In our study, all of the marmosets inoculated intranasally had severe rhinitis with intranuclear inclusions, and EHV-9 antigen was detected in the olfactory epithelium and glands. From these findings, the EHV-9 inoculated into the nasal cavity presumably multiplied in the olfactory mucosa, and then intruded into the nerve sheath connected to the olfactory bulb, going through the foramina in the cribriform plate of the ethmoid bone. As the olfactory epithelium is usually covered by secreta produced in the olfactory glands, the question remains of how the virus infected the epithelial and glandular cells. The inclusion body formation in the glandular epithelium indicated that a large amount of EHV-9 virus had multiplied in the olfactory glands and shed into the nasal cavity. This suggests that, once EHV-9 has infected the nasal mucosa, the marmoset sheds a large enough quantity of virus for transmission to another animal when contact occurs. In addition, a smaller amount of the virus may cause rhinitis with viral propagation once the virus intrudes into the nasal cavity. However, in the present study, it was not clear how the nerve axons were affected by the EHV-9 in the olfactory mucosa, or how the virus in the nerve sheath migrated to the olfactory bulb.

The study demonstrated that marmosets can be infected by a larger dose of EHV-9 by the intranasal route. It suggests the possibility that EHV-9 might be transmitted to other primates, including macaques, great apes and humans. EHV-9 might also be easily transmitted via the nasal route to immuno-compromised animals and patients such as AIDS patients. A recent study showed that Burchell's zebras (*Equus burchelli*) in Tanzania had a high seroprevalence to EHV-9 or to viruses serologically similar to EHV-9 (Borcher et al., 2005), which suggested that EHV-9 is present in zebras permanently residing in East Africa. Also, there has been some possibility of an outbreak of EHV-9 infection as an emerging infection in immuno-compromised animals and patients.

3. Cynomolgus macaques

One male and four female cynomolgus macaques were obtained from a commercial breeder (Kodama et al., 2011). All of the animals were free from pathogens such as salmonella and *Mycobacterium spp.* and passed the viral antibody tests for B virus and measles virus. The animals were divided into two groups consisting of Nos. 1 and 2 in one group and Nos. 3 and 4 in the other, and the two groups were inoculated intranasally with 1 ml of EHV-9 virus solution containing 10^3 and 10^6 plaque-forming units, respectively. The virus fluid was prepared by propagating the fifth passage of the original stock, which is in Madin-Darby bovine kidney (MDCK) cells, in fetal horse kidney cells. The infectivity of the inoculums was confirmed by virus plaque assay with MDCK cells. As a control, cynomolgus monkey No. 5 was inoculated with 1 ml of minimal essential medium. Animals Nos. 1 and 3 were euthanized in accordance with animal welfare regulations on 6 dpi. The other animals were euthanized on 10 dpi.

In contrast with the control animal, the inoculated animals began avoiding light starting from 4 dpi. Blood studies showed no hematological abnormalities in any of the animals.

At necropsy, no significant abnormalities were observed in any organs from any of the animals.

Histopathologically, no significant pathological changes were observed in any of the organs from any of the animals. Immunohistochemistry revealed no positive reactions in any of the organs or tissues, including the nasal cavities or brains of the animals. In the amplification of the gene for gB (ORF33) using specific primers for EHV-9 by PCR, no bands were detected in any of the samples from the right olfactory bulb, right cerebrum or right cerebellum, the blood samples, or the nasal swabs. It was demonstrated that the nasal swabs had no infectivity. The EHV-9 virus was not neutralized by the serum from any of the animals in the neutralization test.

The results in this study suggest that EHV-9 may be non-pathogenic for adult cynomolgus monkeys. The etiology for the clinical symptom was not apparent because there were no histopathological changes. However, the symptom may have been a response to the EHV-9 inoculation.

Although lethal encephalitis was induced via the nasal, oral, intraperitoneal and ocular routes of EHV-9 inoculation in hamsters (El-Habashi et al., 2010), the intranasal route may be the most probable one. In addition, EHV-9 replicated in the olfactory epithelium and olfactory glandular epithelium in common marmosets (Kodama et al., 2007). Based on those results, successful infection to the olfactory epithelium might be among the essential factors for following EHV-9 induced encephalitis. The proportion of surface area covered by the olfactory epithelium in macaques may be considerably smaller than that in rodents and dogs (Herkema, 1991). Thus, there may be constitutional barriers to the entrance of the EHV-9 into the olfactory epithelium. However, because it has been suggested that the relative amount of the olfactory epithelium in common marmosets is much closer to that of macaques than that of rats, the constitutional distinction may not be associated with EHV-9 infection induced via the intranasal route (Wako et al., 1999).

4. Conclusion: EHV-9 can induce encephalitis in primates, including humans

In assessments of infectivity of EHV-9 in nonhuman primates, there were different results between new world and old world monkeys. While EHV-9 caused fulminant encephalitis, no infectivity was seen in cynomolgus macaques. It is still uncertain whether macaques have barriers to invasion of EHV-9 at the entrance, and this could apply to humans as well. Thus, it has not been determined that EHV-9 can cross the species barrier between new world and old world monkeys and humans. It is also uncertain whether EHV-9 can infect immune-compromised patients like AIDS patients, infants or elderly people. Ocular transmission of viruses to the CNS has been suspected in many viral diseases such as Cercopithecine herpes virus 1 (B-virus) in humans (CDC, 1999). Fatal infection by B-virus in humans via ocular exposure from biological fluid from macaque monkeys has been reported (CDC, 1999). Further studies using nonhuman primates may be needed to assess the risk to infants from the ocular route of infection.

5. References

[1] Adams JH, Graham DI: Virus and other infections. *In*: An Introduction to Neuropathology, second edition, pp. 103-132. Churchill Livingstone, Edinburgh, 1994

[2] Borchers K, Wiik H, Frolich K, Ludwig H, East ML: Antibodies against equine herpesviruses and equine arteritis virus in Burchell's zebras (Equus burchelli) from the Serengeti ecosystem. J Wildl Dis 41: 80-86, 2005

[3] CDC (1999): Hazard ID 5- Cercopithecine herpesvirus 1 (B Virus) infection resulting from ocular exposure. National Institute for Occupational Safety and Health (NIOSH), Publication, 99-100.
[4] El-Habashi N, Murakami M, EL-Nahass E, Hibi D, Sakai H, Fukushi H, Sasseville V, Yanai T: Study on the infectivity of equine herpesvirus 9 (EHV-9) by different routes of inoculation in hamsters. Vet Pathol 47: 1-7, 2010
[5] Fukushi H, Tomita T, Taniguchi A, Ochiai Y, Kirisawa R, Matsumura T, Yanai T, Masegi T, Yamaguchi T, Hirai K: Gazelle herpesvirus 1: a new neurotropic herpesvirus immunologically related to equine herpesvirus 1. Virology 227: 34-44, 1997
[6] Fukushi H, Taniguchi A, Yasuda K, Yanai T, Masegi T, Yamaguchi T, Hirai K: A hamster model of equine herpesvirus 9 induced encephalitis. J Neurovirol 6: 314-319, 2000
[7] Herkema JR: Comparative aspects of nasal airway anatomy; relevance to inhalation toxicology. Toxicol Pathol 19: 321-336, 1991
[8] Kodama A, Yanai T, Yomemaru K, Sakai H, Masegi T, Yamada S, Fukushi H, Kuraishi T, Hattori S, Kai C: Acute neuropathogenicity with experimental infection of equine herpesvirus 9 in common marmosets (*Callithrix jacchus*). J Med Primatol 36 : 335 - 342, 2007
[9] Kodama A, Yanai T, Kubo M, El-Habashi N, Kasem S, Sakai H, Masegi T, Fukushi H, Kuraishi T, Hattori S, Kai C: Cynomolgus monkeys (*Macaca fascicularis*) may not become infected with equine herpesvirus 9. J Med Primatol 40: 18 - 20, 2011
[10] Matz-Rensing K, Jentsch KD, Rensing S, Langenhuyzen S, Verschoor E, Niphuis H, Kaup FJ: Fatal Herpes simplex infection in a group of common marmosets (Callithrix jacchus). Vet Pathol 40: 405-411, 2003
[11] Narita M, Uchimura A, Kimura K, Tanimura N, Yanai T, Masegi T, Fukushi H, Hirai K: Brain lesions and transmission of experimental equine herpesvirus type 9 in pigs. Vet Pathol 37: 476-479, 2000
[12] Narita M, Uchimura A, Kawanabe M, Fukushi H, Hirai K: Invasion and spread of equine herpesvirus 9 in the olfactory pathway of pigs after intranasal inoculation. J Comp Pathol 124: 265-272, 2001
[13] Taniguchi A, Fukushi H, Yanai T, Masegi T, Yamaguchi T, Hirai K: Equine herpesvirus 9 induced lethal encephalomyelitis in experimentally infected goats. Arch Virol 145: 2619-2627, 2000
[14] Wako K, Hiratsuka H, Katsuta O, Tsuchitani M: Anatomical structure and surface epithelial distribution in the nasal cavity of the common cotton-eared marmoset (Callithrix jacchus). Exp Animal 48:31-36, 1999
[15] Weigler BJ: Biology of B virus in macaque and human hosts: a review. Clin Infect Dis 14: 555-567, 1992
[16] Yanai T, Sakai T, Fukushi H, Hirai K, Narita M, Sakai H, Masegi T: Neuropathological study of gazelle herpesvirus 1 (equine herpesvirus 9) infection in Thomson's gazelles (Gazella thomsoni). J Comp Pathol 119: 159-168, 1998
[17] Yanai T, Fujishima N, Fukushi H, Hirata A, Sakai H, Masegi T: Experimental infection of equine herpesvirus 9 in dogs. Vet Pathol 40: 263-267, 2003a
[18] Yanai T, Tujioka S, Sakai H, Fukushi H, Hirai K, Masegi T: Experimental infection with equine herpesvirus 9 (EHV-9) in cats. J Comp Pathol 128: 113-118, 2003b

8

Coronaviruses as Encephalitis - Inducing Infectious Agents

Pierre J. Talbot, Marc Desforges, Elodie Brison and Hélène Jacomy
Laboratory of Neuroimmunovirology,
INRS-Institut Armand-Frappier, Laval (Québec)
Canada

1. Introduction

Encephalitis usually refers to brain inflammation of various possible causes, including viral infections. Overall, viruses represent the most common cause of encephalitis in humans. The U.S. Center for Disease Control and Prevention (CDC) estimates an annual incidence of usually between 150 and 3000 new cases per year of Arboviral encephalitis in the United States (http://www.cdc.gov/). Although several thousand cases of encephalitis of various viral origins are reported each year, the CDC suspects that many more cases may go unreported. Indeed, encephalitis can follow or accompany common viral illnesses, such as infectious respiratory diseases, and sometimes signs and symptoms of the latter may mask concurrent encephalitis. Most commonly, clinically relevant viral encephalitis affects children, young adults, or elderly patients. The involvement of other determinants, such as the nature of the specific viral agent, the host immune status, and various genetic and environmental factors, is also of importance.

The pathophysiology of viral encephalitis varies according to the virus family involved. Encephalitis occurs in two forms: primary encephalitis involving direct viral infection of the central nervous system (CNS; brain and spinal cord) and secondary encephalitis involving a viral infection which first occurs elsewhere in the body and then travels to the brain. Viruses may enter the CNS through two distinct routes: hematogenous dissemination or neuronal retrograde dissemination. The hematogenous spread, which is the most common path, involves the presence of a given virus in the blood (viremia), where it can either remain free for a period of time or infect leukocytes that will become some sort of viral reservoir. This latter situation, called the Trojan horse, is the route taken by human immunodeficiency virus (HIV) to disseminate to the CNS in humans. Arboviruses also use the hematogenous route to gain access to the CNS, where they can induce a zoonotic encephalitis, with the virus surviving in infection cycles involving bites by arthropods and various vertebrates, especially birds and rodents. After an insect bite, the virus can be transmitted in the blood of a susceptible animal after local replication in the skin.

Another form of viral spread towards the CNS is through retrograde neuronal dissemination, where a given virus infects neurons in the periphery and uses the transport machinery within those cells in order to gain access to the CNS.

Neuroinvasive viruses can damage the CNS as a result of misdirected host immune responses (virus-induced neuroimmunopathology) and/or viral replication, which will directly induce damage to CNS cells (virus-induced neuropathology). In acute encephalitis, viral replication occurs in the brain tissue itself, possibly causing destructive lesions of the gray matter, as was described after herpes simplex virus (HSV), rabies, or some arbovirus infections. Rabies virus usually spreads to the CNS through retrograde peripheral nerve dissemination and one of the possible routes of HSV spread to the CNS is through the olfactory tracts.

Encephalitis caused by viruses generally can be classified into four different groups. (1) *Arboviruses* which appear to be the primary cause of acute encephalitis (Eastern Equine Encephalitis, Japanese Encephalitis, La Crosse Encephalitis, St. Louis Encephalitis, Western Equine Encephalitis, West Nile Virus Encephalitis). These viruses are transmitted to humans by the bite of infected mosquitoes and/or ticks. (2) *Enteroviruses*, such as coxsackievirus or polioviruses. These viruses spread through the fecal-oral route. Infection can result in a wide variety of symptoms ranging from mild respiratory illness (common cold), to, foot-and-mouth disease, acute hemorrhagic conjunctivitis, aseptic meningitis, myocarditis, severe neonatal sepsis-like disease, and acute flaccid paralysis. (3) *Herpes viruses* constitute another major cause of encephalitis in North America. Members of this virus family include HSV, Epstein-Barr virus (EBV), cytomegalovirus (CMV), and varicella-zoster virus (VZV). They are highly contagious as they can be spread when an infected person is producing the virus. (4) Other viruses, following childhood viral diseases such as measles, mumps, and rubella can in rare cases develop secondary encephalitis. More recently, respiratory viruses were closely associated with encephalitis as reported for influenza virus (for reviews, see Maurizi, 2010 and Wang et al., 2010) or occasionally for coronaviruses (Yeh et al., 2004).

2. Coronavirus

Coronaviruses are ubiquitous respiratory and enteric pathogens. They also represent one family of viruses that bear neurotropic and neuroinvasive properties in various hosts including humans, pigs, and rodents. Coronaviruses form a group of enveloped, positive-sense, single-stranded polyadenylated RNA viruses that have the largest genome (~30 kb) among RNA viruses. They replicate in the cytoplasm of infected cells using a viral RNA-dependent RNA polymerase that is translated from the genomic RNA very early after viral entry in the host cell. Coronaviruses first target respiratory and mucosal surfaces and then, depending of host and virus strain, may spread to other tissues (brain, eyes, liver, kidneys and spleen) and cause a range of pathologies such as pneumonia, encephalitis, neurodegenerative demyelination, hepatitis, enteritis, and nephritis among others (Resta et al., 1985; Riski & Hovi, 1980).

Human coronaviruses (HCoV) are represented by five different strains; HCoV-229E, HCoV-OC43, HCoV-NL63, HCoV-HKU1 and the causative agent of the severe acute respiratory syndrome (SARS), named SARS-CoV. Among these five strains, at least HCoV-229E and HCoV-OC43, as well as SARS-CoV possess neuroinvasive properties as viral RNA can be detected in human brains (Arbour et al., 2000; Gu et al., 2005; Xu et al., 2005).

However, these human coronaviruses are not well characterized as to their capacity to invade and infect the CNS. On the other hand, the murine counterpart of HCoV-OC43, which is designated Mouse Hepatitis Virus (MHV), represents one of the best-characterized models of this family. MHV infects mice and rats and some strains are neurotropic and neuroinvasive, causing a large spectrum of diseases from hepatitis to encephalitis and chronic demyelination (Stohlman & Hinton, 2001; for reviews, see also Bender & Weiss, 2010 and Lane & Hosking, 2010).

2.1 Murine Hepatitis Virus: An agent of encephalitis

MHV exhibits various organ tropisms as well as pathogenic potentials. The most common strains used for pathogenesis studies are the neurotropic MHV-JHM (previously called MHV-4), the hepatotropic/neurotropic MHV-A59 and the hepatotropic MHV-3. Experimental infections of rodents with these strains provide animal models for human diseases such as hepatitis, encephalitis, and demyelinating diseases such as multiple sclerosis. Infection of mice by the intranasal or intracerebral route with MHV-JHM or MHV-A59 serves as a model for studying encephalitis and determinants of neurovirulence.
MHV is part of the family *Coronaviridae* and the genus betacoronavirus. Its genome is 32-kilobases long and comprises different open reading frames (ORFs), which encode four structural proteins: spike (S), envelope (E), membrane (M), nucleocapsid (N), with some strains also expressing a gene encoding two other structural proteins: hemagglutinin-esterase (HE) and internal protein (I). The genome also encodes three nonstructural proteins, which functions remain poorly understood. The assembly of coronavirus virions needs a concerted action of three structural proteins: the membrane protein (M), the small envelope protein (E), and the nucleocapsid protein (N) (de Haan & Rottier, 2005; Masters 2006). Among these three proteins, no role in pathogenesis has been reported for M and E.

2.2 Viral molecular determinants of encephalitis

While the molecular determinants of pathogenesis remain poorly understood, there is evidence that both host and viral factors play a role in coronavirus-induced disease. Experiments completed during the last decade have used infectious cDNA clones to produce viruses of high and low virulence to investigate, by the mean of reciprocal chimeric viruses, the molecular determinants of neurovirulence. Viral genes responsible for high MHV neuropathogenesis contribute to viral spread, replication and activation of innate/adaptive immunity.

2.2.1 Spike glycoprotein: S

The S protein mediates attachment of the virus to its receptor on the target cell and viral fusion with the cell membrane, as well as viral entry and cell to cell spread (Collins et al., 1982; Williams et al., 1991). Based on previous studies, which used numerous variant viruses selected for resistance to neutralizing monoclonal antibodies, an association was made between various mutations or deletions in the S gene and neuroattenuation of the different strains of MHV (Gallagher et al., 1990; Wege et al., 1988). More recently, the use of recombinant MHV viruses with a modified spike (S) glycoprotein has definitively identified the S protein as a major determinant of neurovirulence. The recombinant A59 (rA59) virus which contains the S gene of JHM (S_{JHM}) confers a highly neurovirulent phenotype. The viral infectious dose inoculated into mouse brain to induce a 50% lethal dose (LD_{50}) is decreased by more than 1000-fold, demonstrating the role of S in neurovirulence (Phillips et al., 1999). Neuronal infection has long been proposed to be a major determinant of MHV neurovirulence (Dubois-Dalcq et al., 1982), and the recent use of recombinant viruses demonstrated that even if neurovirulence is increased, cellular tropism remained the same, as rA59 and rA59/S_{JHM} recombinant viruses target equally neurons and astrocytes (Phillips et al., 2002). The degree of neurovirulence is associated with the degree of spread through the brain. The faster the spread, the higher will be the neurovirulence. This increased viral spread and dissemination also induces a greater immune response to infection. The magnitude of lymphocytic infiltration in mouse brain following infection by rA59 with S_{JHM} and rA59 with S_{A59} is different, as S_{JHM} induced a more efficient CNS invasion of lymphocytes than S_{A59} and a significant increase in the percentage of $CD8^+$ T cells (Phillips et al., 2002). Increased immune-mediated pathology was associated with rapid viral spread (Miura et al., 2008; Wodarz & Krakauer, 2000). The recombinant virus rA59, harboring the JHM S protein (S_{JHM}) is not as virulent as wild-type recombinant rJHM, indicating that neurovirulence also depends on other background genes. The high neurovirulence of JHM is also associated with an increased innate immune response characterized by high numbers of infiltrating neutrophils and macrophages, demonstrated by comparing rJHM bearing S_{A59} to rJHM bearing S_{JHM} during the acute phase of encephalitis (Iacono et al., 2006). Nevertheless, the viral strain background also plays a strong role, as viruses containing the rA59 genes demonstrated markedly increased levels of CD8+ and CD4+ T-cell infiltration compared to the rJHM background-containing viruses (Iacono et al., 2006). Virus-specific $CD8^+$ T cells are critical for protection against neurotropic coronaviruses. On the other hand, the combination of a rapid and extensive spread through the CNS with the lack of induction of a significant T-cell response results in the high lethality of JHM-infected mice (MacNamara et al., 2005; 2008).

2.2.2 Nucleocapsid protein: N

Structural proteins are transmembrane proteins located in the viral envelope, except for the N protein, which is associated with the viral RNA genome (Baric et al., 1988; Sturman et al., 1980). Replacement of the N gene of rA59 with that of JHM (N_{JHM}) confers to the rA59 background a highly neurovirulent phenotype. The viral infectious dose inoculated into mouse brain to induce a 50% lethal dose (LD_{50}) is decreased between 100- and 1000-fold. Inversely, the rJHM with N_{A59} is attenuated, but this is more evident on the attenuated phenotype (rA59/S_{JHM}), indicating that replacing the MHV-JHM N gene with that of MHV-A59 is attenuating (Cowley et al., 2010). The rA59/N_{JHM} induced a faster spread of virus in the CNS than rA59, whereas the rJHM/N_{A59} demonstrated a restrained viral spread as compare to rJHM. These data illustrated that the N background determined viral spread, which is a constituent of virulence. The N_{JHM} is suspected to be associated to microtubules (Pasick et al., 1994) and then to be able to increase the transport of virus along axons to favor viral spread between neurons to other neurons. Unfortunately, the infection of primary hippocampal neuronal cultures by rA59/N_{JHM} did not demonstrate an increased spread of virus as compared to rA59 (Cowley et al., 2010). Moreover, the N gene influences T-cell infiltration into the brain, as $CD4^+$ and $CD8^+$ T cell response is strong if the virus possesses N_{A59} and weak with the N_{JHM} (Cowley et al., 2010).

2.2.3 Hemagglutinin Esterase glycoprotein (HE)

The hemagglutinin esterase (HE), is an envelope glycoprotein, which is present in some strains of the betacoronaviruses such as the human coronaviruses (HCoV-OC43 and HCoV-HKU1), as well as the bovine coronavirus (BCoV). The JHM strain of MHV expresses the HE glycoprotein, whereas MHV-A59 does not, due to a defective HE gene (Shieh et al.,

1989). Nevertheless, MHV-A59 is able to induce an encephalitis in infected mice but the disease is less important as this strain is less neurovirulent than MHV-JHM. By using targeted RNA recombination to introduce the HE gene of MHV-JHM into the genome of MHV-A59, the role of the HE gene in neurovirulence was addressed. The expression of HE on the MHV-A59 background neither increased virulence in mice (as evaluated by the LD_{50}), nor the production of infectious virus (in brain or liver tissue), or virus spread (revealed by the distribution of viral antigen) (Kazi et al., 2005). Whereas, Kazi and collaborators demonstrated that the expression of HE in combination with the MHV-JHM spike protein in rA59 enhances the disease outcome and increased viral spread in the brain, without changing viral replication, their results suggest that a structurally intact HE, in combination with the MHV-JHM spike protein, has a significant impact on the neurovirulence. In fact, even though the S protein is the main viral factor, which determines tissue tropism and infection of target cell, the HE viral protein appears to serve as a second receptor-binding protein, which increases infection and viral dissemination in the brain (Kazi et al., 2005).

2.3 Human coronaviruses (HCoV)

Human coronaviruses (HCoV) are recognized respiratory pathogens but, in rare cases, they may be associated with encephalitis. As previously mentioned, five different strains of human coronaviruses are currently described: HCoV-OC43, HCoV-229E, HCoV-NL-63, HCoV-HKU1 and SARS-CoV, and neuroinvasive properties were reported for at least three of these five strains. Indeed, our laboratory has demonstrated that HCoV-OC43 and HCoV-229E can infect human neural cells (neurons and glial cells) and does persist in human brains (Bonavia et al., 1997; Arbour et al., 1999a; 1999b; 2000). Others have reported the presence of HCoV-OC43 in a child with acute disseminated encephalomyelitis (Yeh et al., 2004). Moreover, the SARS-CoV epidemics reported in China in the fall of 2002, strongly illustrated the potentially fatal illness caused by a coronavirus (Drosten et al., 2003; Fouchier et al., 2003; Ksiazek et al., 2003). The severe acute respiratory syndrome described was usually transmitted by contact with droplets sprayed into the air by an infected person's coughing. Other symptoms can include high fever, headache, body aches, and pneumonia. A few years after the 2002-2003 epidemics, scientists found that SARS-CoV was able to also infiltrate brain tissue and cause significant CNS problems associated with edema, degeneration of neuronal cells and gliosis, and SARS-CoV RNA could be detected in the brain of patients who died of SARS (Gu et al., 2005; Xu et al., 2005). Moreover, the use of a transgenic mouse model expressing the recognized viral receptor, human angiotensin-converting enzyme 2 (hACE-2), showed that SARS-CoV possesses neuroinvasive properties, as the virus reached the brain by the olfactory bulbs, infecting neuronal cells and induced a lethal disease, with a restrained immune infiltration (Netland et al., 2008).

2.3.1 Animal model to understand the human coronavirus infection

We have characterized the neurotropic, neuroinvasive and neurovirulent properties of HCoV-OC43 through the development of an experimental animal model. We have reported that intranasal (IN) infection of mice with HCoV-OC43 led to acute encephalitis and to a generalized infection of the whole CNS, demonstrating HCoV-OC43 neuroinvasiveness and neurovirulence (Jacomy & Talbot, 2003). Damage to the CNS appeared to be mainly a consequence of direct virus-mediated neuronal injury. Indeed, as illustrated in Figure 1, this acute infection targeted neurons, which underwent vacuolation and degeneration. We were also able to demonstrate that caspase-related virus-induced apoptosis of neuronal cells both *in vitro* and *in vivo* (Jacomy and Talbot, 2006). This type of virus-induced apoptosis is of particular interest as in the human brain, activation of caspase 3 is involved in pathologic pathway of influenza encephalopathy (Nakai et al., 2003), reovirus-induced encephalitis (Beckham et al., 2010) and Japanese-encephalitis virus-induced pathology (Yang et al., 2009).

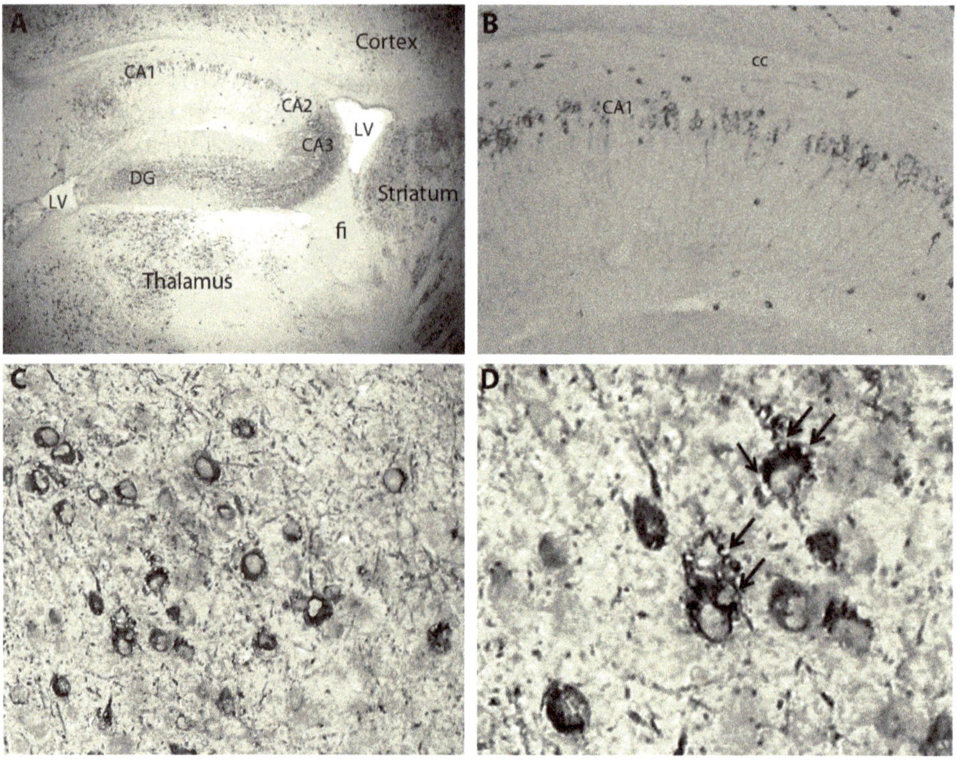

Fig. 1. Infection of neuronal cells by HCoV-OC43. (A) Numerous cells positive for virus antigens at 7 days post-infection (DPI) in the CNS. Virus was present in hippocampal region (especially in pyramidal cell layers CA1, CA2 and CA3, as well as in dentate gyrus (DG)), in cortical area (Cortex), in Striatum as well as in Thalamus. (B) Magnification of pyramidal cell layers CA1, illustrating numerous infected cells stained in black. (C) Infected neurons in the Striatum, at higher magnification (D), numerous vacuolation were present in the cytoplasm of infected neurons (arrows). LV: Lateral ventricle; cc: corpus callosum; fi: fimbria of hippocampus.

While neurons are the primary target of HCoV-OC43, infected regions presented strong microglial reactivity and inflammatory reactions (neuroinflammation). Although initiation of immune responses by microglial cells is normally an important protective mechanism in the CNS, unrestrained inflammatory responses may result in irreversible brain damage. It is likely that strong microglial activation can trigger bystander damage, as they can release large amounts of cytokines and chemokines. In fact, we have recently shown that infection of susceptible mice by HCoV-OC43 induced the production of high level of numerous pro-inflammatory cytokines such as tumor necrosing factor (TNF)-alpha, interleukin (IL)-1 beta and IL-6, released in the CNS, as well as chemokines and strong infiltration of immune cells (Jacomy et al., 2010). This is again of particular interest since accumulating evidence show that these types of factors may influence the degree of encephalitis. For instance, the mortality rate following JEV encephalitis is directly linked to the concentration of cytokine in serum and cerebrospinal fluid (CSF) in patients (Winter et al., 2004). Furthermore, neuronal cell death in a mice model of Japanese Encephalitis Virus (JEV) infection was demonstrated to be related to the activation of microglia and subsequent production of multiple proinflammatory mediators (Ghoshal et al., 2007). We also reported that apoptosis of neurons occurred in infected and non-infected cells, suggesting that it is independent of the presence of virus (Jacomy et al., 2006). Host adaptive immune response was demonstrated to contribute to HCoV-OC43-induced encephalitis (Butler et al., 2006). We also reported that mice surviving encephalitis developed motor dysfunctions as the result of viral persistence in the CNS (Jacomy et al., 2006). In addition to the direct effect of the viral pathogen, acute encephalopathy may be associated with viral infections and increased plasma concentrations of CXCL8/IL-8 and CCL2/MCP-1, CXCL10/IP-10 and IL-6, without viral neuroinvasion (hyperactivated cytokine/chemokine response) as demonstrated following infection by another respiratory virus, Influenza virus, which can cause encephalitis (Lee et al., 2010). JEV also induces a rapid inflammatory response, which is accompanied by an increased level of cytokines and chemokines in the serum and cerebrospinal fluid of infected patients. Moreover, levels of interferon (IFN)-alpha, TNF-alpha, and the cytokines IL-8 and IL-6 have been associated with a bad outcome (Burke & Morill, 1987; Singh et al., 2000, Winter et al., 2004)

Excitotoxic neurotransmission, which is an excessive stimulation by the neurotransmitter glutamate on its specific receptors (AMPAr and NMDAr), seems to play an important role in neuronal damage during encephalitis as concentration of glutamate in CSF is significantly increased in acute encephalitis (Launes et al., 1998). Moreover, the concentration of glutamate was also correlated with a poor outcome during encephalitis in humans, as well as in an animal model of human encephalitis (Carmen et al., 2009; Launes et al., 1998). During the HCoV-OC43-induced encephalitis, we recently found that hippocampal neurons died in part by this pathological process (Brison et al., submitted for publication). Indeed, treatment of infected mice with the AMPA receptor antagonist (GYKI-52466) did not affect the survival rate of mice but histological analysis revealed that mice treated by the GYKI-52466 presented less neurodegeneration compared to infected mice without the AMPA antagonist, as determined by Neurosilver staining (Figure 2) (Brison et al., submitted for publication). Again, this is of particular interest since glutamate excitotoxicity was demonstrated to be involved in several viral infection such as West Nile virus, Sindbis virus, JEV, HIV and HSV (Blakely et al., 2009; Golembewski et al., 2007; Haughey et al., 2001; Mishra et al., 2007; Nargi-Aizenman et al., 2004). The loss of neuronal subpopulations in the brain during HIV dementia was also related to an indirect mechanism conjugating glial activation, cytokines released and excitotoxic transmission (Alirezaei et al., 2008; Masliah & Mucke, 1996).

We have also demonstrated that the severity of the HCoV-OC43 induced-encephalitis depended on a number of factors such as the genetic background (Jacomy & Talbot, 2003) and the gender of the mice, as revealed by inoculation of male and female animals of different mouse strains, aged 21 days post-natal (DPN). At the equal infectious viral dose, male animals are more susceptible than female animals. For all strains of mice tested, male animals appeared more susceptible than female animals to encephalitis, as illustrated for strains C57BL/6 and BALB/c in Figure 3.

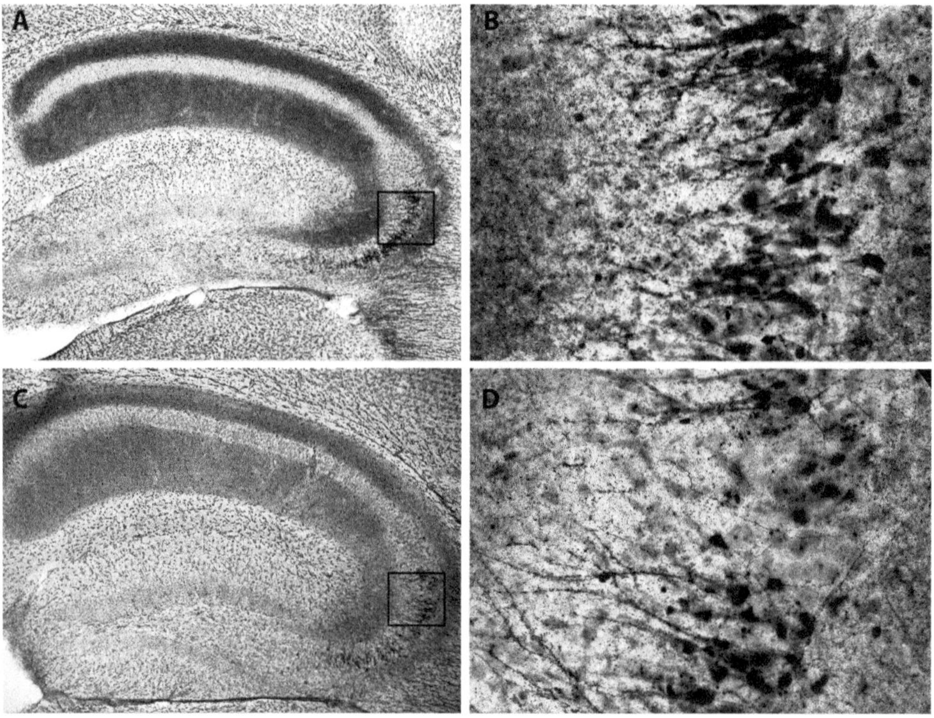

Fig. 2. Hippocampus of mice following HCoV-OC43 infection treated or not treated by the GYKI-52466 antagonist. Following infection, neurodegeneration was investigated with Silver staining in non-treated (A and higher magnification B) and AMPA receptor antagonist-treated mice (C and higher magnification D). Neurons that underwent degeneration appear in black. As illustrated at higher magnification, non-treated mice present more numerous dark CA3 neurons (B) as compared to mice treated with GYKI-52466 (D).

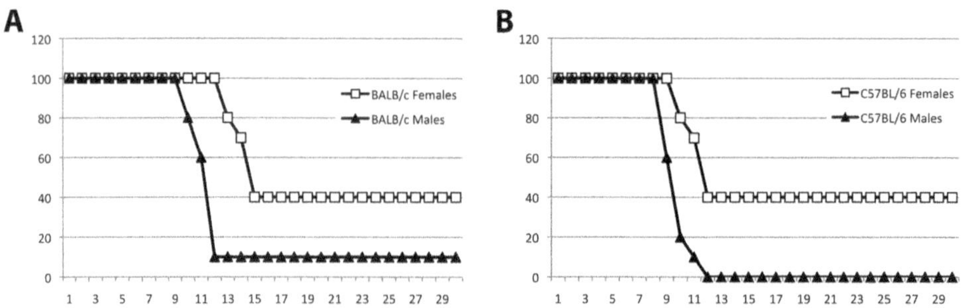

Fig. 3. Survival rate of female versus male mice to a same infectious dose. Mice were monitored for 30 days for mortality following intracerebral infection. C57BL/6 (A) and BALB/c (B) mice were infected, respectively, with $10^{2.5}$ $TCID_{50}$ or $10^{0.5}$ $TCID_{50}$ of virus. For the same infectious dose, male mice were more susceptible to viral infection than female.

How immunological, hormonal, and or genetic differences between males and females could affect gender differences in susceptibility to infection? Males and females are differentially susceptible to several pathogens including viruses (Fish, 2008; Klein, 2000). In fact, in the case of viral infection in general, this difference in susceptibility between males and females was shown for different viruses including Seoul Virus (Klein et al., 2000), and Influenza virus (Avitsur et al., 2011) and this is also true in the particular case of viral infection of the CNS, which leads to encephalitis, for other viruses such as HIV-1 (Wilson et al., 2006), and vesicular stomatitis virus (VSV) (Barna et al., 1996). The concept of sex-based (or gender-based) differences in host response to infection has been studied for many years and appears to be highly related to differences in immunological capacities between males and females (Purtilo & Sullivan, 1979; Fish, 2008). Furthermore, it appears now that even though the relative importance of different factors may vary with the type of infection, X-linked genes, hormones, immunity and, at least in humans, societal context are among the factors that explain this sex-based difference (Fish, 2008; Klein, 2000). Even though it remains difficult to clarify evidence on how the different factors make a difference between genders, studies aimed to addressing the question appear to more and more link specific hormones such as androgens in males and estrogens in females (Klein, 2000; Wilson et al., 2006), host innate immunity (expression of cytokines and of pattern recognition receptors such as toll-like receptors (TLR)) (Hannah et al., 2008; Hill et al., 1998) as well as acquired immunity involving T and B lymphocytes (reviewed in Klein, 2000) to explain part of the puzzle.

As already published in our model, C57BL/6 were more susceptible than BALB/c mice and CD1 mice were in between, being more resistant than C57BL/6 mice and more susceptible than BALB/c mice. As already described, susceptibility to intracellular pathogens depends on human genetics (for review, see Vannberg et al., 2011). Therefore, susceptibility to infectious diseases could be linked to loci or alleles that could favor clearance of virus, such as for hepatitis C virus (Ge et al., 2009; Thomas et al., 2009). In the contrary, genetics may determine persistence of infection, such as in the case of Hepatitis B virus (Kamatani et al., 2009) or restrict viral loads as shown in HIV-1 infections (Fellay et al., 2007; 2009) Furthermore, we also showed that susceptibility to intranasal infection diminished with age (Figure 4), as adult mice became resistant to intranasal infection. All infected mice (21 days post natal (DPN) and more) survived to intranasal infection, no infectious virus was detected in the brain even though viral RNA could be detected in the CNS, demonstrating neuroinvasive properties without evident signs of pathology. This is an interesting fact considering that this restrictive susceptibility to CNS infection and encephalitis appear to exist in humans, where mostly children, the elderly and immuno-compromised individuals are more susceptible (Schneider & Higgs, 2008; Wang et al., 2010).

We also reported that mice became less susceptible to intracerebral infection with the age of mice, as illustrated in Figure 5.

2.4 Other non human coronaviruses as encephalitis-inducing agents

Over the years, some coronaviruses, which can infect cattle or domestic animals, were described as agent able to induced encephalitis in certain conditions.

2.4.1 Swine coronaviruses (HEV)

Hemagglutinating encephalitis virus (HEV) was demonstrated to induce disease ranging from gastroenteritis to encephalomyelitis in piglets (Andries & Pensaert, 1980; Siddell et al.,

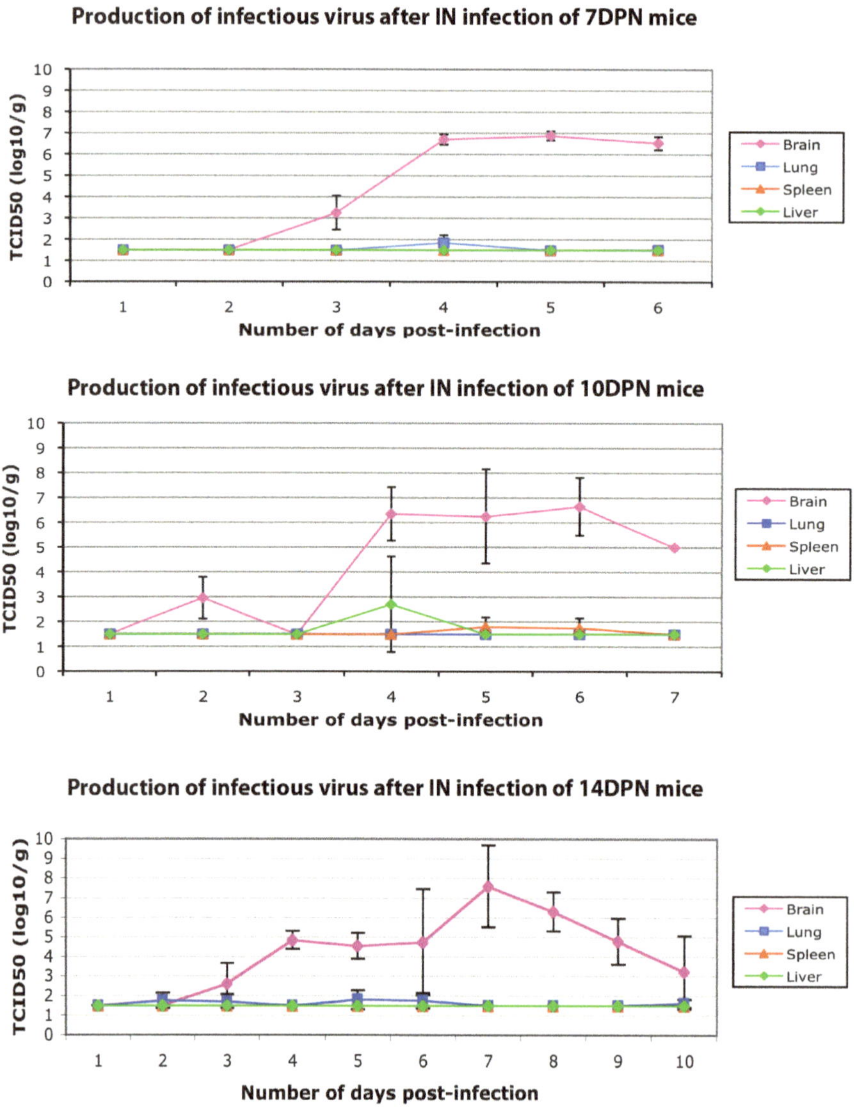

Fig. 4. Neuroinvasive properties following intranasal (IN) inoculation of C57BL/6 aged from 7 to 14 DPN. After inhalation of virus (5000 $TCID_{50}$), 5 mice of each age were sacrificed every 24 hours and the production of infectious virus (virus titers) measured in the CNS, lung, liver and spleen. A detectable level of HCoV-OC43 was found in the brain as early as 2 or 3 DPI (days post-infection), and reached its maximum level a few days later. Infectious virus was occasionally found in lung, spleen or liver (detection limit of the assay: $10^{1.5}$ $TCID_{50}$), especially at times when brain viral titers reached a maximum. Moreover, 7 and 10 DPN mice did not survive HCoV-OC43 inhalation and about 10% of 14 DPN mice did survive.

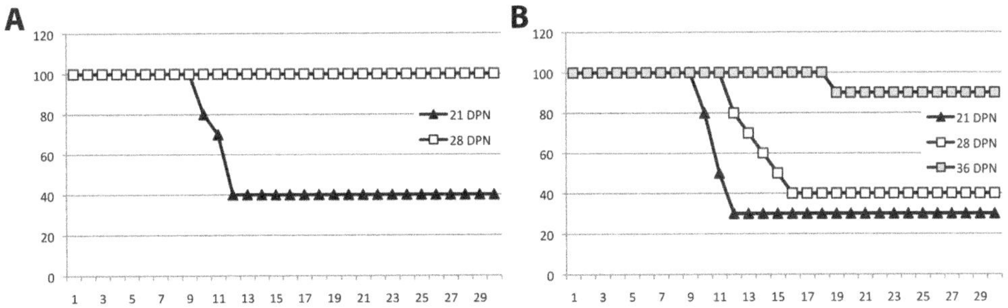

Fig. 5. Susceptibility of mice to the same infectious dose depends of age. (A) C57BL/6 mice became totally unsusceptible to a $10^{0.5}$ infectious dose at 28 days post-natal (DPN), whereas, 60% died following the same infectious dose when they were aged 21 DPN. (B) In the same manner, the susceptibility of CD1 mice to a $10^{1.5}$ infectious doses depended on the age at the time of infection.

1983). The virus was isolated from the brains of suckling pigs suffering from encephalomyelitis several years ago (Greig et al., 1962). The disease could be reproduced experimentally in piglets following intranasal inoculation (Alexander, 1962). A murine model demonstrated that this virus, as other coronaviruses including the HCoV-OC43, is neuroinvasive and neurotropic. In that latter case, neuroinvasion depends on a number of variables such as the route of inoculation and the age of the mice (Yagami et al., 1986; Hirano et al., 1990; 2004). As for the SARS-CoV in mice, HEV induced a poor inflammatory reaction in CNS (Hirano et al., 2004) and unlike HCoV-OC43-infected neurons (Jacomy & Talbot, 2003), HEV-infected cells showed no cytopathological changes.

2.4.2 Feline coronaviruses (FCoV)

Feline infectious peritonitis (FIP) is a common cause of death in cats, caused by a virulent feline coronavirus (FCoV). The virulent form of FCoV, called FIPV, occurs following mutations acquired during a persistent infection (Brown et al., 2009; Rottier et al., 2005; Vennema et al., 1998) and neurologic involvement could occur in FIP disease (Foley et al., 1998; Summers et al., 1995). The colon was identified as the major site of FCoV persistence; nevertheless the virus could also persist in tissue macrophages representing a source for viremia (Kipar et al., 2010). Infected macrophages disseminate systemically and trigger immunological responses resulting in microgranuloma formation, vasculitis, organ failure, and death (Pedersen and Boyle, 1980; Poland et al., 1996 and Vennema et al., 1998). The immunopathogenesis of the disease is poorly understood and often there is little coronavirus present in FIP-affected brain tissue (Foley et al 1998), even though infected phagocytes cells were recovered in CNS of cats (Poncelet et al., 2008), yet inflammatory cells are recruited to the brain and appear to contribute to disease, in part, through secretion of cytokines (Foley et al., 2003).

3. Conclusion

Knowledge of mechanisms and consequences of virus interactions with the nervous system is essential to better understand potentially pathological relevant consequences and design intervention strategies that are highly appropriate to encephalitis. Therefore, collecting new data will be instrumental to our understanding of how a ubiquitous respiratory virus, the human coronavirus, given the proper susceptibility conditions and proper virus evolution and infection conditions, could trigger the neuropathology that is characteristic of at least some forms of encephalitis.

4. Acknowledgment

Work from the Talbot laboratory was funded by operating grants MT-9203 from the Institute of Infection and Immunity, Canadian Institutes of Health Research, and 42619-2009 from the National Sciences and Engineering Research Council of Canada, a Tier-1 Canada Research Chair to P.J.T., as well as a studentship from the Canadian Multiple Sclerosis Society to E.B..

5. References

Alexander, T.J.L. (1962) Viral encephalomyelitis of swine in Ontario. Experimental and natural transmission. Amer. J. Vet. Res. 32, 756–762.

Alirezaei, M., Kiosses, W.B. & Fox, H.S. (2008) Decreased neuronal autophagy in HIV dementia: a mechanism of indirect neurotoxicity. Autophagy 4, 963-966.

Andries, K. & Pensaert, M. (1980) Virus isolation and immunofluorescence in different organs of pigs infected with hemagglutinating encephalomyelitis virus. Amer. J. Vet. Res. 41, 215–218.

Arbour, N., Côté, G., Lachance, C., Tardieu, M., Cashman, N.R. & Talbot, P.J (1999a) Acute and persistent infection of human neural cell lines by human coronavirus OC43. J. Virol. 73, 3338-3350.

Arbour, N., Ekandé, S., Côté, G., Lachance, C., Chagnon, F., Tardieu, M., Cashman, N.R. & Talbot, P.J. (1999b) Persistent infection of human oligodendrocytic and neuroglial cell lines by human coronavirus 229E. J. Virol. 74, 3326-3337.

Arbour, N., Day, R., Newcombe, J. & Talbot, P.J. (2000) Neuroinvasion by human respiratory coronaviruses and association with multiple sclerosis. J. Virol. 74, 8913-8921.

Avitsur, R., Mays, J.W. & Sheridan, J.F. (2011) Sex differences in the response to influenza virus infection: modulation by stress. Horm. Behav. 59, 257-264.

Baric, R.S., Nelson, G.W., Fleming, J.O., Deans, R.J., Keck, J.G., Casteel, N. & Stohlman, S.A. (1988) Interactions between coronavirus nucleocapsid protein and viral RNAs: implications for viral transcription. J. Virol. 62, 4280-4287.

Barna, M., Komatsu, T., Bi, Z. & Reiss, C.S. (1996) Sex differences in susceptibility to viral infection of the central nervous system. J. Neuroimmunol. 67, 31-39.

Beckham, J.D., Tuttle, K.D. & Tyler, K.L. (2010) Caspase-3 activation is required for reovirus-induced encephalitis in vivo. J. Neurovirol. 16, 306-317.

Bender, S.J. & Weiss, S.R. (2010) Pathogenesis of murine coronavirus in the central nervous system. J Neuroimmune Pharmacol. 5, 336-354.

Blakely, P.K., Kleinschmidt-DeMasters, B.K., Tyler, K.L. & Irani, D.N. (2009) Disrupted glutamate transporter expression in the spinal cord with acute flaccid paralysis caused by West Nile virus infection. J. Neuropathol. Exp. Neurol. 68, 1061-1072.

Bonavia, A., Arbour, N., Wee Yong, V. & Talbot, P.J. (1997) Infection of primary cultures of human neural cells by human coronavirus 229E and OC43. J.Virol. 71, 800-806.

Brown, M. A., Troyer, J. L., Pecon-Slattery, J., Roelke, M. E. & O'Brien, S. J. (2009). Genetics and pathogenesis of feline infectious peritonitis virus. Emerg. Infect. Dis. 15, 1445–1452.

Butler, N., Pewe, L., Trandem, K. & Perlman, S. (2006) Murine encephalitis caused by HCoV-OC43, a human coronavirus with broad species specificity, is partly immune-mediated. Virology 347, 410-421.

Burke, D.S. & Morill, J.C. (1987) Levels of interferon in the plasma and cerebrospinal fluid of patients with acute Japanese encephalitis. J. Infect. Dis. 155, 797-799.

Carmen, J., Rothstein, J.D. & Kerr, D.A. (2009) Tumor necrosis factor-alpha modulates glutamate transport in the CNS and is a critical determinant of outcome from viral encephalomyelitis. Brain Res. 1263, 143-154.

Collins, A.R., Knobler, R.L., Powell, H. & Buchmeier, M.J. (1982) Monoclonal antibodies to murine hepatitis virus-4 (strain JHM) define the viral glycoprotein responsible for attachment and cell--cell fusion. Virology 119, 358-371.

Cowley, T.J., Long, S.Y. & Weiss, S.R. (2010) The murine coronavirus nucleocapsid gene is a determinant of virulence. J. Virol. 84, 1752-1763.

de Haan, C.A.M. & Rottier, P.J.M. (2005) Molecular interactions in the assembly of coronaviruses. Adv. Virus Res. 64, 165-230.

Drosten, C., Günther, S., Preiser, W., van der Werf, S., Brodt, H.R., Becker, S., Rabenau, H., Panning, M., Kolesnikova, L., Fouchier, R.A., Berger, A., Burguière, A.M., Cinatl, J., Eickmann, M., Escriou, N., Grywna, K., Kramme, S., Manuguerra, J.C., Müller, S., Rickerts, V., Stürmer, M., Vieth, S., Klenk, H.D., Osterhaus, A.D., Schmitz, H. & Doerr, H.W. (2003) Identification of a novel coronavirus in patients with severe acute respiratory syndrome. N. Engl. J. Med. 348, 1967-1976.

Dubois-Dalcq, M.E., Doller, E.W., Haspel, M.V., & Holmes, K.V. (1982). Cell tropism and expression ofmouse hepatitis viruses (MHV) in mouse spinal cord cultures. Virology 119, 317–331.

Fellay, J., Shianna, K.V., Ge, D., Colombo, S., Ledergerber, B., Weale, M., Zhang, K., Gumbs, C., Castagna, A., Cossarizza, A., Cozzi-Lepri, A., De Luca, A., Easterbrook, P., Francioli, P., Mallal, S., Martinez-Picado, J., Miro, J.M., Obel, N., Smith, J.P., Wyniger, J., Descombes, P., Antonarakis, S.E., Letvin, N.L., McMichael, A.J., Haynes, B.F., Telenti, A., & Goldstein, D.B. (2007) A whole-genome association study of major determinants for host control of HIV-1. Science 317, 944-947.

Fellay, J., Ge, D., Shianna, K.V., Colombo, S., Ledergerber, B., Cirulli, E.T., Urban, T.J., Zhang, K., Gumbs, C.E., Smith, J.P., Castagna, A., Cozzi-Lepri, A., De Luca, A., Easterbrook, P., Günthard, H.F., Mallal, S., Mussini, C., Dalmau, J., Martinez-Picado, J., Miro, J.M., Obel, N., Wolinsky, S.M., Martinson, J.J., Detels, R., Margolick, J.B., Jacobson, L.P., Descombes, P., Antonarakis, S.E., Beckmann, J.S., O'Brien, S.J., Letvin, N.L., McMichael, A.J., Haynes, B.F., Carrington, M., Feng, S., Telenti, A., Goldstein, D.B.& NIAID Center for HIV/AIDS Vaccine Immunology (CHAVI). (2009) Common genetic variation and the control of HIV-1 in humans. PLoS Genet. 5, e1000791.

Fish, E.N. (2008) The X-files in immunity: sex-based differences predispose immune responses. Nat. Rev. Immunol. 8, 737-744.

Foley, J., Lapointe, J.-M., Koblik, P., Poland, A. & Pedersen, N. 1998. Diagnostic features of neurologic feline infectious peritonitis. J. Vet. Int. Med. 12, 36–63.

Foley, J.E., Rand, C. & Leutenegger, C. (2003) Inflammation and changes in cytokine levels in neurological feline infectious peritonitis. J. Feline Med. Surg. 5, 313-322.

Fouchier, R.A., Kuiken, T., Schutten, M., van Amerongen, G., van Doornum, G.J., van den Hoogen, B.G., Peiris, M., Lim, W., Stöhr, K. & Osterhaus, A.D. (2003) Aetiology: Koch's postulates fulfilled for SARS virus. Nature 423, 240.

Gallagher, T.M., Parker, S.E. & Buchmeier, M.J. (1990) Neutralization-resistant variants of a neurotropic coronavirus are generated by deletions within the amino-terminal half of the spike glycoprotein. J. Virol. 64, 731-741.

Ge, D., Fellay, J., Thompson, A.J., Simon, J.S., Shianna, K.V., Urban, T.J., Heinzen, E.L., Qiu, P., Bertelsen, A.H., Muir, A.J., Sulkowski, M., McHutchison, J.G. & Goldstein, D.B. (2009) Genetic variation in IL28B predicts hepatitis C treatment-induced viral clearance. Nature 461, 399-401.

Ghoshal, A., Das, S., Ghosh, S., Mishra, M.K., Sharma, V., Koli, P., Sen, E. & Basu, A. (2007) Proinflammatory mediators released by activated microglia induces neuronal death in Japanese encephalitis. Glia 55, 483-496.

Golembewski, E.K., Wales, S.Q., Aurelian, L. & Yarowsky, P.J. (2007) The HSV-2 protein ICP10PK prevents neuronal apoptosis and loss of function in an in vivo model of neurodegeneration associated with glutamate excitotoxicity. Exp. Neurol. 203, 381-393.

Greig, A.S., Mitchell, D., Cormer, A.H., Bannister, G.L., Meads, E.B. & Julian, R.J. (1962) Hemagglutinating virus producing encephalomyelitis in baby pigs. Can J Comp Med. Vet. Sci. 26, 49-56.

Gu, J., Gong, E., Zhang, B., Zheng, J., Gao, Z., Zhong, Y., Zou, W., Zhan, J,. Wang, S., Xie, Z., Zhuang, H., Wu, B., Zhong, H., Shao, H., Fang, W., Gao, D., Pei, F., Li, X., He, Z., Xu, D., Shi, X., Anderson, V.M. & Leong, A.S. (2005) Multiple organ infection and the pathogenesis of SARS. J. Exp. Med. 202, 415-424.

Hannah, M.F., Bajic, V.B. & Klein, S.L. (2008) Sex differences in the recognition of and innate antiviral responses to Seoul virus in Norway rats. Brain Behav. Immun. 22, 503-516.

Haughey, N.J., Nath, A., Mattson, M.P., Slevin, J.T. & Geiger, J.D. (2001) HIV-1 Tat through phosphorylation of NMDA receptors potentiates glutamate excitotoxicity. J. Neurochem. 78, 457-467.

Hill, K.E., Pigmans, M., Fujinami, R.S. & Rose, J.W. (1998) Gender variations in early Theiler's virus induced demyelinating disease: differential susceptibility and effects of IL-4, IL-10 and combined IL-4 with IL-10. J. Neuroimmunol. 85, 44-51.

Hirano, K., Ona, T., Takasawa, T., Murakami & Haga, S. (1990) Replication and plaque formation of swine hemagglutinating encephalomyelitis virus (67N) in swine cell line, SK-K culture. J. Virol. Methods 27, 91–100.

Hirano, N., Nomura, R., Tawara, T. & Tohyama, K. (2004) Neurotropism of swine haemagglutinating encephalomyelitis virus (coronavirus) in mice depending upon host age and route of infection. J. Comp. Pathol. 130, 58-65.

Iacono, K. T., L. Kazi, & Weiss, S.R. (2006) Both spike and background genes contribute to murine coronavirus neurovirulence. J. Virol. 80, 6834–6843.

Jacomy, H. & Talbot, P.J. 2003. Vacuolating encephalitis in mice infected by human coronavirus OC43. Virology 315, 20-33.

Jacomy, H., Fragoso, G., Almazan, G., Mushynski, W.E. & Talbot, P.J. (2006) Human coronavirus OC43 infection induces chronic encephalitis leading to disabilities in BALB/c mice. Virology 349, 335-346.

Jacomy, H. & Talbot, P.J. (2006) HCoV-OC43-induced apoptosis of murine neuronal cells. Adv. Exp. Med. Biol. 581, 473-478.

Jacomy, H., St-Jean, J.R., Brison, E., Marceau, G., Desforges, M. & Talbot, P.J. (2010) Mutations in the spike glycoprotein of human coronavirus OC43 modulate disease in BALB/c mice from encephalitis to flaccid paralysis and demyelination. J. Neurovirol. 16, 279-293.

Kamatani, Y., Wattanapokayakit, S., Ochi, H., Kawaguchi, T., Takahashi, A., Hosono, N., Kubo, M., Tsunoda, T., Kamatani, N., Kumada, H., Puseenam, A., Sura, T., Daigo, Y., Chayama, K., Chantratita, W., Nakamura, Y. & Matsuda, K. (2009) A genome-wide association study identifies variants in the HLA-DP locus associated with chronic hepatitis B in Asians. Nat. Genet. 41, 591-595.

Kazi, L., Lissenberg, A., Watson, R., de Groot, R.J. & Weiss, S.R. (2005) Expression of hemagglutinin esterase protein from recombinant mouse hepatitis virus enhances neurovirulence. J. Virol. 79, 15064-15073.

Kipar, A., Meli, M.L., Baptiste, K.E., Bowker, L.J. & Lutz, H. (2010) Sites of feline coronavirus persistence in healthy cats. J. Gen. Virol. 91, 1698-1707.

Klein S.L. (2000) The effects of hormones on sex differences in infection: from genes to behavior. Neurosci. Biobehav. Rev. 24, 627-638.

Ksiazek, T.G., Erdman, D., Goldsmith, C.S., Zaki, S.R., Peret, T., Emery, S., Tong, S., Urbani, C., Comer, J.A., Lim, W., Rollin, P.E., Dowell, S.F., Ling, A.E., Humphrey, C.D., Shieh, W.J., Guarner, J., Paddock, C.D., Rota, P., Fields, B., DeRisi, J., Yang, J.Y., Cox, N., Hughes, J.M., LeDuc, J.W., Bellini, W.J., Anderson, L.J. & SARS Working Group. (2003). A novel coronavirus associated with severe acute respiratory syndrome. N. Engl. J. Med. 348:1953-1966.

Lane, T.E. & Hosking, M.P. (2010) The pathogenesis of murine coronavirus infection of the central nervous system. Crit. Rev. Immunol. 30:119-130.

Launes, J., Sirén, J., Viinikka, L., Hokkanen, L. & Lindsberg, P.J. (1998) Does glutamate mediate brain damage in acute encephalitis? Neuroreport 9, 577-581.

Lee, N., Wong, C.K., Chan, P.K., Lindegardh, N., White, N.J., Hayden, F.G., Wong, E.H., Wong, K.S., Cockram, C.S., Sung, J.J. & Hui, D.S. (2010) Acute encephalopathy associated with influenza A infection in adults. Emerg. Infect. Dis. 16, 139-142.

MacNamara, K.C., Chua, M.M., Nelson, P.T., Shen, H., & Weiss, S.R. (2005) Increased epitope-specific CD8+ T cells prevent murine coronavirus spread to the spinal cord and subsequent demyelination. J. Virol. 79, 3370-3381.

MacNamara, K.C., Bender, S.J., Chua,M.M., Watson, R. & Weiss, S.R. (2008) Priming of CD8 T cells during central nervous system infection with a murine coronavirus is strain-dependent. J. Virol. 82, 6150–6160.

Masliah, E., Ge, N. & Mucke, L. (1996) Pathogenesis of HIV-1 associated neurodegeneration. Crit. Rev. Neurobiol. 10, 57-67.

Masters, P. S. (2006) The molecular biology of coronaviruses. Adv. Virus Res. 66, 193-292.

Maurizi, C.P., (2010) Influenza caused epidemic encephalitis (encephalitis lethargica): the circumstantial evidence and a challenge to the nonbelievers. Med. Hypotheses. 74, 798-801.

Mishra, M.K., Koli, P., Bhowmick, S. & Basu, A. (2007) Neuroprotection conferred by astrocytes is insufficient to protect animals from succumbing to Japanese encephalitis. Neurochem Int. 50, 764-773.

Miura, T.A., Travanty, E.A., Oko, L., Bielefeldt-Ohmann, H., Weiss, S.R., Beauchemin, N. & Holmes, K.V. (2008) The spike glycoprotein of murine coronavirus MHV-JHM mediates receptor-independent infection and spread in the central nervous system of Ceacam1a-/- mice. J. Virol. 82, 755–763.

Nakai, Y., Itoh, M., Mizuguchi, M., Ozawa, H., Okazaki, E., Kobayashi, Y., Takahashi, M., Ohtani, K., Ogawa, A., Narita, M., Togashi, T. & Takashima, S. (2003) Apoptosis and microglial activation in influenza encephalopathy. Acta Neuropathol. 105, 233-239.

Nargi-Aizenman, J.L., Havert, M.B., Zhang, M., Irani, D.N., Rothstein, J.D. & Griffin, D.E. (2004) Glutamate receptor antagonists protect from virus-induced neural degeneration. Ann. Neurol. 55, 541-549.

Netland, J., Meyerholz, D.K., Moore, S., Cassell, M. & Perlman, S. (2008) Severe acute respiratory syndrome coronavirus infection causes neuronal death in the absence of encephalitis in mice transgenic for human ACE2. J. Virol. 82, 7264-7275.

Pasick, J.M., Kalicharran, K. & Dales, S. (1994) Distribution and trafficking of JHM coronavirus structural proteins and virions in primary neurons and the OBL-21 neuronal cell line. J. Virol. 68, 2915-2928.

Pedersen, N. & Boyle, J. (1980) Immunologic phenomena in the effusive form of feline infectious peritonitis. Amer. J. Vet. Res. 41, 868–876.

Phillips, J.J., Chua, M.M., Lavi, E., & Weiss, S.R. (1999) Pathogenesis of chimeric MHV4/MHV-A59 recombinant viruses: the murine coronavirus spike protein is a major determinant of neurovirulence. J. Virol. 73, 7752-7760.

Phillips, J.J., Chua, M.M., Rall, G.F. & Weiss, S.R. (2002) Murine coronavirus spike glycoprotein mediates degree of viral spread, inflammation, and virus-induced immunopathology in the central nervous system. Virology 301, 109-120.

Poland, A.M., Vennema, H., Foley, J.E. & Pedersen, N.C., (1996) Two related strains of feline infectious peritonitis virus isolated from immunocompromised cats infected with a feline enteric coronavirus. J. Clin. Microbiol. 34, 3180–3184.

Poncelet, L., Coppens, A., Peeters, D., Bianchi, E., Grant, C.K. & Kadhim, H. (2008) Detection of antigenic heterogeneity in feline coronavirus nucleocapsid in feline pyogranulomatous meningoencephalitis. Vet. Pathol. 45, 140-153.

Purtilo, D.T. & Sullivan, J.L. (1979) Immunological bases for superior survival of females. Amer. J. Dis. Child. 133, 1251-1253.

Resta, S., Luby, J.P., Rosenfeld, C.R. & Siegel, J.D. (1985). Isolation and propagation of a human enteric coronavirus. Science 229, 978-981.

Riski, N., & Hovi, T. (1980). Coronavirus infections of man associated with diseases other than the common cold. J. Med. Virol. 6, 259–265.

Rottier, P.J.M., Nakamura, K., Schellen, P., Volders, H. & Haijema, B.J. (2005) Acquisition of macrophage tropism during the pathogenesis of feline infectious peritonitis is determined by mutations in the feline coronavirus spike protein. J. Virol. 79, 14122–14130.

Schneider, B.S. & Higgs, S. (2008) The enhancement of arbovirus transmission and disease by mosquito saliva is associated with modulation of the host immune response. Trans. R. Soc. Trop. Med. Hyg. 102, 400-408.

Shieh, C.K., Lee, H.J., Yokomori, K., La Monica, N., Makino, S. & Lai, M.M. (1989) Identification of a new transcriptional initiation site and the corresponding functional gene 2b in the murine coronavirus RNA genome. J. Virol. 63, 3729-3736.

Siddell, S.G., Anderson, R., Cavanagh, D., Fujiwara, K., Klenk, H.D., Macnaughton, M.R.. Pensaert, M., Stohlman S.A. & van der Zeijist B.A.M. (1983) Coronaviridae. Intervirology 20, 181-189.

Singh, A., Kulshreshtha, R., & Mathur, A. (2000) Secretion of the chemokine interleukin- 8 during Japanese encephalitis virus infection. J. Med. Microbiol. 49, 607-612.

Stohlman, S.A. & Hinton, D.R. (2001) Viral induced demyelination. Brain Pathol. 11, 92-106.

Sturman, L.S., Holmes, K.V. & Behnke, J. (1980) Isolation of coronavirus envelope glycoproteins and interaction with the viral nucleocapsid. J. Virol. 33, 4494-4462.

Summers, B.A., Cummings, J.F. & deLahunta, A. (1995) Inflammatory diseases of the central nervous system. In: *Veterinary Pathology*, Summers, B.A., Cummings, J.F. & deLahunta, A., eds., pp. 95-188. Mosby, St. Louis, MO.

Thomas, D.L., Thio, C.L., Martin, M.P., Qi, Y., Ge, D., O'Huigin, C., Kidd, J., Kidd, K., Khakoo, S.I., Alexander, G., Goedert, J.J., Kirk, G.D., Donfield, S.M., Rosen, H.R., Tobler, L.H., Busch, M.P., McHutchison, J.G., Goldstein, D.B. & Carrington, M. (2009) Genetic variation in IL28B and spontaneous clearance of hepatitis C virus. Nature 461, 798-801.

Vannberg, F.O., Chapman, S.J. & Hill, A.V.S (2011) Human genetic susceptibility to intracellular pathogens. Immunol. Rev. 240, 105-116.

Vennema, H., Poland, A., Foley, J. & Pedersen, N. C. (1998) Feline infectious peritonitis viruses arise by mutation from endemic feline enteric coronaviruses. Virology 243, 150-157.

Wang, G.F., Li, W. & Li, K. (2010) Acute encephalopathy and encephalitis caused by influenza virus infection. Curr. Opin. Neurol. 23, 305-311.

Wege, H., Winter, J. & Meyermann, R. (1988) The peplomer protein E2 of coronavirus JHM as a determinant of neurovirulence: definition of critical epitopes by variant analysis. J. Gen. Virol. 69, 87-98.

Williams, R.K., Jiang, G.S. & Holmes, K.V. (1991) Receptor for mouse hepatitis virus is a member of the carcinoembryonic antigen family of glycoproteins. Proc. Natl Acad. Sci . U.S.A. 88, 5533-5536.

Wilson, M.E., Dimayuga, F.O., Reed, J.L., Curry, T.E., Anderson, C.F., Nath, A. & Bruce-Keller, A.J. (2006) Immune modulation by estrogens: role in CNS HIV-1 infection. Endocrine 29, 289-297.

Winter, P.M., Dung, N.M., Loan, H.T., Kneen, R., Wills, B., Thu le, T., House, D., White, N.J, Farrar, J.J., Hart, C.A. & Solomon, T. (2004) Proinflammatory cytokines and chemokines in humans with Japanese encephalitis. J. Infect. Dis. 190, 1618-1626.

Wodarz, D., & Krakauer, D.C. (2000). Defining CTL-induced pathology: Implications for HIV. Virology 274, 94-104.

Xu, J., Zhong, S., Liu, J., Li, L., Li, Y., Wu, X., Li, Z., Deng, P., Zhang, J., Zhong, N., Ding, Y. & Jiang, Y. (2005) Detection of severe acute respiratory syndrome coronavirus in the brain: potential role of the chemokine mig in pathogenesis. Clin. Infect. Dis. 41, 1089-1096.

Yagami, K., Yagami, K., Hirai, K. & Hirano, N. (1986) Pathogenesis of haemagglutinating encephalomyelitis virus (HEV) in mice experimentally infected by different routes. J. Compar. Pathol. 96, 645–657.

Yang, T.C., Shiu, S.L., Chuang, P.H., Lin, Y.J., Wan, L., Lan, Y.C. & Lin, C.W. (2009) Japanese encephalitis virus NS2B-NS3 protease induces caspase 3 activation and mitochondria-mediated apoptosis in human medulloblastoma cells. Virus Res. 143, 77-85.

Yeh, E.A., Collins, A., Cohen, M.E., Duffner, P.K. & Faden, H. (2004) Detection of coronavirus in the central nervous system of a child with acute disseminated encephalomyelitis. Pediatrics 113, 73-76.

9

Subacute Sclerosing Panencephalitis and Other Lethal Encephalitis Caused by Measles Virus Infection: Pathogenesis and New Approaches to Treatment

Fernandez-Muñoz R.*, Carabaña J.[1], Caballero M.[1], Ortego J.[2], Liton P.B.[1], Duque B.M, Martin-Cortes A.[3], Serrano-Pardo A., Muñoz-Alia M.A., Porras-Mansilla R., Alvarez-Cermeño J.C.[4] and Celma M.L.*

1. Introduction

Measles virus (MV) is a human, negative-stranded RNA virus, member of the Paramyxoviridae family, genus Morbillivirus. The virus enters cells by interaction of viral glycoprotein Hemagglutinin (H) with cellular receptors (CD46, CD150, CD147/EMMPRIN) and membrane fusion is mediated by viral fusion glycoprotein (F); helical nucleocapsids replicate in the cytoplasm on replication-transcription complexes formed by the viral catalytic subunit (L), the phosphoproteín (P) and the RNA wrapped in the viral nucleoprotein (N); virus particles bud out from plasmatic cell membrane patches internally lined by viral matrix protein(M). MV causes cytopathic effects by cell fusion forming syncytia, by inducing apoptosis, or both together, and may produce persistent infections in cultured cells and in the infected host. MV is highly lymphotropic infecting macrophages, lymphocytes and dendritic cells; causes systemic acute infections after cell-associated viremia generating life-long immunity (Griffin, 2007 for a review).

Despite the availability of an efficient live attenuated vaccine, MV still remains an important global pathogen infecting over 25 millions individuals and causing over 250.000 deaths per year, being one of the main causes of child death worldwide. Plans for the global eradication of measles are hindered by a number of factors: 1. high contagiousness of MeV (it is the most transmissible respiratory virus known, and it is needed a 95% to 98% protection in a population to avoid measles out-brakes), 2. vaccination fails in over 5% of the general population (non-responders), 3. vaccination has a low efficiency in infants under 9 months, 4. poor health care in some countries, and 5. objection to vaccination in sectors of the population.

Virology Unit (Madrid and Nacional Reference Laboratory for Measles Virus) Ramón y Cajal University Hospital, Madrid, Spain

1 Present address: Duke University Medical Center, Durham, NC, USA

2 Present address: Animal Health Research Center (CISA-INIA), Valdeolmos, Madrid, Spain

3 Present address: Complutense University of Madrid. Madrid, Spain

4 Neurology Department, Ramón y Cajal University Hospital, Madrid, Spain

** Corresponding authors*

During acute measles, MV produces a transient clinical significant immunosuppression that can contribute to some complications as measles interstitial pneumonitis and giant cell pneumonia, otitis media and diarrhoea. Unfrequently, MV may cause Central Nervous System lethal complications as Acute measles post-infection disseminated encephalomyelitis (ADEM), Measles inclusion body encephalitis (MIBE), and Subacute sclerosing panencephalitis (SSPE) Figure 1 and Table1. In this chapter we will briefly review the epidemiology, clinical course, pathogenesis, treatment, and prevention of these encephalitis with emphasis on SSPE, and present some results from our group concerning pathogenesis and possible therapeutics approaches to this fatal disease.

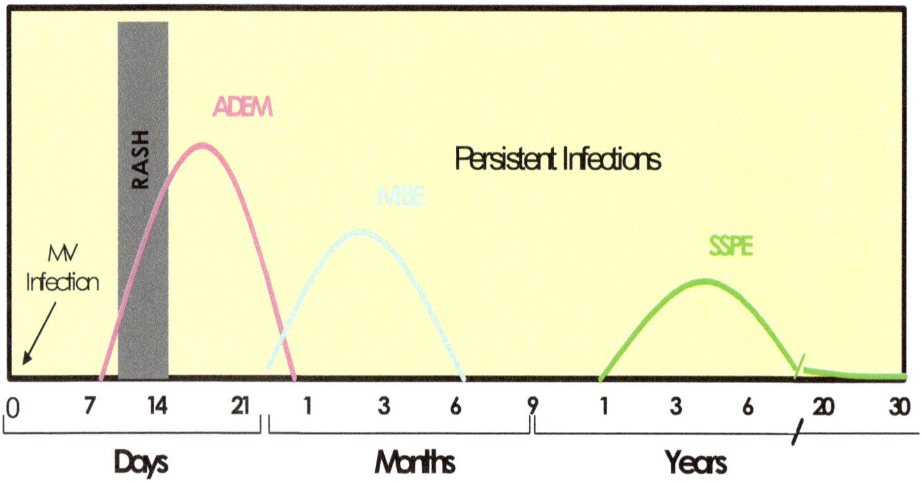

Fig. 1. Neurological complications of Measles Virus Infections. Onset and time course of encephalitis after MV infection (ADEM, MIBE, and SSPE)

2. Acute post-infectious measles disseminated encephalomyelitis (ADEM)

Onset occurs about one to 2 weeks after the appearance of the rash (in some rare cases, coincident with rash) in approximately one case in 10^3 cases of measles, usually in children older than 2 years and adults. In contrast, the incidence drops to one in one million after measles vaccination. The onset is typically abrupt, starting with irritability fever, headache, vomiting, and confusion and progressing rapidly to seizures impaired consciousness and coma, Present a monophasic clinical course over weeks and the mortality rate is 10 to 20%. The majority of survivors have neurological sequelae, in one quarter of them permanent. Neither MeV virus, or viral RNA has been found in the brain of patients with ADEM at autopsy, and not intrathecal synthesis of anti-MV antibodies have been demonstrated. Among other pathology changes, perivascular inflammation and demyelination are observed. Possibly it is an autoimmune parainfectious disease. Molecular mimicry between myelin basic protein and MV proteins has been conjectured. Antibodies to myelin basic protein are found in CSF, but no cross-reacting antibodies or T cells have been identified. Besides supportive therapy, immunomodulatory treatment with intravenous (i.v.) corticosteroids, i.v. immunoglobulin or plasmapheresis have been employed in monitored patients with variable results. Current live measles virus vaccine has reduced the incidence of ADEM after vaccination campaigns.

Disease	Host	Virus	Epidemiology	Onset, and Course	Clinical features	Pathogenesis	Treatment	Prevention
ADEM Acute Disseminated Encephalomyelitis	Otherwise healthy. Tipically older than 2 years.	Wild-type or Vaccinal MV.	Incidence: Approximately $1/10^3$ cases of measles, and $1/10^6$ MV vaccinations.	Onset within the first week of rash. Monophasic over weeks. Mortality rate is 10 to 20%. Mayority of survivors with neurological sequelae.	Abrupt onset with headache, vomiting, irritabitliy confusion, frequently recurrence of fever, and seizures. Progressing rapidly to obtundation and coma.	No MV particles, RNA, or proteins detected in the brain, or intrathecal synthesis of MV antibodies. Possibly an acute parainfectious encephalomyelitis without evidence of MV brain invasion. Perivascular inflammation and demyelination.	Besides supportive therapy, iv corticosteroids, iv. immuno globulin and plasmapheresis have been used with variable results.	Current live attenuated MV vaccine has reduced the incidence of ADEM.
MIBE Measles Inclusion Body Encephalitis	Inmuno-deficient patients of any age. (with deficient cell-mediated immunity).	Wild-type MV. Vaccinal MV in severily immuno-deficient infants.	Patients with congenital or adquired immuno-deficiency after exposure to MV.	Onset tipically months after infection or exposure to MV. Progressive course over months. Mortality rate is 75 to 85%.	Patients usually present with afebrile refractory focal seizures and altered mentation and progress to generalized seizures, coma, and death.	Brain biopsia or autopsia show gliosis, focal necrosis, perivascular cuffing , in neurons and glia nuclear and cytoplsmic MV inclusion bodies, MV RNA and nucleocapsids . In general no infectious MV virus can be isolated from brain. No detectable anti-MV immune response.	No effective specific treatment exist for MIBE. Early iv. ribavirin could improve symptoms. There is not evidedence of IFN-alfa benefit.	Routine MV vaccination of all children may be the best available strategy to reduce the incidence of MIBE.

Disease	Host	Virus	Epidemiology	Onset, and Course	Clinical features	Pathogenesis	Treatment	Prevention
SSPE Subacute Sclerosing Panencephalitis	Otherwise healthy individuals with previous infection or exposure to MV, in the majority of cases under 2 years of age. Genetic pre-disposition, and environmental factors, as coincident infection by other pathogens, might be involved.	Wild-type MV belonging to different genotypes. There is no evidence of MV vaccine causing SSPE.	SSPE incidence is 4 to 11 per 10^5 cases of measles (18 per 10^5, when measles at age under 2 years) The incidence of SSPE has declined dramatically years after the introduction of MV vaccination programmes. SSPE predominates in males at approximately a 2.5 ratio. Very rarely, small clusters of SSPE has been described. SSPE development in only one of identical twins after coincident measles.	Onset on the average 8 years after MV acute infection. The incubation period ranging from one year to several decades after MV acute infection. The course is progressive from one to 20 years (some times with transient remission periods), but in most cases death occur within 3 years of onset.	Insidious onset with symptoms of progressive cortical dysfunction (deterioration of intellectual capacity, and some times awkwardness, stumbling and symptoms of retinitis). Later, motor disability and paroxysmal disorders develop: myoclonic jerks, convulsive seizures and ataxia. Next stage is characterized by coma and decerebrate rigidity and subsequently athony and death.	Pathological changes are usually diffuse and involve grey and white matter: Neuronal loss, gliosis, immflamation and demyelination. MV virus invades CNS and a key feature is the presence of both cytoplasmic (MV nucleoapsid) and nuclear inclusion bodies. Virus proteins are mutated and functionally defective, and no virus budding or syncytia are observed. Neurons, oligodendrocytes, lymphocytes and microglia infected by MV undergoing apoptosis. Hyper humoral immune response and intrathecal synthesis of MV antibodies.	Much of therapy in SSPE is symptom-based. To date there is not antiviral therapy of proven efficacy for SSPE. Several therapeutic agents have been used to treat SSPE, including IFN-alfa, ribavirin, Isoprinosine and levamasole. Experience has been anecdotal (due to the low frequency and variability of disease course it is hard to perform controlled clinical trials) benefit has been transient at best.	Today the only effective prevention of SSPE is to implement MV vaccination. It has been observed a marked reduction of SSPE incidence decades following MV vaccination campaigns in many countries.

Table 1. Encephalitis Caused by Measles Virus

3. Measles Inclusion Body Encephalitis (MIBE)

The disease occurs at any age in immunocompromised patients after MV exposition. MIBE affects persons with congenital or adquired cell-mediated immunodeficiency as oncologic (approximately 70% of MIBE cases occurring in acute lymphocytic leukaemia), transplanted or HIV-infected patients. In severily inmmunodeficient patients the live attenuated measles vaccine in use may also cause MIBE. It has been described one fatal case of MIBE in a boy with chronic granulomatous disease after stem cell transplant without a history of recent clinical measles in the donor or the receptor (Bitnum et al.1999).
Typically, the onset occurs within one year of MV infection. MIBE may accompany or follows measles giant cell pneumonia, but more often occurs as the sole clinical manifestation, two to six months after MV infection or vaccination. Patients usually present with afebrile refractory focal seizures and altered mentation, and progress to generalized seizures, coma and death. CSF parameters are often normal and unlike SSPE hyperimmune antibody response to MV and oligoclonal bands may be not detected. EEG are abnormal, but unspecific; head computed tomography (CT) and Nuclear Magnetic Images (MRI) scans are normal. The mortality exceeds 85%, and survivors have severe neurological sequelae. At autopsia or biopsia the brain show gliosis and focal necropsia, lymphocyte perivascular cuffing, and intranuclear and intracytoplasmic inclusions in glial cells and neurons. MV nucleocapsids can be detected by electron microscopy, MV antigens by immuno-assays, and MV RNA by in situ hybridization or RT-PCR.
The virus persists and progressively invades the brain over months. At a brain autopsia from a patient with MIBE, R. Cattaneo, M. Billeter and collaborators first reported the phenomena of biased U to C RNA hypermutation in the MeV genome (Cattaneo et al, 1988). This hypermutation may take place by the enzyme Adenosine deaminasa ADAR present in nervous tissue which would transform Adenosine into Inosine in the replicative intermediary RNA (see below).

4. Subacute Sclerosing Panencephalitis (SSPE)

SSPE is a rare delayed progressive encephalitis that occurs in 4 to 11 cases per 10^5 cases of measles in apparently immunocompetent children after an acute uncomplicated measles. Under 2 years of age, the risk to develop SSPE is higher, 18 per 10^5 cases of measles. The incidence has fallen drastically after successful measles vaccination campaigns. Recent epidemiological data suggest that measles vaccination protects against SSPE, and MV vaccine strain does not cause SSPE (Bellini et al, 2005; WHO, 2006; Campbell et al, 2007; Garg, 2008). The disease is caused by a persistent MeV infection that progressively invades the brain, possibly with a clonal origin, in the presence of a potent humoral response anti-MeV. The mean period from acute measles to onset of SSPE symptoms is eight years, ranging from one to over thirty years (adult onset SSPE). After a progressive course with sporadic relapses in some cases the patients usually die from few months to twenty years after the onset, although the majority of patients die between one to four years after onset of symptoms. In this chapter we describe some previous and undergoing work from our laboratory on samples obtained at autopsy from three SSPE patients (Figure 2) who presented short (3 to 4 months, SMa79), average (3.5 years, SMa84), and long (18 years, SMa94) disease course (Figure 3).

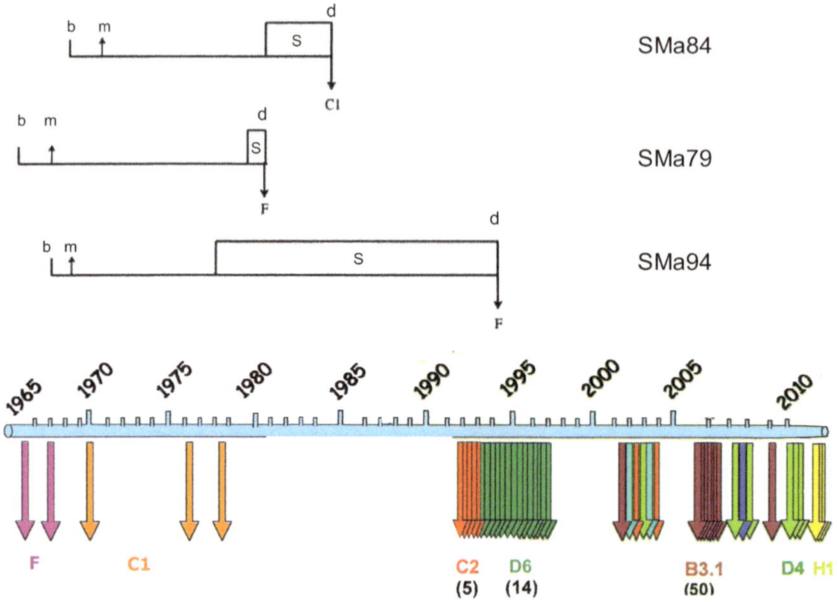

Fig. 2. Temporal distribution of measles virus genotypes circulating in a geographic area (Madrid) in the MV pre-vacccination and vaccination periods and SSPE cases. Superimposed the time-course of 3 cases of SSPE from Madrid with short duration (SMa79, 3-4 months), average duration (SMa84, 3.5 years) and long duration (SMa94, 18 years) of disease. For each patient birth date (b), date of measles acute infection (m) and dates of SSPE from onset to death are boxed (S). At autopsy, brain samples were separated and from them the whole genome sequence (15894 nucleotides for each one) was determined in our laboratory. The genotype of MV present in the brain at autopsy from each SSPE case is indicated with an arrow at the right end of the respective box. In brackets, number of isolates.

4.1 The SSPE virus

To date, MV strains present in SSPE brain tissue are wild-type strains belonging to different genotypes and no MV vaccinal strain (A genotype) has been found (Rima et al. 1995; Jin et al, 2002; Forcic et al, 2004; Mahadevan et al, 2008; Souraud et al, 2009). It is an open question the existence of circulating MV strains with high ability to establish persistent infections and cause SSPE. The epidemiological data indicate that although has been described some clusters of SSPE cases they are small and very rare, and some of them are familiar clusters (Beersma et al. 1992; Sharma et al, 2008). Reported simultaneous measles infections in identical twins with subsequent development of SSPE in only one twin do not point to the existence of "SSPE prone" MV strains (Houff and al. 1979). These data suggest it is unlikely the existence of circulating SSPE measles virus strains prone to cause SSPE, but does not exclude they could play a co-factor role in conjunction with environmental and genetic predisposing traits in the host. In this context our group has reported a MV strain produced by a long-term persistent infection which, in contrast with the cytocidal parental virus, establishes an immediate persistence in the original human lymphoblastoid cell line (Celma & Fernandez-Muñoz, 1992). This MV strain of "persistent" phenotype establishes an immediate persistence without cytocidal effect on a number of human cell lines of different lineages (Fernandez-Muñoz & Celma , 1988). We have also observed a MV primary isolate from a clinical sample of a patient with measles that when inoculated in a human B lymphoblastoid cell line has established directly an immediate steady-state persistent infection in absence of cytopatic effects. (Fernandez-Muñoz and collaborators, unpublished results).

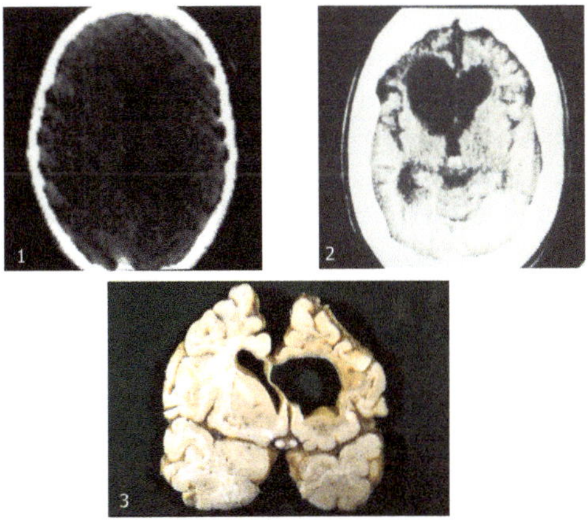

Fig. 3. Brain images of a long-course case of Subacute Sclerosing Panencephalitis (case SMa94, diagnosed and autopsied in Ramón y Cajal Hospital in Madrid). Panel 1 shows a Brain Computed Tomography (CT) image at the time the patient was 9 years old and presented a retinitis with high serum titre of anti-MV antibodies by Complement fixation and Hemagglutinin Inhibition assays, whereas serology for other neurotropic viruses was normal. One year later she presented neurologic symptoms and signs of subacute encephalitis and of intrathecal synthesis of MV antibodies was demonstrated confirming the diagnosis of SSPE. After a 20 years progressive course with transient relapses, she was hospitalized and died at Ramon y Cajal Hospital in Madrid. Panel 2 shows a brain CT image shortly before death and panel 3 shows at autopsy a sliced cerebrum from the patient. Brain atrophy with loss of white and grey matter, and ventricular dilatation were observed
(Courtesy from Dr M. García-Villanueva, Dept. Anatomía Patologica, Hospital Ramon y Cajal)

The absence of detectable virus budding and infective viral particles in the SSPE and MIBE brain and the slow course of infection indicated a defective nature of these MV strains. Studies on MV persistent infections in animal models and cultured neural and lymphoid human cells in the in 1970s and 1980s, analysis of MV genomic and mRNAs present in SSPE after the development of nucleic acid amplification by PCR studies, and the rescue of infective MV from cloned genomic cDNA by M.Billeter and collaborators (Radecke et al, 1995) have provided valuable information on the pathogenesis of SSPE. Thus, amplification and sequencing of MV genomic and transcripts RNAs from diseased brain has revealed a range of mutations that could explain defective expression and functionality for several viral genes (Cattaneo et al 1988). Despite the hyperimmune response to MV antigens in SSPE patients, early observations of selective absence of antibodies to matrix protein (M) pointed to a defective expression of this protein which is necessary, among other steps, for the budding of viral particles. The search for mutation that may lead to defective budding and absence of syncytia observed in the diseased brains are concentrated in the MV viral membrane proteins: H glycoprotein, F glycoprotein, and M matrix protein.

F protein from three SSPE cases studied by Billeter et al. and two cases studied by our group (SMa79 and SMa84) presents mutational alterations in their cytoplasmic tail(Billeter et al.1994) , region which have been found involved in cell fusion (Caballero et al.1998). In all 5 cases the SSPE F glycoprotein shows fusion activity after transfection in cultured cells (Cattaneo & Rose 1993; Carabaña,1997).

Viral glycoprotein H from 2 of the 3 SSPE cases from Madrid (SMa79 and SMa94) showed mutations in their distal cytoplasmic region with extension of 4 amino acids due to mutation in the stop translation codon (Carabaña, 1997, and Celma et al unpublished results).

In a MV matrix gene from brain of a child with MIBE, M. Billeter and collaborators described for the first time the phenomenon of biased hypermutation, a cluster of exceptional point mutations (50% of U residues were changed to C); these biased mutations found only in the M gene could confer to the MV an selective advantage in the brain (Cattaneo et al. 1988). Wong and collaborators (Wong et al. 1989) shortly afterwards, found a non-random M gene hypermutation, similar to the one identified by Billeter, in a SSPE virus strain (Yamagata-1) passaged in human neuroblastoma cells.

Biased hypermutation was reported for the first time in the brain of a SSPE case by Celma and collaborators in the matrix protein M gene of SMa84 (Carabaña et al., IX International Congress of Virology, Glasgow, 1993). 38% of the U residues mutated to C, generating 59 amino acids changes in M protein, 18 of the changes being Leu to Pro, which probably altered drastically its secondary structure. Figure 4 shows a map of the different type point mutations found across the entire genome sequence in 3 SSPE cases. In SMa94 we observed biased hypermutation U to C at a lower lever, 10% U to C, producing 12 aminoacid changes; besides the hypermutation, there is a loss of the 83 amino acids at the C-end. In contrast, in SMa79, there is not biased hypermutation, and we found the creation of a premature stop triplet that caused the loss of 40 residues at the C-end of M protein. In this SSPE case, M protein presented a drastically impaired interaction with MV nucleocapsids tested by binding of radio-labelled cloned M proteins to purified MV nucleoprotein (Carabaña,1997, and unpublished results). Thus in SSPE, 1. biased hypermutation was not dependent of MV genotype, 2. bias hipermutation may requires several years course of disease, and 3. the level of final hypermutation do not increase necessarily with the length of the disease (Figure 4).

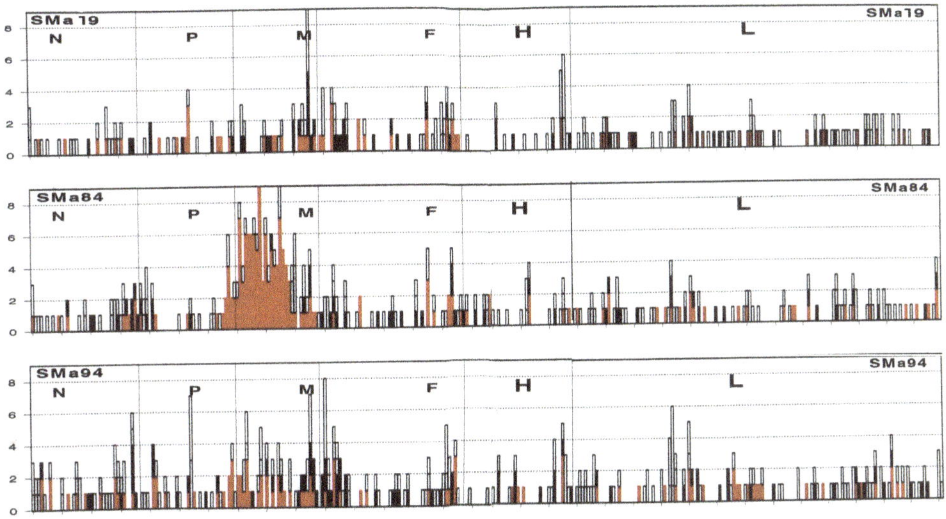

Fig. 4. Distribution of mutation events in MV Genome of SSPE cases with short, average and long disease course. The antigenome of SMa79, SMa84 and SMa94 are represented. Point mutations U to C (red boxes), C to U (black boxes), G to A (grey boxes) and others (white) are indicated. The height of boxes correspond to the number of mutated bases. On the horizontal axis, groups of 50 consecutive nucleotides were taken as a unit. Gene junctions are indicated by vertical lines. The methodology used for determination of intergenomic regions and whole genes were as described for analyzing MV genotypes (Rima et al.1995). RT-PCR products were sequenced directly in both directions by dideoxynucleotide chain-terminating sequencing with primers constructed at 400-500 base intervals and manual analysis or by using an automated DNA sequencer (model ABI PRISM 377 Applied Biosystems). Sequences of 5´and 3´end of the SSPE genomes were determined by a ligation method (Sidhu et al. 1993) and a modification of the 5´RACE method (Frohman et al. 1988, Baron et al. 1995, Carabaña,1997).

The same hypermutation pattern was observed in distant zones of brain for each case, in agreement with previous results form Billeter, ter Meulen and collaborators (Bazko et al. 1993), suggesting a clonal origin of brain infection in SSPE. Biased hypermutation was not observed outside the M gene in any of the studied cases. (Carabaña,1997, and Celma and cols, unpublished results). It remains unknown whether the M gene transcription is particularly susceptible to hypermutation or the process is frequent for every MV gene, but hypermutation in other viral genes generates unfit genomes which are counter-selected in the brain environment. A possible mechanism for this biased hypermutation was proposed by M. Billeter group in collaboration with H. Weintraub group (Bass et al , 1988). Essentially, the mechanism consist in the action of Adenosin-deaminase that convert in double stranded RNA Adenosine into Inosine resulting in a transition A to G or U to C. This enzyme found by Weintraub group has been later identifided as ADAR1, a member of ADAR protein family inducible by Interferon I. While ADAR1 activity in cell culture has been reported to be barely detectable (Horikami & Moyer, 1995), recent studies in transgenic mice indicate that ADAR1 is a restriction factor controlling the replication of MV and other Paramyxovirus. On the other hand there are indications that ADAR1 is a proviral antiapoptotic host factor in the context of MV infection (Ward et al, 2011; Toth et al. 2009; and Samuel, 2011 for a recent review).

Since 1954 when von Magnus first described in influenza virus subgenomic nucleic acid particles, defective interfering particles (DI) have been found in a variety of viruses. In 1970 Alice Huang and David Baltimore suggested that DI particles play a role the establishment of viral persistent infections. E. Norrby described MV DI particles, and in 1977 Rima, Martin and collaborators demonstrate a role of DIs in establishment of MV persistence in cultured cells (Rima et al, 1977). DI particles were detected in measles vaccine pharmaceutical preparations by Roux and coll. (Calain & Roux, 1988). In 1992 Fernandez-Muñoz and Celma did not found evidence the subgenomic RNAs at detectable level in MV metabolically radio-labelled nucleocapsids by denaturating formaldehyde gels from a long-term steady-state MV persistent infection in human lymphoblastoide cells with reduced level of infective virus (Fernandez-Muñoz & Celma, 1992). In 1994 Dowling, Udem and collaborators with dot-blot hybridization and RT-PCR experiments found over representation (2 to 5 times) of MV genomic 5´end sequences and the presence of copy-back type DI particles in MV nucleocapsids from brain material of 3 SSPE cases (Sidhu et al, 1994).

In post mortem obtained brain samples from 3 SSPE cases of short (SMa79), average (SMa84) and long (SMa94) course of disease (Figure 2), we have searched for MV defective particles. Genomic RNA (-) from purified nucleocapsids was hybridized with radio-labelled (32P) RNA probes with polarity (+) designed to recognize different MV genes along the viral genome to determinate de abundance in the brain of the regions of MV genome. As shown in Figure 5 no detectable overrepresentation of 5´or 3´ ends of MV genome was observed in any of the 3 SSPE cases, indicating that no abundant DI particles of deletion type were present. To assay specifically for the presence of copy-back type MV DI particles we amplify by RT-PCR MV nucleocapsid RNA with suitable primers of the same polarity and products were detected by liquid hyridization with radio-labelled probes. Only in one SSPE case, SMa84 with clinical course of average length, were detected copy-back DI particles (Figure 6). Sequencing of amplified cDNA corroborated de copy-back structure of the subgenomic RNA and determined the polymerase jump point. Thus, the presence of copy-back DI particles in the brain is not universal in SSPE cases, and its presence is not associated with long clinical course of disease. The possible functional interfering ability of these copy-back DI particles that could modulate MV replication in SSPE remains conjectural.

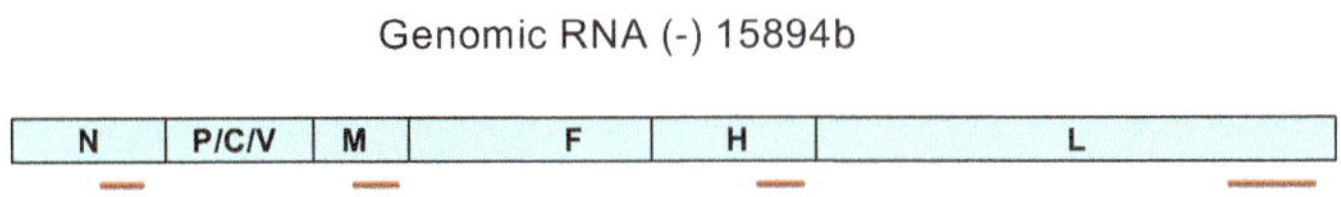

(32P) probes RNA(+)	850 b	520 b	787 b	850 b
SMa79	0.41	0.7	0.47	0.37
SMa94	0.54	1.22	0.76	0.46
SMa81	0.08	0.2	0.25	0.16

Fig. 5. Search for possible subgenomic MV in SSPE brains. Hybridization with labelled probes across MV genome show that different regions are similarly represented in genomic RNA (-) from brain material of SSPE cases with short (SMa79), long (SMa94), and average (SMa84) disease course. Positions of the RNA probes for four MV genes (top) and the fentomoles of each gene hybridized per 10µg of Brain Nucleocapsid RNA (bottom). Genomic RNA and labelled RNA standards of antisense polarity were slot blot hybridized with P^{32} sense polarity probes and radioactivity estimated by densitometry analysis (Carabaña 1997). Genomic RNA from postmortem SSPE brain tissue was purified from nucleocapsids isolated by CsCl gradients. Probes and standards RNA specific for nucleoprotein (N), Matrix (M), Hemagglutinin (H), and polymerase (L) was of obtained by transcription with T7 and SP6 polymerases of Gemini vectors (Celma and Fernandez-Muñoz 1992) containing from nucleotide 825 to 1676 for N gene, from 4215 to 4719 for M gene, from 7669 to 8456 for H gene (generous gift from Dr.M.A.Billeter) and a clone obtained in our laboratory containing a 3´terminal fragment of gene L from nucleotide 14892 to 15742.

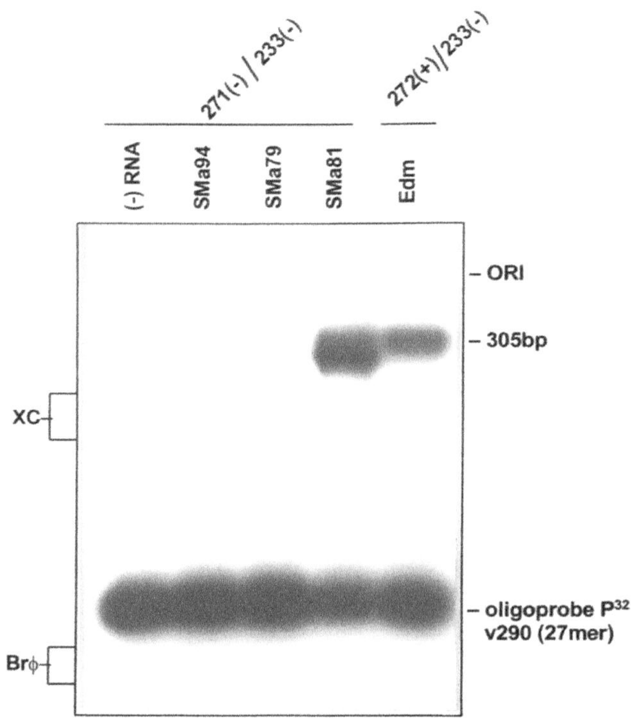

Fig. 6. Copy-back defective measles virus particles in SSPE brain. Liquid Hybrydization autoradiograph of 5´copy-back genome specific PCR products synthesized with primers designed to amplified copy-back DIs. The determination in our laboratory of the entire sequence of MV genomes from brain of 3 SSPE cases allowed us to synthesize transcription vectors from which riboprobes specific for their genomic 5´end region were synthesized (Carabaña J. 1997). Defective viral products were amplified by RT-PCR of Nucleocapside RNA with primers of same polarity as described by Calain et al.1992 and Sidhu et al.1994. Products amplified with primers V233 (antigenome nucleotide numbers15894 to 15866) and V271 (15648 to 15621) were detected by liquid hybridization with internal probe V290(15783 to 15812). Positive control hybridization from Edmonston measles virus RNA amplified with primers of both polarity V272 (15588 to 15613) and V233 is shown. Based on the sequence of amplified DI copy back, the polymerase jump point position is 15764 and15570. Assuming the DIs follow a precise copy-back mechanism and their generation assumes complete complementarity of the ends, the size of the detected SMa84 DI particles were 456 nucleotides. Detection of copy-back DI particles was observed in only one of the three SSPE cases studied.

4.2 The SSPE patient

The SSPE patients were otherwise healthy individuals who has a history of past acute measles, typically uncomplicated and before the age of two; SSPE affects males preferentially, ratio 2.5:1. Several hypothesis have been proposed to explain the epidemiological data of early MV infection as a predisposing factor for SSPE development;

for instance it has been suggested, un still immature immune response, anatomical factors that favor viral invasion of CNS, or the presence of maternal anti-measles antibodies which could modulate the MV infection. So far these hypotesis remains unproven. Another conceivable possibility would be the coincidence of the acute MV infection with another infection by a different pathogen which could facilitate the MV persistence and invasion of the CNS. Were this the case, as coincident infections may be more frequent at an early age, the coinfection hypothesis could explain the association of SSPE development with an acute measles early in life. In our laboratory we have been testing during the last three decades this hypothesis in a collection of samples from SSPE patients diagnosed along those years, but so far we found no conclusive results. In 2005, based on the association between the development of SSPE and the immunodepression by intensive immunosuppressive therapy in unimmunized subjects, or on the early age immaturity of immune system, M. Oldstone and collaboratos proposed SSPE likely arises after MV infects an transiently immunosuppressed individual; these authors developed an SSPE transgenic mouse model expressing CD46 MV-receptor transiently immunodepressed by prior infection with lymphocytic coriomeningitis virus (LCM -Cl 13), proposing a dual viral hit playing a role in causation of SSPE (Oldstone et al, 2005; Oldstone, 2009). This model promises to be useful for pathogenesis studies and assays in search of effective new therapeutic approaches to SSPE and MIBE.

It is conceivable that some individuals have genetic traits that predispose them to develop SSPE after MV exposure. In recent years several polymorphisms have been associated with SSPE from different populations. Thus, several functional polymorphisms in the regulatory regions of genes for the expression of proteins involved in the immune response as MxA (protein associated to the anti-viral response induced by Interferon I), Interferon Regulatory Factor 1 (IRF-1), Interlekin-4 (IL-4), Toll-like receptor 3 and granulysin are associated with development of SSPE in the Japanese and Filipino populations. On the other hand polymorphisms in IL-12, IL-2, Interferon-gamma, Angiotensin-converting enzyme (ACE) and Angiotensin II type 1 receptor have been associated with SSPE in Turkish population (Kusuhara et al, 2007). More recently these authors have obtained results in Japanese and Filipino populations suggesting that PD1 gene may contribute to genetic susceptibility to SSPE. Due to the small size of some of these samples, further studies are needed to confirm these associations and their significance for the development of SSPE.

4.3 SSPE onset, clinical course and pathogenesis

Onset occurs on the average 8 years after MV acute infection, ranging from one year to decades in adult-onset SSPE; in rare cases onset occurs during pregnancy and it is often fulminant. The course of SSPE is progressive for one to twenty years, sometimes with transient remission periods, but in most cases death occur within 3 to 4 years of onset. The course of SSPE use to be divided in 4 stages with rare transient remissions periods (Garg, 2008). Stage 1. The onset is insidious with symptoms of progressive cortical dysfunction, behavioural changes, deterioration of intellectual capacity, and some times awkwardness, stumbling or visual symptoms of retinitis, optical neuritis or cortical blindness, over months. Stage2, Later, manifest motor disability and paroxysmal disorder develop: mioclonus jerks (pathognomonic electroencephalographic alterations-Rodermacker complexes). Stage 3. Pyramidal and extrapyramidal manifestations, disappearance of myoclonus, alteration in sensorium. Stage 4. Vegetative state, and death.

The diagnosis of SSPE can be established with the compliance of the following diagnostic Dyken´s criteria: 1. Atypical clinical picture of progressive subacute mental deterioration with stereotyped generalized myoclonus. 2. Characteristic electroencephalogram changes. 3 Elevated CSF globulin levels greater than 20% of total protein. 4. Raised CSF anti-MV antibody titers (intrathecal synthesis of measles antibodies) 5. Typical histopathologic findings in brain biopsia or autopsy; pathological changes are usually diffuse and involve grey and white matter: neural loss (Figure 3), gliosis, inflammation, and demyelination. A key feature is the presence of both cytoplasmic and nuclear inclusion bodies, predominantly in neurons and oligodendrocytes. No budding of MV particles or syncytia cytoplasmic effects are observed, and scarce neurons, oligodendrocytes, microglia, and lymphocytes infected by MV undergo apoptosis.

When and how MV enter into the CNS in SSPE remain unknown questions, but molecular epidemiology and *in situ*_studies have provided some likely answers. A basic question is whether the MV causing SSPE is the same virus that caused the acute measles in the patient years before. This is a difficult question to answer, especially in SSPE presenting a long course, since is improbable to have for one patient both the primary MV isolate causing the acute infection and the virus recovered from his brain years to decades later. The recognition of MV genotypes, and their geographical and temporal distribution pattern (rapid "endemic" genotype replacement after years of circulation) in the pre-vaccination period provided an answer to this question (Rima et al, 1995). Thus, studying the MV genotypes that circulated in a large city like Madrid from 1960s to 1990s and 3 local SSPE cases from this period (Figure 2), we observed that the genotype of the MV recovered at autopsy from the brain of each SSPE patient was the same genotype circulating in Madrid at the documented date of his acute infection at early infancy, and not the one circulating in Madrid at the date of onset of SSPE years later. This was the first confirmation that a SSPE is long-term infection by MV, and that it is not caused by a MV re-infection, representing the prime example for a long-term persistent human infection by an RNA virus, (Rima et al, 1995; Carabaña, 1997).

The question arises, where MV resides and replicates in an individual during the intervening years between acute infection and onset of SSPE symptoms. One possibility would be that during acute measles the virus enter into the CNS of the subjects who will develop SSPE. This hypothesis is based on data from post-mortem brain samples from SSPE cases where cerebral vascular endothelial cells showed infection by MV (Kirk et al.1991), and in acute fatal infection cases where MV infected cerebral endothelial cells were found by in situ hybridization and in situ RT-PCR (Esolen et al, 1995). This site of infection may provide a portal of entry for MV in subjects who subsequently would develop SSPE or MIBE or a target for immunological reaction in ADEM. Although these epithelial cells do not express the CD150(SLAM) receptor, they could be infected through recently discovered CD147/EMMPRIN receptor expressed in epithelial cells (Watanabe et al, 2010).

MV is highly lymphotropic (Moench et al, 1989) and the virus infect monocytes, lymphocytes and possibly dendritic cells early in the natural acute infection and in experimental animal infections. The data after aerosol infection of non-human primates strongly suggest that MV entered the host at the alveolus by infecting macrophages or dendritic cells which traffic the virus to local lymph nodes, resulting in a primary local amplification and subsequent systemic dissemination by cell-associated viremia (Ferreira et al, 2010; Lemon et al, 2011). In patients with measles the clearance of detectable RNA by RT-

PCR in MV-infected blood cells may occur after several months of acute infection (Ridell et al, 2007). From these results, it is conceivable that MV infecting mononuclear cells as monocytes could survive as long-lived macrophages for months or years invading by a troyan horse mechanism different organs, including the brain in some patients. In our laboratory we have established long-term steady-state persistent infection in a number of human monocytic cell lines (Ortego, 1994); in some of them we observed cell-surface over-expression of cell adhesion molecules as Intercellular Adhesion Molecule 1 (ICAM-1) or integrin LFA-1, which could facilitate the attachment of infected leukocytes to endothelial cells (Fernandez-Muñoz et al. unpublished results). On the other hand, we differenciated in vitro the MV-persistently infected human monocytic cell lines to macrophage-like cells by means of PMA or GM-CSF which kept expressing high levels of MV proteins for weeks in the follow-up (Ortego, 1994, and Fernandez-Muñoz et al. unpublished results). These results suggest that MV infected monocytes may be converted to macrophages which could remain infected by MV and might harbour the virus for years. Previous results suggesting that MV was present in peripheral blood mononuclear cells (PBMC) and lymphoid organs from some SSPE patients (Brown et al, 1989), have not been confirmed (Schneider-Schaulies et al, 1991, Rima & Duprex 2005 for a review). In an early study by J. Sever and collaborators MV was isolated in mixed cultures of HeLa cells with lymph node biopsies from 2 out of 5 SSPE patients (Horta-Barbosa et al, 1971). As the isolated MV hemagglutinated macacus rhesus erythrocytes, it is possible that the isolates were a MV vaccine strain contamination (Lecouturier et al 1996). As we had the opportunity to be present at the time autopsy was performed for patients SMa84 and SMa94, we could collect "clean" extra cranial tissues before the braincase was opened to obtain brain samples. Thus, among other samples, we collected separately thoracic and mesenteric lymph nodes from these SSPE patients. From every lymph node we amplified by RT-PCR MV genomic (-) RNA from N, P, M, F and H genes (Figure 7). The MV in lymph nodes belongs to the same genotype that the MV in the respective brain, C1 in SMa84, and F in SMa94, and had high sequence homology with the respective MV in the respective brain. In both patients we have detected differential mutations between lymph nodes and brain in genes N, P and M, some of them resulting in aminoacid change. Interestingly, in both patients MV found in lymph nodes showed biased hypermutation U to C in the M gene, and in the SMa94 lymph nodes M gene, besides having all mutation found in brain, there are 10 additional mutations, all of them T to C mutations, and 7 resulting in change of aminoacid (Carabaña 1977, Celma et al. unpublished results). Although the separate collection of extra brain tissues and the diversity of sequences obtained, did not indicated possible contamination with brain RNA, to further exclude it we designed and performed in parallel amplification from lymph nodes RNA of Glial fibrillar acidic protein, abundant protein in nervous tissue, that resulted lower than amplification from PBMC from a control sample (Fig. 7). Although our results indicate that MV is present in lymph nodes of SSPE patients at the late stages of the disease, so far can not answer the question where the virus resides and replicate in the patient the years elapsing between the acute infection and the onset of encephalitis. The comparative analysis of genome sequence of two coetaneous MV belonging to the same genotype, F , one causing a short course (months) SSPE (SMa79) and the other one causing a very long course(twenty years) SSPE (SMa94) might shed some light on this issue (Celma et al, work in course). The study of MV sequences present in different zones of brain from one SSPE patient suggest that the invasion of CNS by MV has a clonal origin (Bazcko et al. 1993; Carabaña, 1997).

MV dissemination through brain in SSPE. The presence of MV nucleocapsids and MV Hemagglutinin in the neuronal axonal processes suggest that MV spreads transneuronally (Rima & Duprex, 2005 for a review). In 1990 D.Payan and collaborators found that a lymphoblastoid cell line that constitutively express the neuropeptide, (substance P) receptor, neurokinin-1, facilitate MV fusion (Harrowe et al, 1990). M. Billeter and cols in slice cultures demonstrated neuron-to-neuron polarized spread of a recombinant autoflurescent MV (Ehrengruber et al, 2002). More recently, G.Rall showed in a transgenic mice model implication of neurokinin-1 in infection and spread of MV, serving as viral receptor, or co-receptor in neurons, allowing MV synapsis (Makhortova N et al, 2007). No doubt the integration of these approaches will shed light on the pathogenesis of SSPE and other viral encephalitis.

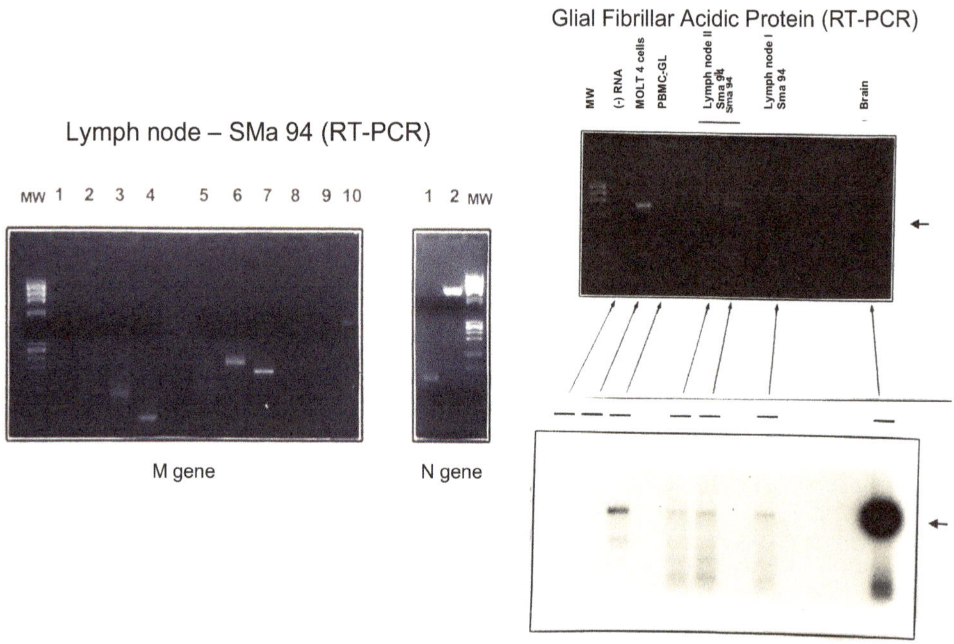

Fig. 7. Detection of genomic MV RNA in lymph nodes of SSPE patients. Agarose gel electrophoresis of cDNA amplified for MV M and N genes of a lymph node from SMa 94(left). Analysis of fibrillary acidic protein gene in SMa94 lymph nodes I and II by amplification and hybridization with specific primers (right).

Left panel. At autopsy mesenteric lymph nodes were obtained before opening the braincase. RNA was extracted using guanidinium isothiocyanate technique, reverse transcribed, amplified (1,2,3,4) and re-amplified (5,6,7,8,9,10) with specific genes for different regions of gene M and N (1,2). Negative controls 1M, 5M and 1N and MW markers. Sequencing the amplified DNA for N gene, besides the nucleotide changes characteristic of brain genotype there is one aminoacid change Ser432 to Leu. For M gene, from 1 to 135 residue, there are 8 aminoacid changes with respect to the brain sequence.

Right panel. To further exclude any MV RNA from brain samples glial fibrillary acidic protein mRNA was amplified. This transcripts are abundantly represented in brain RNA and scarcely in lymphoid tissue; agarose gel electrophoresis of RT-PCR amplification with fibrillary acidic protein gene specific primers (Reves et al. 1989) (top) of RNA from MOLT4 as negative control , RNA from a control sample of peripheral blood mononuclear cells (PBMC), RNA from two lymph nodes (I,II) and SMa 94brain RNA. Analysis of the amplified material by hybridization with specific radiolabelled probe (bottom). Carabaña1997.

5. Antiviral therapeutic approaches to encephalitis caused by measles virus infection of the central nervous nystem: SSPE and MIBE

Multiple therapeutic agents, including Interferons, Ribavirine, Isoprinosine, vitamin A have been used to treat measles complications, including SSPE and MIBE, but benefit has been transient at best. Today there is not antiviral therapy of proven efficacy for MV. We will briefly review past experience, some times necessarily anecdotal, given the low frequency and highly variable course of these diseases that hinder controlled clinical trials. We will discuss new potential anti-MV therapies including, RNA interference, inhibitors of virus entry and MV RNA polymerase, (reviews by Garg, 2008; Pempler & Snyder, 2009; Reuter & Schneider-Schaulies, 2010) and a novel therapeutic approaches including selective induction of apoptosis in MV infected cells as a potential early treatment of SSPE and MIBE.

5.1 Small molecules and natural products with anti measles activity

Ribavirin. This pro-drug analogue of ribonucleosides with a broad antiviral spectrum has been used alone or combined with Interferon-alfa by intra-ventricular administration for SSPE patients with variable results, transient benefit at best, and undesired effects. Experimental results in MV intra-cranial infected hamsters and mice have shown that complexation of ribavirin with cyclodextrin-alfa reduced five-fold the 50% inhibitory dose and improved crossing of the brain-blood-barrier (Jeulin et al., 2009), and could improve the treatment with ribavirin in MV encephalitis.

Vitamin A. Supplements of Vitamin A significantly reduce measles mortality and morbidity, especially in children younger than 2 years of age, and it is the treatment recommended by WHO for children suffering from acute measles (Joint WHO-UNICEF statement-1987-Vitamin A for measles. Wkly Epidemiol Rec 19,133-134). There are indications of Vitamin A playing a role in the innate immune response, particularly in Interferon I signalling pathway, and it has been reported that retinoids directly inhibit MV replication in cultured cells (Trottier et al, 2009). On the other hand, it has been reported about one third of a SSPE (6 of 21) and (0 of 20 matched controls) showed low levels (<20micrograms per dL) of vitamin A (Gugor et al, 2007). It remains an open question whether Vitamin A supplements might implement the Intereferon treatment in some SSPE patients.

Inhibitors of MV entry or MV RNA-polymerase. During the last decade a number of small molecules strong inhibitors of MV entry or viral RNA-dependent RNA polymerase as AS-136A have being designed by R. Compans, R. Plemper & collaborators. Targets in MV RNA-polymerase L protein catalytic subunit were identified studying in cell cultures MV escape mutants to the antiviral. The emergence of MV escape mutants could be a draw-back in potential long treatments as for SSPE. It remains to test these drugs in MV persistent infections in animal models for SSPE (for a review, Plemper & Snyder, 2009).

5.2 Interferon-α

In SSPE patients treatments with intraventricular Interferon-α alone or in combination with ribavirine or isoprinosine produce at best transient effects, and in some cases severe toxic effects (for review, Garg, 2008; Nacagawa et al 2009). Possibly, the low antiviral effect of Interferon-α treatment could be explained by the MV inhibition of antiviral response to exogenous Interferon I in the infected cell (Ortego, 1994 Fernandez-Muñoz et al, 2000). We found that MV inhibited the antiviral response to IFN I by blocking the signal transduction from the IFN I-receptor (Liton, 2001), and that MV non-structural protein V is associated with this inhibition (Celma and collaborators, unpublished results; Palosaari et al. 2003)). Silencing the V protein expression by anti-sense RNA oligonucleotides or RNA interference may be a way to increase IFN I antiviral effect in SSPE treatment. With this aim we have designed siRNAs that block MV P gene expression that could render MV persistently infected cells sensitive to IFN-α (see below). Another possible factor for the low antiviral response to Interferon I in SSPE patients could be the functional MxA promoter polymorphisms associated with SSPE (Torisu et al, 2004).

5.3 RNA interference to control progression of SSPE and MIBE

The gene suppression effects mediated transiently by short interfering RNA molecules (siRNA) or stably by intracellular expression of short hairpin RNAs (shRNAs) wich are processed by the cellular RNAi machinery (for a review Dykxhoorn et al. 2008) into effective siRNAs, are currently being tested as therapy for acute virus infections such as RSV end for chronic infections as HIV, Hepatitis B virus and Hepatitis C virus. To determine whether exogenous siRNA could inhibit the expression of MV genes and suppress viral replication during acute and persistent infections, we have designed siRNA molecules targeting conserved sequences in the genome of MV in brain of SSPE patients which inhibit the expression of MV Phosphoprotein gene, involved in viral RNA transcription, replication, and IFN response, and Hemagglutinin gene(H), playing a critical role in adsorption, cell fusion, assembly and budding of viral particles (Martín-Cortes et al, 2004 and Celma and coll. unpublished results). As shown in Figure 8 these siRNAs efficiently inhibit the production of MV infective particles in acute and persistently infected cells and indicates could be an useful tool for antiviral therapies by themselves or in combination with others MV specific siRNAs (Reuter et al. 2006; Otaki et al. 2007; Keita et al. 2008). For an efficient siRNA therapy besides a high gene target specificity it will be necsesary to solve problems of siRNA delivery and undesirable toxic site effects, as discussed by Rossi et al 2009.

5.4 Inducers of apoptosis in MV infected cells as a potential early treatment of SSPE and MIBE

Formation of syncitia by inducing cell fusion is the prominent cytopathic effect of MV in cultured cells (Enders, 1954) and in patients with measles giant cell pneumonia. In our laboratory by infecting a series of human lymphoblastoid cell lines with a MV strain showing low cell fusion activity, we observed that infected MOLT3 cell line underwent an atypical rapid cytopathic effect without a significant formation of syncytia that we described at the 1988 Negative Strand Viruses Conference (Fernandez-Muñoz et al. 1988).

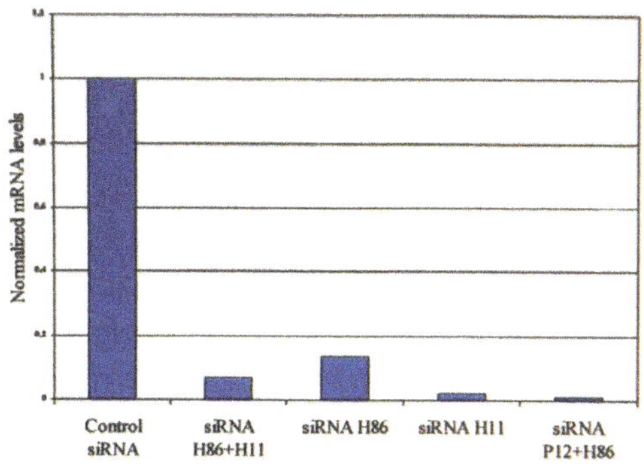

Titer of extracellular virus (%inhibition)

	Control siRNA	siRNA-P12	siRNA-H86
Lytic infection (293+EdMeV)	1:192	1:24 (87%)	1:48 (75%)
Persistent infection (293-FV-P)	1:1024	1:128 (87%)	ND

Table 1: Effect of siRNA-P12 and siRNA-H86 on production of infective extracellular MeV in lytic and persistently infected 293 cells.

Fig. 8. Inhibition by small interfering RNAs (siRNAs) of MV gene expression and viral replication during acute and persistent infections. Based on conserved sequences among MV primary isolates from patients with acute measles or SSPE we have designed siRNAs ds-oligonucleotides complementary to MV Phosphoprotein (siRNA P12) and Hemagglutinin (siRNA H86 and H11). Human epithelial 293 cells lytically infected with Edmonston virus or persistently infected with MV isolates were transfected with chemically synthesized siRNAs using Lipofectamin 2000. Upper panel. Quantitative assay to measure hemagglutinin gene silencing by siRNA. MV-H mRNA was assayed by quantitative reverse-transcriptase-polymerase-chain-reaction using SYBR Green core reagents from Applied Biosystems after primer optimization and Actine or GAPDH as endogenous controls in a ABI Prism7000 Sequence Detection System. Each column shows the relative quantification for Hemagglutinin mRNA following transfection of 293-FV-P persistently infected infected cells with the indicated siRNA.Lower panel. Effects of siRNA-P12 and siRNA H86 on production of infective extracellular MV during acute and persistent infections. Cell supernatants were titrated by plaque assay on B95 cells adapted in our laboratory to grow in monolayers.

Attempting to characterize this previously un-recognized MV cytopathic effect we found in MOLT3 infected cells chromatin condensation and DNA inter-nucleosoma fragmentation, hallmarks of the cell death mechanism described and named apoptosis by J.Kerr and collaborators in 1972. Measles virus can induce apoptotic cell death in cultured human cells and this process is mediated by over-expression of Fas membrane protein in MV infected lymphoid cells (Fernandez-Muñoz et al., Ninth International Conference on Negative Strand Viruses, Estoril, 1994). At this conference apoptosis induced by MV was also present by Dr D. Griffin in Vero cultured cells (Esolen et al, 1995; Caballero et al, 1996). Based in our previous observation of Fas (CD95) involvement in apoptosis caused by MV, we studied the effect of Fas ligand (FasL) and other analogs as TRAIL (TNF-related apoptosis-inducing ligand) on acute and persistently infected human cells. We observed that MV persistently infected cells were more sensitive to apoptosis induced by exogenous TRAIL than uninfected cells (Figure 9). This sensitization could be explained by the up-regulation of functional TRAIL receptors TRAIL-R1 and TRAIL-R2, and down-regulation of anti-apoptotic factor bcl-2 and activation of protein-kinase Akt and NFkB (Duque et al, 2007, and unpublished results by Celma and collaborators). Since has been generally observed that cancer cells are more sensitive than normal cells to apoptosis induced by recombinant TRAIL this molecule has been object of numerous clinical trials. Although phase I trials have shown low TRAIL toxicity, the efficiency tests got mixed results, largely due to the development of tumours resistence to the action of TRAIL (Yagita et al 2004 for a review, Kim et al. 2008; Eaton et al, 2011). Given the lack of efficient therapies for the encephalitis caused by persistent infection for MV, MIBE and SSPE, we have proposed the potential use of TRAIL as an early treatment of these diseases with the object to kill selectively the cells where MV resides before the virus disseminates across the brain.

TRAIL and its receptors have been shown to play important roles in the immune response to viral infections and in immune surveillance of tumours and metastasis (Falschlehener et al, 2009). During the last decade several studies have shown that different viral infections sensitize cells to apoptosis induced by TRAIL. Thus, TRAIL-resistant fibroblasts could be sensitized to TRAIL-induced apoptosis by infection with human cytomegalovirus (Sedger et al. 1999). On the other hand, it was observed and strong up-regulation of TRAIL, TRAIL-R1, and TRAIL-R2 in response to respiratory syncytial virus in primary tracheal-bronchial cells, A549 and HEP-2 cells and, RSV-infected cells could be eliminated by TRAIL-expressing immune cells in vivo (Kotelkin et al 2003). Furthermore, TRAIL has been implicated in chronic HCV infection and HCV has been shown to sensitize human hepatocytes to TRAIL induced apoptosis (Lan et al, 2008). Thus, the approach of an early treatment with TRAIL could help to control persistent infections by different viruses. However, there are some motives for concern after recent results showing that TRAIL, in addition to anti-tumour activity, has immunomodulatory functions and it has been demonstrated that TRAIL can eliminate plasma cells in vitro and suppress antibody production in vivo. Therefore, it should be noted that a strategy to over-express endogenous TRAIL, as well as administration of rTRAIL may impair host defense against infection (Faschlehener et al, 2009). For treatments of SNC diseases, some findings in cultured brain slices raise concern about neuro-toxicity and argue against the use of TRAIL for therapy of human brain tumours (Nitsch et al, 2000). A recent study obtained successful results combining anti-papillomavirus E6/E7 siRNA and TRAIL induction of apoptosis in cancer cells being refractory to TRAIL treatment (Eaton et al 2011).

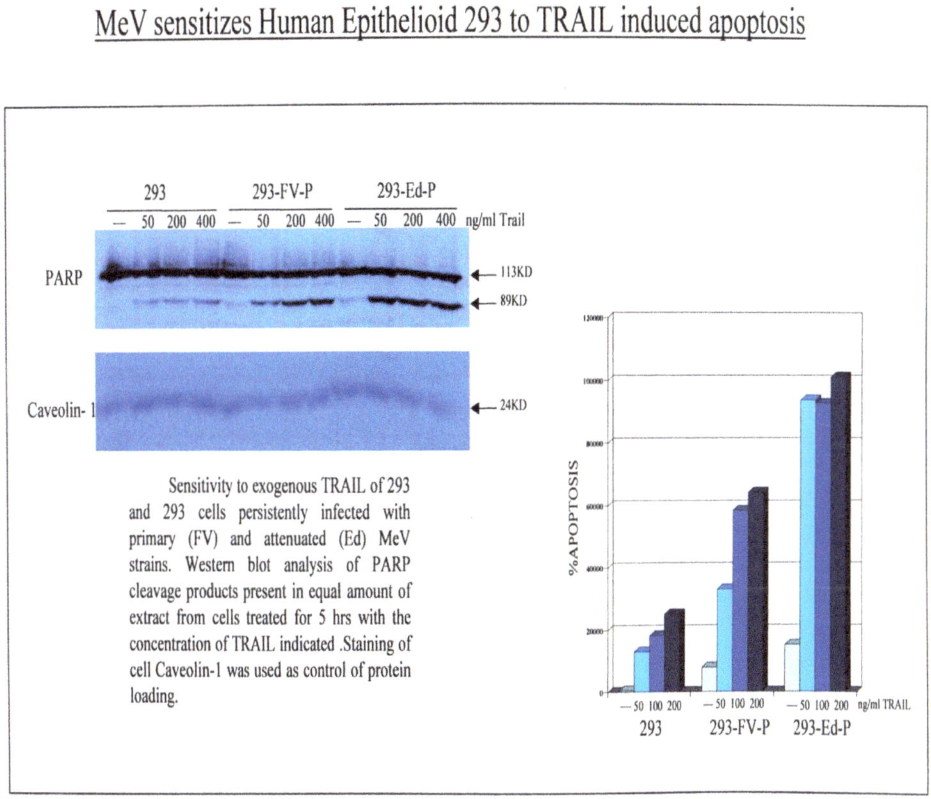

Fig. 9. Apoptosis in MV persistently infected cells treated with recombinant TRAIL.

Left panel. To measure the sensitivity of cells to recombinant TRAIL (tumour-necrosis-factor-related apoptosis inducing ligand) the expression of the uncleaved poly (ADP-ribose) polymerase (PARP)(113KD) substrate for apoptosis specific ICE-family proteases, and its cleaved product 89KD fragment were used as specific markers for apoptosis. Cells were untreated or treated with soluble human recombinant TRAIL with cross-linking enhancer or the killer TRAIL (His-tag) from Alexis, at concentrations and time indicated. Western blot analysis were performed in RIPA-cell extracts, normalized for protein concentration, run in SDS-PAGE , transferred to membranes end developed with specific antibodies. Staining of cell caveolin was used as control of protein loading.

293 cells were less sensitive to PARP cleavage induced by TRAIL than their persistent infected cell lines established with a vaccine strain or with a primary isolate. These finding in epithelial cells were further extended to human lymphoid B (Dakiki) and T (MOLT3) cells.

Right panel. To study the sensitivity to exogenous TRAIL of 293 and 293 cells persistently infected with primary (FV) and attenuated (Ed) MV strains, cell apoptosis was stimated as chromatine condensation in more than 200 nuclei after acridine orange staining. The specificity of acridine orange assay has been previously established in MV infected cells by DNA fragmentation detection techniques.

6. Conclusions

The comparison of the MV genomic sequence corresponding to Madrid SSPE cases SMa79, SMa84, and SMa94 with those of MV genotypes circulating in Madrid during the last 5 decades provided the first confirmation that the MV causing SSPE corresponds to the virus producing the measles acute infection and not to a possible re-infection years later at onset of the encephalitis. This was the first example of a human persistent infection by an RNA virus.

2. Concerning the question of where the virus could persist and replicate during the long latent period, we have observed that at least in the final stages of SSPE, MV is also present in abdominal and thoracic lymph nodes. The comparison of MV genomic RNA from brain and lymph nodes for each patient showed both viruses belong to the same genotype.

3. In two SSPE cases, those presenting an average and long disease course, but not in the short disease course case, biased hypermutation U to C was observed in the matrix M gene at a high level (38% U to C) and low level (10%U to C) respectively. The mutation map across the entire genome was the same from distant parts of each brain, supporting the indication of clonal origin of MV brain invasion proposed by V. ter Meulen, M. Billeter and collaborators. After the first decription of biased U to C hypermutation phenomena by M.Billeter and collaborators in one brain from a MIBE case, our results were the first description of biased hypermutation in SSPE brain. Our results indicate that biased hypermutation U to C are found at autopsia in brain of SSPE patients after years of disease, and it is not proportional to the length of the disease. Biased hypermutation U to C is present in MV localized in lymph nodes at similar or higher level than in the respective brain, suggesting that biased hypermutation may take place also in infected lymphoid cells. In the three cases the transcription of M, F and H genes were down-regulated, and M protein ability to bind to MV nucleocapsids was impaired by deletion or biased hypermutation.

4. The length of MV genome found in the brain of SSPE remains constant, 15894 after years to decades of persitent infection, and no evidence of significant proportion of nucleocapsid subgenomic RNAs was found in the brains of the SSPE cases studied. Copy-back subgenomic RNAs were found in MV nucleocapsids only in one of the three brains, indicating that the presence of MV defective interfering particles is not an universal feature in SSPE.

5. Currently, no efficient treatment for SSPE o MIBE patients is available. New approaches to therapy of these lethal encephalitis are underway in several laboratories, and possibly the future treatments will combine several therapies to control MV infection by specific antiviral designed drugs and molecules that would counteract virus escape to host immune response. Today, the only effective way to prevent MV encephalitis is the implementation of measles vaccination programs.

7. Acknowledgements

Work from authors's laboratory was funded by grants from Comunidad de Madrid, Ministerio de Ciencia e Innovación, Fondo de Investigaciones Sanitarias, Fundación MAPFRE Medicina, Fundación Española de Esclerosis Multiple to M.L.Celma and R. Fernandez-Muñoz. We thank Purnell Choppin, Erling Norrby, George Klein, Fabian Wild, Albert Osterhaus, Martin Billeter and Roberto Cattaneo for valuable materials and Concepción Muela and Ricardo Vázquez for skilful art work.

8. References

Agamanolis D.P., Tam J.S., & Parker D.L.(1979) Immunosuppresive measles encephalitis in a patient with a renal transplant (1979) Arch Neurol ,36,686-690.

Ayata M., Takeuchi K., Takeda M., Ohgimoto S., Kato S., Sharma L.B., Tanaka M., Kuwamura M., Ishida H., & Ogura I. (2010) The F gene of the Osaka-2 strain of measles virus derived from a case of subacute sclerosing panencephalitis is a major determinant of neurovirulence. J Virol , 84, 11189-11199.

Ayata M., Hayashi K., Seto T.,Murata R. & Ogura H. (1998) The matrix gen expresión of subacute sclerosing panencephalitis (SSPE) virus (Osaka-1 strain): A comparison of two sibling viruses isolated from different lobes of an SSPE brain. Microbiol Immunol 42, 773-780.

Baczko K., Lampe J., Liebert U.G., ter meulen V., Pardowitz I., Budka H., Cosby S.L., Isserte S., & Rima B.K. (1993) Clonal expansion of hypermutated measles virus in a SSPE brain. Virology 197, 188-195.

BaricevicM., Forcic D., Santak M., & Maruran R (2007). A comparison of complete untranslated regions of measles virus genomes derived from wild-type viruses and SSPE brain tissues. Virus Genes 35,17-27.

Bass B.L., Weintraub H., Cattaneo R., & Billeter M:A.,(1988)Biased hypermutation of viral RNA genomes could be due to unwinding/modification of double-stranded RNA. Cell, 56, 331.

Becker D., Patel A., Abou-Kahlil B.W., & Pina-Garza J.E. (2009) Successful treatment of encephalopathy and myoclonus with levetiracetam in a case of subacute sclerosing panencephalitis, J Child Neurol 24, 763-767.

Beersma M.F., Galama J.M. van Drulen H.A., Reñiré W.O., Lucas C.G. & Kapsenberg J.G. (1992) Suabcute sclerosing panencephalitis in The Netherlands-1976-1990. Int J Epidemiol 21, 583-588.

Bellini W.J., Rota J.S., Lowe L.E., Katz R.S., Dyken P.R., Zaki, S.R., ShiehW.J., & Rota P.A. (2005) Subacute sclerosing panencephalitis: More cases of this fatal disease are prevented by measles immunization than was previously rcognized. J Infec Dis 192,1686-1693.

Bellock C., Mottet G., & Roux L. (1990) Wide occurrence of measles virus subgenomic RNAs in attenuated live-virus vaccines. Biologicals 18, 337-343.

Billeter M, Cattaneo R.,Spielhofer P., Kaelin K., Huber M., Scnmid A., Baczko K. & ter Meulen V.(1994) Generation and properties of mutations typically associated with Subacute Sclerosing Panencephalitis. Annals of the N.York Acad Sci , 724, 367-377.

Bitnun A., Shannon P., Durward A., Rota P.A., Bellini W.J., Graham C., Wang E., Ford-Jones E.L., Cox P., Becker L., Fearon M., Petric M., & Tellier R. (1999) Measles inclusion-body encephalitis caused by the vaccine strain of measles virus. Clin Infet Dis 29, 855-861.

Brown H.R., Goller N.L., Rudelli R.D., Dymecki J., & Wisnieski H.M. (1989) Postmortem detection of measles virus in non-neural tissues in subacute sclerosing panencephalitis. Ann Neurol 26, 263-268.

Caballero M. (1996) Molecular mechanisms of viral persistence and cell death in measles virus infections. Doctoral Thesis, Universidad Autonoma de Madrid, Spain

Caballero M,, Carabaña J., Ortego J., Fernandez-Muñoz R., & Celma M.L. (1998) Measles virus Fusion protein is palmitoylated on transmembrane-cytoplasmic cystein residues which participate in cell fusion. J Virol 72, 8198-8204.

Calain P., & Roux L. (1988) Generation of Defective Interfering particles and their presence in a preparation of attenuated live-virus vaccine. J Virol 62,2859-2866.

Campbell H., Andrews N., Brown K.E. & Millar E. (2007) Review of the effect of measles vaccination on the epidemiology of SSPE. Int J Epidemiol 36, 1334-1348.

Carabaña J. (1997) Genomic and phenotypic studies of measles virus wild-types and subacute sclerosing panencephalitis virus. Doctoral Thesis Universidad Autonoma de Madrid, Spain.

Cattaneo R., Schmid A., Eschle D., Baczko K., ter Meulen V. & Billeter M.A. (1988) Biased hipermutation and other genetic changes in defective measles viruses in human brain infections. Cell 55, 255-265.

Cattaneo R. & Rose J.K. (1993) Cell fusion by the envelope glycoproteins of persistent measles vituses wich caused lethal human brain disease. J Virol 67, 1493-1502.

Celma M.L. & Fernandez-Muñoz R. (1992) Measles virus gene expression in lytic and persistent infections of a human lymphoblastoid cell line. J Gen Virol 73,2203-2209.

Dykxhoorn DM, Chowdhury D & Lieberman J. (2008). RNA interference and cancer: endogenous pathways and therapeutic approaches. Adv.Exp.Med.Biol. 615, 299-329.

Duque B.M., Martin-Cortes A., Fernandez-Muñoz R. & Celma M.L. (2004) Measles virus persistent infection sensitize cells to apoptosis mediated by Tumor Necrosis Factor -Related Apoptosis Inducing ligand (TRAIL): basis for a possible treatment for SSPE and other subacute measles virus encephalitis. II European Congress of Virology, Madrid,

Duque B.M., Martin-Cortes A., Fernandez-Muñoz R., & Celma M.L. (2007) Measles virus persistently infected cells are more sensitive to apoptosis induction by TRAIL: Basis for a potential therapy in SSPE and other measles virus encephalitis. Mapfre Medicina 18, 249-258.

Eaton S., Wiktor P., Thirstup D., Lake D., & Nagaraj V.J. (2011) Efficacy of TRAIL treatment against HPV16 infected cervical cancer cells undergoing senescence following siRNA knockdown of E6/E7 genes. Biochem Biophis Res Commun ,405,1-8.

Enami M., Kohama T., & Sugiura A (1989) A measles virus subgenomic RNA: structure and generation mechanism.. Virology 171, 427-433.

Ehrengruber M.U., Ehler E., Billeter M.A. & NainH.Y.(2002) Measles virus spread in rat hypocampal neuron by cell-to-cell contact in a polarized fashion. J. Virol, 76.5720-5728.

Esolen L.M., Takahashi K., Jonhnson R.T., Vaisberg A., Moench T.R., Wesselingh S.L., & Griffin D.E. (1995) Brain endothelial cell infection in children with acute fatal disease. J Clin Invest, 96,2478-2481.

Esolen L.M., Park S.W., Hardwick J.M., & Griffin D.E. (1995) Apoptosis as a cause of death in measles virus-infected cells. J Virol. 69, 3955-3958.

Falschleherner C., Schaefer U., & Walczak H. (2009) Following TRAIL`s path in the immune system. Immunology,127, 145-154.

Fernandez-Muñoz R. & Celma M.L. (1988) Host cell and viral factors in the establishment of persistent infections and cell fusion cytopathology by measles virus in human lymphoblastoid cell lines. Virus Reseach Supl. 2, 80.

Fernandez-Muñoz R. & Celma M.L.(1992) Measles virus from a long-term persistently infected human T lymphoblastoid cell line, in contrast to the cytocidal parental virus, establishes an immediate persistence in the original cell line. J Gen Virol 73,2195-2202.

Fernandez-Muñoz R., Liton P.B., Ortego J., Villal6n M.D., Duque B.M., & Celma M.L. (2000) Clinical isolates of measles virus , in contrast to vaccinal Edmonston strain, do not induce detectable secretion of alpha Interferon in lytic and persistent infections of human lymphoblastoid cell lines. J Clin Virol 18,189-190.

Ferreira C.S., Frenzkle M., Leonard V.H., Welstead G:G., Richardson C.D. & Cattaneo R.(2010) Measles virus infection of alveolar macrophages and dendritic cells precedes spread to lymphatic organs in transgenic mice expressing human signalling lymphocytic activation molecule (SLAM, CD150). J Virol 84, 3033-3042.

Forcic D., Baricevic M., Zgorelec R., Kruzic V., Kaic B., Marina B.M., Sojat L.C., Tesovic´ G., & Mazuran R. (2004) Detection and characterizatio of measles virus strains in cases of subacute sclerosing panencephalitis in Croatia. Virus Res 88, 51-56.

Freeman A.F. Jacobson D.A., Shulman S.T., Bellini W.J., Jaggi P., de Leon G., Keating G.F., Kim F., Pachman L.M., Kletzel M. , & Duerst R.E. (2004) A New Complication of Stem Cell Transplantation: Measles Inclusion Body Encephalitis, Pediatrics,114, 657-660.

Furusaki A., Jodo S., Yamashita Y., Amasaki yY., Atsumi T., & Koike T. (2006) TRAIL-mediated Cytotoxicity: Impact of s`TRAIL and v`TRAIL Microvesicles. J Biol Sci, 6, 150-159.

Garg R.K. Subacute sclerosing panencephalitis. (2008) J Neurol 255, 1861-1871.

Griffin D.E. (2007) Measles Virus. In Fields Virology. Fifth edition. Editors Knipe D.M., Howley P.M., Griffin D.E., Martin M.A., Lamb R.A., Roizman B., Straus S.E.. Lippincott Williams & WilkinsPhiladelphia, USA, 1551-1585.

Harrowe G., Mitsuhashi M. & Payan D.G. (1990) Measles virus-substance P receptor interactions.Possible novel mechanism of viral fusion. J Clin Invest 85,1324-1327.

Horikami S.M. & Moyer S.A. (1995) Double-stranded RNAadenosine deaminase activity during measles virus infection. Virus Res, 36, 87-96.

Horta-Barbosa L., Fucillo D.A., Sever J.L., & Zeman W. (1969) Subacute Sclerosing Panencephalitis: Isolation of measles virus from a brain biopsia. Nature 221, 974.

Horta-Barbosa L., Hamilton R., Witting B., Fucillo D.A., Sever J.L., & Vernon M.l. (1971) Subacute sclerosing panencephalitis:Isolation of suppressed measles virus from lymph node biopsies. Science 173, 840-841.

Houff S.A., Madden D.L., & Sever J.L. (1979) Subacute sclerosing panencephalitis in only one of identical twins. A seven -years follow-up. Arch Neurol 36, 854-856.

Jeulin H., Venard V., Carapito D., & Financeand Kedzierenvicz F. (2009) Effective ribavirinconcentration in mice brain using Cyclodextrin as a drug carrier: evaluation in a measles encephalitis model. Antiviral Res ,81, 261-266.

Jin L., Beard S., Hunjan R., Brown D.V., & Miller E. (2002) Characterization of measles virus strains causing SSPE: a study of 11 cases J Neurovirol 8, 335-349.

Kim S-H., Ricci S., & El-Deiry W.S. Mcl-1: A gateway to TRAIL sensitizacion. Cancer Res , 68, 2062-2064.

Keita D, Servan de Almeida R, Libeau G, & Albina E. (2008) Identification and mapping of a region on the mRNA of Morbillivirus nucleoprotein susceptible to RNA interferente. Antiviral Res. 80, 158-167.

Kirk J, Zhou AL, McQuaid S, Cosby SL, & Allen IV. (1991) Cerebral endothelial cell infection by measles virus in subacute sclerosing panencephalitis: ultrastructural and in situ hybridization evidence. Neuropathol Appl Neurobiol.17, 289-297.

Kolakofsky D., Pelet T., Garin D., Housmann S., Curran J., & Roux L. (1998) Paramyxovirus RNA synthesis and the requirement for hexamer genome length: the rule of six revisited. J Virol 72, 891-899.

Koschel K., Brinckmann U. & Hoyningen-Huene V.V. (1995) Measles virus antisense sequences specifically cure cells persistently infected with measles virus. Virology 207, 168-178.

Kühne Simmonds M.,Brown D.W.G., & Lin J. (2006) Measles viral load may reflect SSPE disease progression. Virology Journal 10.1, 1-9.

Kusuhara K.,Torisu H., Kira R., & Hara T. (2007) Host genetic factors for the development of SSPE. Nippon Rinsho, 65, 1467-1474.

Lan I., Gorke S., & Rau S.J. (2008) Hepatitis C virus infection sensitizes human hepatocytes to Trail-induced apoptosis in a caspase9-dependent manner. J Immunol ,181, 4926-4935.

Lecouturier V, Fayolle J., Caballero M., Celma M.L., Fernandez-Muñoz R., Wild F.T., & Auckland R. (1996) Identification of two aminoacids in the hemagglutinin glycoprotein of measles virus that govern hemadsortion, HeLa cells fusion and CD46 down regulation. J Virol 70, 4200-4204.

Lemon K, de Vries R.D., Mesman A.W., McQuaid S., van Amerongen G., Yüksel S., Ludlow M., Rennick L.J., Kuiken T., Rima B.K., Geijtenbeek T.B., Osterhaus A.D., Duprex W.P., & Swart R.L. (2011) Early target cells of measles virus after aerosol infection on non-human primates. Plos Pathol , Jan 27;7(1):e1001263.

Mahadevan A., Vaidya S.R., Wairagkar N.S., Khedekar D., Kovoor J.M., Santosh V., Yasha T.C., Saithchandra P., Ravi V., & Shankar S.K. (2008) Case of fulminant-SSPE associated with measles genotype D7 from India: An autopsy study. Neuropathology,28,621-626.

Makhortova N., Askovich P., Patterson C.E., Gechman L.A., Gerard N.P., & Rall G.F.,(2007) Neurokinin-1 enables measles virus trans-synaptic spread in neurones. Virology, 362,235-244.

Manchester M. , Valmasakis A., Liton P.B.,Fernandez-Muñoz R., Rota P., Bellini W.J., Forthal D.N. & Oldstone M.B.A. (2000) Clinical isolates of measles virus use CD6 as a cellular receptor. J Virol , 74, 3967-3974.

Martin-Cortes A., Duque B.M., Fernandez-Muñoz R & Celma M.L. (2004) Inhibition of measles virus replication by small interfering RNAs (siRNAs), II European Congress of Virology,Madrid,

Moench T.R., Griffin D.E., Obriecht C.R., Vaisberg A.J., & Johnson R.T. (1989) Acute measles in patients with and without neurological involvement: distribution of measles virus antigen and RNA. J Infect Dis , 158,433-442.

MottetG., CurranJ., & Roux L. (1990) Intracellular stability of nonreplicating paramyxovirus nucleocapsisds, Virology 176, 1-7.

Nitsch R., Bechmann I., Deisz R., Haas d., Lehmann T., Wending U., & Zipp F. (2000) Human brain-cell death induced by tumor-necrosis-factor-related apoptosis-inducing ligand (TRAIL). The Lancet, 356,827-828)

Norrby E., & Kristensson K. (1997) Measles in the brain. Brain Res Bull , 44, 213-220.

Ogata S., Ogata A., Schneider-Schulies S. & Schneider-Schaulies J. (2004) Expression of the interferon-alpha/beta-inducible MxA protein in brain lesions of subacute sclerosing panencephalitis. J Neurol Sci 223, 113-119.

Oldstone M.B.A., Dales S., Tishon A., Lewicki H. & Martin L. (2005) A role for dual viral hits in causation of subacute sclerosing panencephalitis. J Exp Med ,202, 1185-1190.

Oldstone M.B.A.(2009) Modelling Subacute Sclerosing Panencephalitis in a Transgenic Mouse System: Uncoding Pathogenesis of Disease and Illuminating Componenets of Immune Control. In Measles Pathogenesis and Control: Editors Griffin D.E. and Oldstone M.B.A., Springer-Verlag, Berlin, CTMI 330,31-54.

Ortego J. (1994) Studies on the molecular mechanisms of measles virus pathogenesis. Doctoral Thesis , Universidad Autonoma de Madrid, Spain.

Otaki M., Jiang D.P., Sasayama M., Nagano-Fuji M & Ota H.(2007) Generation of recombinant adenovirus expressing siRNA against the L mRNA of measles virus and subacute sclerosing panencephalitis virus. Microbial Immunol ,51,985-991.

Pan C.H., Greer C.E.,Hauer D., Legg H.S., Bergen M.J. , Lau B., Adams R.J., Polo J.M. & Griffin D.E. (2010)A chimeric alphavirus replicon particle vaccine expressing the hemagglutinin and fusion proteins protects juvenile and infant rhesus macaques from measles. J Virol 84, 3798-3807.

Plemper R.K. & Snyder J.P. (2009) Measles control, Can measles virus inhibitors make a difference? , Curr Opin Investig Drugs, 10, 811-820.

Radecke F., Spielhofer P., Schneider H., Kaelin K., Huber M., Dotsch C., Christiansen G., & Billeter M.A. (1995) Rescue of measles virus from cloned DNA. EMBO J , 14, 5773-5784.

Reuter D. & Schneider-Schaulies J. (2010) Measles virus infection of the CNS: human disease, animal models, and approaches to therapy. Med Microbiol Immunol, 99, 261-271.

Reuter T., Wessbrich B., Scneider-Schaulies S. & Schneider-Schaulies J. (2006) RNA Interference with measles virus N, P, and L mRNAs efficiently prevents and with matrix protein mRNA enhance viral transcription. J Virol 80,5951-5957.

Ridell M.A., Moss W.J., Hauer D., Monze M., & Griffin D.E. (2007) Slow clearance of measles virus RNA after acute infection. J Clin Virol , 39, 312-317.

Rima B.K., Davidson W.B., & Martin S.J. (1977) The role of Defective Interfering Particles in Persistent Infection of Vero Cells with Measles Virus. J Gen Virol 35:89-97.

Rima B.K., Earle J.A.P., Yeo R.P., Herlihy L., Backo K., ter Meulen V., Carabaña J., Caballero M., Celma M.L. & Fernandez-Muñoz R. (1995). Temporal and Geographic distribution of measles virus genotypes. J Gen Virol., 76, 1173-1180.

Rima B.K., Earle A.P., Backo K., Liebert V.G., Carsten C., Carabaña J,, Caballero M., Celma M.l. & Fernandez-Muñoz R., (1997) Sequence divergence of measles virus hemagglutinin during natural evolution and adaptation to cell culture, J Gen Virol, 78,97-106.

Rima B.K. & Duprex W.P.(2005) Molecular mechanisms of measles virus persistence. Virus Research, 111, 132-147.

Rima B. K. & Duprex W.P. (2006) Morbilliviruses and Human disease. J Pathol, 208, 199-214.

Rossi J., Gait M.J., & Eckstein F. edt. (2009) Oligonucleotide Therapeutics. Four Annual Meeting. Ann NY ACAD SCI. vol 1175.

Samuel C.E. (2011) Adenosine deaminases acting on RNA (ADARs) are both antiviral and proviral. Virology, 411, 180-193.

Sato K., Nakagawa E., Arai A., Sakuma H., Komaki H., Sugai K., & Sasaki M. (2009) Serious complications of interferon-alfa and ribavirine in the treatment of subacute sclerosing panencephalitis. No To Hattatsu, 41, 224-228.

Schneider-Schaulies S.,Kreth H.W., Hofman G.,,Billeter M., & ter Meulen V. (1991) Expression of measles virus RNA in peripheral blood mononuclear cells of patients with measles , SSPE,and autoimmune diseases. Virology, 182, 703-711.

Sedger L.M., Shows R.A., Blanton J.J., Pechon R.G., Goodwin D., Cosman D., & Wiley S.R. (1999) IFN-gamma mediates a novel antiviral activity through dynamic modulation of TRAIL and TRAIL receptor expression. J Immunol, 163, 920-926.

Sharma V., Gupta V.B. & Eisenhut M. (2008) Familial subacute sclerosing panencephalitis associated with short latency. Pediatr Neurol., 38, 215-217.

Sidhu M.S., Husar W., Cook S.D.,, Dowling P.C., & Udem S. (1993) Canine Distemper terminal an intergenic non-protein coding nucleotide sequences: completion of the entire CDV genome sequence. Virology, 193, 66-72.

Sidhu M.S., Crowley J, Lowenthal A. Karchen D.Mennona J.,Cook S, Udem S. & Dowling P. (1994) Defective measles virus in human subacute sclerosing brain. Virology, 202, 631-641.

SleemanK., Stein D.A., Tamin A., Reddish M.,Iversen P.L., & Rota P.A. (2009) Inhibition of measles virus infectionsin cell cultures by peptide-conjugated morpholin oligomers. Virus Res., 140, 49-56.

Souraud J.B., Faivre a., Waku-KouomouD., Gaillard T., Aouad N., Meaudre E., Wild F.T., & Fouet (2009) Adult fulminant subacute sclerosing panencephalitis: Pathological and molecular studies-a case report. Clin Neuropathol, 28,213-218.

Tatli B.,Ekici B. & Ozmen M. (2010) Flupirtine may stop the progressive course of subacute sclerosing panencephalitis. Med Hypotheses 75, 576-577.

Titomanlio L., Soyah N., Guerin V., Delante C., Sterkers G. Evrard P. & Husson I. (2007) Rituximab in subacute sclerosing panencehalitis. Eur J Paediatr Neurol, 11, 43-45.

Torisu H., Kusuhara k., Kira R., Bassuny W.M., Sakai Y., Sanefugi M., Takemoto M., & Hara T. (2004) FunctionalMxA promoter polymorphism associated with subacute sclerosing panencephalitis., Nerology,62, 457-460.

Toro-Riera M., Macaya-Ruiz A., Raspall-Chaure M., Tallada-Serra M., Pasqual-Lopez I. & Roig-Quilis M. (2006) Subacute sclerosing panencephalitis: Combined treatment with Interferon alpha and intraventricular ribavirin. Rev Neurol 42,277-281.

Toth A.M., Li Z,, Cattaneo R., & Samuel C.E.(2009) RNA-specific adenosine deaminase ADR1 suppress measles virus-induced apoptosis and activation of protein kinase PKR. J Biol Chem, 284, 29350-29356.

Trottier C., Colombo M., Mann K., Miller W., & Ward B.J. (2009) Retinoids inhibit measles virus through a type 1 IFN-dependent bystander effect. Faseb J , 80, 45-53.

Ward S.V., George C.X., Welch M.J., Liou L.Y., Hahm B., Lewicky H., de la Torre J.C., Samuel C.E.& Oldstone M.B. (2011) RNA editing enzyme adenosine deaminase is a restriction factor for controlling measles virus replication that is also required for embryogenesis. Proc Natl Acad Sci U S A , 108, 331-336.

Watanabe A., Yoneda M., IkedaF., Terao-Muto Y., Sato H. & Kai C. (2010) CD147/EMMPRIN acts as a fundamental entry receptor for measles virus on epithelial cells. J Virol , 84,4183-4193.

Wong T.C., Ayata M., Hirano A., Yoshikawa Y., Tsruoka H, & Yamanouchi K. (1989) Generalized and localized biased hypermutation affecting the matrix gene of measles virus strain that causes subacute sclerosing panencephalitis. J Virol ,63, 5464-5468

World Health Organization (2006) Global Advisory Committee on Vaccine Safety. (1-2 December 2005) Wkly Epidemiol Rec 81, 15-19.

Yagita h., Takeda K., Hayakawa Y., Smyth M.J., & Okumura k. (2004) TRAIL and its receptors as targets for cancer therapy. Cance Sci ,95, 777-783.

Young V.A, & Rall G.F. (2009) Making it to the Synapse: Measles virus Spread in and among Neurons. In Measles Virus Pathogenesis and Control, editors GriffinD.E. and Oldstone M.B.A., Springer, Berlin, CTMI, 330, 3-30.

Zinke M., Kendl S., Singethan K., Fehrholz M., Reuter D., Rennick L., Herold M.J., & Schneider-Schaulies J. (2009) Clearance of measles virus from persistently infected cells by shot hairpin RNA. J Virol 83,9423-9431.

10

Encephalitic Development in Alphaviral Infection

Slobodan Paessler and Katherine Taylor
University of Texas Medical Branch
United States of America

1. Introduction

Viruses are currently the most common cause of encephalitis. With more than 20 viruses known to cause human encephalitis, arboviruses, arthropod-borne viruses, represent a significant number of emerging infectious diseases both in the United States and worldwide. The *Alphavirus* genus in the family *Togaviridae* contains three viruses capable of causing human encephalitis: Venezuelan equine encephalitis virus (VEEV), eastern equine encephalitis virus (EEEV), and western equine encephalitis virus (WEEV). WEEV and EEEV are endemic to the United States and South America while VEEV circulates in Central and South America; however, spread of epidemic outbreaks has resulted in disease in North America. No specific therapy or vaccine is currently available against these viruses. In this review, we summarize the development and progression of alphavirus encephalitis in both human populations and murine models of alphavirus infection. We concentrate on the host response that characterizes the development of central nervous system (CNS) disease following alphaviral infection. In addition, we focus on immune factors that influence successful resolution of infection.

Alphaviruses represent a significant public health threat as both emerging infectious diseases and possible agents of bioterrorism. Natural, endemic infections of alphavirus disease are currently absent in certain areas of the globe where the mosquito vector capable of transmitting alphaviruses exists making potential virus introduction into such unaffected areas a significant public health concern (Calisher, 1994; Hawley & Eitzen, 2001; Weaver & Barrett, 2004; Zacks & Paessler, 2010). Additionally, many of the encephalitic alphaviruses are highly stable as an aerosol, cause significant mortality or incapacitating disease, and grow rapidly in easily utilized, readily available cell culture systems. This combination of factors makes this group of viruses of significant interest for biodefense in the United States (Hawley & Eitzen, 2001; Weaver, 2005).

One of three of the original serological groups of arboviruses, the group A complex became the *Alphavirus* genus within the *Togaviridae* family representing enveloped, plus-strand RNA viruses (Porterfield, 1975; Porterfield, 1986). Pathogenic alphaviruses can be roughly grouped further by a combination of phylogenetics, geographical circulation, and disease manifestation into two groups. Viruses circulating in the Old World (Europe, Asia, and Africa) typically cause arthralgia, malaise or a rash. (Griffin, 2007; Zacks & Paessler, 2010). New World alphaviruses' infections result in a flu-like syndrome that may progress to neurological involvement. New World encephalitic alphaviruses include EEE, WEE, and

VEE complex viruses. Of these the primary causes of neurological involvement and lethal encephalitis are WEE, EEE, and VEE viruses. More rarely, Highlands J virus, a member of the WEE antigenic complex, and some Old World alphaviruses may be neuroinvasive (Zacks & Paessler, 2010).

Neurovirulence of the viruses associates with efficient and rapid spread of virus throughout the neurons of the central nervous system (CNS) resulting in pathogenesis and death of neuronal cells; however, the host response also represents significant determinant of pathogenesis and mortality (Griffin, 2007; Ryman & Klimstra, 2008). This chapter will briefly describe basic viral dissemination and spread in natural cycles, both enzootic and epizootic, followed by a more in-depth overview of the primary encephalitic alphavirus, EEE, WEE, and VEE encompassing the description of disease in animal and man with an emphasis on the host response.

2. Overview of encephalitic alphaviruses

2.1 History and Medical Importance

Records of fatal encephalitis in horses in the northeastern United States date to the 19th century and reports of *peste loca* in South America exist back further though etiology of these infections is uncertain (Groot, 1971; Hanson, 1957). Throughout the early 20th century, sporadic outbreaks of encephalitis in horses continued to occur along the Atlantic seaboard of the United States as well as in regions of South America (Groot, 1971; Sabattini, et al., 1985). In 1930, WEEV became the first of the encephalitic alphaviruses isolated from the brain of an infected equine, and isolation of EEEV closely followed(Meyer, et al., 1931; Tenbroeck, et al., 1935; Tenbroeck & Merrill, 1933). In 1936, an outbreak of equine disease in Venezuela similar to that found in conjunction with EEE and WEE presented isolates not neutralized by either EEE or WEE antisera. VEEV was subsequently discovered as a causative pathogen of equine disease (Kubes & Rios, 1939a; 1939b). Isolation of virus from human cases of encephalitis associated with epizootic outbreaks followed for all three of the viruses (Casals, et al., 1943; Feemster, 1938; Howitt, 1938).

The largely summer occurrence of epidemic disease and disappearance in fall and winter months suggested a mosquito vector and Kelser subsequently demonstrated transmission of WEE virus by mosquitoes (Kelser, 1937). Since that time the EEE, WEE, and VEE viruses have been isolated from mosquitoes, horses, humans, and other vertebrate species, namely birds and rodents (Griffin, 2007). A more detailed history of each virus will be presenting in the sections below.

2.2 Molecular biology of the *Alphavirus* genus

The virions of the encephalitic alphaviruses contain a single-stranded, positive sense RNA genome composed of 5′ non structural proteins (NsP) and 3′ structural proteins totalling 12 kilobases. The first two-thirds of the genome encode non-structural proteins NsP1, NsP2, NsP3 and NsP4 (Frolov, 2004; Griffin, 2007). The structural proteins are encoded in the 3′ third of the genome and translated from a 26S subgenomic promoter resulting in production of the five protein products, the capsid (C), and envelope proteins 1-3 (E1-E3) and 6K (Griffin, 2007). The structural proteins are considered the primary targets for adaptive, antigen specific immunity, both humoral and cell-mediated, and are also capable of interfering with host defense mechanisms (Aguilar, et al., 2008a; Simmons, et al., 2009). A more detailed description of specific viruses will be included in the sections below.

2.3 Transmission cycles

Alphaviruses circulate in enzootic and epizootic cycles between hematophagous arthropods and vertebrate animals. The nature of the vertebrate host determines the maintenance of virus in epizootic or enzootic cycles. As such, vertebrate hosts can be loosely divided into two groups: the natural vertebrate host acting as the primary source of mosquito infection in which the virus replicates, but no symptomatic disease presents and vertebrates that develop symptomatic disease where ability to transmit the virus back to mosquito populations varies based on strain and infected host species. For the encephalitic alphaviruses, the primary host is typically murine or avian (Calisher, 1994). In epizootic or epidemic cycles, infected mosquitoes transmit the virus to a secondary host, usually man or equine. Large outbreaks of disease occur when infected secondary hosts act to amplify viral replication and transmission generating a high titer viremia permitting further infection of mosquito, and, subsequently, host populations. The ability of the secondary host to amplify the virus furthering epidemic spread varies based on virus and host, and is detailed specifically below (Weaver, 2005; Weaver & Barrett, 2004; Zacks & Paessler, 2010). Epizootic outbreaks in equines frequently signal the beginning of epidemic spread of virus followed by subsequent disease in human populations.

2.4 Virus spread

Due to the nature of infection and prevalence of asymptomatic infections, much of what is known about the virus spread has been determined utilizing murine models. As the mosquito feeds on the experimental host, virus is deposited in infected saliva extravascularly (Turell, et al., 1995). Virus initially replicates at the site of inoculation, typically skeletal muscle or immune cells, and dissemination to dendritic cells or Langerhans cells of the skin closely follows (Grimley & Friedman, 1970; Johnston, et al., 2000; Liu, et al., 1970; Murphy & Whitfield, 1970). As these infected cell populations migrate to the draining lymph nodes (DLN) for the site of inoculation, the virus spreads through the blood to other skeletal muscles and through lymph and blood to lymphatic tissue. As the virus continues replication, spread occurs to secondary sites of replication which include the brain and spinal cord neurons (Griffin, 2007). While tropism of other cells of the CNS apart from neurons is uncertain, alphaviruses may be capable of replication in the meningeal cells, ependymal cells, and other glial cell populations (Ehrengruber, et al., 2003; Mims, et al., 1973; Schoneboom, et al., 1999a).

2.5 Pathogenic sequence of alphaviral infection in humans

Upon virus infection the disease progression in humans typically follows a biphasic disease process characterized by a mild, flu-like illness potentially associated with replication at the primary site of infection, viremia, and initiation of the immune response (Calisher, 1994). Length of acute disease varies with virus, but patients typically improve slightly following initial illness then develop a second febrile episode congruent with dissemination of virus to target tissues and development of an adaptive immune response (Brown, 1993; CFSPH, 2008; Zacks & Paessler, 2010). During this second phase, a subset of patients progress to neurological involvement associated with mortality. Typical lesions in fatal cases appear as severe inflammation of the gray matter with neuronal degeneration, infiltration of inflammatory cells, gliosis, perivascular cuffing and hemorrhages (Griffin, 2007). Despite the close phylogenetic relation of VEE, WEE and EEE complex viruses, the genotypes vary significantly in disease, mortality rates, severity of sequelae, and location and pattern of lesions in the brain as detailed below for individual viruses (Luers, et al., 2005; Steele & Twenhafel, 2010; Weaver & Barrett, 2004).

2.6 Host response

Again, as with viral transmission most of what is known regarding the host response has been determined in small animal and non-human primate (NHP) models. The host response has been primarily characterized by the early production of type I interferon (IFN) and the later production of virus-specific neutralizing antibody (Adler & Rabinowitz, 1973; Grieder & Vogel, 1999; Houston, et al., 1977; Konopka, et al., 2009; Schoneboom, et al., 2000d). This set of viruses is sensitive to the effects of the type I IFNs, IFN-α and IFN-β, and, as a result, have developed evasive mechanisms of interference with type I IFN signaling. Thus, the ability to resist type I IFN is considered a factor for the level of virulence of WEE, EEE, and VEE virus strains, and mutations altering type I IFN resistance result in attenuation of the virus. Early control of viral replication is dependent on type I IFN production and the absence of type I IFN signaling is typically fatal in murine models (Aguilar, et al., 2008a; Aguilar, et al., 2005; Frolov, 2004; Grieder & Vogel, 1999; Jahrling, et al., 1976; Spotts, et al., 1998). Conversely, prophylactic treatment with type I IFN or artificial induction of type I IFN prior to infection provides protection or extended time to death in murine models (Julander, et al., 2008a; Julander, et al., 2007; Julander, et al., 2008b). Viral load in target organs and viremia typically correlates with amount of IFN produced (Ryman, 2008).

Interestingly, other models of CNS pathogenesis with no viral etiology demonstrate a role for type I IFN in an anti-inflammatory capacity capable of modulating the early, acute response and altering the adaptive immune response in the CNS (Galligan, et al., 2010; Plosker, 2011). The overwhelming pro-inflammatory cytokine response associated with initiation of the immune response to the encephalitic alphaviruses has been loosely linked to neuropathogenesis apart from viral load and replication in neuronal cell populations (Dikii, et al., 1976; Koterski, et al., 2007; Mokhtarian, et al., 1996; Phillpotts, et al., 2003; Ryman, 2008; Schoneboom, et al., 2000b; Valerol, et al., 2008). Thus, the pleiotropic nature of type I IFN may induce a more forgiving environment in the CNS, reducing levels of proinflammatory cytokines, altering the adaptive response, and buffering the microenviroment of the CNS during alphaviral infection (Plosker, 2011). However, other effects of type I IFN in the CNS pathologies of alphavirus infection remain to be explored.

Resolution of infection and disease has focused on the neutralizing antibody response to infection. Antibody is undoubtedly significant in recovery from peripheral infection and in blocking neuroinvasion (Bedenice, et al., 2009; Burke, et al., 1977; Calisher, et al., 1986a; DeMeio, et al., 1979). However, its effectiveness once neuroinvasion occurs is not well understood. Peripheral passive transfer of antibody has little effect following neuroinvasion; however, production of antibody from B-cells resident in the CNS may impact course of neurological disease though little is known about the presence or role of B-cells in the CNS microenviroment (Yun, et al., 2009). More recently, T-cells, particularly CD4+ T-cells, have been implicated in resolution of CNS infection with these neurotropic viruses (Brooke, et al., 2010; Paessler, et al., 2007; Yun, et al., 2009). Additionally, the early production of TNF-alpha, IL-1, and IL-6 indicates a T-helper 1 (Th1) bias to the adaptive immune response following alphavirus infection (Valerol, et al., 2008). The Th1 response is characterized by predominately IFN-γ producing CD4+ T-cells (Brooke, et al., 2010; Yun, et al., 2009). As a corollary, IFN-γ secretion associated with a Th1 response may be partially protective following entry of virus to the CNS (Paessler, et al., 2007).

3. Western equine encephalitis

3.1 History and significance

Initially isolated from the brain of an infected equine in 1930 in California, WEE virus was the first of the encephalitic alphaviruses to be discovered(Meyer, et al., 1931). However, the virus was not recognized as a cause of human illness till isolation from the brain of an infected child in 1938 (Howitt, 1938). According to the United States Center for Disease Control (CDC) and the Center for Food Security and Public Health (CFSPH), 640 confirmed or probable human cases of WEE occurred between 1964 and 2009 in the United States alone (CDC, 2009b; CFSPH, 2008). Overall case fatality rates are estimated at 3-7%, but mortality rates depend on both age and other factors such as virus strain, dose, and route of infection (Calisher, 1994; CFSPH, 2008; Hanson, et al., 1967; Ryzhikov, et al., 1991; Steele, et al., 1998; Steele & Twenhafel, 2010; Zacks & Paessler, 2010). Accidental, artificial exposure of aerosolized virus in laboratory settings has been documented with the few cases demonstrating a 40% fatality rate (Fothergill, et al., 1939; Gold & Hampil, 1942; Hanson, et al., 1967; Helwig, 1940). As with all the encephalitic alphaviruses, higher mortality rates and incidence of neurological complications are associated with pediatric patients. For WEE, an estimated 90% of children under one year of age show severe CNS signs; additionally, an estimated 15-30% of pediatric and adult patients that survive neurological involvement are left with severe, permanent sequelae (Zacks & Paessler, 2010). Children older than one year of age show a steep increase in numbers of asymptomatic infections (Bruyn & Lennette, 1953; Cohen, et al., 1953). Transplacental transmission has been documented with all know instances surviving acute encephalitis, but developing subsequent neurological sequelae (Bruyn & Lennette, 1953; CFSPH, 2008; Copps & Giddings, 1959; Romero & Newland, 2006; Shinefield & Townsend, 1953). Thus, while overall mortality rates due to WEE infection are low, sequelae are significant and costly particularly in pediatric patients (CFSPH, 2008). A steady decline in cases since the middle of the 20th century has been partially attributed to changes in the natural habitat for the common mosquito vector due to altered irrigation practices and mosquito control programs though the true cause of decline remains in question (Calisher, 1994; Forrester, et al., 2008).

3.2 Transmission cycles and geographic range

WEE acts over a broad geographic range throughout North and South America as an equine pathogen; however, despite the isolation of WEE strains throughout the Americas, human disease appears less frequently and with decreased severity in South America (Calisher, 1994; Sulkin, 1946; Tsai, 1991). Neither equines or humans act as amplifying hosts. Strains of WEE virus have been isolated from humans, horses, wild birds, and vertebrates from western Canada to Argentina (Calisher, et al., 1985; Reisen, 1988). Specifically, infection of bobwhite quails, house finches, sparrows, and domestic chickens has been demonstrated (Hardy, 1987; O'Brien, et al.,; Watts & Williams, 1972; Williams, et al., 1971). The virus can also infect some small mammals including opossum, squirrels, bats, rabbits, and hares. Like horses and humans, a number of these species exhibit a tangential infection and do not act as amplifying hosts (CFSPH, 2008; Fastier, 1952; Hardy, 1987; Kiorpes & Yuill, 1975; Reisen, et al., 2004; Ubico & McLean, 1995; Yuill & Hanson, 1964) Isolations of WEE viruses have been reported in the Veracruz region of Mexico and South America and the genetic analyses of isolates from Brazil and northern Argentina revealed a level of nucleotide identity >90% in the E2/6K/E1 coding region when compared to isolates from the US. This data suggests a monophyletic nature of the WEEV lineage, with an overall slow evolution (Weaver, 2005; Weaver & Barrett, 2004; Zacks & Paessler, 2010)

WEE is maintained in an enzootic cycle between a number of passerine birds and its most common mosquito vector, *Culex;* however, the virus has also been isolated from mites (Hammon & Reeves, 1946; Hammon, et al., 1941; Hammon, et al., 1943; Reeves, et al., 1947; Zacks & Paessler, 2010). The avian host is likely responsible for the distribution of virus strains from North to South America, and explains the widespread geographic range of the virus (Reisen 2010, Calisher 1994). Transmission to humans and horses occurs via bridging mosquito vector species whose habitat and nature results in feeding on these specific vertebrate hosts (Calisher, 1994; Zacks & Paessler, 2010). Bridging vectors include *Ochlerotatus melanimon* in California, *Aedes dorsalis* in Utah and New Mexcio and *Ae. Campestris* in New Mexico (Clark, et al., 1986; Reisen, et al., 1998; Zacks & Paessler, 2010). In temperate climates, the transmission cycle may be maintained through the year, but in less mild climates WEE may either overwinter in unidentified hosts or be reintroduced annually through passerine bird. Isolates of WEE have been obtained from some amphibious species, garter snakes and leopard frogs, indicating that WEE may be able to overwinter in such hosts (Burton, et al., 1966; Gebhardt, et al., 1966; Gebhardt, et al., 1964). Transovarial transmission of the virus in mosquitoes has also been proposed as an overwintering mechanism. However, current literature on the subject is inconclusive (Reeves, et al., 1954; Thomas & Eklund, 1960; Watts & Eldridge, 1975).

3.3 Disease manifestations in humans

WEEV infections tend to have more in common with EEEV infections than with VEEV though infection is associated with less severe disease and lower mortality than EEE. As with both other viruses, WEE infections predominately are either asymptomatic or cause mild disease. Disease appears after a short incubation period of two to seven days and associates with general flu like symptoms and often times an altered mental status (CFSPH, 2008; Hoke, 2005; Zacks & Paessler, 2010). Typical recovery begins after approximately ten days of symptomatic illness (Calisher, 1994). When lethal disease occurs, mortality happens within seven days of symptomatic disease . A minority of infected individual will develop encephalitis and associated neurological symptoms: neck stiffness, confusion, tonic-clonic seizures, somnolence, coma and death (CFSPH, 2008; Steele & Twenhafel, 2010; Zacks & Paessler, 2010). Abnormal reflex responses in adults depend largely on stage of illness and typically consist of weakness and hyporeflexia. Disease progression is slower in adults than in infants which develop sudden onset of illness with fever and seizures. Both adolescents and older children have a prodromal phase typified by severe headaches and fever of two to three days followed by CNS manifestations. Unsurprisingly given the higher mortality rates, children display far more severe neurological symptoms with muscular rigidity, involuntary movements, and paralysis (Calisher, 1994; Steele & Twenhafel, 2010).

Cerebral spinal fluid (CSF) pressure may be mildly elevated with normal glucose, protein and elevated leukocyte counts ($<500/mm^3$) (Calisher, 1994; Rozdilsky, et al., 1968). While typical CSF white blood cell counts are in this range, they have been reported to be as high as $2000/mm^3$, (Romero & Newland, 2003; 2006). Early infection is characterized by polymorphonuclear cells with mononuclear cells dominating later in infection (Calisher, 1994). A computed tomography scan (CT) of one case of neonatal WEE revealed multiple, symmetrical, calcifications in both hemispheres in both the insular cortex and the thalamus as well as dilatation of the temporal ventricles and compression of the peritroncal and sylvian cisterns. Electroencephalogram (EEG) showed diffuse cerebral suffering mimicking pathologies similar to HSV-1 encephalitis (Delfraro, et al., 2011; Romero & Newland, 2003; Somekh, et al., 1991).

Gross pathologies are limited to the CNS in lethal infections and do not appear in the periphery (Calisher, 1994; Steele & Twenhafel, 2010). The brain is typically edematous, but pathologies are primarily characterized by focal hemorrhages. These hemorrhages are observed in the white and gray matter throughout the brain though the basal nuclei, thalamus, and brain stem are the most often severely affected. Lesions also appear in the spinal cord (Steele & Twenhafel, 2010; Zacks & Paessler, 2010).

Histopathologically, the brains of infected individuals demonstrate wide spread perivascular cuffs of lymphocytes and neutrophils. Additionally, smaller areas of focal necrosis with and without cellular infiltrate are found throughout the brain in the striatum, globus pallidus, susbtantia nigra, cerebral cortex, thalamus, and pons. A subset of lethally infected patients displayed predominant concentrations of brain lesions in the subcortical white matter (Anderson, 1984; Rozdilsky, et al., 1968).

3.4 Disease manifestations in experimental models

WEE has not been extensively studied in animal models. While limited and often not precisely representative of human infection, the span of studies in small animal models and non-human primates (NHP) resulted in a general idea of the pathologies and host response to WEE. Animal models used include mice, hamsters, cynomolgus macaques, gerbils, guinea pigs and rabbits (Hayles, 1972; Hayles, et al., 1970; Hayles, et al., 1972; Holbrook & Gowen, 2008; Hurst, 1934; Reed, et al., 2005).

3.4.1 Mouse model

Like in humans, age and strain of mouse infected, route of inoculations, and virulence of virus strain all influence the susceptibility of the host (Aguilar, 1970; Bianchi, et al., 1993; Logue, et al., 2009; Monath, et al., 1978; Nagata, et al., 2006). Peripheral routes of infection result in approximately 50% mortality with intracerebral (IC) or intranasal (IN) challenge resulting in more uniform, dose-dependent mortality depending on strain of virus and background of murine model (Hardy, et al., 1997; Julander, et al., 2007; Liu, et al., 1970).

In suckling mice, subcutaneous (SC) inoculation results in rapid, acute disease with uniform mortality by 48 hours post-infection (PI). Interestingly, in infant animals, mice developed pathologies largely in mesodermally derived tissues, and not in the CNS or other peripheral organs such as the lung, liver, or heart. Histologically, these mice displayed necrotic degeneration of the bone marrow. Despite showing no clinical signs of illness, young adult mice (three to four weeks) develop widespread viral encephomeningitis associated with focal necrosis and perivascular cuffs similar to human disease. Additional pathological changes were noted in the lung, liver, kidney and brown fat though no clinical evidence of disease was present throughout disease course indicating the resilience of the host in the presence of significant CNS pathologies. (Aguilar, 1970). This age group of mice also develop myocardial infection and necrosis as well as peripheral lesions in the heart (Monath, et al., 1978). Thus, tissue tropism and susceptibility to WEE vary with age of the animal.

Comparison of WEEV isolates McMillan (McM) vs. Imperial 181(IMP) in outbred CD1 mice, demonstrated changes time to death and mortality rates varying by route of infection and strain of virus used though both strains are neuroinvasive. More virulent McM causes 100% mortality within five days following SC injection. In contrast, IMP causes no death in infected animals. A similar trend was noted for aerosol, IN and intravenous routes (IV). Thus, while both strains are neuroinvasive, only McM is also neurovirulent. McM when administered IN also causes extensive damage to the neurons of the CNS. The alterations in pathogenicity between the two strains are possible attributed to either slower replication of the attenuated strain or changes in the response to the innate immune system (Logue, et al., 2009). Accumulated data from EEE and VEE indicate that alterations in response of the host and susceptibility of the virus to the immune response are a strong determinant of outcome.

3.4.2 Hamster and guinea pig models

Virulent strains of WEE administered by multiple routes demonstrated lethal disease in hamster models. Hamsters have been postulated as a working model for WEE disease due to high mortality observed and lesions of encephalitis found following infection. Characteristic pathologies associate with lethality include tachypnea, conjunctivitis, incoordination, and seizures (Zlotnik, et al., 1972). Both IC and peripheral infection leads to high viral load in the brain and severe neurological disease characterized by neuronal necrosis and infiltration of the meninges and Virchow-Robins space by lymphocytes (Holbrook & Gowen, 2008; Julander, et al., 2007; Zlotnik, et al., 1972). These pathologies are diffuse throughout the brain with olfactory regions begin particularly damaged. Despite the wide-spread nature of CNS pathologies, groups of neurons from the cerebral cortex and in areas of the mid-brain are typically infected with WEE indicative of bystander activation and killing of nearby cells resulting in disseminated pathologies (Julander, et al., 2007). Astrocytes do not appear to be susceptible to infection *in vivo* (Julander, et al., 2007). Guinea pigs demonstrate a severe disease similar to hamster models with death occurring in less than ten days following infection (Bianchi, et al., 1997; Nalca, et al., 2003a).

3.4.3 Nonhuman primate model

WEE causes lethal encephalitis in non-human primates: cynomolgus macaques and rhesus monkeys (Macaca mulatta) (Hurst, 1936; London, et al., 1982; Reed, et al., 2005; Wyckoff & Tesar, 1939). IC and IN challenge with WEE results in severe lethal encephalitis in NHP with IC infection resulting in uniform fatalities and IN or aerosol challenge resulting in severe CNS infection with some associated mortality. Peripheral routes of challenge including endermally, intramuscularly (IM) or IV do not result in consistent CNS infection (Hurst, 1936; Wyckoff & Tesar, 1939).

Following aerosol inoculation, cynomolgus macaques develop a fever between four and five days and show symptomatic disease including reduced appetite, decreased behavior, and tremors. Leukocytosis, serum glucose levels, and fever associated with severity of disease though none accurately predict survival vs. mortality. Viral antigen was only detected in the CNS and not the periphery of lethally infected animals possibly attributed to the later time point of collection following clearance of virus from the periphery by neutralizing, serum antibody. Antigen appeared in the CNS in the neurons, microglia and Purkinje cells. However, virus was focused in areas of inflammation and demyelination. Interestingly, virus was not detectable in the blood or by throat swab during the course of infection suggestive of entry of WEE to the CNS through the olfactory nerves (Reed, et al., 2005). Thus, aerosol inoculation of WEEV in NHPs appears to be limited to the brain.

Gross findings were also limited to the CNS and consisted of meningeal congestion with histological lesions characterized by meningoencephalitis. Microscopic changes included alteration of the Virchow-Robins spaces of the brain and some spinal cord sections by infiltrating lymphocytes and monocytes, as well as foci of necrosis containing lymphocytes, microglia, and some neutrophils, discrete glial nodules and areas of neuronal demyelination

(Reed, et al., 2005; Wyckoff, 1939). These studies combined with clinical findings in man indicate that aerosolized WEEV is infectious through the olfactory neurons, and likely does not affect the peripheral organs.

3.5 Host response in experimental models

Due to the limitations of WEE studies and lack of clinical cases, little is known about the pathogenic and protective mechanisms mediating WEE in natural infections, and experimental models are responsible for most of the current knowledge of WEE pathogenesis and immunology. This section details the innate immune response to WEE and related therapeutics followed by knowledge of the adaptive immune response and effective vaccination measures to induce a useful memory response.

3.5.1 Innate immune response to WEE

The innate antiviral immune response is a crucial mechanism to control viral replication prior to induction of an adaptive immune response. In addition, the early immune response also molds the quality and phenotype of later immune responses and may be critical in control of pro-inflammatory pathogenic mechanisms following infection. Unfortunately, little is known about innate immune mechanisms important in alphavirus infection apart from a role for type I IFN Like other alphaviruses, WEE is sensitive to the effects of IFN-α and IFN-β. Recombination events that lead to the formation of the WEE from SIN- and EEE-like ancestors was essential for the virus to gain the ability to shut off transcription of anti-viral IFN factors, and likely lead to the emergence of WEE as a pathogenic virus (Garmashova, et al., 2007a; Garmashova, et al., 2007b; Weaver, et al., 1997). *In vitro* examination of human neuronal cells response to WEE indicates that virus cytopathology is reduced depending on maturation state of neurons in a manner independent of autocrine type I IFN activity and may explain the age related susceptibility to WEE infection. Additionally, mature neuronal cells were more sensitive with five to ten-fold less type I IFN needed to reduce viral cytopathology and replication. Type I IFN treatment is unable to completely eliminate WEEV cytopathogenicity in neuronal cells lines indicating factors apart for type I IFN may be important in control of viral replication (Castorena, et al., 2008).

Pre-treatment of hamsters IP with either a consensus type IFN-α , or with Ampligen®, a stimulator of Toll-like receptor 3 and subsequently type I IFN expression, resulted in complete survival compared to 100% lethality in controls (Julander 2007). Additionally, surviving animals treated with IFN were less symptomatic and lost less weight than controls. Both compounds acted as effective anti-virals significantly reducing the viral load in the brain at four days PI (Julander, et al., 2007).

A single dose of adenovirus-construct expressing transient INF-α (Ad5-mIFN-α) is capable of prophylactic and some therapeutic protection in mice against lethal, intranasal WEE challenge. The construct when administered 24 h, 48 h, or 7 d prior to infection provides 100% protection and when given 6 h PI provides 60% protection associated with delayed progression of disease. Clinical signs of infection were decreased in animals receiving the Ad5-mIFN-α. When animals received the vectored cytokine at 13 weeks prior to infection, survival rates were reduced to 38% and delayed time course of infection compared to sham treated controls. These animals lacked observable IFN in serum. The authors hypothesize that the discrepancy between serum IFN and protection could be due to continued higher levels of IFN in the brain providing protection following decrease of serum IFN (Wu, et al.,

2007b). Thus, when given prior to infection, IFN-α treatment provides rapid, lasting protection, and is indicative of the importance of a rapid, strong innate immune response.

3.5.2 Adaptive immune response

Much of what is known about the adaptive immune response to WEEV is derived utilizing models of pre-existing immunity, particularly regarding the antibody response. Currently, little is known about other mechanisms of cell mediated immunity.

3.5.2.1 Antibody response

Vaccination studies in experimental models provide the main basis of what is currently known about immunoprotection to CNS infection with WEE. Early studies in the 1970's on the efficacy of formalin inactivated WEE vaccine in humans demonstrated immunogenicity following a series of two vaccinations. Recipients developed high levels of serum neutralizing antibody 28 days following final vaccination. High levels of neutralizing antibody were present through day 360 with the exception of one recipient (Bartelloni, et al., 1971). Currently, a similar formalin inactivated vaccine is available under investigational new drug (IND) status for vaccination of at risk laboratory workers and personnel (Hoke, 2005). The poor immunogenicity of the inactivated vaccine however requires three immunizations and annual boosts to be effective (Hoke, 2005; Smith, et al., 1997)

Live-attenuated vaccine candidates generate rapid protection associated with high levels of neutralizing antibody in animal models (Atasheva, et al., 2009; Schoepp, et al., 2002). DNA vaccination is able to completely protect mice against WEE; however, as with the inactive vaccine, three immunizations are required to achieve high levels of protection (Nagata, et al., 2005). A single dose of adenovirus vectored WEE vaccine protects against intranasal challenge of WEE, but use of adenovirus vectors is associated with significant risks (Barabe, et al., 2007; Wu, et al., 2007a). Chimeric alphavirus vaccine candidates combining the non-structural proteins of one alphavirus with the structural proteins of WEE provide protection in mice from IN challenge with WEE. Vaccination studies indicate that high level, long-lasting neutralizing antibody is capable of protecting mice from a variety of routes of WEE infection (Atasheva, et al., 2009).

Early studies focused on antibody and complement. Yoshino, et al. showed both early and late forming antibodies demonstrated enhanced virus neutralizing activity when in the presence of complement (Yoshino, et al., 1971). Jahrling et al. demonstrated that immune elimination from immunized hamsters involved formation of virus/antibody aggregates cleared by the reticuloendothelial system. Virulent strains of WEE were cleared slowly from the circulation of non-immune hamsters, but were rapidly cleared when inoculated into immunized hamsters. Mixtures of virus and specific immune sera and from inoculated animals formed aggregates of virus and antibody. Further studies showing more efficient adsorption of WEE by macrophages in the presence of complement led the group to hypothesize that immune clearance of the virus in the intact hamster involves a complement dependent interaction of virus/antibody complexes with cells with Fc and complement receptors (Jahrling, et al., 1983). Thus, the role of antibody dependent cytotoxicity of infected cells remains unclear based on these early studies. However, antibody is well-established as an important factor in the clearance of virus.

Furth studies utilizing hyperimmune sera clarified the role of antibody production in the periphery. Hyperimmune sera from rabbits or equines was experimentally tested and appeared to be efficacious in certain scenarios, again indicating the importance of a robust antibody response in limiting viral pathologies (De Boer, et al., 1955). Hyperimmune horse sera administered to rhesus monkeys at time of development of symptomatic disease had no effect on disease course following IN infection. However, prophylactic or early (within 24 h) administration provided passive protection, but not sterilizing immunity(Wyckoff & Tesar, 1939). Some mouse monoclonal antibodies were shown some of these antibodies were shown to provide protection from infection following passive transfer of antibody (Long, et al., 2000; Long, et al., 2001). Mice were protected from challenge with WEE when injected with antibodies against E1 and E2 in passive transfer studies (Hunt & Roehrig, 1985; Yamamoto, 1986). Administration of an *E. coli* expressed E2 protein into mice demonstrated that immunization of this structural component of E2 could partially protect mice from lethal challenge with WEE, and was associated with a strong cell mediated immune response (Das, et al., 2007). The E1 protein has also been successfully developed as a vaccine target. Delivery of both E1 and E2 proteins by an adenovirus delivery vector offer complete protection against lethal challenge from WEE. Mice given a single dose of vectored E1 alone were also completely protected (Swayze, et al., 2010). The B-cell antibody mediated response and the T-cell responses are intertwined and quite likely both play significant roles in the mediation of infection. However, their specific place following infection of the CNS remains.

3.5.2.2 Other cell-mediated immune responses

In an early paper published in the late 1980's on the Th immune response, stimulation of both primed T-helper cells and B-cells resulted in a virus specific proliferative responses against the immunizing virus. Proliferating T cells were primarily IL-2 secreting Thy-I positive, Lyt-l positive, Lyt-2 negative, and L3T4 positive. This study indicated a Th1 bias to the immune response as well as suggesting highly specific WEE T-cell epitopes mediated the generation humoral immunity and neutralizing antibody. (Mathews & Roehrig, 1989).

Prophylactic administration of cationic liposome-DNA complexes in CD-1 outbred mice challenged with WEEV-McM by either SC or aerosol routes results in significant protection. Protection is associated with increased serum and brain levels of IFN-gamma, TNF-alpha, and IL-12 as well as increases in MCP-1 and IL-10 in the brain after neuroinvasion. Thus, a strong-non specific activation of the innate immune system with a distinct Th1 bias elicits protection in the absence of pre-exisiting memory response (Logue, et al., 2010). Administration of an E1 adenovirus vectored antibody also induced a strong WEE specific T-cell response associated with increased secretion of IFN-γ (Swayze, et al., 2010). The current literature indicates that a predominate Th1 response characterizes the adaptive immune response; however, much work remains to determine specific phenotypes of T-cell populations and to further corroborate the direct and indirect contributions of both antibody and T-cells.

4. Eastern equine encephalitis

4.1 History and significance

EEE is considers the most severe of the arboviral encephalids in North America with mortality from encephalitis in epidemics ranging from 30-75% (CFSPH, 2008; Zacks & Paessler, 2010). Even in the absence of immediate mortality, CNS infections typically result in death following recovery from acute disease with initial mortality rates of 74% progressing to 90% by 9 years after infection with only 3% recovering completely. Intitial survival following CNS symptoms leaves most patients with disabling sequela and neurological impairment. However, in the absence of neurological symptoms, infections typically resolve within one to two weeks (Morris, 1988).

In the US and Canada, a steady decline in number of cases since 1955 has occurred (Zacks & Paessler, 2010). From 1964 to 2009, an estimated 260 cases of EEE occurred in the United States with an average of four to five cases yearly though the number can vary markedly from year to year. Additionally, only 83 cases were reported from 1998 to 2009 (CDC, 2009a). As with the other encephalids, risk of symptomatic EEE infection with neurological complications is higher in children, particularly infants (<1 year of age), and the elderly (Calisher, 1994; CFSPH, 2008; Zacks & Paessler, 2010). Early reports indicated symptomatic cases are primarily pediatric with a large portion (42%) being younger than one year of age (Feemster, 1938; 1957; Feemster & Haymaker, 1958). However as with WEE, decline in EEE indicative of changes in mosquito control practices and living conditions has altered the phenotype of cases and later reports indicate overall pediatric cases likely account for 20% of reported cases (Deresiewicz, et al., 1997; Przelomski, et al., 1988; Romero & Newland, 2003). However, the presence of both vector and host populations throughout North America indicated that cases of asymptomatic infection may be underreported (Weaver, 2005).

Given the preceding discovery of WEE, EEE likely existed in natural cycles long before its first isolation in 1933 from the brain of an infected equine (Tenbroeck, 1933). Corroborating this, reports of outbreaks of equine disease similar to EEE exist as early as 1831 (Feemster, 1957). The virus was first isolated from human brain tissue in 1938, and since that time has been attributed to epizootics and as a cause of avian disease (Brown, et al., 1993; Webster & Wright, 1938; Zacks & Paessler, 2010). While EEE was suspected to cause epidemic human disease following isolation, an outbreak involving 38 infants, children and adults formally linked EEE to epidemic disease (Farber, 1940; Feemster & Haymaker, 1958).

4.2 Transmission cycles and geographic range

The virus is found primarily on the Atlantic seaboard, but infections have been noted in the upper Midwest United States and southeastern Canada (Calisher, 1994). The virus has been isolated from birds and other mammals such as equines, sheep, cattle, and deer as well as mosquitoes throughout these regions (Carman, et al., 1995; Gibbs, 1976; McGee, et al., 1992; Schmitt, et al., 2007). Cotton rats and house sparrows have been proposed as other hosts for the virus (Arrigo, et al., 2010). Annual or recurrence of virus in enzoonotic habitats represents typical transmission with extension to other ranges based on the primary avian host range (Calisher, 1994). Overwintering mechanisms have been poorly studied, but vertical transmission from mosquitoes or, as with WEE, reptiles may explain persistence during the winter months (Cupp, et al., 2004; LeDuc, et al., 1975; Morris & Srihongse, 1978). Alternatively, the virus may be reintroduced annually from passerine birds. Horses and humans, as with WEE, are considered dead end hosts, though equines may act as an amplifying host in regions where they are high concentrations of both equines and mosquitoes(CFSPH, 2008; Zacks & Paessler, 2010). *Cs. melanura* mosquitoes are the accepted primary enzootic vector transmitting EEE between passerine birds, but rarely transmit the virus to equines or humans (Andreadis, et al., 1998). The transmission of EEE to humans and equine occurs via other mosquito populations such as *Coquillettidia, Aedes,* and *Culex* due to their more common feeding on mammals (Andreadis, et al., 1998; Armstrong & Andreadis, ; Moncayo, et al., 2000; Vaidyanathan, et al., 1997).

4.3 Disease manifestations in humans

As with WEE, geographic location is indicative of severity of epidemic disease in humans with southern isolates of disease typically causing mild or subclinical symptoms in humans, though outbreaks of equine disease are still associated with the South American strains (Causey, 1968). EEE presents as either a systemic or encephalitic syndrome depending on a number of external factors, but age correlates with prevalence and severity of neurological symptoms (Calisher, 1994; Zacks & Paessler, 2010). Infections are characterized by general malaise, fever and chills. Presentation includes headache of increasing severity, irritability, restlessness drowsiness, anorexia,, vomiting, diarrhea, cyanosis, convulsion, and coma. Antibody is present at time of onset of symptomatic illness, but virus can rarely be isolated from blood or cerebral spinal fluid (CSF) at this time point (Hauser, 1948; Steele & Twenhafel, 2010; Zacks & Paessler, 2010). The incubation period is thought to be somewhat more protracted that WEE, but reports vary and range from five to ten days. Typical systemic illness lasts one to two weeks and recovery is typically complete with no CNS involvement (CFSPH, 2008; Zacks & Paessler, 2010). In the 33% of patients exhibiting neurological symptoms, lethality usually occurs between two to ten days after disease presentation (CFSPH, 2008; Steele & Twenhafel, 2010; Zacks & Paessler, 2010).

In infants, EEE typically results in abrupt encephalitic involvement while in older children and adults the disease is manifested after systemic infection that is often subclinical (Calisher, 1994; Farber, 1940; Morse, et al., 1992; Winter, 1956). Paralysis develops during the acute phase of illness with tremors and muscle twitching proceeding to continuous nuchal rigidity. Young children present with edema and increased CSF pressure with enhanced cellular presence of neutrophils. During encephalitis, fever, headache, vomiting, respiratory symptoms, leukocytosis, hematuria, seizures and coma may occur (Calisher, 1994). Cause of death is typically attributed to encephalitis, but some patients evidence myocardial damage and impairment of pulmonary functions, unique to EEE and differentiating pathogenesis from that of WEE or VEE (Deresiewicz, et al., 1997; Gutierrez & Prober, 1998; Lury & Castillo, 2004; Zacks & Paessler, 2010). Magnetic resonance imaging and CT images of infected brains demonstrate early changes in basal ganglia and thalami suggestive of edema, ischemia, and hypoperfusion following early, symptomatic disease (Deresiewicz, et al., 1997; Gutierrez & Prober, 1998; Lury & Castillo, 2004).

Gross pathological examination of organs reveals brain edema with necrosis, facial and generalized edema, vascular congestion and hemorrhage in the brain and visceral organs. Examination of brain lesions reveals neuronal destruction and vasculitis both perivascular and parenchymous at the forebrain, basal ganglia, cortex, midbrain, and brain stem. Neither cerebellum nor spinal cord are greatly involved in infection (Bastian, et al., 1975; Calisher, 1994; Zacks & Paessler, 2010) Histopathological changes are consistent with vasculitis, hemorrhage, and encephalitis and represent the primary manifestations of encephalitis (Deresiewicz, et al., 1997). Virus appears in oligodendroglia though primary tropism is neuronal (Gardner, et al., 2008; Kim, et al., 1985). Virus can also be isolated from other tissues post mortem.

4.4 Disease manifestations in experimental models

EEE causes disease in a number of animals including mice, guinea pigs, hamsters, NHP and some bird species such as chickens (Adams, et al., 2008; Cole & McKinney, 1969; King, 1940; Liu, et al., 1970; Ogata & Byrne, 1961; Olitsky & Cox, 1936; Steele & Twenhafel, 2010;

Wyckoff & Tesar, 1939). Experimental infections of mice, guinea pigs and rhesus monkeys provide the primary understanding of EEE pathogenesis (Hurst, 1934; King, 1938; 1939; Nathanson, et al., 1969; Olitsky & Cox, 1936; Pursell, et al., 1972; Sorrentino, et al., 1968; Wyckoff & Tesar, 1939).

4.4.1 Mouse model

While mice are an accepted model for many alphaviruses infections, they fail to reproduce the vascular component of disease typical for human infections making, in this case, the hamster model more representative to study acute vasculitis and encephalitis for EEE (Zacks & Paessler, 2010). However, multiple studies have been conducting in mice with valuable information on the pathogenesis of EEE derived from these experimental infections. Mice are susceptible to infection with EEE virus by cutaneous, JN, and IC inoculation as well as aerosol administration. Mice infected with the virus reproduce a typical biphasic disease course exemplified by viral replication the peripheral tissues followed by viremia, CNS invasion, and encephalitis. While infected mice exhibit seizures, they do not exhibit paralysis as seen in humans (Gardner, et al., 2008; Steele & Twenhafel, 2010). Interestingly no differences in mortality between 15 or 21 day and 1 year old mice are observed following IN infection with EEE, unlike the age dependent resistance seen in WEE infections. Infection by a more rigorous IC route ablates these differences in mortality(Olitsky, et al., 1936).

EEE causes lethal encephalitis in suckling and adult Swiss albino mice following IC infection and causes a pantropic infection with encephalitis following SC inoculations (Liu, et al., 1970). EEE infected mice develop minimal clinical signs of febrile illness early after peripheral inoculation, but progress directly and rapidly to neurological disease though severity varies by age of animal, route of infection, and strain of virus used . Following footpad inoculation, neuroinvasion results in rapid, efficient replication in the CNS inducing widespread infection, direct cytopathogenicity of neurons, and severe encephalitis. In young mice, abnormal bone formation characterized by loss of osteoblasts, reduced osteoid production and cartilage hypertrophy is a defining feature (Steele & Twenhafel, 2010; Vogel, et al., 2005). By four days PI, the virus presents in neurons and glial cells throughout the brain with the caudate nucleus, thalamus, and pons being the most strongly infected areas. Major histological changes in the brains of mice are associated with rarefaction of neuropil in the gray matter as well as some white matter tracks and mild inflammation characterized by neutrophil and eosinophil like infiltrates. In the periphery, EEE targets fibroblasts, skeletal muscle, and cardiac myocytes, osteoblasts, ovarian stromals cells, keratinocytes, sebaceous gland epithelium, odontoblasts, and ameloblast in the teeth, retinal ganglion in the eyes and a few olfactory neuroepithelial cells (Steele & Twenhafel, 2010; Vogel, et al., 2005). Lymphocyte apoptosis throughout the thymus and secondary lymphoid tissues is widespread, but is likely not associated with active viral replication due to failure to replicate in these cells *in vitro* situations unlike WEE (Gardner, et al., 2008; Steele & Twenhafel, 2010).

Rather than entry through olfactory routes as has been suggested for WEE and VEE, EEE appears to enter the brain directly from the bloodstream based on very rapid onset of disease (24 h PI), widely dispersed infection in the CNS, and absence of pathology in the olfactory neuroepithelium (Vogel, et al., 2005). Aerosol infection of animals indicated that mice infected with EEE show neuronal tropism and brain lesions similar to peripherally infected mice. In these animals, infection is presented at 24 hours as with peripheral infection, but only presented in the olfactory bulbs and evidence of infection of the olfactory neuroepithelium suggesting neuroinvasion via direct infection of the neuroepithelium in contrast to peripherally infected animals (Roy, et al., 2009; Steele & Twenhafel, 2010). Thus, route of infection likely plays a significant role in mechanism of CNS entry.

4.4.2 Hamster and guinea pig models

Like mice, EEE also causes lethal encephalitis in hamsters and guinea pigs (Liu, et al., 1970; Morgan, 1941; Morgan, et al., 1942; Murphy & Whitfield, 1970). Hamsters develop biphasic illness like humans when infected with virulent EEE strains, and have the advantage of reproducing the vascular component of disease not present in mouse models (Dremov, et al., 1978; Paessler, et al., 2004).

Peripheral infection results in an early visceral phase, with accompanying virema, then neuroinvasion, and subsequent death caused by encephalitis within four to six days post infection. Fever, appears within 24 hours and clinical signs of neurological systems namely head pressing, stupor and coma follow. However, unlike in mice targeting of the osteoblasts has not been reports. Virus is cleared from blood and peripheral tissues but not the brain following development of neutralizing antibodies(Paessler, et al., 2004).

As with the mouse model, virus appears to be blood-borne as evidence by first appearance of antigen in the neuronal cells of the basal ganglia and brain stem by two days post-infection (Dremov, et al., 1978). This early infection of periventricular and perivascular neuronal cells in the basal ganglia and hippocampus characterize experimental infection and may be due to the hypothesized blood borne nature of the virus, though data is inconclusive (Paessler, et al., 2004). The virus penetrates the brain rapidly and neuronal phase of disease develops quickly with a disseminated virus infection throughout the brain . Though peripheral organ infection develops with early targets including the heart, liver, lungs, kidneys, lymphoid tissues, and skeletal muscles, viral load in the brain is typically much higher (Dremov, et al., 1978; Paessler, et al., 2004).

Peripherally affected organs may display pathological changes such as congestion and micro-hemorrhages as described in fatal human EEE cases (Dremov, et al., 1978; Paessler, et al., 2004). In animals surviving five days or more, inflammatory pathology in the brain is characterized by infiltrates of macrophages, lymphocytes and neutrophils (Cole & McKinney, 1969; Dremov, et al., 1978). Given the early presence of antigen in the basal nuclei, hippocampus, and brainstem, these areas are more severely affected. However, the cerebral cortex and cerebellum also demonstrate severe pathologies. Histopathological features include destruction, of neurons, inflammatory cell infiltration of the neuropil, gliosis, and microhemorrahages as well as vasculitis (Dremov, et al., 1978; Paessler, et al., 2004).

Guinea pigs infected via aerosol by EEE develop clinical signs within 24 hours (Paessler, et al., 2004; Roy, et al., 2009). Symptomatic disease includes decreased activity, dorsal tremors, and progress to coma and death. Virus infection of the neuroepithelium and appearance of the virus in the olfactory bulbs occurs by 24 h PI, and the virus spreads to the remainder of the brain by four day PI. In the brain, neurons again represent the primary viral target of infection, and brain lesions are typified by neuronal necrosis and the presence of perivascular cuffs and infiltrates in the neuropil of macrophages and neutrophils. Vasculitis is evident in some late stage cases and characterized by fragmentation of the vessel walls, intramural infiltrates of inflammatory cells, and fibrinoid necrosis. No peripheral organs examined had detectable infectious virus, and osteoblasts were only rarely infected again in contrast to mice (King, 1938; Olitsky & Cox, 1936; Roy, et al., 2009; Sorrentino, et al., 1968).

4.4.3 Nonhuman primate model

IC inoculation of non human primates results in lethal illness, but by peripheral routs causes subclinical infection (Steele & Twenhafel, 2010; Wyckoff & Tesar, 1939). In cynomolgus macaques, IN or aerosol infections result in lethal neurologic disease (Holbrook & Gowen, 2008; Reed, et al., 2007). Aerosol infection of older cynomolgus macaques resulted in clinical disease characterized by fever, neurological signs, and death within five to nine days after challenge in 66% of infected animals. Symptomatic animals also displayed elevated white blood cell (WBC) counts and elevated liver enzymes indicative of infection and systemic dysfunction. Viremia levels varied and some animals failed to develop detectable levels. Pathology indicated severe meningoencephalomyelitis with widespread neuronal necrosis and strong signs of inflammation including perivascular cuffs, cellular debris, gliosis, satellitosis, edema, and hemorrhage. Reproduction of the vascular component of disease also occurred with vasculitis affected cerebral blood vessels. Unsurprisingly, EEE antigen was disseminated throughout the brain (Reed, et al., 2007). An early study performed in the 1960's utilized virus isolated from a fatal human case to inoculate the thalamus of rhesus macaques. All animals developed acute encephalitis and were euthanized by four day PI. Histology evidenced severe encephalitis with neuronal necrosis and loss of neurons in the forebrain. Inflammation was mild in comparison to the effects on neuronal cells populations and consisted of leptomeningitis and perivascular cuffs (Nathanson, et al., 1969; Steele & Twenhafel, 2010). Adult marmosets inoculated IN with an attenuated strain of EEE responded with asymptomatic disease following administration, and meningeoencephalitis when inoculated with virulent strain. Again animals did not develop detectable viremia, but signs of perivascular hemorrhage affecting the cerebral cortex were present (Adams, et al., 2008). Owl monkeys are also susceptible to infection (Espinosa, et al., 2009).

4.5 Host response in experimental models

As with the other alphaviruses, the mechanism of host defense against EEE is poorly understood. However, data from experimental models corroborates the importance of type I IFN, but indicates that type II IFN (IFN-γ) is not crucial for protection. Furthermore, mechanisms of attenuation related to the type I IFN response are well understood for EEE and require exploration in the other alphaviruses.

4.5.1 Innate immune response to EEE

The discovery that cellular infection with EEE virus was suppressed in the presence of type I IFN led to a body of research on the effect of IFN on EEE infection and vice-versa (Wagner, 1961). A subsequent study examining the temporal effects of IFN and EEE infection of chick embryo and L-cells at a high multiplicity of infection showed production of high levels of IFN occurring with peak viral production and extensive cytopathogenecity (Wagner, 1963). Corroborating the protective, antiviral effects of type I IFN, studies in murine models determined that mice deficient in type I IFN receptors developed higher viremia and had a more rapid time to death. Additionally, pre-treatment of mice with type I IFN inducer (poly(I-C)) results in dose dependent protection (Aguilar, et al., 2005). Unlike VEE, EEE does not induce high levels of IFN rapidly in the serum of infected CD-1 mice. The ability of EEE to antagonize type I IFN induction is cell-dependent, and the failure of EEE to quickly induce IFN production may be due to its inability to replicate in myeloid lineages (Burke, et al., 2009; Ryman & Klimstra, 2008).

Type I IFN's mode of action was pinpointed as antiviral and the cytokine demonstrated the ability to interfere with synthesis of EEE viral RNA (Armstrong, et al., 1971). Mechanistic studies demonstrated that artificial attenuation of EEE results in a marked increase in sensitivity to type I IFN associated with decreased virulence of the virus (Aguilar, et al., 2005; Brown & Officer, 1975; Brown, et al., 1975; Gardner, et al., 2009; Murphy, 1975; Wagner, 1963). Combined with studies in WEE, this led researchers to hypothesize that differences in disease presentation and incidence in humans between South American and North American isolates could be attributed to IFN sensitivity (Brown & Officer, 1975; Brown, et al., 1975). Indeed, comparison of replication of North American and South American strains in IFN pre-treated Vero cells showed a depressive effect on replication of the South American isolates. However, *in vivo*, no differences in IFN induction were observed (Aguilar, et al., 2005). Identification of an avirulent, IFN type I and II sensitive South American strain capable of replication more efficient than virulent strains in mice brains unlike IFN resistant North American strains, identified both structural and non-structural genes as important to generation of virulence and IFN sensitivity (Aguilar, et al., 2008a; Aguilar, et al., 2008b). More specifically, the C protein is associated with host cell gene shut-off likely resulting in cell toxicity (Aguilar, et al., 2007). Amino acids 55 to 75 were critical to the capsid's ability and associated with viral evasion of the anti-viral type I IFN mechanisms (Aguilar, et al., 2008a; Aguilar, et al., 2008b). In addition to inference with host cell systems, EEE may partially avoid the IFN response due to its failure to replicate in myeloid lineages (Ryman & Klimstra, 2008). Thus, host response and viral susceptibility to the host response appears to be a critical determinants of outcome

Mice with a deficiency in the type II IFN (IFN-γ) receptor demonstrate equivalent levels of viremia and mortality rates to wild type animals indicating that IFN-γ is not crucial to control of murine EEE infection (Aguilar, et al., 2008a; Aguilar, et al., 2008b). Induction and modulation of the innate immune response helps to modulate the adaptive immune response, and may have unexplored downstream effects following infection.

4.5.2 Adaptive immune response to EEE

4.5.2.1 Antibody response

Humans develop neutralizing antibody following infection or vaccination (Eklund, et al., 1951). Horses, chickens, and other avian hosts develop neutralizing antibody as well following infection or vaccination (Barber, et al., 1978; Bedenice, et al., 2009; Calisher, et al., 1986c; Clark, et al., 1987; Cole, et al., 1972; Edelman, et al., 1979; Elvinger, et al., 1996). High levels of neutralizing antibody result in mice vaccinated with EEE virion proteins. Humans develop diagnostically useful IgM levels allowing discrimination of different arbovirus populations for serological determination of infection (Calisher, et al., 1986a; Calisher, et al., 1986b). In humans, virus specific IgM antibodies can develop as early as 24 h following onset of disease and persist for upwards of 3 months. IgG cannot be detected till the middle of the 2nd week of disease (Calisher, et al., 1986b; Calisher, et al., 1986c; Knoroz, et al., 1986). Individuals immunized with investigational inactivated EEE (PE-6) develop high titer neutralizing antibodies against E1 and E2 glycoproteins of the parent strain. However, the neutralizing antibody titers against a related South American strain are minimal for these

epitopes (Strizki & Repik, 1995). Taken together data indicated that humoral viral immunity is highly specific for different EEE strains.
Immunization of guinea pig and hamster models results in protection and vaccination of certain avian populations has been reported to reduce numbers of infected birds (Clark, et al., 1987; Olsen, et al., 1997). Chimeric vaccines of EEE and WEE have also been proposed as have trivalent vaccines utilizing immunogens from all three encephalitic alphaviruses or recombinant genetic systems (Atasheva, et al., 2009; Barber, et al., 1978; Pedersen, 1976; Schoepp, et al., 2002). In murine models with pre-existing immunity generated via vaccination, neutralizing antibody is typically detected ten days following infection (Brown & Officer, 1975; Brown, et al., 1975). Neutralizing antibody also develops in the spinal fluid of rabbits vaccinated with either a live or formalin-inactivated vaccine, and such animals are able to resist vigorous challenge routes by IC injection of active virus. Interestingly, failure to resist CNS infection occurred in animals with detectable levels of neutralizing antibody in the serum, but lacking antibody in the cerebral spinal fluid (Morgan, 1941; Morgan, et al., 1942). Such data indicates the importance of the immune responses in the microenvironment of the CNS and indicate that once virus reaches the CNS peripheral measures of protection may be insufficient to determine prevention of disease.

4.5.2.2 Other cell-mediated immune responses

Early studies in T-cell mediated immunity indicate that T-cells proliferate in a virus-specific manner and are predominately of a Th1 phenotype. (Mathews, et al., 1994). As mentioned previously EEE virus replicates poorly in lymphoid tissues, but preferentially infects osteoblasts in murine models. Compared to VEE, the ability of EEE to infected dendritic cells (DC) or macrophage populations is severely limited. However, both viruses replicate efficiently in other cell populations of mesenchymal lineage. Translation of EEE is inhibited in lymphoid tissues of myeloid lineage, but not other cells. This inhibition was shown to be independent of IFN responses both *in vitro* and *in vivo*. (Gardner, et al., 2008; Gardner, et al., 2009).
EEEV does not replicate well in lymphoid tissues *in vivo* on in *vitro*. Specifically, EEE fails to replicate in either macrophages or dendritic cells (Gardner, et al., 2008). Additionally, replication is restricted in human leukocytes *in vitro* (Levitt, et al., 1979). This corroborates with evidence from mouse models demonstrating the primary site of EEE replication occurs in fibroblasts, skeletal muscle and osteoblasts. Failure to replicate in lymphoid organs may explain the later appearance of EEE symptoms than the WEE or VEE (Gardner, et al., 2008; Vogel, et al., 2005). Thus, the failure of EEE to initiate significant signs of early febrile disease may be due to this primary tropism for the oesteoblast lineage of cells rather than lymphotropic nature of the VEE or WEE virus. In fact, while antigen is noted in the draining lymph node (DLN), serum viremia is low (Vogel, et al., 2005).

5. Venezuelan equine encephalitis

5.1 History and significance

Despite lower mortality rates of VEEV compared to EEEV, of the New World alphaviruses, VEEV is the most important human and equine pathogen due to large epizootic and epidemic outbreaks associated with the virus (Weaver, et al., 2004). Isolated in 1938 from the brain of an infected equine, VEEV was not recognized as a significant cause of illness in man till the 1950's though the virus was isolated from a lethal case of encephalitis in the early 1930s (Beck &

Wyckoff, 1938; Kubes & Rios, 1939b; Saleh, et al., 2009; Sanmartin & Arbelaez, 1965; Sanmartin, et al., 1973). Since that time, the virus has been identified as the causative agent for epizootic outbreaks occurring sporadically at approximately 10 year intervals from time of discovery through the early 1970's. One of the largest outbreaks of VEE originated in South America, spread through Central America, and reached southern Texas in 1971 causing thousands of equine and human cases of disease (Franck & Johnson, 1971; Gibbs, 1976). Circumstantial evidence and isolation of vaccine strain from mosquitoes in Louisiana led to speculation that inoculation of equines with incompletely inactivated live-attenuated vaccine, or the presence of mixed virus populations in vaccine preparations led to the extensive disease spread (Brown, 1993; Pedersen, et al., 1972). However, evidence remains inconclusive. Following this outbreak, epidemics and epizootics ceased only to reappear in the early 1990's. The most recent major outbreak occurred in 1995 in Venezuela and Colombia in which 75,000 to 100,000 human cases were reported (Weaver, et al., 2004).The sporadic nature of these outbreaks is likely related to the viability of virus transmission to equine amplifying hosts. In the presence of sterilizing immunity in survivors of outbreaks or following vaccination, viral spread in amplifying hosts is greatly limited. Thus, the interepoozotic periods can be partially explained by resistance of the amplifying host as can the disappearance of epizootic or epidemic outbreaks following 1972 through effective vaccination campaigns. However, changes in mosquito control programs and alterations in rural and urban living conditions impacting the mosquito vector may also be partially responsible for the long hiatus of epidemic outbreaks though true cause is uncertain(Calisher, 1994; Forrester, et al., 2008; Weaver, et al., 2004).

While the majority of VEE cases from natural disease outbreaks are asymptomatic, approximately 10% of infected individuals develop an apparent infection. Of apparent infections less than 1% are lethal, but 14% develop neurological disease and, in pediatric populations mortality in apparent infections is higher (~4%) (Sanmartin-Barberi, et al., 1954; Sanmartin, et al., 1973; Steele & Twenhafel, 2010). In cases with CNS manifestations, mortality increases to as high as 35% in children and 10% in adults (Bowen & Calisher, 1976; Bowen, et al., 1976; Gibbs, 1976; Steele & Twenhafel, 2010). As with the other encephalitic alphaviruses, the prevalence of severe infections greatly increases at the extremes of the age spectrum with the majority of deaths seen in pediatric patients. Virus is highly infectious via aerosol and the virus has been responsible for numerous laboratory related exposures (CFSPH, 2008; Hanson, et al., 1967; Weaver, et al., 2004).

5.2 Transmission on cycles and geographic range

VEEV circulates in an enzootic cycle between a mosquito vector and vertebrate host, namely rodents and humans. In epidemic or epizootic cycle, the virus transmits between horses, humans and mosquitos (Watts, et al., 1998; Zacks & Paessler, 2010). Typically, multiple mosquito(Weaver, et al., 2004) vectors present during epizootic outbreaks, but, *Ochlerotatus taeniorhynchus*, *Aedes* and *Psorphora*, are believed to be the principal vectors responsible for transmission in this scenario with *Culex (Melanconion)* species believed to transmit the enzootic strains (Weaver, et al., 2004). Domestic goats, sheep, and pigs can be infected, but rarely show disease. Dogs and domestic rabbits are susceptible to infection and develop symptomatic disease though none of these hosts develop high titer viremia. The primary, enzootic host is thought to be rodents such as the cotton rat, but species likely vary based on geographic location (Johnson and Martin 1974; Johnson 1974; Gibbs 1976; Johnson and Varma 1976). Horses act as amplifying hosts generating a very high titer viremia, and are capable of transmitting the virus back to mosquitoe-to-human populations (Gibbs, 1976;

Paessler & Weaver, 2009; Zacks & Paessler, 2010). Long thought to be a dead end host with levels of viremia below the limit able to reinfect mosquito populations, humans may be capable of acting as the primary vertebrate host for some strains of VEEV. Namely, VEEV ID strains circulate in an urban cycle in Peru with transmission occurring in a primary cycle between humans and mosquitoes. Restriction to geographic range is based primarily on habitat of the mosquito vector and primary vertebrate host (Watts, et al., 1998).

5.3 Disease manifestations in humans

Humans present with a spectrum of diseases ranging from inapparent infections to lethal encephalitis. However, human infections are typically mild or asymptomatic, and severe encephalitis is less commonly seen. Fever, headache, convulsions, disorientation, ataxia, and mental depression appear in a subset of symptomatic cases, but primarily in patients under 15 years of age (de la Monte, et al., 1985; Rivas, et al., 1997; Weaver, et al., 1996). In the event neurological symptoms occur and the patient survives, sequelae are common (Weaver, et al., 2004). Virus has been isolated from throat swabs, serum and brains. Most of what is known of onset of disease has been determined based on accidental infection of laboratory workers where incubation period appears to be two to five days followed by sudden appearance of flu like symptoms though reports from natural disease outbreaks vary (CFSPH, 2008; Steele & Twenhafel, 2010). Acute disease typically lasts approximately four to six days. However, the disease can be biphasic with a secondary fever developing four to eight days after onset. During this second phase, neurological symptoms develop, though again a range is present from somnolence and mild confusion to seizures, ataxia, paralysis, and coma (Tsai, 1991). Following recovery from acute disease, patients develop generalized asthenia lasting one to two weeks. CSF protein and liver enzymes are typically elevated with cell counts in the CSF ranging from 12 to 900 WBC/mm^3. An EEG tracing in one patient identified diffuse irregular slowing (Johnson, et al., 1968).

Gross findings in neurological cases include cerebral edema, but gross pathology of infections is poorly described in the literature (de la Monte, et al., 1985; Johnson, et al., 1968; Steele & Twenhafel, 2010). Fatal human cases are histopathologically characterized by edema, congestion, meningitis, and encephalitis in the brain. Vasculitis and hemorrhage are more rarely found (Johnson & Martin, 1974; Paessler & Weaver, 2009; Weaver, et al., 2004). Lymphocytes, mononuclear cells, and neutrophils infiltrate the meninges with cells extending into the Virchow Robins space and neuropil in a subset of cases. In the peripheral organs in the majority of cases, interstitial pneumonia associated with cellular infiltration, alveolar hemorrhage, congestion and edema present in the lung with diffuse hepatocellular degeneration and few infiltrates presenting in the liver (Walton & Grayson, 1988). In lymphoid tissues, lymphocyte degeneration, lymphoid depletion and follicular necrosis are accompanied by infiltrates of neutrophils as well as vasculitis (Steele & Twenhafel, 2010).

5.4 Disease manifestations in experimental models

Mouse and NHP models make the largest contribution to the understanding of VEE pathogenesis. However, hamsters and guinea pigs are also susceptible to infection, and early studies in these models initiated understanding of the host response to infection.

5.4.1 Mouse model

Mice are highly susceptible to VEEV infection (Holbrook & Gowen, 2008; Paessler & Weaver, 2009; Walton & Grayson, 1988; Zacks & Paessler, 2010). The mouse model mimics both human and equine disease with mice developing neurotropic disease characterized by lethal encephalitis and lymphotropism following a biphasic disease course (Gardner, et al., 2008; Gleiser, et al., 1962; Steele, et al., 1998). Following peripheral routes of infection, mice display human like disease with progression from infection of the lymphoid tissue and ultimate destruction of CNS tissues. Clinical symptoms in mice include: lethargy, huddling, dehydration, weight loss, tremors, and paralysis or paresis with a minority of animals developing seizures (Davis, et al., 1994; Grieder, et al., 1995).

The lymphotropic nature of VEE results in severe myeloid depletion in rodents and lymphocyte destruction in lymph nodes and spleen (Davis, et al., 1994; Grieder, et al., 1995; Steele & Twenhafel, 2010; Zacks & Paessler, 2010). Peripheral infection is not present late in disease, but high levels of infectious virus are found in the CNS with death in immunocompetent mice occurring five to seven days after infection (Ludwig, et al., 2001; Vogel, et al., 1996).

Encephalitic pathologies vary based on background of mouse, route of inoculation and strain of virus (Ludwig, et al., 2001; Ryzhikov, et al., 1991; Steele, et al., 1998; Steele, et al., 2006; Stephenson, et al., 1988; Vogel, et al., 1996). Thus, based on study design, encephalitic pathologies range from mild neutrophilic infiltration to neuronal degeneration, necrotizing vascultis and Purkinje cell destruction. Lesions appear that are surrounded by necrotic cellular debris, perivascular cuffs composed of mononuclear cells, rarefaction of the neuropil and infiltration of neutrophils lymphocytes and macrophages. These lesions spread following the virus by an approximately 24 h delay from olfactory bulb to more caudal regions (Jackson, et al., 1991; Jensen & Jackson, 1966; Ludwig, et al., 2001; Ryzhikov, et al., 1991; Steele, et al., 1998; Steele, et al., 2006; Stephenson, et al., 1988; Vogel, et al., 1996). Once in the CNS viral tropism is primarily neuronal though CNS macrophages as well as astrocytes may become infected with VEEV, but do not appear to be a primary target (Jackson & Rossiter, 1997a; Schoneboom, et al., 2000b; Steele, et al., 1998; Steele, et al., 2006). As a result, neuronal damage is extensive and has been ascribed to both necrosis and apoptosis (Jackson & Rossiter, 1997b; Jensen & Jackson, 1966; Schoneboom, et al., 2000b; Schoneboom, et al., 2000d; Steele, et al., 2006). Neuropathology may also be attributed to bystander activation and death as damage to glial cells, lympohcytolysis and astrocytosis are reported in areas where virus is not detected (Davis, et al., 1994; Grieder, et al., 1995; MacDonald & Johnston, 2000b; Schoneboom, et al., 2000a; Schoneboom, et al., 2000c).

Routes of infection mimicking natural, mosquito borne infection utilize SC or footpad inoculation results in infection of DC, the primary cell type for VEE infection, at the site of inoculation. These cells then carry the virus to the DLN where VEE begins replication approximately four hours after infection (Aronson, et al., 2000; Davis, et al., 1994; Grieder, et al., 1997; Grieder, et al., 1995; Grieder & Nguyen, 1996b; MacDonald & Johnston, 2000a). The virus enters the blood stream by 12 hours and reaches high levels of serum viremia followed by infection of other tissues, particularly lymphoid. As such, VEEV presents in the spleen, gut and nasal-associated lymphoid tissues, thymus, bone marrow, and non-draining lymph nodes(Grieder & Nguyen, 1996a; Vogel, et al., 1996). Histological lesions found in peripherally infected animals are both neuronal and non-neuronal (Aronson, et al., 2000; Grieder, et al., 1997; Grieder, et al., 1995; Grieder & Nguyen, 1996a; Steele & Twenhafel, 2010).

Aerosol or IN infection results in a direct infection of the olfactory epithelium (Pratt, et al., 2003; Steele, et al., 1998; Vogel, et al., 1996). Other nasal epithelia tissues (respiratory or squamous) do not appear to become infected (Charles, et al., 1995; Davis, et al., 1995; Griffin, 2007; Pratt, et al., 2003; Steele, et al., 1998). VEEV is proposed to reach the brain via the olfactory nerve, but dental structure involvement has also been proposed (Charles, et al., 1995; Steele, et al., 1998; Steele & Twenhafel, 2010). Direct invasion of the brain via the bloodstream does not seem to be significant in VEE infection. Neuroinvasion results in caudal spread of the virus, and ultimately, overwhelming disseminated brain infection (Julander, et al., 2007; Julander, et al., 2008b). Thus, all routes of infection in mice with virulent forms of the virus result in neuroinvasion. However, infection of the nasal cavity, by either aerosol or IN infection, results in more rapid entry to the CNS depending on strain of virus used.

Strain of mice also is an important determinant of outcome. C3H/HeN and BALB/C mice vaccinated dermally with TC-83, the live attenuated vaccine strain, survive. However, aerosol or IN infection with TC83 results in 90-100% mortality in C3H/HeN animals unlike inbred counterparts BALB/C that respond with no evidence of mortality (Julander, et al., 2007; Julander, et al., 2008c; Steele, et al., 2007; Steele, et al., 1998; Steele, et al., 2006). Similar experiences have shown that route of administration can alter neuroinvasion with nonpathogenic viruses failing to enter the CNS by peripheral routes, but exhibiting the ability to enter the CNS by IC, IN, or aerosol administration. However, neuroinvasion, regardless of route, does not always correlate with mortality and virus strains avirulent in the periphery may remain so once in the CNS (Grieder, et al., 1995; MacDonald & Johnston, 2000a; Steele, et al., 1998; Steele, et al., 2006). This creates an interesting dichotomy between neuroinvasiveness and neurovirulence of the virus and indicates that outcome depends on factors beyond neuroinvasion or viral replication to generate mortality.

5.4.2 Hamster and guinea pig models

In guinea pigs and hamsters, VEEV causes acute, fulminant disease associated with extensive necrosis of lymphoid tissues, and death typically occurs prior to development of CNS disease making these models limited for studies of human infections and encephalitis (Gorelkin & Jahrling, 1975; Jackson, et al., 1991; Jahrling & Scherer, 1973a; Jahrling & Scherer, 1973b; 1973c; Walker, et al., 1976)

5.4.3 Nonhuman primate model

Like the majority of symptomatic human infections, infection in NHP represents an acute biphasic, nonspecific febrile disease with infection of lymphoid organs (Danes, et al., 1973; Gleiser, et al., 1962; Monath, et al., 1974a; Nalca, et al., 2003b; Pratt, et al., 1998; Reed, et al., 2007; Verlinde, 1968; Victor, et al., 1956) . In a comprehensive study with rhesus macaques infected IP, animals developed a transient viremia and biphasic fever, but otherwise displayed no clinical signs of disease with complete resolution of pathologies by five weeks PI. Lymphoid depletion occurred rapidly by two days post-infection with extensive lymphoid necrosis, later followed by lymphoid hyperplasia as the animals recovered from infection. Lesions in the brain characterized by perivascular cuffs associated with lymphocytes and gliosis were also apparent and developed around six days post-infection starting at the olfactory bulb and spread caudally throughout the brain (Danes, et al., 1973; Gleiser, et al., 1961; 1962; Monath, et al., 1974b; Pratt, et al., 1998; Reed, et al., 2007; Verlinde, 1968; Victor, et al., 1956). A range of CNS involvement presents depending on strain of virus utilized and route of inoculation with IN and IC inoculation being particularly severe. In cynomolgus macaques similar findings were reported except in the case of IN or aerosol infection where CNS damage is more severe and, in the case of IC infection, lethal (Danes, et al., 1973; Monath, et al., 1974b; Pratt, et al., 1998; Reed, et al., 2007; Steele & Twenhafel, 2010;

Verlinde, 1968; Victor, et al., 1956). Thus, IN inoculation results in disease ranging from simply clinical signs of encephalitis and subsequent recovery to fulminant lethal encephalitis (Gleiser, et al., 1962; Steele & Twenhafel, 2010).

5.5 Host response in experimental models

Of the three viruses, VEEV has the best characterized animal models, and therefore the most is understood regarding the specific host response to infection. However, significant obstacles due to the high biocontaiment level and the rapid death of the host animal following infection resulted in alternatives to typical infection models. Thus, the majority studies examining host response to VEE has been generated using models of attenuated virus or pre-existing immunity, so to date little is known about the primary host response to virulent infection.

5.5.1 Innate immune response to VEE

Like other alphaviruses, VEEV is highly susceptible to the effects of type I IFN (Jordan, 1973). Attenuation in enzootic strains limits the virus' ability to interfere with type I IFN signaling pathways and partially explains the absence of typical disease symptoms following infection with enzootic strains (Grieder & Vogel, 1999; Jahrling, 1975; Jahrling, et al., 1976; Simmons, et al., 2009; Spotts, et al., 1998; White, et al., 2001). Conversely, epizootic and epidemic strains are able to limit host production of type I IFN through interference with signaling pathways, particularly STAT1 (Simmons, et al., 2009; White, et al., 2001a; Yin, et al., 2009). However, the susceptibility of enzootic and epizootic strains appears to vary significantly based on the virus strain(Anishchenko, et al., 2004). As with EEE, the ability to interfere with host transcription has been ascribed to properties of the capsid protein (Garmashova, et al., 2007a; Garmashova, et al., 2007b). Attenuating mutations in the 5′ untranslated region of the genome are associated with susceptibility of the virus to the effects of type I IFN. Animals genetically modified with deficiencies in type I IFN signaling are highly susceptible to VEE infection and, even attenuated strains are uniformly lethal in these animals(White, et al., 2001). Additionally, artificial induction of type I IFN or prophylactic administration of type I IFN delays or prevents death in animal models (Julander, et al., 2008b). In the case of IN or aerosol infection, the rapid entry of virus to the CNS results in earlier neuroinvasion and may limit or alter the effectiveness of early innate immune mechanisms such as IFN or other as yet other unexplored mechanisms.

Vaccination of immunocompromised mice genetically deficient in the IFN-γ receptor is only partially protective unlike complete protection observed in wild-type counterparts indicating type 2 IFN signaling is not required for complete protection unlike type I IFN signaling (Paessler, et al., 2007).

5.5.2 Adaptive immune response to VEE

5.5.2.1 Antibody response

Current knowledge of the humoral response of the host is largely derived using models of pre-existing immunity (vaccination) or using attenuated strains of the virus. Early work identified high-level neutralizing serum antibody as essential following peripheral infection, and the production of neutralizing antibody is utilized as an endpoint in vaccine studies as well as marking efficacy of the IND vaccine, TC83, to vaccinate at risk laboratory personnel (Alevizatos, et al., 1967; Berge, et al., 1961; Eddy, et al., 1972; Engler, et al., 1992; Feigin, et al.,

1967; Jochim & Barber, 1974; Pittman, et al., 1996; Walton, et al., 1972). However, more recent research efforts indicate that circulating antibody may be irrelevant once virus reaches, invades, and begins replicating in the CNS and the role of antibody produced in the endogenous micro-environment of the CNS has been poorly explored (Paessler, et al., 2007; Yun, et al., 2009). Research from Sindbis models using neuroadapted strains of this particular alphavirus indicate that neutralizing antibody is capable of non-cytolytic clearance of virus from neurons (Burdeinick-Kerr, et al., 2009; Griffin, et al., 1997; Griffin, 2010). Primary tropism of VEE in the periphery is for dendritic cells; however, in the CNS it replicates in neurons where non-cytolytic clearance may be of great importance(MacDonald & Johnston, 2000a; Schoneboom, et al., 1999b).

Monoclonal antibodies against specific surface glycoproteins, particularly E1 and E2, may act as useful therapeutic agents and may provide passive immunity to infected animals (Hart, et al., 2000; Hart, et al., 2001; Hart, et al., 1997; Mathews & Roehrig, 1982; Roehrig, et al., 1988; Roehrig & Mathews, 1985). Alterations in the E2 protein are capable of altering the pathogenesis of the virus and preventing neuroinvasion (Davis, et al., 1995). Since aerosol and IN infection bypasses the need to develop viremia to be neuroinvasive, the IgG peripheral neutralizing antibodies may not afford protection against nasal routes of infection. Studies of the antibody response indicate that not all species are equally protected by the same vaccines and specific IgA production at the nasal mucosal surfaces may play a critical role in prevention from aerosol infection (Hart, et al., 1997). More recent studies indicate that administration of hyperimmune sera is only effective against peripheral infection, and has little effect once virus invades the CNS though transfer is able to prolong survival probably due to depression of peripheral infection (Hart, et al., 1997). However, the role of plasma cells or locally produced antibody in the brain by memory B-cells remains to be determined for this infection (Paessler, et al., 2007; Yun, et al., 2009). Research efforts in the 1970's indicated that Fc-dependent clearance of the virus does not rely on complement (Mathews, et al., 1985). Vaccinated mice with non-functional B-cells (μMT deficient) are highly susceptible to intranasal infection, and when infected with attenuated strains develop persistent viral infection (Brooke, et al., 2010; Paessler, et al., 2007; Yun, et al., 2009).

5.5.2.2 Other cell-mediated immune responses

Recent research indicates that T-cells are crucial in recovery from VEE. Specifically, CD4+ T-cells contribute to resolution of infection. While adoptive transfer of primed CD3+ and CD4+ T-cells generated via vaccination ameliorates encephalitis in vaccinated αβ T-cell receptor deficient animals, CD8+ T-cells fail to generate protection. Vaccination of γδ T-cell receptor deficient animals is partially protective, but animals develop a persistent viral infection to 28 days. Thus, while αβ T-cell subsets appear to be required for protection, γδ T-cells do not and viral persistence in these animals may be an indirect effect of a deficit in T-cell help for B cells in these animals (Paessler, et al., 2007; Yun, et al., 2009). Earlier studies of the immune response to the attenuated, live vaccine strain TC83 identified a Th 1 mediate immune response with local activation of CD4+ and CD8+ T-cells (Bennett, et al., 2000; Jahrling & Stephenson, 1984; Phillpotts, 1999; Phillpotts, et al., 2003; Phillpotts & Wright, 1999). Later data examining transcriptional profiles in the brain and sera corroborate an overwhelming proinflammatory response and support the Th1 bias in response to infection(Davis, et al., 1994; Grieder, et al., 1997; Grieder & Vogel, 1999; Koterski, et al., 2007). These studies indicated that T-cells are critical to the host defense against infection, survival, encephalitis, and the repair of neural damage and homeostasis in the brain(Paessler & Weaver, 2009; Paessler, et al., 2007; Yun, et al., 2009; Zacks & Paessler, 2010). The role of CD8+ T-cells explored previously by Jones et al. and arrived at much the same conclusion that CD8+ T-cells were not cytolytic or immunoprotective in VEE encephalitis (Jones, et al., 2003). However, given the pleiotropic roles of CD8+ T-cells and their significance in other viral infections the elimination of a role in VEE infection is doubtful.

Functional antibody production is not required for recovery from infection with an genetically modified, attenuated VEE virus while T-cells were critical to complete protection and survival of the animals. Persistence, as seen previously in γδ deficient mice, was present in mice deficient in functional B-cell response (μMT knock out) and infection was less controlled in animals depleted of CD3, CD4 or CD8 T-cells with CD4 cells appearing to contribute the most significantly in viral control (Brooke, et al., 2010).

Additionally data indicate that IFN-y secretion from these cell populations contributes to survival. However, their role in primary infection has not been well defined. The ability of animals to sustain high levels of virus in the CNS calls into question the importance of viral replication in host pathogenesis. Vaccinated animals maintain equivalent levels of virus to uninfected counterparts with differential outcome indicated that viral load is not the best discriminator for mortality(Paessler, et al., 2007; Yun, et al., 2009). Additionally, such evidence indicates that the efficacy of antivirals once the virus invades the CNS may be limited and therapeutic efforts may be better focused on limiting or altering the host response to generate a non-pathogenic response. However, further understanding of the host response and pathogenic and protective mechanisms of resolution of infection are integral to effective therapeutics development.

6. References

Adams, A.P., Aronson, J.F., Tardif, S.D., Patterson, J.L., Brasky, K.M., Geiger, R., de la Garza, M., Carrion, R., Jr. & Weaver, S.C. (2008). Common marmosets (Callithrix jacchus) as a nonhuman primate model to assess the virulence of eastern equine encephalitis virus strains. *J Virol*, 82, 18, 9035-9042,

Adler, W.H. & Rabinowitz, S.G. (1973). Host defenses during primary Venezuelan equine encephalomyelitis virus infection in mice. II. In vitro methods for the measurement and qualitation of the immune response. *J Immunol*, 110, 5, 1354-1362,

Aguilar, M.J. (1970). Pathological changes in brain and other target organs of infant and weanling mice after infection with non-neuroadapted Western equine encephalitis virus. *Infect Immun*, 2, 5, 533-542,

Aguilar, P.V., Paessler, S., Carrara, A.-S., Baron, S., Poast, J., Wang, E., Moncayo, A.C., Anishchenko, M., Watts, D., Tesh, R.B. & Weaver, S.C. (2005). Variation in Interferon Sensitivity and Induction among Strains of Eastern Equine Encephalitis Virus. *J. Virol.*, 79, 17, 11300-11310,

Aguilar, P.V., Weaver, S.C. & Basler, C.F. (2007). Capsid protein of eastern equine encephalitis virus inhibits host cell gene expression. *J Virol*, 81, 8, 3866-3876,

Aguilar, P.V., Adams, A.P., Wang, E., Kang, W., Carrara, A.-S., Anishchenko, M., Frolov, I. & Weaver, S.C. (2008a). Structural and Nonstructural Protein Genome Regions of

Eastern Equine Encephalitis Virus Are Determinants of Interferon Sensitivity and Murine Virulence. *J. Virol.*, 82, 10, 4920-4930,

Aguilar, P.V., Leung, L.W., Wang, E., Weaver, S.C. & Basler, C.F. (2008b). A five-amino-acid deletion of the eastern equine encephalitis virus capsid protein attenuates replication in mammalian systems but not in mosquito cells. *J Virol*, 82, 14, 6972-6983,

Alevizatos, A.C., McKinney, R.W. & Feigin, R.D. (1967). Live, attenuated Venezuelan equine encephalomyelitis virus vaccine. I. Clinical effects in man. *Am J Trop Med Hyg*, 16, 6, 762-768,

Anderson, B.A. (1984). Focal neurologic signs in western equine encephalitis. *Can Med Assoc J*, 130, 8, 1019-1021,

Andreadis, T.G., Anderson, J.F. & Tirrell-Peck, S.J. (1998). Multiple isolations of eastern equine encephalitis and highlands J viruses from mosquitoes (Diptera: Culicidae) during a 1996 epizootic in southeastern Connecticut. *J Med Entomol*, 35, 3, 296-302,

Anishchenko, M., Paessler, S., Greene, I.P., Aguilar, P.V., Carrara, A.S. & Weaver, S.C. (2004). Generation and characterization of closely related epizootic and enzootic infectious cDNA clones for studying interferon sensitivity and emergence mechanisms of Venezuelan equine encephalitis virus. *J Virol*, 78, 1, 1-8,

Armstrong, J.A., Freeburg, L.C. & Ho, M. (1971). Effect of interferon on synthesis of Eastern equine encephalitis virus RNA. *Proc Soc Exp Biol Med*, 137, 1, 13-18,

Armstrong, P.M. & Andreadis, T.G. Eastern equine encephalitis virus in mosquitoes and their role as bridge vectors. *Emerg Infect Dis*, 16, 12, 1869-1874,

Aronson, J.F., Grieder, F.B., Davis, N.L., Charles, P.C., Knott, T., Brown, K. & Johnston, R.E. (2000). A single-site mutant and revertants arising in vivo define early steps in the pathogenesis of Venezuelan equine encephalitis virus. *Virology*, 270, 1, 111-123,

Arrigo, N.C., Adams, A.P., Watts, D.M., Newman, P.C. & Weaver, S.C. (2010). Cotton rats and house sparrows as hosts for North and South American strains of eastern equine encephalitis virus. *Emerg Infect Dis*, 16, 9, 1373-1380,

Atasheva, S., Wang, E., Adams, A.P., Plante, K.S., Ni, S., Taylor, K., Miller, M.E., Frolov, I. & Weaver, S.C. (2009). Chimeric alphavirus vaccine candidates protect mice from intranasal challenge with western equine encephalitis virus. *Vaccine*, 27, 32, 4309-4319,

Barabe, N.D., Rayner, G.A., Christopher, M.E., Nagata, L.P. & Wu, J.Q. (2007). Single-dose, fast-acting vaccine candidate against western equine encephalitis virus completely protects mice from intranasal challenge with different strains of the virus. *Vaccine*, 25, 33, 6271-6276,

Barber, T.L., Walton, T.E. & Lewis, K.J. (1978). Efficacy of trivalent inactivated encephalomyelitis virus vaccine in horses. *Am J Vet Res*, 39, 4, 621-625,

Bartelloni, P.J., McKinney, R.W., Calia, F.M., Ramsburg, H.H. & Cole, F.E., Jr. (1971). Inactivated western equine encephalomyelitis vaccine propagated in chick embryo cell culture. Clinical and serological evaluation in man. *Am J Trop Med Hyg*, 20, 1, 146-149,

Bastian, F.O., Wende, R.D., Singer, D.B. & Zeller, R.S. (1975). Eastern equine encephalomyelitis. Histopathologic and ultrastructural changes with isolation of the virus in a human case. *Am J Clin Pathol*, 64, 1, 10-13,

Beck, C.E. & Wyckoff, R.W. (1938). Venezuelan Equine Encephalomyelitis. *Science*, 88, 2292, 530,

Bedenice, D., Bright, A., Pedersen, D.D. & Dibb, J. (2009). Humoral response to an equine encephalitis vaccine in healthy alpacas. *J Am Vet Med Assoc*, 234, 4, 530-534,

Berge, T.O., Banks, I.S. & Tigertt, W.D. (1961). Attenuation of Venezuelan equine encephalomyelitis virus by in vitro cultivation in guinea pig heart cells. *Am. J. Hyg.*, 73, 209,

Bianchi, T.I., Aviles, G., Monath, T.P. & Sabattini, M.S. (1993). Western equine encephalomyelitis: virulence markers and their epidemiologic significance. *Am J Trop Med Hyg*, 49, 3, 322-328,

Bianchi, T.I., Aviles, G. & Sabattini, M.S. (1997). Biological characteristics of an enzootic subtype of western equine encephalomyelitis virus from Argentina. *Acta Virol*, 41, 1, 13-20,

Bowen, G.S. & Calisher, C.H. (1976). Virological and serological studies of Venezuelan equine encephalomyelitis in humans. *J Clin Microbiol*, 4, 1, 22-27,

Bowen, G.S., Fashinell, T.R., Dean, P.B. & Gregg, M.B. (1976). Clinical aspects of human Venezuelan equine encephalitis in Texas. *Bull Pan Am Health Organ*, 10, 1, 46-57,

Brooke, C.B., Deming, D.J., Whitmore, A.C., White, L.J. & Johnston, R.E. (2010). T cells facilitate recovery from Venezuelan equine encephalitis virus-induced encephalomyelitis in the absence of antibody. *J Virol*, 84, 9, 4556-4568,

Brown, A. & Officer, J.E. (1975). An attenuated variant of Eastern encephalitis virus: biological properties and protection induced in mice. *Arch Virol*, 47, 2, 123-138,

Brown, A., Vosdingh, R. & Zebovitz, E. (1975). Attenuation and immunogenicity of ts mutants of Eastern encephalitis virus for mice. *J Gen Virol*, 27, 1, 111-116,

Brown, F. (1993). Review of accidents caused by incomplete inactivation of viruses. *Dev Biol Stand*, 81, 103-107,

Brown, T.P., Roberts, W. & Page, R.K. (1993). Acute hemorrhagic enterocolitis in ratites: isolation of eastern equine encephalomyelitis virus and reproduction of the disease in ostriches and turkey poults. *Avian Dis*, 37, 2, 602-605,

Bruyn, H.B. & Lennette, E.H. (1953). Western equine encephalitis in infants; a report on three cases with sequelae. *Calif Med*, 79, 5, 362-366,

Burdeinick-Kerr, R., Govindarajan, D. & Griffin, D.E. (2009). Noncytolytic clearance of sindbis virus infection from neurons by gamma interferon is dependent on Jak/STAT signaling. *J Virol*, 83, 8, 3429-3435,

Burke, C.W., Gardner, C.L., Steffan, J.J., Ryman, K.D. & Klimstra, W.B. (2009). Characteristics of alpha/beta interferon induction after infection of murine fibroblasts with wild-type and mutant alphaviruses. *Virology*, 395, 1, 121-132,

Burke, D.S., Ramsburg, H.H. & Edelman, R. (1977). Persistence in humans of antibody to subtypes of Venezuelan equine encephalomyelitis (VEE) virus after immunization with attenuated (TC-83) VEE virus vaccine. *J Infect Dis*, 136, 3, 354-359,

Burton, A.N., McLintock, J. & Rempel, J.G. (1966). Western equine encephalitis virus in Saskatchewan garter snakes and leopard frogs. *Science*, 154, 752, 1029-1031,

Calisher, C.H., Monath, T.P., Mitchell, C.J., Sabattini, M.S., Cropp, C.B., Kerschner, J., Hunt, A.R. & Lazuick, J.S. (1985). Arbovirus investigations in Argentina, 1977-1980. III. Identification and characterization of viruses isolated, including new subtypes of western and Venezuelan equine encephalitis viruses and four new bunyaviruses

(Las Maloyas, Resistencia, Barranqueras, and Antequera). *Am J Trop Med Hyg*, 34, 5, 956-965,

Calisher, C.H., Berardi, V.P., Muth, D.J. & Buff, E.E. (1986a). Specificity of immunoglobulin M and G antibody responses in humans infected with eastern and western equine encephalitis viruses: application to rapid serodiagnosis. *J Clin Microbiol*, 23, 2, 369-372,

Calisher, C.H., el-Kafrawi, A.O., Al-Deen Mahmud, M.I., Travassos da Rosa, A.P., Bartz, C.R., Brummer-Korvenkontio, M., Haksohusodo, S. & Suharyono, W. (1986b). Complex-specific immunoglobulin M antibody patterns in humans infected with alphaviruses. *J Clin Microbiol*, 23, 1, 155-159,

Calisher, C.H., Fremount, H.N., Vesely, W.L., el-Kafrawi, A.O. & Mahmud, M.I. (1986c). Relevance of detection of immunoglobulin M antibody response in birds used for arbovirus surveillance. *J Clin Microbiol*, 24, 5, 770-774,

Calisher, C.H. (1994). Medically important arboviruses of the United States and Canada. *Clin Microbiol Rev*, 7, 1, 89-116,

Carman, P.S., Artsob, H., Emery, S., Maxie, M.G., Pooley, D., Barker, I.K., Surgeoner, G.A. & Mahdy, M.S. (1995). Eastern equine encephalitis in a horse from southwestern Ontario. *Can Vet J*, 36, 3, 170-172,

Casals, J., Curnen, E.C. & Thomas, L. (1943). Venezuelan Equine Encephalomyelitis in Man. *J Exp Med*, 77, 6, 521-530,

Castorena, K.M., Peltier, D.C., Peng, W. & Miller, D.J. (2008). Maturation-dependent responses of human neuronal cells to western equine encephalitis virus infection and type I interferons. *Virology*, 372, 1, 208-220,

Causey, O.S., RE, Sutmoller, P; Laemmert, H (1968). Epizootic eastern equine encephalitis in Bragança, Region of Pari, Brazil. *Rev Seri Esp Saiíde Publ*, 12, 39-45,

Charles, P.C., Walters, E., Margolis, F. & Johnston, R.E. (1995). Mechanism of neuroinvasion of Venezuelan equine encephalitis virus in the mouse. *Virology*, 208, 2, 662-671,

Clark, G.G., Crabbs, C.L., Bailey, C.L., Calisher, C.H. & Craig, G.B., Jr. (1986). Identification of Aedes campestris from New Mexico: with notes on the isolation of western equine encephalitis and other arboviruses. *J Am Mosq Control Assoc*, 2, 4, 529-534,

Clark, G.G., Dein, F.J., Crabbs, C.L., Carpenter, J.W. & Watts, D.M. (1987). Antibody response of sandhill and whooping cranes to an eastern equine encephalitis virus vaccine. *J Wildl Dis*, 23, 4, 539-544,

Cohen, R., O'Connor, R.E., Townsend, T.E., Webb, P.A. & McKey, R.W. (1953). Western equine encephalomyelitis; clinical observations in infants and children. *J Pediatr*, 43, 1, 26-34,

Cole, F.E., Jr. & McKinney, R.W. (1969). Use of hamsters of potency assay of Eastern and Western equine encephalitis vaccines. *Appl Microbiol*, 17, 6, 927-928,

Cole, F.E., Jr., Pedersen, C.E., Jr. & Robinson, D.M. (1972). Early protection in hamsters immunized with attenuated Venezuelan equine encephalomyelitis vaccine. *Appl Microbiol*, 24, 4, 604-608,

Copps, S.C. & Giddings, L.E. (1959). Transplacental transmission of western equine encephalitis; report of a case. *Pediatrics*, 24, 1, 31-33,

Cupp, E.W., Zhang, D., Yue, X., Cupp, M.S., Guyer, C., Sprenger, T.R. & Unnasch, T.R. (2004). Identification of reptilian and amphibian blood meals from mosquitoes in an eastern equine encephalomyelitis virus focus in central Alabama. *Am J Trop Med Hyg*, 71, 3, 272-276,

Danes, L., Kufner, J., Hruskova, J. & Rychterova, V. (1973). The role of the olfactory route on infection of the respiratory tract with Venezuelan equine encephalomyelitis virus in normal and operated Macaca rhesus monkeys. I. Results of virological examination. *Acta Virol*, 17, 1, 50-56,

Das, D., Nagata, L.P. & Suresh, M.R. (2007). Immunological evaluation of Escherichia coli expressed E2 protein of Western equine encephalitis virus. *Virus Res*, 128, 1-2, 26-33,

Davis, N.L., Grieder, F.B., Smith, J.F., Greenwald, G.F., Valenski, M.L., Sellon, D.C., Charles, P.C. & Johnston, R.E. (1994). A molecular genetic approach to the study of Venezuelan equine encephalitis virus pathogenesis. *Arch Virol Suppl*, 9, 99-109,

Davis, N.L., Brown, K.W., Greenwald, G.F., Zajac, A.J., Zacny, V.L., Smith, J.F. & Johnston, R.E. (1995). Attenuated mutants of Venezuelan equine encephalitis virus containing lethal mutations in the PE2 cleavage signal combined with a second-site suppressor mutation in E1. *Virology*, 212, 1, 102-110,

De Boer, C.J., Cadilek, A.E. & Walters, S.R. (1955). The use of hyperimmune antiserum concentrates in experimental western equine encephalomyelitis. *J Immunol*, 75, 4, 308-314,

de la Monte, S., Castro, F., Bonilla, N.J., Gaskin de Urdaneta, A. & Hutchins, G.M. (1985). The systemic pathology of Venezuelan equine encephalitis virus infection in humans. *Am J Trop Med Hyg*, 34, 1, 194-202,

Delfraro, A., Burgueno, A., Morel, N., Gonzalez, G., Garcia, A., Morelli, J., Perez, W., Chiparelli, H. & Arbiza, J. (2011). Fatal human case of Western equine encephalitis, Uruguay. *Emerg Infect Dis*, 17, 5, 952-954,

DeMeio, J.L., DeSanctis, A.N. & Thomas, W.J. (1979). Persistence in humans of antibody after immunization with four alphavirus vaccines. *Asian J Infect Dis*, 3, 3, 119-124,

Deresiewicz, R.L., Thaler, S.J., Hsu, L. & Zamani, A.A. (1997). Clinical and neuroradiographic manifestations of eastern equine encephalitis. *N Engl J Med*, 336, 26, 1867-1874,

Dikii, V.V., Petkevich, A.S., Leont'eva, N.A. & Galegov, G.A. (1976). [Effect of rimantadine on the synthesis of virus-specific RNA in the culture of cells infected with Sindbis virus]. *Vopr Med Khim*, 22, 6, 844-848,

Dremov, D.P., Solyanik, R.G., Miryutova, T.L. & Laptakova, L.M. (1978). Attenuated variants of eastern equine encephalomyelitis virus: pathomorphological, immunofluorescence and virological studies of infection in Syrian hamsters. *Acta Virol*, 22, 2, 139-145,

Eddy, G.A., Martin, D.H., Reeves, W.C. & Johnson, K.M. (1972). Field studies of an attenuated Venezuelan equine encephalomyelitis vaccine (strain TC-83). *Infect Immun*, 5, 2, 160-163,

Edelman, R., Ascher, M.S., Oster, C.N., Ramsburg, H.H., Cole, F.E. & Eddy, G.A. (1979). Evaluation in humans of a new, inactivated vaccine for Venezuelan equine encephalitis virus (C-84). *J Infect Dis*, 140, 5, 708-715,

Ehrengruber, M.U., Renggli, M., Raineteau, O., Hennou, S., Vaha-Koskela, M.J., Hinkkanen, A.E. & Lundstrom, K. (2003). Semliki Forest virus A7(74) transduces hippocampal neurons and glial cells in a temperature-dependent dual manner. *J Neurovirol*, 9, 1, 16-28,

Eklund, C.M., Bell, J.F. & Brennan, J.M. (1951). Antibody survey following an outbreak of human and equine disease in the Dominican Republic, caused by the eastern strain of equine encephalomyelitis virus. *Am J Trop Med Hyg*, 31, 3, 312-328,

Elvinger, F., Baldwin, C.A., Liggett, A.D., Tang, K.N. & Dove, C.R. (1996). Protection of pigs by vaccination of pregnant sows against eastern equine encephalomyelitis virus. *Vet Microbiol*, 51, 3-4, 229-239,

Engler, R.J., Mangiafico, J.A., Jahrling, P., Ksiazek, T.G., Pedrotti-Krueger, M. & Peters, C.J. (1992). Venezuelan equine encephalitis-specific immunoglobulin responses: live attenuated TC-83 versus inactivated C-84 vaccine. *J Med Virol*, 38, 4, 305-310,

Espinosa, B.J., Weaver, S.C., Paessler, S., Brining, D., Salazar, M. & Kochel, T. (2009). Susceptibility of the Aotus nancymaae owl monkey to eastern equine encephalitis. *Vaccine*, 27, 11, 1729-1734,

Farber, A.H.C., M.L;Dingle, J.H. (1940). Encephalitis in infants and children caused by the virus of Eastern variety of equine encephalitis

Journal of the American Medical Association, 1725-1731,

Fastier, L.B. (1952). Toxic manifestations in rabbits and mice associated with the virus of Western equine encephalomyelitis. *J Immunol*, 68, 5, 531-541,

Feemster, R.F. (1938). Outbreak of Encephalitis in Man Due to the Eastern Virus of Equine Encephalomyelitis. *Am J Public Health Nations Health*, 28, 12, 1403-1410,

Feemster, R.F. (1957). Equine encephalitis in Massachusetts. *N Engl J Med*, 257, 15, 701-704,

Feemster, R.F. & Haymaker, W. (1958). [Eastern equine encephalitis]. *Neurology*, 8, 11, 882-883,

Feigin, R.D., Jaeger, R.F., McKinney, R.W. & Alevizatos, A.C. (1967). Live, attenuated Venezuelan equine encephalomyelitis virus vaccine. II. Whole-blood amino-acid and fluorescent-antibody studies following immunization. *Am J Trop Med Hyg*, 16, 6, 769-777,

Forrester, N.L., Kenney, J.L., Deardorff, E., Wang, E. & Weaver, S.C. (2008). Western Equine Encephalitis submergence: lack of evidence for a decline in virus virulence. *Virology*, 380, 2, 170-172,

Fothergill, L., Holden, M. & Wyckoff, R. (1939). Western equine encephalomyelitis in a laboratory worker. *JAMA*, 113, 206-207,

Franck, P.T. & Johnson, K.M. (1971). An outbreak of Venezuelan equine encephalomeylitis in Central America. Evidence for exogenous source of a virulent virus subtype. *Am J Epidemiol*, 94, 5, 487-495,

Frolov, I. (2004). Persistent infection and suppression of host response by alphaviruses. *Arch Virol Suppl*, 18, 139-147,

Galligan, C.L., Pennell, L.M., Murooka, T.T., Baig, E., Majchrzak-Kita, B., Rahbar, R. & Fish, E.N. (2010). Interferon-beta is a key regulator of proinflammatory events in experimental autoimmune encephalomyelitis. *Mult Scler*, 16, 12, 1458-1473,

Gardner, C.L., Burke, C.W., Tesfay, M.Z., Glass, P.J., Klimstra, W.B. & Ryman, K.D. (2008). Eastern and Venezuelan equine encephalitis viruses differ in their ability to infect dendritic cells and macrophages: impact of altered cell tropism on pathogenesis. *J Virol*, 82, 21, 10634-10646,

Gardner, C.L., Yin, J., Burke, C.W., Klimstra, W.B. & Ryman, K.D. (2009). Type I interferon induction is correlated with attenuation of a South American eastern equine encephalitis virus strain in mice. *Virology*, 390, 2, 338-347,

Garmashova, N., Atasheva, S., Kang, W., Weaver, S.C., Frolova, E. & Frolov, I. (2007a). Analysis of Venezuelan equine encephalitis virus capsid protein function in the inhibition of cellular transcription. *J Virol*, 81, 24, 13552-13565,

Garmashova, N., Gorchakov, R., Volkova, E., Paessler, S., Frolova, E. & Frolov, I. (2007b). The Old World and New World alphaviruses use different virus-specific proteins for induction of transcriptional shutoff. *J Virol*, 81, 5, 2472-2484,

Gebhardt, L.P., Stanton, G.J., Hill, D.W. & Collett, G.C. (1964). Natural Overwintering Hosts of the Virus of Western Equine Encephalitis. *N Engl J Med*, 271, 172-177,

Gebhardt, L.P., Stanton, G.J. & De St Jeor, S. (1966). Transmission of WEE virus to snakes by infected Culex tarsalis mosquitoes. *Proc Soc Exp Biol Med*, 123, 1, 233-235,

Gibbs, E.P. (1976). Equine viral encephalitis. *Equine Vet J*, 8, 2, 66-71,

Gleiser, C.A., Gochenour, W.S., Jr., Berge, T.O. & Tigertt, W.D. (1961). Studies on the virus of Venezuelan equine encephalomyelitis. I. Modification by cortisone of the response of the central nervous system of Macaca mulatta. *Journal of Immunology*, 87, 504-508,

Gleiser, C.A., Gochenour, W.S., Jr., Berge, T.O. & Tigertt, W.D. (1962). The comparative pathology of experimental Venezuelan equine encephalomyelitis infection in different animal hosts. *Journal of Infectious Disease*, 110, 80-97,

Gold, H. & Hampil, B. (1942). Equine encephalomyelitis in a laboratory technician with recovery. *Annals of Internal Medicine*, 16, 556-569,

Gorelkin, L. & Jahrling, P.B. (1975). Virus-initiated septic shock. Acute death of Venezuelan encephalitis virus-infected hamsters. *Lab Invest*, 32, 1, 78-85,

Grieder, F.B., Davis, N.L., Aronson, J.F., Charles, P.C., Sellon, D.C., Suzuki, K. & Johnston, R.E. (1995). Specific restrictions in the progression of Venezuelan equine encephalitis virus-induced disease resulting from single amino acid changes in the glycoproteins. *Virology*, 206, 2, 994-1006,

Grieder, F.B. & Nguyen, H.T. (1996a). Virulent and attenuated mutant Venezuelan equine encephalitis virus show marked differences in replication in infection in murine macrophages. *Microbial Pathogenesis*, 21, 2, 85-95,

Grieder, F.B. & Nguyen, H.T. (1996b). Virulent and attenuated mutant Venezuelan equine encephalitis virus show marked differences in replication in infection in murine macrophages. *Microb Pathog*, 21, 2, 85-95,

Grieder, F.B., Davis, B.K., Zhou, X.D., Chen, S.J., Finkelman, F.D. & Gause, W.C. (1997). Kinetics of cytokine expression and regulation of host protection following infection with molecularly cloned Venezuelan equine encephalitis virus. *Virology*, 233, 2, 302-312,

Grieder, F.B. & Vogel, S.N. (1999). Role of interferon and interferon regulatory factors in early protection against Venezuelan equine encephalitis virus infection. *Virology*, 257, 1, 106-118,

Griffin, D., Levine, B., Tyor, W., Ubol, S. & Despres, P. (1997). The role of antibody in recovery from alphavirus encephalitis. *Immunological Reviews*, 159, 155-161,

Griffin, D.E. (2007). Alphaviruses, In: *Fields Virology*, D.M.H. Knipe, P., 1023-1054, Wolters Kluwer Health/Lippincott Williams & Wilkins, Philadelphia

Griffin, D.E. (2010). Recovery from viral encephalomyelitis: immune-mediated noncytolytic virus clearance from neurons. *Immunologic Research*, 47, 1-3, 123-133,

Grimley, P.M. & Friedman, R.M. (1970). Arboviral infection of voluntary striated muscles. *J Infect Dis*, 122, 1, 45-52,

Groot, H. The Health and Economic Impact of Venezuelan Equine Encephalitis, *Venezuelan Encephalitis: Proceedings of a Workshop-Symposium on Venezuelan Encephalitis Virus*, Washington, D.C. , 1971

Gutierrez, K.M. & Prober, C.G. (1998). Encephalitis. Identifying the specific cause is key to effective management. *Postgrad Med*, 103, 3, 123-125, 129-130, 140-123,

Hammon, W.M., Reeves, W.C., Brookman, B., Izumi, E.M. & Gjullin, C.M. (1941). Isolation of the Viruses of Western Equine and St. Louis Encephalitis from Culex Tarsalis Mosquitoes. *Science*, 94, 2440, 328-330,

Hammon, W.M., Reeves, W.C. & Gray, M. (1943). Mosquito Vectors and Inapparent Animal Reservoirs of St. Louis and Western Equine Encephalitis Viruses. *Am J Public Health Nations Health*, 33, 3, 201-207,

Hammon, W.M. & Reeves, W.C. (1946). Western Equine Encephalomyelitis Virus in the Blood of Experimentally Inoculated Chickens. *J Exp Med*, 83, 3, 163-173,

Hanson, R.P. (1957). An epizootic of equine encephalomyelitis that occurred in Massachusetts in 1831. *American Journal of Tropical Medicine and Hygiene*, 6, 5, 858-862,

Hanson, R.P., Sulkin, S.E., Beuscher, E.L., Hammon, W.M., McKinney, R.W. & Work, T.H. (1967). Arbovirus infections of laboratory workers. Extent of problem emphasizes the need for more effective measures to reduce hazards. *Science*, 158, 806, 1283-1286,

Hardy, J.L. (1987). The ecology of western equine encephalomyelitis virus in the Central Valley of California, 1945-1985. *Am J Trop Med Hyg*, 37, 3 Suppl, 18S-32S,

Hardy, J.L., Presser, S.B., Chiles, R.E. & Reeves, W.C. (1997). Mouse and baby chicken virulence of enzootic strains of western equine encephalomyelitis virus from California. *Am J Trop Med Hyg*, 57, 2, 240-244,

Hart, M.K., Pratt, W., Panelo, F., Tammariello, R. & Dertzbaugh, M. (1997). Venezuelan equine encephalitis virus vaccines induce mucosal IgA responses and protection from airborne infection in BALB/c, but not C3H/HeN mice. *Vaccine*, 15, 4, 363-369,

Hart, M.K., Caswell-Stephan, K., Bakken, R., Tammariello, R., Pratt, W., Davis, N., Johnston, R.E., Smith, J. & Steele, K. (2000). Improved mucosal protection against Venezuelan equine encephalitis virus is induced by the molecularly defined, live-attenuated V3526 vaccine candidate. *Vaccine*, 18, 26, 3067-3075,

Hart, M.K., Lind, C., Bakken, R., Robertson, M., Tammariello, R. & Ludwig, G.V. (2001). Onset and duration of protective immunity to IA/IB and IE strains of Venezuelan equine encephalitis virus in vaccinated mice. *Vaccine*, 20, 3-4, 616-622,

Hauser, G.H. (1948). Human equine encephalomyelitis, eastern type, in Louisiana. *New Orleans Med Surg J*, 100, 12, 551-558,

Hawley, R.J. & Eitzen, E.M. (2001). Biological weapons: A primer for microbiologists. *Annual Review of Microbiology*, 55, 235,

Hayles, L.B., Saunders, J.R. & Bigland, C.H. (1970). Demonstration of western equine encephalitis virus in mouse brain by immunofluorescence. *Can J Microbiol*, 16, 12, 1167-1169,

Hayles, L.B. (1972). Susceptibility of the Mongolian gerbil (Meriones unguiculatus) to Western equine encephalitis. *Can J Microbiol*, 18, 6, 941-944,

Hayles, L.B., Saunders, J.R. & McLintock, J. (1972). Some aspects of diagnosis of western equine encephalitis in chicks and mice by immunofluorescence. *Can J Comp Med*, 36, 2, 180-182,

Helwig, F. (1940). Western equine encephalomyelitis following accidental inoculation with chick embryo virus. *Journal of the American Medical Association*, 115, 291-292,

Hoke, C.H., Jr. (2005). History of U.S. military contributions to the study of viral encephalitis. *Mil Med*, 170, 4 Suppl, 92-105,

Holbrook, M.R. & Gowen, B.B. (2008). Animal models of highly pathogenic RNA viral infections: encephalitis viruses. *Antiviral Research*, 78, 1, 69-78,

Houston, W.E., Kremer, R.J., Crabbs, C.L. & Spertzel, R.O. (1977). Inactivated Venezuelan equine encephalomyelitis virus vaccine complexed with specific antibody: enhanced primary immune response and altered pattern of antibody class elicited. *J Infect Dis*, 135, 4, 600-610,

Howitt, B. (1938). Recovery of the Virus of Equine Encephalomyelitis from the Brain of a Child. *Science*, 88, 2289, 455-456,

Hunt, A.R. & Roehrig, J.T. (1985). Biochemical and biological characteristics of epitopes on the E1 glycoprotein of western equine encephalitis virus. *Virology*, 142, 2, 334-346,

Hurst, E.W. (1934). The Histology of Equine Encephalomyelitis. *J Exp Med*, 59, 5, 529-542,

Hurst, E.W. (1936). Infection of the rhesus monkey (Macaca mulatta) and the guinea-pig with the virus of equine encephalomyelitis. *The Journal of Pathology and Bacteriology*, 42, 1, 271-302,

Jackson, A.C., SenGupta, S.K. & Smith, J.F. (1991). Pathogenesis of Venezuelan equine encephalitis virus infection in mice and hamsters. *Vet Pathol*, 28, 5, 410-418,

Jackson, A.C. & Rossiter, J.P. (1997a). Apoptotic cell death is an important cause of neuronal injury in experimental Venezuelan equine encephalitis virus infection of mice. *Acta Neuropathol*, 93, 4, 349-353,

Jackson, A.C. & Rossiter, J.P. (1997b). Apoptotic cell death is an important cause of neuronal injury in experimental Venezuelan equine encephalitis virus infection of mice. *Acta Neuropathololologica*, 93, 4, 349-353,

Jahrling, P.B. & Scherer, F. (1973a). Histopathology and distribution of viral antigens in hamsters infected with virulent and benign Venezuelan encephalitis viruses. *Am J Pathol*, 72, 1, 25-38,

Jahrling, P.B. & Scherer, W.F. (1973b). Growth curves and clearance rates of virulent and benign Venezuelan encephalitis viruses in hamsters. *Infect Immun*, 8, 3, 456-462,

Jahrling, P.B. & Scherer, W.F. (1973c). Homegeneity of Venezuelan encephalitis virion populations of hamster-virulent and benign strains, including the attenuated TC83 vaccine. *Infect Immun*, 7, 6, 905-910,

Jahrling, P.B. (1975). Interference Between Virulent and Vaccine Strains of Venezuelan Encephalitis Virus in Mixed Infections of Hamsters. *J Gen Virol*, 28, 1, 1-8,

Jahrling, P.B., Navarro, E. & Scherer, W.F. (1976). Interferon induction and sensitivity as correlates to virulence of Venezuelan encephalitis viruses for hamsters. *Arch. Virol.*, 51, 23,

Jahrling, P.B., Hesse, R.A., Anderson, A.O. & Gangemi, J.D. (1983). Opsonization of alphaviruses in hamsters. *J Med Virol*, 12, 1, 1-16,

Jensen, M.M. & Jackson, N.L. (1966). Influence of urine on viruses. *Journal of Urology*, 95, 1, 87-89,

Jochim, M.M. & Barber, T.L. (1974). Immune response of horses after simultaneous or sequential vaccination against eastern, western, and Venezuelan equine encephalomyelitis. *J Am Vet Med Assoc*, 165, 7, 621-625,

Johnson, K.M., Shelokov, A., Peralta, P.H., Dammin, G.J. & Young, N.A. (1968). Recovery of Venezuelan equine encephalomyelitis virus in Panama. A fatal case in man. *Am J Trop Med Hyg*, 17, 3, 432-440,

Johnson, K.M. & Martin, D.H. (1974). Venezuelan equine encephalitis. *Adv Vet Sci Comp Med*, 18, 0, 79-116,

Johnston, L.J., Halliday, G.M. & King, N.J. (2000). Langerhans cells migrate to local lymph nodes following cutaneous infection with an arbovirus. *J Invest Dermatol*, 114, 3, 560-568,

Jones, L.D., Bennett, A.M., Moss, S.R., Gould, E.A. & Phillpotts, R.J. (2003). Cytotoxic T-cell activity is not detectable in Venezuelan equine encephalitis virus-infected mice. *Virus Res*, 91, 2, 255-259,

Jordan, G.W. (1973). Interferon sensitivity of Venezuelan equine encephalomyelitis virus. *Infection and Immunity*, 7, 6, 911-917,

Julander, J.G., Siddharthan, V., Blatt, L.M., Schafer, K., Sidwell, R.W. & Morrey, J.D. (2007). Effect of exogenous interferon and an interferon inducer on western equine encephalitis virus disease in a hamster model. *Virology*, 360, 2, 454-460,

Julander, J.G., Bowen, R.A., Rao, J.R., Day, C., Shafer, K., Smee, D.F., Morrey, J.D. & Chu, C.K. (2008a). Treatment of Venezuelan equine encephalitis virus infection with (-)-carbodine. *Antiviral Res*, 80, 3, 309-315,

Julander, J.G., Skirpstunas, R., Siddharthan, V., Shafer, K., Hoopes, J.D., Smee, D.F. & Morrey, J.D. (2008b). C3H/HeN mouse model for the evaluation of antiviral agents for the treatment of Venezuelan equine encephalitis virus infection. *Antiviral Res*, 78, 3, 230-241,

Julander, J.G., Skirpstunas, R., Siddharthan, V., Shafer, K., Hoopes, J.D., Smee, D.F. & Morrey, J.D. (2008c). C3H/HeN mouse model for the evaluation of antiviral agents for the treatment of Venezuelan equine encephalitis virus infection. *Antiviral Research*, 78, 3, 230-241,

Kelser, R.A. (1937). Transmission of the Virus of Equine Encephalomyelitis by Aedes Taeniorhynchus. *Science*, 85, 2198, 178,

Kim, J.H., Booss, J., Manuelidis, E.E. & Duncan, C.C. (1985). Human eastern equine encephalitis. Electron microscopic study of a brain biopsy. *Am J Clin Pathol*, 84, 2, 223-227,

King, L.S. (1938). Studies on Eastern Equine Encephalomyelitis : I. Histopathology of the Nervous System in the Guinea Pig. *J Exp Med*, 68, 5, 677-692,

King, L.S. (1939). Studies on Eastern Equine Encephalomyelitis : Ii. Pathogenesis of the Disease in the Guinea Pig. *J Exp Med*, 69, 5, 675-690,

King, L.S. (1940). Studies on Eastern Equine Encephalomyelitis : Iv. Infection in the Mouse with Fresh and Fixed Virus. *J Exp Med*, 71, 1, 95-106,

Kiorpes, A.L. & Yuill, T.M. (1975). Environmental modification of western equine encephalomyelitis infection in the snowshoe hare (Lepus americanus). *Infect Immun*, 11, 5, 986-990,

Knoroz, M., Davydova, A.A., Eremian, L.K. & Barinskii, I.F. (1986). [Virus-specific antibodies in persons inoculated with a bivaccine against eastern and western equine encephalomyelitis]. *Vopr Virusol*, 31, 3, 353-354,

Konopka, J.L., Thompson, J.M., Whitmore, A.C., Webb, D.L. & Johnston, R.E. (2009). Acute infection with venezuelan equine encephalitis virus replicon particles catalyzes a systemic antiviral state and protects from lethal virus challenge. *J Virol*, 83, 23, 12432-12442,

Koterski, J., Twenhafel, N., Porter, A., Reed, D.S., Martino-Catt, S., Sobral, B., Crasta, O., Downey, T. & DaSilva, L. (2007). Gene expression profiling of nonhuman primates exposed to aerosolized Venezuelan equine encephalitis virus. *FEMS Immunol Med Microbiol*, 51, 3, 462-472,

Kubes, V. & Rios, F.A. (1939a). The Causative Agent of Infectious Equine Encephalomyelitis in Venezuela. *Science*, 90, 2323, 20-21,

Kubes, V. & Rios, F.A. (1939b). Equine Encephalomyelitis in Venezuela: Advance Data Concerning the Causative Agent. *Canadian Medical Association Journal*, 3, 2, 43-44,

LeDuc, J.W., Burger, J.F., Eldridge, B.F. & Russell, P.K. (1975). Ecology of Keystone virus, a transovarially maintained arbovirus. *Ann N Y Acad Sci*, 266, 144-151,

Levitt, N.H., Miller, H.V. & Edelman, R. (1979). Interaction of alphaviruses with human peripheral leukocytes: in vitro replication of Venezuelan equine encephalomyelitis virus in monocyte cultures. *Infect Immun*, 24, 3, 642-646,

Liu, C., Voth, D.W., Rodina, P., Shauf, L.R. & Gonzalez, G. (1970). A comparative study of the pathogenesis of western equine and eastern equine encephalomyelitis viral infections in mice by intracerebral and subcutaneous inoculations. *J Infect Dis*, 122, 1, 53-63,

Logue, C.H., Bosio, C.F., Welte, T., Keene, K.M., Ledermann, J.P., Phillips, A., Sheahan, B.J., Pierro, D.J., Marlenee, N., Brault, A.C., Bosio, C.M., Singh, A.J., Powers, A.M. & Olson, K.E. (2009). Virulence variation among isolates of western equine encephalitis virus in an outbred mouse model. *J Gen Virol*, 90, Pt 8, 1848-1858,

Logue, C.H., Phillips, A.T., Mossel, E.C., Ledermann, J.P., Welte, T., Dow, S.W., Olson, K.E. & Powers, A.M. (2010). Treatment with cationic liposome-DNA complexes (CLDCs) protects mice from lethal Western equine encephalitis virus (WEEV) challenge. *Antiviral Research*, 87, 2, 195-203,

London, W.T., Levitt, N.H., Altshuler, G., Curfman, B.L., Kent, S.G., Palmer, A.E., Sever, J.L. & Houff, S.A. (1982). Teratological effects of western equine encephalitis virus on the fetal nervous system of Macaca mulatta. *Teratology*, 25, 1, 71-79,

Long, M.C., Jager, S., Mah, D.C., Jebailey, L., Mah, M.A., Masri, S.A. & Nagata, L.P. (2000). Construction and characterization of a novel recombinant single-chain variable fragment antibody against Western equine encephalitis virus. *Hybridoma*, 19, 1, 1-13,

Long, M.C., Marshall, K.E., Kearney, B.J., Ludwig, G.V., Wong, J.P. & Nagata, L.P. (2001). Pharmacokinetics study of a novel chimeric single-chain variable fragment antibody against western equine encephalitis virus. *Hybridoma*, 20, 1, 1-10,

Ludwig, G.V., Turell, M.J., Vogel, P., Kondig, J.P., Kell, W.K., Smith, J.F. & Pratt, W.D. (2001). Comparative neurovirulence of attenuated and non-attenuated strains of Venezuelan equine encephalitis virus in mice. *The American Journal of Tropical Medicine and Hygiene*, 64, 1-2, 49-55,

Luers, A.J., Adams, S.D., Smalley, J.V. & Campanella, J.J. (2005). A phylogenomic study of the genus Alphavirus employing whole genome comparison. *Comp Funct Genomics*, 6, 4, 217-227,

Lury, K.M. & Castillo, M. (2004). Eastern equine encephalitis: CT and MRI findings in one case. *Emerg Radiol*, 11, 1, 46-48,

MacDonald, G.H. & Johnston, R.E. (2000a). Role of dendritic cell targeting in Venezuelan equine encephalitis virus pathogenesis. *Journal of Virology*, 74, 2, 914-922,

MacDonald, G.H. & Johnston, R.E. (2000b). Role of dendritic cell targeting in Venezuelan equine encephalitis virus pathogenesis. *J Virol*, 74, 2, 914-922,

Mathews, J.H. & Roehrig, J.T. (1982). Determination of the protective epitopes on the glycoproteins of Venezuelan equine encephalomyelitis virus by passive transfer of monoclonal antibodies. *J Immunol*, 129, 6, 2763-2767,

Mathews, J.H., Roehrig, J.T. & Trent, D.W. (1985). Role of complement and the Fc portion of immunoglobulin G in immunity to Venezuelan equine encephalomyelitis virus infection with glycoprotein-specific monoclonal antibodies. *Journal of Virology*, 55, 3, 594-600,

Mathews, J.H. & Roehrig, J.T. (1989). Specificity of the murine T helper cell immune response to various alphaviruses. *J Gen Virol*, 70 (Pt 11), 2877-2886,

Mathews, J.H., Kinney, R.M., Roehrig, J.T., Barrett, A.D. & Trent, D.W. (1994). Murine T-helper cell immune response to recombinant vaccinia-Venezuelan equine encephalitis virus. *Vaccine*, 12, 7, 620-624,

McGee, E.D., Littleton, C.H., Mapp, J.B. & Brown, R.J. (1992). Eastern equine encephalomyelitis in an adult cow. *Vet Pathol*, 29, 4, 361-363,

Meyer, K.F., Haring, C.M. & Howitt, B. (1931). THE ETIOLOGY OF EPIZOOTIC ENCEPHALOMYELITIS OF HORSES IN THE SAN JOAQUIN VALLEY, 1930. *Science*, 74, 1913, 227-228,

Mims, C.A., Murphy, F.A., Taylor, W.P. & Marshall, I.D. (1973). Pathogenesis of Ross River virus infection in mice. I. Ependymal infection, cortical thinning, and hydrocephalus. *J Infect Dis*, 127, 2, 121-128,

Mokhtarian, F., Wesselingh, S.L., Choi, S., Maeda, A., Griffin, D.E., Sobel, R.A. & Grob, D. (1996). Production and role of cytokines in the CNS of mice with acute viral encephalomyelitis. *J Neuroimmunol*, 66, 1-2, 11-22,

Monath, T.P., Calisher, C.H., Davis, M., Bowen, G.S. & White, J. (1974a). Experimental studies of rhesus monkeys infected with epizootic and enzootic subtypes of Venezuelan equine encephalitis virus. *Journal of Infectious Disease*, 129, 2, 194-200,

Monath, T.P., Calisher, C.H., Davis, M., Bowen, G.S. & White, J. (1974b). Experimental studies of rhesus monkeys infected with epizootic and enzootic subtypes of Venezuelan equine encephalitis virus. *J Infect Dis*, 129, 2, 194-200,

Monath, T.P., Kemp, G.E., Cropp, C.B. & Chandler, F.W. (1978). Necrotizing myocarditis in mice infected with Western equine encephalitis virus: Clinical, electrocardiographic, and histopathologic correlations. *J Infect Dis*, 138, 1, 59-66,

Moncayo, A.C., Edman, J.D. & Turell, M.J. (2000). Effect of eastern equine encephalomyelitis virus on the survival of Aedes albopictus, Anopheles quadrimaculatus, and Coquillettidia perturbans (Diptera: Culicidae). *J Med Entomol*, 37, 5, 701-706,

Morgan, I.M. (1941). Influence of Age on Susceptibility and on Immune Response of Mice to Eastern Equine Encephalomyelitis Virus. *J Exp Med*, 74, 2, 115-132,

Morgan, I.M., Schlesinger, R.W. & Olitsky, P.K. (1942). Induced Resistance of the Central Nervous System to Experimental Infection with Equine Encephalomyelitis Virus : I. Neutralizing Antibody in the Central Nervous System in Relation to Cerebral Resistance. *J Exp Med*, 76, 4, 357-369,

Morris, C. (1988). In: *The Arboviruses: Epidemiology and Ecology*, T.P. Monath, 1-20, CRC Press, Boca Raton, FLorida

Morris, C.D. & Srihongse, S. (1978). An evaluation of the hypothesis of transovarial transmission of eastern equine encephalomyelitis virus by Culiseta melanura. *Am J Trop Med Hyg*, 27, 6, 1246-1250,

Morse, R.P., Bennish, M.L. & Darras, B.T. (1992). Eastern equine encephalitis presenting with a focal brain lesion. *Pediatr Neurol*, 8, 6, 473-475,

Murphy, F.A. & Whitfield, S.G. (1970). Eastern equine encephalitis virus infection: electron microscopic studies of mouse central nervous system. *Exp Mol Pathol*, 13, 2, 131-146,

Murphy, F.A. (1975). Cellular resistance to arbovirus infection. *Ann N Y Acad Sci*, 266, 197-203,

Nagata, L.P., Hu, W.G., Masri, S.A., Rayner, G.A., Schmaltz, F.L., Das, D., Wu, J., Long, M.C., Chan, C., Proll, D., Jager, S., Jebailey, L., Suresh, M.R. & Wong, J.P. (2005). Efficacy of DNA vaccination against western equine encephalitis virus infection. *Vaccine*, 23, 17-18, 2280-2283,

Nagata, L.P., Hu, W.G., Parker, M., Chau, D., Rayner, G.A., Schmaltz, F.L. & Wong, J.P. (2006). Infectivity variation and genetic diversity among strains of Western equine encephalitis virus. *J Gen Virol*, 87, Pt 8, 2353-2361,

Nalca, A., Fellows, P.F. & Whitehouse, C.A. (2003a). Vaccines and animal models for arboviral encephalitides. *Antiviral Res*, 60, 3, 153-174,

Nalca, A., Fellows, P.F. & Whitehouse, C.A. (2003b). Vaccines and animal models for arboviral encephalitides. *Antiviral Research*, 60, 3, 153-174,

Nathanson, N., Stolley, P.D. & Boolukos, P.J. (1969). Eastern equine encephalitis. Distribution of central nervous system lesions in man and Rhesus monkey. *J Comp Pathol*, 79, 1, 109-115,

O'Brien, V.A., Meteyer, C.U., Ip, H.S., Long, R.R. & Brown, C.R. Pathology and virus detection in tissues of nestling house sparrows naturally infected with Buggy Creek virus (Togaviridae). *J Wildl Dis*, 46, 1, 23-32,

Ogata, M. & Byrne, R.J. (1961). Relationships between eastern and western equine encephalomyelitis viruses as demonstrated by the hemagglutination-inhibition antibody response of experimentally infected chickens. *Am J Vet Res*, 22, 266-270,

Olitsky, P.K. & Cox, H.R. (1936). Active Immunication of Guinea Pigs with the Virus of Equine Encephalomyelitis : I. Quantitative Experiments with Various Preparations of Active Virus. *J Exp Med*, 63, 3, 311-324,

Olitsky, P.K., Sabin, A.B. & Cox, H.R. (1936). An Acquired Resistance of Growing Animals to Certain Neurotropic Viruses in the Absence of Humoral Antibodies or Previous Exposure to Infection. *J Exp Med*, 64, 5, 723-737,

Olsen, G.H., Turell, M.J. & Pagac, B.B. (1997). Efficacy of eastern equine encephalitis immunization in whooping cranes. *J Wildl Dis*, 33, 2, 312-315,

Paessler, S., Aguilar, P., Anishchenko, M., Wang, H.Q., Aronson, J., Campbell, G., Cararra, A.S. & Weaver, S.C. (2004). The hamster as an animal model for eastern equine encephalitis--and its use in studies of virus entrance into the brain. *Journal of Infectious Disease*, 189, 11, 2072-2076,

Paessler, S., Yun, N.E., Judy, B.M., Dziuba, N., Zacks, M.A., Grund, A.H., Frolov, I., Campbell, G.A., Weaver, S.C. & Estes, D.M. (2007). Alpha-beta T cells provide protection against lethal encephalitis in the murine model of VEEV infection. *Virology*, 367, 2, 307-323,

Paessler, S. & Weaver, S.C. (2009). Vaccines for Venezuelan equine encephalitis. *Vaccine*, 27 Suppl 4, D80-85,

Pedersen, C.E., Jr., Robinson, D.M. & Cole, F.E., Jr. (1972). Isolation of the vaccine strain of Venezuelan equine encephalomyelitis virus from mosquitoes in Louisiana. *Am J Epidemiol*, 95, 5, 490-496,

Pedersen, C.E., Jr. (1976). Preparation and testing of vaccines prepared from the envelopes of Venezuelan, eastern, and western equine encephalomyelitis viruses. *Journal of Clinical Microbiology*, 3, 2, 113-118,

Phillpotts, R.J., Jones, L.D., Lukaszewski, R.A., Lawrie, C. & Brooks, T.J. (2003). Antibody and interleukin-12 treatment in murine models of encephalitogenic flavivirus (St. Louis encephalitis, tick-borne encephalitis) and alphavirus (Venezuelan equine encephalitis) infection. *J Interferon Cytokine Res*, 23, 1, 47-50,

Pittman, P.R., Makuch, R.S., Mangiafico, J.A., Cannon, T.L. & Gibbs, P.H. (1996). Long-term duration of detectable neutralizing antibodies after administration of live-attenuated VEE vaccine and following booster vaccination with inactivated VEE vaccine. *Vaccine*, 14, 337,

Plosker, G.L. (2011). Interferon-beta-1b: a review of its use in multiple sclerosis. *CNS Drugs*, 25, 1, 67-88,

Porterfield, J.S. (1975). The basis of arbovirus classification. *Medical Biology*, 53, 5, 400-405,

Porterfield, J.S. (1986). Comparative and historical aspects of the Togaviridae and Flaviviridae, In: *The Togaviridae and Flaviviridae*, S.S. Schlesinger, M.J., Plenum Press, New York

Pratt, W.D., Gibbs, P., Pitt, M.L. & Schmaljohn, A.L. (1998). Use of telemetry to assess vaccine-induced protection against parenteral and aerosol infections of Venezuelan equine encephalitis virus in non-human primates. *Vaccine*, 16, 9-10, 1056-1064,

Pratt, W.D., Davis, N.L., Johnston, R.E. & Smith, J.F. (2003). Genetically engineered, live attenuated vaccines for Venezuelan equine encephalitis: testing in animal models. *Vaccine*, 21, 25-26, 3854-3862,

Przelomski, M.M., O'Rourke, E., Grady, G.F., Berardi, V.P. & Markley, H.G. (1988). Eastern equine encephalitis in Massachusetts: a report of 16 cases, 1970-1984. *Neurology*, 38, 5, 736-739,

Pursell, A.R., Peckham, J.C., Cole, J.R., Jr., Stewart, W.C. & Mitchell, F.E. (1972). Naturally occurring and artificially induced eastern encephalomyelitis in pigs. *J Am Vet Med Assoc*, 161, 10, 1143-1147,

Reed, D.S., Larsen, T., Sullivan, L.J., Lind, C.M., Lackemeyer, M.G., Pratt, W.D. & Parker, M.D. (2005). Aerosol exposure to western equine encephalitis virus causes fever and encephalitis in cynomolgus macaques. *Journal of Infectious Disease*, 192, 7, 1173-1182,

Reed, D.S., Lackemeyer, M.G., Garza, N.L., Norris, S., Gamble, S., Sullivan, L.J., Lind, C.M. & Raymond, J.L. (2007). Severe encephalitis in cynomolgus macaques exposed to aerosolized Eastern equine encephalitis virus. *J Infect Dis*, 196, 3, 441-450,

Reeves, W.C., Hammon, W.M., Furman, D.P., McClure, H.E. & Brookman, B. (1947). Recovery of Western Equine Encephalomyelitis Virus From Wild Bird Mites (Liponyssus sylviarum) in Kern County, California. *Science*, 105, 2729, 411-412,

Reeves, W.C., Sturgeon, J.M., French, E.M. & Brookman, B. (1954). Transovarian transmission of neutralizing substances to western equine and St. Louis encephalitis viruses by avian hosts. *J Infect Dis*, 95, 2, 168-178,

Reisen, W.K., Lothrop, H.D. & Chiles, R.E. (1998). Ecology of Aedes dorsalis (Diptera: Culicidae) in relation to western equine encephalomyelitis virus in the Coachella Valley of California. *J Med Entomol*, 35, 4, 561-566,

Reisen, W.K., Chiles, R.E., Martinez, V.M., Fang, Y. & Green, E.N. (2004). Encephalitis virus persistence in California birds: experimental infections in mourning doves (Zenaidura macroura). *J Med Entomol*, 41, 3, 462-466,

Reisen, W.M., TP. (1988). Western Equine Encephalomyelitis, In: *The Arboviruses: Epidemiology and Ecology.*, T.P. Monath, 89-137, CRC Press, Boca Raton

Rivas, F., Diaz, L.A., Cardenas, V.M., Daza, E., Bruzon, L., Alcala, A., De la Hoz, O., Caceres, F.M., Aristizabal, G., Martinez, J.W., Revelo, D., De la Hoz, F., Boshell, J., Camacho, T., Calderon, L., Olano, V.A., Villarreal, L.I., Roselli, D., Alvarez, G., Ludwig, G. & Tsai, T. (1997). Epidemic Venezuelan equine encephalitis in La Guajira, Colombia, 1995. *J Infect Dis*, 175, 4, 828-832,

Roehrig, J.T. & Mathews, J.H. (1985). The neutralization site on the E2 glycoprotein of Venezuelan equine encephalomyelitis (TC-83) virus is composed of multiple conformationally stable epitopes. *Virology*, 142, 2, 347-356,

Roehrig, J.T., Hunt, A.R., Kinney, R.M. & Mathews, J.H. (1988). In vitro mechanisms of monoclonal antibody neutralization of alphaviruses. *Virology*, 165, 1, 66-73,

Romero, J.R. & Newland, J.G. (2003). Viral meningitis and encephalitis: traditional and emerging viral agents. *Semin Pediatr Infect Dis*, 14, 2, 72-82,

Romero, J.R. & Newland, J.G. (2006). Diagnosis of viral encephalitides: zoonotic-associated viruses. *Pediatr Infect Dis J*, 25, 8, 741-742,

Roy, C.J., Reed, D.S., Wilhelmsen, C.L., Hartings, J., Norris, S. & Steele, K.E. (2009). Pathogenesis of aerosolized Eastern Equine Encephalitis virus infection in guinea pigs. *Virology*, 6, 170,

Rozdilsky, B., Robertson, H.E. & Chorney, J. (1968). Western encephalitis: report of eight fatal cases. Saskatchewan epidemic, 1965. *Can Med Assoc J*, 98, 2, 79-86,

Ryman, K.D. & Klimstra, W.B. (2008). Host responses to alphavirus infection. *Immunol Rev*, 225, 27-45,

Ryman, K.D.K.W.B. (2008). Host responses to alphavirus infection. *Immunological Reviews*, 225, 1, 27-45,

Ryzhikov, A.B., Tkacheva, N.V., Sergeev, A.N. & Ryabchikova, E.I. (1991). Venezuelan equine encephalitis virus propagation in the olfactory tract of normal and immunized mice. *Journal of Biomedical Science*, 2, 6, 607-614,

Sabattini, M.S., Monath, T.P., Mitchell, C.J., Daffner, J.F., Bowen, G.S., Pauli, R. & Contigiani, M.S. (1985). Arbovirus investigations in Argentina, 1977-1980. I. Historical aspects and description of study sites. *The American Journal of Tropical Medicine and Hygiene*, 34, 5, 937-944,

Saleh, M.C., Tassetto, M., van Rij, R.P., Goic, B., Gausson, V., Berry, B., Jacquier, C., Antoniewski, C. & Andino, R. (2009). Antiviral immunity in Drosophila requires systemic RNA interference spread. *Nature*, 458, 7236, 346-350,

Sanmartin-Barberi, C., Groot, H. & Osorno-Mesa, E. (1954). Human epidemic in Colombia caused by the Venezuelan equine encephalomyelitis virus. *Am J Trop Med Hyg*, 3, 2, 283-293,

Sanmartin, C. & Arbelaez, N. (1965). [Immunity of the population of La Guajira, Colombia, in April 1963, to Venezuelan encephalitis virus]. *Bol Oficina Sanit Panam*, 59, 6, 516-525,

Sanmartin, C., Mackenzie, R.B., Trapido, H., Barreto, P., Mullenax, C.H., Gutierrez, E. & Lesmes, C. (1973). [Venezuelan equine encephalitis in Colombia, 1967]. *Bol Oficina Sanit Panam*, 74, 2, 108-137,

Schmitt, S.M., Cooley, T.M., Fitzgerald, S.D., Bolin, S.R., Lim, A., Schaefer, S.M., Kiupel, M., Maes, R.K., Hogle, S.A. & O'Brien, D.J. (2007). An outbreak of Eastern equine encephalitis virus in free-ranging white-tailed deer in Michigan. *J Wildl Dis*, 43, 4, 635-644,

Schoepp, R.J., Smith, J.F. & Parker, M.D. (2002). Recombinant chimeric western and eastern equine encephalitis viruses as potential vaccine candidates. *Virology*, 302, 2, 299-309,

Schoneboom, B.A., Fultz, M.J., Miller, T.H., McKinney, L.C. & Grieder, F.B. (1999a). Astrocytes as targets for Venezuelan equine encephalitis virus infection. *J Neurovirol*, 5, 4, 342-354,

Schoneboom, B.A., Fultz, M.J., Miller, T.H., McKinney, L.C. & Grieder, F.B. (1999b). Astrocytes as targets for Venezuelan equine encephalitis virus infection. *Journal of Neurovirology*, 5, 4, 342-354,

Schoneboom, B.A., Catlin, K.M., Marty, A.M. & Grieder, F.B. (2000a). Inflammation is a component of neurodegeneration in response to Venezuelan equine encephalitis virus infection in mice. *Journal of Neuroimmunology*, 109, 2, 132-146,

Schoneboom, B.A., Catlin, K.M., Marty, A.M. & Grieder, F.B. (2000b). Inflammation is a component of neurodegeneration in response to Venezuelan equine encephalitis virus infection in mice. *J Neuroimmunol*, 109, 2, 132-146,

Schoneboom, B.A., Lee, J.S. & Grieder, F.B. (2000c). Early expression of IFN-alpha/beta and iNOS in the brains of Venezuelan equine encephalitis virus-infected mice. *Journal of Interferon & Cytokine Research*, 20, 2, 205-215,

Schoneboom, B.A., Lee, J.S. & Grieder, F.B. (2000d). Early expression of IFN-alpha/beta and iNOS in the brains of Venezuelan equine encephalitis virus-infected mice. *J Interferon Cytokine Res*, 20, 2, 205-215,

Shinefield, H.R. & Townsend, T.E. (1953). Transplacental transmission of western equine encephalomyelitis. *J Pediatr*, 43, 1, 21-25,

Simmons, J.D., White, L.J., Morrison, T.E., Montgomery, S.A., Whitmore, A.C., Johnston, R.E. & Heise, M.T. (2009). Venezuelan equine encephalitis virus disrupts STAT1 signaling by distinct mechanisms independent of host shutoff. *Journal of Virology*, 83, 20, 10571-10581,

Smith, R.K., Zunino, L., Webbon, P.M. & Heinegard, D. (1997). The distribution of cartilage oligomeric matrix protein (COMP) in tendon and its variation with tendon site, age and load. *Matrix Biol*, 16, 5, 255-271,

Somekh, E., Glode, M.P., Reiley, T.T. & Tsai, T.F. (1991). Multiple intracranial calcifications after western equine encephalitis. *Pediatr Infect Dis J*, 10, 5, 408-409,

Sorrentino, J.V., Berman, S., Lowenthal, J.P. & Cutchins, E. (1968). The immunologic response of the guinea pig to Eastern equine encephalomyelitis vaccines. *Am J Trop Med Hyg*, 17, 4, 619-624,

Spotts, D.R., Reich, R.M., Kalkhan, M.A., Kinney, R.M. & Roehrig, J.T. (1998). Resistance to alpha/beta interferons correlates with the epizootic and virulence potential of Venezuelan equine encephalitis viruses and is determined by the 5' noncoding region and glycoproteins. *J. Virol.*, 72, 10286,

Steele, K.E., Davis, K.J., Stephan, K., Kell, W., Vogel, P. & Hart, M.K. (1998). Comparative neurovirulence and tissue tropism of wild-type and attenuated strains of Venezuelan equine encephalitis virus administered by aerosol in C3H/HeN and BALB/c mice. *Veterinary Pathology*, 35, 5, 386-397,

Steele, K.E., Seth, P., Catlin-Lebaron, K.M., Schoneboom, B.A., Husain, M.M., Grieder, F. & Maheshwari, R.K. (2006). Tunicamycin enhances neuroinvasion and encephalitis in mice infected with Venezuelan equine encephalitis virus. *Veterinary Pathology*, 43, 6, 904-913,

Steele, K.E., Alves, D.A. & Chapman, J.L. (2007). Challenges in biodefense research and the role of US Army veterinary pathologists. *US Army Med Dep J*, 28-37,

Steele, K.E. & Twenhafel, N.A. (2010). REVIEW PAPER: pathology of animal models of alphavirus encephalitis. *Veterinary Pathology*, 47, 5, 790-805,

Stephenson, E.H., Moeller, R.B., York, C.G. & Young, H.W. (1988). Nose-only versus whole-body aerosol exposure for induction of upper respiratory infections of laboratory mice. *American Industrial Hygiene Association Journal*, 49, 3, 128-135,

Strizki, J.M. & Repik, P.M. (1995). Differential reactivity of immune sera from human vaccinees with field strains of eastern equine encephalitis virus. *Am J Trop Med Hyg*, 53, 5, 564-570,

Sulkin, S.E. (1946). Human encephalitis due to the Western equine encephalomyelitis virus. *Tex State J Med*, 41, 455-458,

Swayze, R.D., Bhogal, H.S., Barabe, N.D., McLaws, L.J. & Wu, J.Q. (2010). Envelope protein E1 as vaccine target for western equine encephalitis virus. *Vaccine*, 29, 4, 813-820,

Tenbroeck, C. & Merrill, M.H. *Proceedings of the Society for Experimental Biology and Medicine*, 1933

Tenbroeck, C., Hurst, E.W. & Traub, E. (1935). Epidemiology of Equine Encephalomyelitis in the Eastern United States. *Journal of Experimental Medicine*, 62, 5, 677-685,

Tenbroeck, C.M., M. H. *Proceedings of the Society for Experimental Biology and Medicine*, 1933

Thomas, L.A. & Eklund, C.M. (1960). Overwintering of western equine encephalomyelitis virus in experimentally infected garter snakes and transmission to mosquitoes. *Proc Soc Exp Biol Med*, 105, 52-55,

Tsai, T.F. (1991). Arboviral infections in the United States. *Infect Dis Clin North Am*, 5, 1, 73-102,

Turell, M.J., Tammariello, R.F. & Spielman, A. (1995). Nonvascular delivery of St. Louis encephalitis and Venezuelan equine encephalitis viruses by infected mosquitoes (Diptera: Culicidae) feeding on a vertebrate host. *J Med Entomol*, 32, 4, 563-568,

Ubico, S.R. & McLean, R.G. (1995). Serologic survey of neotropical bats in Guatemala for virus antibodies. *J Wildl Dis*, 31, 1, 1-9,

Vaidyanathan, R., Edman, J.D., Cooper, L.A. & Scott, T.W. (1997). Vector competence of mosquitoes (Diptera:Culicidae) from Massachusetts for a sympatric isolate of eastern equine encephalomyelitis virus. *J Med Entomol*, 34, 3, 346-352,

Valerol, N., Bonilla, E., Espina, L.M., Maldonado, M., Montero, E., Anez, F., Levy, A., Bermudez, J., Melean, E. & Nery, A. (2008). [Increase of interleukin-1 beta, gamma interferon and tumor necrosis factor alpha in serum and brain of mice infected with the Venezuelan Equine Encephalitis virus]. *Invest Clin*, 49, 4, 457-467,

Verlinde, J.D. (1968). Susceptibility of cynomolgus monkeys to experimental infection with arboviruses of group A (Mayaro and Mucambo), group C (Oriboca and Restan) and an unidentified arbovirus (Kwatta) originating from Surinam. *Trop Geogr Med*, 20, 4, 385-390,

Victor, J., Smith, D.G. & Pollack, A.D. (1956). The comparative pathology of Venezuelan equine encephalomyelitis. *J Infect Dis*, 98, 1, 55-66,

Vogel, P., Abplanalp, D., Kell, W., Ibrahim, M.S., Downs, M.B., Pratt, W.D. & Davis, K.J. (1996). Venezuelan equine encephalitis in BALB/c mice: kinetic analysis of central nervous system infection following aerosol or subcutaneous inoculation. *Archives of Pathology and Laboratory Medicine*, 120, 2, 164-172,

Vogel, P., Kell, W.M., Fritz, D.L., Parker, M.D. & Schoepp, R.J. (2005). Early events in the pathogenesis of eastern equine encephalitis virus in mice. *The American Journal of Pathology*, 166, 1, 159-171,

Wagner, R.R. (1961). Biological studies of interferon. I. Suppression of cellular infection with eastern equine encephalomyelitis virus. *Virology*, 13, 323-337,

Wagner, R.R. (1963). Biological studies of interferon. II. Temporal relationships of virus and interferon production by cells infected with Eastern equine encephalomyelitis and influenza viruses. *Virology*, 19, 215-224,

Walker, D.H., Harrison, A., Murphy, K., Flemister, M. & Murphy, F.A. (1976). Lymphoreticular and myeloid pathogenesis of Venezuelan equine encephalitis in hamsters. *Am J Pathol*, 84, 2, 351-370,

Walton, T.E., Alvarez, O., Jr., Buckwalter, R.M. & Johnson, K.M. (1972). Experimental infection of horses with an attenuated Venezuelan equine encephalomyelitis vaccine (strain TC-83). *Infect Immun*, 5, 5, 750-756,

Watts, D.M. & Williams, J.E. (1972). Experimental infection of bobwhite quail (Colinus virginianus) with western equine encephalitis (WEE) virus. *J Wildl Dis*, 8, 1, 44-48,

Watts, D.M. & Eldridge, B.F. (1975). Transovarial transmission of arboviruses by mosquitoes: a review. *Med Biol*, 53, 5, 271-278,

Watts, D.M., Callahan, J., Rossi, C., Oberste, M.S., Roehrig, J.T., Wooster, M.T., Smith, J.F., Cropp, C.B., Gentrau, E.M., Karabatsos, N., Gubler, D. & Hayes, C.G. (1998). Venezuelan equine encephalitis febrile cases among humans in the Peruvian Amazon River region. *The American Journal of Tropical Medicine and Hygiene*, 58, 1, 35-40,

Weaver, S.C., Salas, R., Rico-Hesse, R., Ludwig, G.V., Oberste, M.S., Boshell, J. & Tesh, R.B. (1996). Re-emergence of epidemic Venezuelan equine encephalomyelitis in South America. VEE Study Group. *Lancet*, 348, 9025, 436-440,

Weaver, S.C., Kang, W., Shirako, Y., Rumenapf, T., Strauss, E.G. & Strauss, J.H. (1997). Recombinational history and molecular evolution of western equine encephalomyelitis complex alphaviruses. *Journal of Virology*, 71, 1, 613-623,

Weaver, S.C. & Barrett, A.D. (2004). Transmission cycles, host range, evolution and emergence of arboviral disease. *Nature Reviews Microbiology*, 2, 10, 789-801,

Weaver, S.C., Ferro, C., Barrera, R., Boshell, J. & Navarro, J. (2004). Venezuelan equine encephalitis. *Annu. Rev. Entomol.*, 49, 141-174,

Weaver, S.C. (2005). Host range, amplification and arboviral disease emergence. *Archives of Virology, Supplement*, 19, 33-44,

Webster, L.T. & Wright, F.H. (1938). Recovery of Eastern Equine Encephalomyelitis Virus from Brain Tissue of Human Cases of Encephalitis in Massachusetts. *Science*, 88, 2283, 305-306,

White, L.J., Wang, J.G., Davis, N.L. & Johnston, R.E. (2001). Role of alpha/beta interferon in Venezuelan equine encephalitis virus pathogenesis: effect of an attenuating mutation in the 5' untranslated region. *J Virol*, 75, 8, 3706-3718,

Williams, J.E., Young, O.P., Watts, D.M. & Reed, T.J. (1971). Wild birds as eastern (EEE) and western (WEE) equine encephalitis sentinels. *J Wildl Dis*, 7, 3, 188-194,

Winter, W.D., Jr. (1956). Eastern equine encephalomyelitis in Massachusetts in 1955; report of two cases in infants. *N Engl J Med*, 255, 6, 262-267,

Wu, J.Q., Barabe, N.D., Chau, D., Wong, C., Rayner, G.R., Hu, W.G. & Nagata, L.P. (2007a). Complete protection of mice against a lethal dose challenge of western equine encephalitis virus after immunization with an adenovirus-vectored vaccine. *Vaccine*, 25, 22, 4368-4375,

Wu, J.Q., Barabe, N.D., Huang, Y.M., Rayner, G.A., Christopher, M.E. & Schmaltz, F.L. (2007b). Pre- and post-exposure protection against Western equine encephalitis virus after single inoculation with adenovirus vector expressing interferon alpha. *Virology*, 369, 1, 206-213,

Wyckoff, R.W. (1939). ENCEPHALOMYELITIS IN MONKEYS. *Science*, 89, 2319, 542-543,

Wyckoff, R.W.G. & Tesar, W.C. (1939). Equine Encephalomyelitis in Monkeys. *The Journal of Immunology*, 37, 4, 329-343,

Yamamoto, K. (1986). Properties of monospecific antibodies to the glycoprotein of western equine encephalitis virus. *Microbiol Immunol*, 30, 4, 343-351,

Yoshino, K., Morishima, T. & Aoki, Y. (1971). Absence of an all-or-none type of complement requirement in early neutralizing antibody against western equine encephalitis virus. *Jpn J Microbiol*, 15, 1, 63-72,

Yuill, T.M. & Hanson, R.P. (1964). Serologic evidence of California encephalitis virus and western equine encephalitis virus in snowshoe hares. *Zoonoses Res*, 3, 3, 153-164,

Yun, N.E., Peng, B.H., Bertke, A.S., Borisevich, V., Smith, J.K., Smith, J.N., Poussard, A.L., Salazar, M., Judy, B.M., Zacks, M.A., Estes, D.M. & Paessler, S. (2009). CD4+ T cells provide protection against acute lethal encephalitis caused by Venezuelan equine encephalitis virus. *Vaccine*, 27, 30, 4064-4073,

Zacks, M.A. & Paessler, S. (2010). Encephalitic alphaviruses. *Vet Microbiol*, 140, 3-4, 281-286,

Zlotnik, I., Peacock, S., Grant, D.P. & Batter-Hatton, D. (1972). The pathogenesis of western equine encephalitis virus (W.E.E.) in adult hamsters with special reference to the long and short term effects on the C.N.S. of the attenuated clone 15 variant. *Br J Exp Pathol*, 53, 1, 59-77,

11

Human Rabies Epidemiology and Diagnosis

Brett W. Petersen and Charles E. Rupprecht
Centers for Disease Control and Prevention, Atlanta, GA USA

1. Introduction

Rabies is a fatal viral infection that is most commonly spread to humans through the bite of an infected animal. The disease is an acute progressive encephalitis caused by highly neurotropic zoonotic viruses belonging to the *Lyssavirus* genus in the *Rhabdoviridae* family (Kuzmin, 2009). Of the twelve species of lyssaviruses, rabies virus (RABV) is the most important with respect to its impact on public health. RABV is distributed globally and found on all continents except Australia and Antarctica. In the United States, multiple RABV variants circulate in wild mammalian reservoir populations including raccoons, skunks, foxes, and bats. Rabies has the highest case fatality rate of any infectious disease and kills an estimated 55,000 people annually, primarily in developing countries within Africa and Asia (Knobel, 2005). However, rabies is a preventable disease. Postexposure prophylaxis (PEP) consisting of rabies immune globulin and rabies vaccine is successful in preventing the disease when administered promptly after an exposure to the virus has occurred. Additionally, vaccination of domestic animals against rabies and stray animal control programs greatly reduce the risk of RABV transmission to humans. Implementation of these measures in developed countries such as the United States has led to drastic declines in the incidence of human rabies. Despite this success, rabies remains a significant public health issue. Each year approximately 7,000 rabid animals are reported in the United States (Blanton, 2010). Up to 35,000 people annually are estimated to receive PEP due to exposures to suspect rabid animals (Christian, 2009). Given the high cost of rabies PEP, this represents a substantial economic burden as well. A clear understanding of the epidemiology of human rabies in the United States can help to manage these human exposures using the best available evidence. In this way, the risk of infection can be assessed more precisely and ensure rabies PEP is administered more judiciously. The identification of epidemiologic patterns can also be used to focus educational messages for human rabies prevention and thereby increase public awareness of rabies and the importance of seeking medical care after a potential exposure occurs. Furthermore, providing accurate descriptions of the clinical presentation of human rabies is essential in recognizing and diagnosing the disease in a timely fashion. Delayed or missed diagnoses place others at risk of exposure if appropriate infection control precautions are not instituted, exposures are not treated appropriately, or organs or tissues from an infected individual are used for transplantation (Houff, 1979; Javadi, 1996; Hellenbrand, 2005; Kusne, 2005; Srinivasan, 2005). An early diagnosis also provides the patient with the opportunity for treatment and possible survival. Insights gained from each attempt at treatment further our understanding of the disease and add to the body of knowledge that can be applied to future cases. When rabies is ruled out, efforts can be focused on identifying more treatable causes of encephalitis. With these goals in mind, this review will describe the epidemiology of human rabies, examine the signs and symptoms of disease, and review the laboratory diagnostic testing and results for all reported human rabies cases in the United States between 1960 and 2010.

2. Methods

2.1 Case definition and data sources

This review includes all cases of human rabies reported to the Centers for Disease Control and Prevention (CDC) that occurred within the United States and its territories between the years 1960–2010. These cases include both indigenous cases occurring in United States nationals as well as imported cases in foreign nationals diagnosed and treated within the United States and it territories. All cases were confirmed using standard diagnostic laboratory tests performed by CDC or by a state laboratory and were reported by health authorities as part of ongoing national surveillance. The clinical and laboratory findings were taken from CDC's Morbidity and Mortality Reports, published journal articles, and unpublished CDC notes. In addition, this review contains clinical data from patients with suspected rabies submitted to the CDC for laboratory diagnostic testing between the years 2007–2010 for whom rabies was subsequently ruled out (non-rabies cases).

2.2 Variable definitions

Onset of illness was defined as either the first day of reported symptoms attributable to rabies or, when this date was unknown, the date when medical care was first sought prior to the confirmation of rabies. Signs and symptoms attributable to rabies included aerophobia, hydrophobia, paresthesia or localized pain, priapism or spontaneous ejaculation, dysphagia, localized weakness, fever, muscle spasm, hypersalivation, anxiety, hallucinations, autonomic instability, agitation or combativeness, nausea or vomiting, ataxia, anorexia, insomnia, seizures, confusion or delirium, malaise or fatigue, and headache. When a bite from a known species, laboratory RABV exposure, or transplantation of infected organs or tissue was reported the species of biting animal or type of exposure and the location of the exposure incident are indicated in the exposure history. Probable exposures where no known bite occurred but physical contact with an animal or close proximity to an animal was reported are also indicated. All other exposures were defined as "unknown." The RABV variant determined by antigenic or molecular typing also provides evidence of the likely source of infection and is particularly useful when no exposure history is known. The type of case was defined as indigenous if the bite incident occurred in the United States or its territories or if the RABV variant identified matched an indigenous source. Imported cases were defined by an exposure occurring outside of the United States or its territories or by identification of a RABV variant not found within the United States. The diagnosis of rabies was considered antemortem when samples were obtained specifically for rabies diagnostic testing before death or when the signs, symptoms, and clinical history were deemed sufficient by the clinicians involved to establish the diagnosis.

2.3 Statistical analysis

Data analyses were performed using SAS version 9.2 (SAS Institute Inc., Cary, North Carolina). Data were summarized using descriptive statistics and comparisons between human rabies cases and cases of encephalopathy with negative rabies diagnostic testing were made using Chi-square or Fisher's exact test. Some variables were dichotomized before statistical comparisons for determination of odds ratios (OR) and 95% confidence intervals (CI). Associations were considered statistically significant at p-values less than 0.05.

2.4 Diagnostic laboratory testing

2.4.1 Detection of antigen

RABV antigens were detected using the direct fluorescent antibody (DFA) test of skin biopsy specimens, touch impressions of corneal epithelial cells, or fresh brain tissue as described (CDC, 2006). Skin biopsy specimens were taken from the nuchal area of the neck where viral antigens can be present in hair follicles containing cutaneous nerves, as described previously (Noah, 1998).

2.4.2 Serology

RABV antibody testing for cases reported before 1973 utilized the mouse neutralization test (Jackson, 2003). After 1973, serology was determined using the rapid fluorescent focus inhibition test (RFFIT) or the indirect fluorescence assay (IFA), as described previously (Noah, 1998). The RFFIT measures RABV neutralizing antibodies while the IFA detects serum reactive with RABV antigen in infected cell cultures. Antibodies in serum were considered diagnostic if there was no history of rabies immunization prior to sample collection. Antibodies in cerebrospinal fluid (CSF) were considered diagnostic regardless of rabies immunization history.

2.4.3 Virus isolation

RABV was isolated through intracerebral inoculation of suckling mice or by addition of suspensions of brain or saliva specimens to cultured mouse neuroblastoma cells, as described previously (Noah, 1998).

2.4.4 RNA detection

Viral nucleic acids were obtained using standard extraction procedures and reagents. Samples used for nucleic acid extraction included saliva, fresh brain, paraffin-embedded brain, and nuchal skin. Reverse transcription polymerase chain reaction (RT-PCR) was performed using primers targeting the sequence of the nucleoprotein gene. Standard dideoxynucleotide sequencing methods were utilized to determine the nucleotide sequences of all PCR products obtained, as described previously (Noah, 1998).

2.4.5 Identification of rabies virus variants

RABV variants were identified through antigenic and/or molecular typing. Antigenic typing uses a reference panel of monoclonal antibodies directed against the nucleoprotein to determine the variant of RABV isolates. Molecular typing methods identify the RABV variant by comparing the nucleotide sequence obtained by RT-PCR with a database of sequences from known reservoirs within the United States as well as foreign countries throughout the world.

Patient	Date of Death	Date of Onset	Age (yrs)	Sex	State / Territory of Death	Exposure History	Variant*	Type	Diagnosis	PEP (n)	Ref.
1	5/21/1960	5/19/1960	9	Male	Georgia	Dog-Georgia	--	Indigenous	Postmortem	--	1
2	8/6/1960	8/1/1960	19	Female	Ohio	Cat-Guatemala	--	Imported	Postmortem	--	2
3	1/6/1961	12/30/1960	53	Female	Kentucky	Fox-Kentucky	--	Indigenous	Postmortem	--	3
4	1/20/1961	1/7/1961	76	Male	California	Dog-California	--	Indigenous	Postmortem	--	4
5	6/26/1961	6/22/1961	74	Male	Kentucky	Fox-Kentucky	--	Indigenous	Postmortem	--	5
6	7/25/1962	7/16/1962	3	Male	Texas	Dog†-Texas	--	Indigenous	Postmortem	--	6
7	10/8/1962	10/1/1962	11	Male	Idaho	Bat†-Idaho	--	Indigenous	Postmortem	--	7
8	9/4/1963	8/29/1963	52	Female	Alabama	Dog†-Alabama	--	Indigenous	Postmortem	--	8
9	9/1/1964	8/24/1964	10	Male	Minnesota	Skunk-Minnesota	--	Indigenous	Postmortem	--	9
10	5/21/1965	5/14/1965	60	Male	West Virginia	Dog-West Virginia	--	Indigenous	Postmortem	--	10
11	9/5/1966	8/27/1966	10	Male	South Dakota	Skunk-South Dakota	--	Indigenous	Postmortem	--	11
12	7/25/1967	7/16/1967	58	Female	New York	Dog-Guinea	--	Imported	Postmortem	--	12
13	7/31/1967	7/21/1967	8	Male	Oregon	Dog-Egypt	--	Imported	Antemortem‡	--	13
14	10/10/1968	8/7/1968	14	Male	Kansas	Dog-Kansas	--	Indigenous	Antemortem	--	14
15	8/29/1969	4/18/1969	2	Male	California	Bobcat-California	--	Indigenous	Antemortem	--	15
16	7/31/1970	7/20/1970	11	Male	Arizona	Skunk-Arizona	--	Indigenous	Postmortem	--	16
17	8/2/1970	7/25/1970	4	Male	South Dakota	Skunk-South Dakota	--	Indigenous	Antemortem‡	--	16
18	Survived	10/30/1970	6	Male	Ohio	Bat-Ohio	--	Indigenous	Antemortem	--	17
19	4/23/1971	3/27/1971	6	Male	California	Dog-Mexico	--	Imported	Antemortem	--	18
20	11/25/1971	11/17/1971	64	Male	New Jersey	Bat-New Jersey	--	Indigenous	Postmortem	--	19
21	2/22/1972	2/9/1972	70	Male	California	Dog-Philippines	--	Imported	Postmortem	8	20
22	3/9/1972	3/1/1972	56	Male	Texas	Lab aerosol-Texas	--	Indigenous	Postmortem	18	21
23	9/22/1973	9/7/1973	26	Male	Kentucky	Bat-Kentucky	--	Indigenous	Antemortem	--	22
24	1/15/1975	1/1/1975	60	Male	Minnesota	Cat-Minnesota	Skunk§	Indigenous	Postmortem	--	23
25	8/2/1975	7/27/1975	51	Male	Puerto Rico	Dog-Puerto Rico	--	Indigenous	Postmortem	--	24
26	8/30/1975	8/11/1975	16	Female	California	Dog-Mexico	--	Imported	Antemortem	--	25
27	6/27/1976	6/4/1976	55	Female	Maryland	Bat-Maryland	Bat§	Indigenous	Antemortem	--	26
28	9/3/1976	8/30/1976	17	Male	Texas	Dog-Mexico	--	Imported	Postmortem	19	27
29	Survived	4/14/1977	32	Male	New York	Lab-NY	--	Indigenous	Antemortem	--	28
30	7/22/1978	7/1/1978	39	Male	Oregon	Unknown	Bat§	Indigenous	Postmortem	--	29

Patient	Date of Death	Date of Onset	Age (yrs)	Sex	State / Territory of Death	Exposure History	Variant*	Type	Diagnosis	PEP (n)	Ref.
31	9/17/1978	9/1/1978	37	Female	Idaho	Transplant-ID	Bat§	Indigenous	Postmortem	--	29
32	6/17/1978	6/13/1978	25	Male	Texas	Unknown	--	Imported	Postmortem	14	30
33	1/4/1979	12/1/1978	50	Male	Pennsylvania	Unknown	--	Indigenous	Postmortem	180	31
34	7/15/1979	6/5/1979	8	Male	Texas	Dog†-Mexico	--	Imported	Antemortem	31	32
35	7/3/1979	6/24/1979	7	Female	Texas	Dog-Texas	Dog§	Indigenous	Antemortem	--	33
36	8/5/1979	7/18/1979	37	Male	California	Dog-Mexico	--	Imported	Postmortem	37	34
37	10/4/1979	9/15/1979	24	Male	Oklahoma	Unknown	Bat§	Indigenous	Antemortem	52	35
38	11/30/1979	11/20/1979	45	Male	Kentucky	Unknown	Bat§	Indigenous	Antemortem	--	36
39	7/4/1981	6/21/1981	27	Male	Oklahoma	Unknown	Skunk§	Indigenous	Postmortem	102	37
40	9/11/1981	8/19/1981	40	Male	Arizona	Dog-Mexico	Dog	Imported	Antemortem	41	38
41	1/28/1983	1/1/1983	30	Male	Massachusetts	Dog-Nigeria	Dog	Imported	Antemortem	28	39
42	3/9/1983	2/5/1983	5	Female	Michigan	Bat†-Michigan	No Isolate	Indigenous	Antemortem	54	40
43	8/8/1984	7/11/1984	12	Female	Texas	Unknown	Dog	Imported	Antemortem	142	41,42
44	9/29/1984	9/14/1984	12	Male	Pennsylvania	Unknown	Bat§	Indigenous	Antemortem	46	43
45	10/1/1984	9/3/1984	72	Female	California	Dog-Guatemala	Dog	Imported	Postmortem	179	44
46	5/20/1985	5/2/1985	19	Male	Texas	Unknown	Dog	Imported	Postmortem	85	45
47	12/15/1987	11/26/1987	13	Male	California	Unknown	Dog	Imported	Postmortem	87	42,46,47
48	2/3/1989	1/17/1989	18	Male	Oregon	Unknown	Dog	Imported	Postmortem	9	42,48
49	6/5/1990	5/30/1990	22	Male	Texas	Bat-Texas	Tb	Indigenous	Antemortem	67	49
50	8/20/1991	8/7/1991	55	Female	Texas	Unknown	Dog	Indigenous	Antemortem	43	50
51	8/25/1991	8/17/1991	29	Male	Arkansas	Bat†-Arkansas	Ln/Ps	Indigenous	Postmortem	99	50
52	10/8/1991	10/2/1991	27	Female	Georgia	Unknown	Ln/Ps	Indigenous	Postmortem	--	50
53	5/8/1992	4/21/1992	11	Male	California	Dog-India	Dog	Imported	Antemortem	17	51
54	7/11/1993	7/5/1993	11	Female	New York	Unknown	Ln/Ps	Indigenous	Postmortem	55	52
55	11/9/1993	11/3/1993	82	Male	Texas	Unknown	Ln/Ps	Indigenous	Antemortem	73	53
56	11/21/1993	11/7/1993	69	Male	California	Dog-Mexico	Dog	Imported	Antemortem	34	53
57	1/18/1994	1/1/1994	44	Male	California	Unknown	Ln/Ps	Indigenous	Postmortem	26	54
58	6/21/1994	6/3/1994	40	Male	Florida	Unknown	Dog	Imported	Postmortem	16	55
59	10/11/1994	9/29/1994	24	Female	Alabama	Bat†-Alabama	Tb	Indigenous	Postmortem	99	56
60	10/15/1994	10/3/1994	41	Male	West Virginia	Bat†-West Virginia	Ln/Ps	Indigenous	Antemortem	48	57
61	11/23/1994	11/8/1994	42	Female	Tennessee	Unknown	Ln/Ps	Indigenous	Antemortem	47	56

Patient	Date of Death	Date of Onset	Age (yrs)	Sex	State / Territory of Death	Exposure History	Variant*	Type	Diagnosis	PEP (n)	Ref.
62	11/27/1994	11/13/1994	14	Male	Texas	Dog†-Texas	Dog	Indigenous	Antemortem	54	56
63	3/15/1995	3/6/1995	4	Female	Washington	Bat†-Washington	Msp	Indigenous	Antemortem	72	58
64	9/21/1995	9/8/1995	27	Male	California	Bat†-California	Tb	Indigenous	Antemortem	12	59
65	10/3/1995	9/18/1995	13	Female	Connecticut	Bat†-Connecticut	Ln/Ps	Indigenous	Antemortem	83	60
66	11/9/1995	10/26/1995	74	Male	California	Bat†-California	Ln/Ps	Indigenous	Postmortem	76	59
67	2/8/1996	12/29/1995	26	Male	Florida	Dog†-Mexico	Dog	Imported	Antemortem	4	61
68	8/20/1996	8/10/1996	32	Female	New Hampshire	Dog-Nepal	Dog	Imported	Antemortem	7	62,63
69	10/15/1996	9/28/1996	42	Female	Kentucky	Unknown	Ln/Ps	Indigenous	Antemortem	87	64
70	12/19/1996	12/4/1996	49	Male	Montana	Unknown	Ln/Ps	Indigenous	Antemortem	26	64
71	1/5/1997	12/20/1996	65	Male	Montana	Bat†-Montana	Ln/Ps	Indigenous	Postmortem	60	65
72	1/18/1997	12/30/1996	64	Male	Washington	Unknown	Ef	Indigenous	Postmortem	55	65
73	10/17/1997	10/3/1997	71	Male	Texas	Bat†-Texas	Ln/Ps	Indigenous	Postmortem	46	66
74	10/23/1998	10/12/1998	32	Male	New Jersey	Bat†-New Jersey	Ln/Ps	Indigenous	Antemortem	50	66
75	12/31/1998	12/14/1998	29	Male	Virginia	Unknown	Ln/Ps	Indigenous	Antemortem	48	67
76	9/20/2000	9/13/2000	49	Male	California	Bat†-California	Tb	Indigenous	Antemortem	37	68
77	10/9/2000	9/26/2000	54	Male	New York	Dog-Ghana	Dog, African	Imported	Antemortem	24	68,69
78	10/10/2000	10/3/2000	26	Male	Georgia	Bat†-Georgia	Tb	Indigenous	Postmortem	71	68
79	10/25/2000	10/8/2000	47	Male	Minnesota	Bat-Minnesota	Ln/Ps	Indigenous	Antemortem	20	68
80	11/1/2000	10/12/2000	69	Male	Wisconsin	Bat†-Wisconsin	Ln/Ps	Indigenous	Postmortem	27	68
81	2/4/2001	1/19/2001	72	Male	California	Unknown	Dog, Philippines	Imported	Postmortem	11	70
82	3/31/2002	3/18/2002	28	Male	California	Bat†-California	Tb	Indigenous	Antemortem	46	71
83	8/31/2002	8/21/2002	13	Male	Tennessee	Bat†-Tennessee	Ln/Ps	Indigenous	Antemortem	23	72
84	9/28/2002	9/16/2002	20	Male	Iowa	Unknown	Ln/Ps	Indigenous	Antemortem	124	73
85	3/10/2003	2/17/2003	25	Male	Virginia	Unknown	Raccoon	Indigenous	Postmortem	8	74
86	6/5/2003	5/28/2003	65	Male	Puerto Rico	Dog-Puerto Rico	Mongoose/ Dog	Indigenous	Postmortem	--	75
87	9/14/2003	8/23/2003	66	Male	California	Bat-California	Ln/Ps	Indigenous	Antemortem	6	76
88	2/15/2004	2/9/2004	41	Male	Florida	Dog-Haiti	Dog, Haiti	Imported	Postmortem	24	77
89	5/4/2004	4/27/2004	20	Male	Arkansas	Bat-Arkansas	Tb	Indigenous	Postmortem	--	78,79

Patient	Date of Death	Date of Onset	Age (yrs)	Sex	State / Territory of Death	Exposure History	Variant*	Type	Diagnosis	PEP (n)	Ref.
90	5/31/2004	5/25/2004	53	Male	Texas	Transplant-Texas	Tb	Indigenous	Postmortem	--	78,79
91	6/9/2004	5/29/2004	50	Female	Texas	Transplant-Texas	Tb	Indigenous	Postmortem	--	78,79
92	6/10/2004	6/2/2004	55	Female	Texas	Tissue Graft-Texas	Tb	Indigenous	Postmortem	--	79
93	6/21/2004	5/31/2004	18	Male	Texas	Transplant-Texas	Tb	Indigenous	Postmortem	--	78,79
94	Survived	10/13/2004	15	Female	Wisconsin	Bat-Wisconsin	No Isolate	Indigenous	Antemortem	37	80,81
95	10/26/2004	10/19/2004	22	Male	California	Unknown	Dog, El Salvador	Imported	Postmortem	39	82
96	9/27/2005	9/11/2005	10	Male	Mississippi	Bat†-Mississippi	No Isolate	Indigenous	Postmortem	32	83
97	5/12/2006	5/4/2006	16	Male	Texas	Bat†-Texas	Tb	Indigenous	Antemortem	53	84,85
98	11/2/2006	9/30/2006	10	Female	Indiana	Bat-Indiana	Ln/Ps	Indigenous	Antemortem	66	86
99	12/13/2006	11/15/2006	11	Male	California	Dog-Philippines	Dog, Philippines	Imported	Antemortem	24	86
100	10/20/2007	9/19/2007	46	Male	Minnesota	Bat-Minnesota	No Isolate	Indigenous	Antemortem	54	87
101	3/18/2008	3/17/2008	16	Male	California	Dog/Fox-Mexico	Tbr Related	Imported	Postmortem	20	88
102	11/30/2008	11/19/2008	55	Male	Missouri	Bat-Missouri	Ln/Ps	Indigenous	Antemortem	5	89
103	Survived	2/25/2009	17	Female	Texas	Bat†-Texas	No Isolate	Indigenous	Antemortem	1	90
104	10/20/2009	10/5/2009	43	Male	Indiana	Unknown	Ln/Ps	Indigenous	Postmortem	20	91
105	11/11/2009	10/20/2009	55	Male	Michigan	Bat†-Michigan	Ln/Ps	Indigenous	Postmortem	17	92
106	11/20/2009	10/23/2009	42	Male	Virginia	Dog-India	Dog, India	Imported	Antemortem	32	93
107	8/21/2010	7/30/2010	19	Male	Louisiana	Bat-Mexico	Ds	Imported	Antemortem	95	94
108	1/8/2011	12/23/2010	70	Male	Wisconsin	Unknown	Ln/Ps	Indigenous	Antemortem	7	95

* Ln/Ps = *Lasionycteris noctivagans* or *Perimyotis subflavus*, the silver-haired bat or the tricolored bat; Msp = *Myotis*, species unknown; Tb = *Tadarida brasiliensis*, the Brazilian (Mexican) free-tailed bat; Ef = *Eptesicus fuscus*, the big brown bat; Ds = *Desmodus rotundus*, the common vampire bat, -- = Not performed or unknown,

† Probable location or source of exposure, ‡ Diagnosis based on signs, symptoms, and clinical history, § RABV variant determined from archived pathological tissue

Table 1. Human Rabies in the United States, 1960–2010

3. Results

A total of 108 cases of human rabies were reported in the United States from 1960 through 2010 (Table 1). One hundred and four cases (96%) died and 4 (4%) survived. Fifty-three cases were diagnosed antemortem while 55 cases were diagnosed postmortem. Fifty-one of the cases diagnosed antemortem had positive laboratory diagnostic test results with the remaining 2 cases diagnosed based on the signs, symptoms, and clinical history alone

3.1 Demographic Information

The median age of patients was 29 years and ranged from 2 to 82 years. Forty cases (37%) were less than 20 years of age and 20 (19%) were 60 years or older. Eighty-three cases (77%) were male and 25 (33%) were female. Cases were reported from 35 states and territories (Figure 1); California and Texas were the only states with more than 5 cases and reported 20 cases (19%) and 19 cases (18%) respectively. Of the states not represented in this series, all had reported a case of human rabies within the last century with the exception of Hawaii, North Dakota, Wyoming and Vermont. Illness onset occurred in all months but was most likely to occur during the fall (August, September, and October) when compared to other seasons (P-value = 0.001). Similarly, definite exposures occurring within the United States were more frequent in fall and summer months though this observation was not statistically significant (P-value = 0.27).

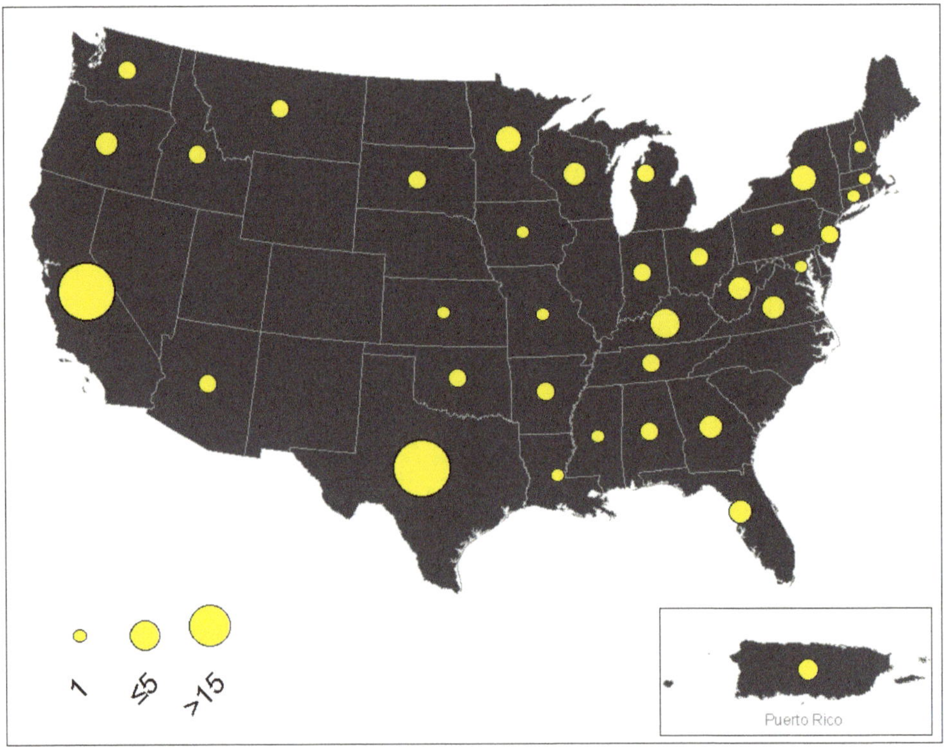

Fig. 1. Geographic Distribution of Human Rabies Cases in the United States, 1960–2010

3.2 Source of infection

The majority of human rabies cases (78/108; 72%) resulted from exposures that occurred within the United States and its territories. However, exposures in 12 foreign countries were responsible for a total of 30 imported cases. Exposures in Mexico were the most common and accounted for 13 imported cases. Animals were linked epidemiologically to 98 cases (91%) either by exposure history or RABV variant typing. Transplantation of infected organs or tissue was responsible for 5 cases (5%) and exposure to a laboratory RABV was implicated in two cases (2%). In 3 cases (3%) there was no history of exposure and no RABV variant identified to suggest a likely source of infection. The animal species linked epidemiologically to human rabies were bats (48/98; 49%), dogs (37/98; 38%), skunks (5/98; 5%), foxes (2/98; 2%), a cat (1/98; 1%), a bobcat (1/98; 1%), and a raccoon (1/98; 1%). The species responsible for infection was unclear in three cases in which the RABV variant identified did not match the exposure history; patient 24 reported a bite from a stray cat while a RABV variant associated with skunks was identified, patient 55 reported contact with a sick cow that later died while a RABV variant associated with bats was identified, and patient 101 had a history of exposure to a dog and a fox while the RABV variant identified was most closely related to viruses found in bats. These appear to have been spillover infection from a primary reservoir species to another animal. In all other cases where an animal exposure was reported the RABV variant identified matched the species of the exposing animal.

3.3 Exposure history

A definite history of exposure to RABV was reported in 54 cases; 47 reported an animal bite, 2 involved exposures to laboratory RABV, and 5 had undergone transplantation of infected organs or tissue. A probable exposure was reported in 26 cases, 21 of which involved a probable exposure to a bat and 5 described a probable exposure to a dog. Of the 28 cases with an unknown exposure, a bat RABV variant was identified in 16 cases, a dog RABV variant was identified in 8 cases, and RABV variants associated with raccoons and skunks were identified in 1 case each. Among the definite exposures involving animal bites, 27 cases were indigenous cases involving bites from 12 bats, 7 dogs, 4 skunks, 2 foxes, 1 cat, and 1 bobcat. Only 2 of the 20 imported cases involved a RABV variant not associated with a domestic animal species. Only 9 animals involved in exposures were available for diagnostic testing, though all tested positive for RABV antigen. With respect to seasonality, rabies cases associated with bats (either by exposure or by identification of a bat RABV variant) were more likely to have onset of illness during the fall when compared to all other cases excluding those acquired through transplantation (OR 3.30; 95% CI 1.45–7.54). Exposures to bats were also more likely to occur during fall months when compared to exposures to other animals (OR 16.50; 95% CI 1.83–148.61).

3.4 Prophylaxis

Sixteen patients received PEP prior to the onset of symptoms. All of these cases occurred prior to 1980 and before the introduction of modern cell culture vaccines. Only two cases completed the PEP regimen according to recommended guidelines and can be considered true failures. The failure of PEP to prevent disease in the remaining 14 patients was attributed to either a delay in administration (i.e. administered greater than 72 hours after exposure), receipt of too few doses of vaccine, or failure to administer rabies immune globulin. Two patients had received rabies vaccine prior to their exposure: patient 22 received four doses of an experimental rabies vaccine 13 years prior to illness onset, however subsequent serologic testing failed to detect antibodies in serum; patient 29 received pre-exposure prophylaxis and regular booster doses with duck embryo vaccine and had a positive RABV antibody titer 6 months before exposure. Patient 22 died of his illness, while patient 29 survived.

3.5 Clinical course

Excluding cases acquired through laboratory exposures and tissue and organ transplantation, specific dates of definite and probable exposures reported for 28 cases were used to calculate a median incubation period of 41.5 days (range 8–701 days). Fifty patients had sought healthcare prior to admission with a median of one day (range 0–6 days) between illness onset and presentation for medical evaluation. Hospital admission dates were reported in 94 cases with a median of 4 days (range 0–16 days) from the onset of illness to hospital admission. Median time from onset of illness to admission to an intensive care unit (ICU) was also 4 days (range 1–13 days) in 14 cases reporting ICU admission date. Similarly, in 65 cases reporting the date of intubation the median time from onset of illness to intubation was 5 days (range 1–19 days). Time from onset of illness to development of fever was reported in 30 cases giving a median of 2 days (range 0–11 days); time from onset of illness to development of coma was reported in 33 cases giving a median of 7 days (range 1–28 days). The median length of illness (defined as days from illness onset until death) was 13.5 days (range 1–133 days).

3.6 Comparison of rabies cases and non-rabies cases

3.6.1 Demographics

Data available from 108 confirmed human rabies cases and 144 encephalitis cases where rabies was ruled out by laboratory diagnostic testing were compared (Table 2). Rabies cases were older on average than non-rabies cases with a mean of 34.4 years (range 2–82 years) versus 30.7 years (range <1–78 years). However, this result was not statistically significant. Male gender was nearly 2 times more likely among rabies cases than non-rabies cases (P-value 0.019).

Variable	Positive, N=108 n (%)	Negative, N=144 n (%)	Odds Ratio (95% CI*)	P-value
Mean age (range)	34.35 (2–82)	30.72 (<1–78)		0.173
Aerophobia	10 (9.3%)	1 (0.7%)	14.59 (1.84–115.83)	0.001†
Hydrophobia	36 (33.3%)	9 (6.3%)	7.50 (3.42–16.43)	<0.001†
Paresthesia or localized pain	54 (50.0%)	21 (14.6%)	5.86 (3.22–10.64)	<0.001†
Priapism or spontaneous ejaculation	4 (3.7%)	2 (1.4%)	2.73 (0.50–15.19)	0.41
Dysphagia	53 (49.1%)	43 (29.9%)	2.26 (1.35–3.80)	0.003†
Localized weakness	44 (40.7%)	34 (23.6%)	2.22 (1.29–3.83)	0.004†
Male gender	83 (76.9%)	87 (62.6%)	1.98 (1.13–3.49)	0.019†
Fever	90 (83.3%)	113 (78.5%)	1.37 (0.72–2.61)	0.422
Muscle spasm	45 (41.7%)	59 (41.0%)	1.03 (0.62–1.71)	1

Variable	Positive, N=108 n (%)	Negative, N=144 n (%)	Odds Ratio (95% CI*)	P-value
Hypersalivation	28 (25.9%)	38 (26.4%)	0.98 (0.55–1.72)	1
Anxiety	33 (30.6%)	51 (35.4%)	0.80 (0.47–1.37)	0.50
Hallucinations	26 (24.1%)	42 (19.2%)	0.77 (0.44–1.36)	0.39
Autonomic instability	29 (26.9%)	47 (32.6%)	0.76 (0.44–1.31)	0.34
Agitation or combativeness	55 (50.9%)	86 (59.7%)	0.70 (0.42–1.16)	0.20
Nausea or vomiting	38 (35.2%)	66 (45.8%)	0.64 (0.38–1.07)	0.09
Ataxia	20 (18.5%)	38 (26.4%)	0.63 (0.34–1.17)	0.17
Anorexia	19 (17.6%)	37 (25.7%)	0.62 (0.33–1.15)	0.17
Insomnia	11 (10.2%)	27 (18.8%)	0.49 (0.23–1.04)	0.08
Confusion or delirium	67 (62.0%)	123 (85.4%)	0.28 (0.15–0.51)	<0.001†
Seizures	27 (25.0%)	79 (54.9%)	0.27 (0.16–0.47)	<0.001†
Malaise or fatigue	39 (36.1%)	101 (70.1%)	0.24 (0.14–0.41)	<0.001†
Headache	29 (26.9%)	90 (62.5%)	0.22 (0.13–0.38)	<0.001†
* CI = Confidence interval, † Statistically significant				

Table 2. Signs and Symptoms Among Cases Testing Positive and Negative for Rabies

3.6.2 Seasonality

The onset of illness of rabies cases was more likely to occur during summer or fall months (May through October) when compared to non-rabies cases (OR 1.77; 95% CI 1.04–3.01). While no significant difference was observed between indigenous rabies cases and non-rabies cases in the seasonal pattern of exposures to animals, the limited number of cases reporting a definite animal exposure was a limiting factor in this analysis.

3.6.3 Signs and symptoms

The presenting signs and symptoms of human rabies in the United States were often nonspecific such as fever, malaise, headache, weakness, fatigue, sore throat, and anorexia. The most commonly reported signs and symptoms reported among rabies cases during the course of illness were fever (83%), confusion or delirium (62%), agitation or combativeness (51%), paresthesia or localized pain (50%), and dysphagia (49%). In contrast, the most common signs and symptoms reported among non-rabies cases were confusion or delirium (85%), fever (78%), malaise or fatigue (70%), headache (63%), and agitation or combativeness (60%). When comparing these two groups, aerophobia, hydrophobia, and paresthesia or localized pain were more likely to be reported among rabies cases than non-rabies cases with an OR of 14.59, 7.50, and 5.86 respectively (P-values ≤ 0.001). Dysphagia and localized weakness were also more likely to occur among rabies cases with ORs of 2.73 and 2.26 (P-values ≤ 0.004). Priapism or spontaneous ejaculation was reported more commonly among rabies cases (OR 2.73) but this finding did not reach statistical significance. Among non-rabies cases, headache, malaise or fatigue, seizures, and confusion or delirium were more frequent than in rabies cases with ORs of 0.22–0.28 (P-values <0.001). Although not statistically significant, insomnia was also seen more often in non-rabies cases. Fever, muscle spasm, hypersalivation, anxiety, hallucinations, autonomic instability, agitation or combativeness, nausea or vomiting, and ataxia all appeared to occur with equal likelihood in rabies and non-rabies cases.

3.6.4 Laboratory values

Laboratory values reported for the first collected samples of serum and CSF from rabies and non-rabies cases were compared. The serum white blood cells of rabies cases were elevated higher than non-rabies cases with mean values of 14.8 x 10^3 cells/µL (range 7.0–46.6 x 10^3 cells/µL) and 12.1 x 10^3 cells/µL (range 2.9–29.4 x 10^3 cells/µL) for rabies and non-rabies cases respectively (P-value 0.009). Over 95% of both rabies and non-rabies cases reporting CSF values had an abnormal CSF white blood cell count, red blood cell count, protein, or glucose. The percentage of abnormal values for each of these tests was similar between rabies and non-rabies cases. The white blood cell count in CSF was elevated in both rabies cases and non-rabies cases with mean values of 61.3 cells/µL (range 0–1000 cells/µL) and 89.0 cells/µL (range 0–980 cells/µL) respectively though this difference was not statistically significant (P-value 0.213). A lymphocytic predominance in CSF was seen in the majority of rabies cases. Rabies cases also demonstrated higher percentages of lymphocytes with a mean of 79% lymphocytes (range 31–100%) compared to a mean of 66% lymphocytes (range 0–100%) in non-rabies cases (P-value 0.034). Segmented neutrophils in CSF were also found to be higher in rabies cases with a mean of 30% (range 1–99%) compared to a mean of 15% (range 0–97%) in non-rabies cases (P-value 0.013). Protein in CSF was elevated in both groups with mean values of 72.8 mg/dL (range 15.0–178.0 mg/dL) in rabies cases and 86.2 mg/dL (range 4.0–1140.0) in non-rabies cases. This difference was not statistically significant (P-value 0.460). The mean value of glucose in CSF was elevated in rabies cases (85.8 mg/dL, range 24.0–211.0 mg/dL) while the mean of non-rabies cases was within the normal range (73.2 mg/dL, range 14.0–157.0 mg/dL) (P-value 0.004). No significant differences between rabies and non-rabies cases were found in CSF red blood cell counts, serum lymphocyte counts, serum segmented neutrophil counts, or serum glucose (P-values 0.193-0.781).

3.7 Treatment

Treatment of human rabies was successful in 4 cases. Of these, 2 had received rabies vaccine before the onset of illness. The first survivor (patient 18) became ill 2 days after completing a 14-day course of duck embryo vaccine following a bat bite. The diagnosis of rabies was based on CSF RABV antibody detection and serum antibody titers most consistent with clinical infection in combination with compatible epidemiologic and clinical histories. This patient required intensive supportive care but recovered fully within 6 months after onset. The second survivor (patient 29) had onset of symptoms ~2 weeks after spraying suspensions of a modified live RABV strain while performing research as a laboratory technician. Diagnosis was confirmed by detection of CSF antibodies and rising RABV serum antibody titers. The patient had received pre-exposure prophylaxis with annual boosters and had demonstrated RABV antibodies in response to these vaccinations. It is hypothesized that the strain he was exposed to may have developed increased infectivity following passage through animal and cell culture systems (Gibbons, 2002). Following intensive medical care, the patient survived but was left with severe neurologic sequelae. The third survivor (patient 94) developed rabies after being bitten by a bat. RABV antibodies were found in both serum and CSF. She was treated with an experimental treatment protocol (later termed the Milwaukee Protocol) involving induction of coma and administration of antiviral agents and recovered with only minor residual deficits (Hu,

2007). The last survivor in this series (patient 103) showed clinical signs and symptoms of encephalitis 2 months after exposure to bats and RABV antibodies were detected in both serum and CSF prior to the administration of a single dose of rabies vaccine and rabies immune globulin. This patient made a full recovery without the need for intensive care. No RABV was identified from any of the surviving patients.

Excluding the surviving cases, a total of 31 cases reported treatment after the onset of symptoms consisting of either administration of rabies immune globulin, immunization with rabies vaccine, induction of coma via the Milwaukee Protocol, or receipt of one or more antiviral medications including acyclovir, ganciclovir, amantadine, ribavirin, interferon, cytarabine, or adenine arabinoside. Thirteen patients were administered rabies immune globulin, 8 patients were immunized with rabies vaccine, 23 patients received antiviral therapy, and 5 patients underwent treatment with the Milwaukee Protocol during the course of illness. The median length of illness among all of those treated was longer when compared to those who did not receive any of the specified treatments (23.0 days vs. 13.0 days, P-value 0.029 by Log-rank test). It may be that those who received treatment were also more likely to receive supportive care which has previously been seen to increase the length of illness (Anderson, 1984). When treatments were compared individually, the median length of illness was longer for patients receiving rabies vaccine (14.0 day versus 13.5 days), the Milwaukee Protocol (28.0 days versus 13.0 days), or antiviral therapy (17.0 day versus 13.0 days) but shorter for patients receiving rabies immune globulin (13.0 days versus 14.0 days). However, none of the differences for individual treatments reached statistical significance (P-value 0.198-0.537 by Log-rank test). Overall, the median length of illness was 13.5 days (range 1-133 days).

3.8 Postexposure prophylaxis of contacts of cases

Data on administration of PEP was available in 71 cases (Table 1). A minimum of 3,359 individuals received PEP due to contact with a human rabies patient with a median of 39 individuals per case (range 1-180). The average number of individuals receiving PEP was greater in cases diagnosed postmortem compared to cases diagnosed antemortem (51 vs. 54) though this result was not statistically significant (P-value 0.453). The number of total risk assessments performed was reported for 22 cases. Typically 33% of individuals evaluated for RABV exposure received PEP per case (range 3-69%).

3.9 Rabies virus diagnostic testing

3.9.1 Antemortem test results

Results of RABV laboratory diagnostic testing were collected and summarized for 62 patients where specimens were collected prior to death (Table 3). When available, the number of days after illness onset the sample was collected (i.e. the sample collection date - illness onset date) is reported in parentheses following the test result. The cutaneous nerves of nuchal skin biopsies were tested for RABV antigen in 41 cases. A positive result was obtained in 24 cases (59%) with the first positive sample occurring a median of 7 days (range 2-12 days) after illness onset. RABV was detected in corneal impressions in 9 of 19 cases (47%) with 3 (16%) reporting inconclusive results and 7 (37%) reporting negative results. RABV antigen was first detected in corneal impressions a median of 11 days (range 2-13 days) after onset of rabies. Samples of brain were tested in 6 cases; 1 was inconclusive, 1 was negative, and 4 were first found positive a median of 12 days (range 7-21 days)

Patient	Detection of Antigen			Saliva Virus Isolation	Saliva RNA Detection	Detection of Antibody	
	Cutaneous Nerve	Cornea	Brain			Serum	CSF
9*	--†	--	--	Negative	--	--	--
13	--	--	--	--	--	Negative	--
14	--	--	--	--	--	Positive (11, 54, 64,65‡)	--
15	--	Negative (18–27)	Positive (21)	Negative (27)	--	Positive (6,13,17,21,45)	Positive (10,21)
16	--	Negative	--	Negative	--	--	--
18	--	--	Negative (16)	Negative (14)	--	Positive (14)	Positive (14)
19	--	--	--	Positive (3–5,7,9,11), Negative(6,13,16)	--	Positive (7–9,11,13,16,20,23), Negative (2,3,5,6)	Negative (4,6,11)
23	--	Positive	--	Positive (13)	--	--	--
26	Positive (9)	Negative (7,8)	--	Positive (7,11), Negative (16)	--	Positive (9–11,14,15,18)	Positive (17)
27	Positive (11)	Positive (11)	--	--	--	Positive (10,12,18)	--
28	Negative	Negative	--	--	--	--	--
29*	Negative (33)	Negative (33)	--	--	--	Positive (7,11,21)	Positive (28)
34*	Negative (6,10)	Positive (10), Negative (6)	--	--	--	Positive (6,10)	Negative (6,10)
35*	--	Inconclusive (5)	--	--	--	Positive (5)	Negative (5)
36	--	--	--	--	--	Positive (7)	Positive (6)
37	--	--	--	--	--	Positive (7,8,13)	Negative (7)
38	Negative (8)	Positive (8)	--	Negative (8)	--	Negative (8)	Negative (8)
40*	Positive (7)	--	--	Positive (10,14)	--	Negative (7–23)	Negative (7–23)
41	Positive (6,11)	Negative (6,18)	Positive (8)	Positive (9–13), Negative (16–25)	--	Positive (16–27), Negative (6–14)	Negative (8–19)
42	Negative (18,22)	--	--	Negative (18)	--	Positive (18,23,27)	Positive (27), Negative (18,23)
43	--	--	Positive (16)	Negative (17)	--	Positive (17), Negative (10)	Positive (14)
44	Positive (6)	--	--	--	Positive	Negative (6)	Negative (6)
49	Negative (5)	--	--	Negative (5)	--	Negative (5)	Negative (5)

Patient	Detection of Antigen			Saliva Virus Isolation	Saliva RNA Detection	Detection of Antibody	
	Cutaneous Nerve	Cornea	Brain			Serum	CSF
50	Positive (12)	--	--	Positive (5)	Positive (5)	Negative (5)	Negative (5)
53*	Positive (7,13), Negative (3)	Negative (2)	--	Negative (7,11,13)	Positive (7,11,13,16)	Positive (7,16), Negative (2)	Negative (13)
55	--	--	--	--	--	Negative (6)	--
56	Positive (5)	Inconclusive (5–9)	--	Positive (5)	Positive (5)	Negative (5–9)	Negative (8)
60	Positive (4)	--	Positive (7)	Negative (4)	Positive (4)	Positive (4)	--
61	--	Positive (13)	--	--	--	--	--
62	Positive (10)	--	--	Positive (10)	Positive (10)	Negative (10)	Negative (10)
63	Positive (7)	--	--	Positive (8)	Positive (8)	--	--
64	Negative (5)	Inconclusive (5)	--	--	--	Positive (11,13), Negative (5)	Negative (4)
Patient	Detection of Antigen			Saliva Virus Isolation	Saliva RNA Detection	Detection of Antibody	
	Cutaneous Nerve	Cornea	Brain			Cutaneous Nerve	Cornea
65	--	Positive (13)	--	Negative (9)	Positive (9)	Positive (7,11,14)	Negative (10)
67	Positive (8)	--	--	Positive (8)	Positive (8)	Negative (8)	--
68	Negative (5,6)	--	--	Positive (5)	Positive (5)	Positive (6), Negative (5)	Negative (5)
69	--	--	--	--	--	Positive (12), Negative (4)	--
70	Negative (13)	--	--	--	Positive (13)	Positive (13)	--
73	--	--	--	--	--	Negative (9)	--
74	Positive (5)	--	--	--	Positive (5)	Negative (5)	Negative (5)
75	Positive (7)	--	--	--	Positive (7)	Positive (7,14)	Positive (7)
76	Positive	Positive	--	--	Positive	--	--
77	Positive	--	--	--	Positive	--	--
79	Positive	--	--	--	Positive	--	--
80	--	--	--	--	--	Negative (6)	--
81	--	--	--	--	Positive	Positive (12,15)	Negative
82	Negative (9)	Positive (11), Inconclusive (9)	--	--	Positive (9)	Positive (12,13), Negative (9)	--
83	Negative (6)	--	--	--	Positive (8)	Positive (8), Negative (6)	Positive (8), Negative (6)

Patient	Detection of Antigen			Saliva Virus Isolation	Saliva RNA Detection	Detection of Antibody	
	Cutaneous Nerve	Cornea	Brain			Serum	CSF
84	Positive (11)	--	Inconclusive (7)	--	--	Positive (9)	Negative (8)
87*	--	--	--	--	Positive	Positive (19,21)	Negative (17)
94	Negative (5)	--	--	Negative (5)	Negative (5,27)	Positive (5,12,20,59,56,70)	Positive (5,12,20,59,56,70)
96	--	--	--	--	--	Positive (5,10)	Positive (10), Negative (5)
97	Positive (2)	--	--	--	Positive (2)	Negative (3)	Negative (2)
98	Positive (10)	--	--	--	Positive (10,19,23,26)	Positive (10,19,23,26)	Positive (19,23,26), Negative (10)
99	Positive (5,21)	Positive (2)	--	--	Positive (4)	Positive (13), Negative (2–12)	Positive (15), Negative (2)
100	Negative	--	--	--	Negative	Positive	Positive (10 or 16)
102	Positive (5)	--	--	--	Positive (5)	Positive (5)	Negative (5)
103	Negative (14)	--	--	--	Negative (14)	Positive (14,18,22,32)	Positive (14,18,22,37)
104	Negative (14)	--	--	--	Positive (14)	Positive (14)	Negative (6)
105	Negative (21)	--	--	--	Negative (21)	Positive (21)	Positive (21)
106	Positive (5)	--	--	--	Positive (5)	Positive (18), Negative (5–17)	Negative
107	Negative (17)	--	--	--	Negative (17)	Positive (12)	Positive (12)
108	Positive (10)	--	--	--	Positive (8)	Negative (8)	--

* Patient received immunization, † -- = Sample not collected, testing not performed, or results not reported, ‡ When known, the number of days after illness onset the sample was collected (i.e. sample collection date – illness onset date) is indicated in parentheses

Table 3. Summary of Antemortem Diagnostic Test Results for 62 Patients with Human Rabies in the United States, 1960–2010 following onset of illness. Virus isolation from saliva was attempted in 23 cases and successful in 11 (48%) in samples collected a median of 8 days (range 3-13 days) after illness onset. RABV RNA was detected in 27 of 32 cases tested (84%) with the first positive results obtained from samples a median of 7 days (range 2-14 days) after the appearance of symptoms. Serum was tested for antibodies in 48 patients with no history of vaccination at the time of sample collection and was positive in 33 cases (69%). Antibodies in serum were first detected a median of 10.5 days (range 4-21 days) from the onset of illness in these unvaccinated patients. In contrast, antibodies in CSF were found in only 17 of 40 cases tested (43%) and first appeared a median of 14 days (range 5-28 days) following illness onset.

3.9.2 Postmortem test results

Confirmation of rabies through laboratory testing of postmortem samples was reported in 81 cases. The confirmation came shortly after death in the majority of cases. However, in at least 14 cases rabies was not suspected prior to death and was diagnosed as part of a postmortem investigation. Notable among these cases were all of the cases involving transplantation of infected organs or tissue (patients 30-31 and 89-93), 2 cases (patient 71 and patient 72) initially evaluated for suspected Creutzfeldt-Jakob disease, 1 case (patient 76) referred for testing of an undiagnosed encephalitis to the California Encephalitis Project, 1 case (patient 96) referred for testing to CDC's Unexplained Deaths Project, and 1 case (patient 59) originally attributed to disseminated candidiasis and mucormycosis in a pregnant female. The delay in diagnosis for these cases ranged from 1 to 6 months after death.

4. Conclusion

Despite being indigenous in wildlife, human rabies was a rarely reported disease in the United States during 1960-2010. An average of 2 cases per year was recorded during this time period, a trend that remained largely stable throughout each decade. While this should be considered a great success of public health efforts towards prevention and control, the true incidence of human rabies is likely higher due to under recognition. The disease occurs so infrequently that most clinicians have little direct experience with rabies and therefore may not consider it in the differential diagnosis of patients presenting with encephalitis. The lack of a clear animal exposure preceding illness in increasing numbers of cases leaves clinicians without a significant clue that might prompt consideration of rabies. The myriad of other possible etiologies of encephalitis further compounds this problem. For these reasons, a clear diagnosis cannot be found in the majority of cases of encephalitis even when extensive testing to identify the cause of illness is employed (Glaser, 2003). In fact, between 1979 and 1998 there was an average of over 1,000 deaths per year from encephalitis due to unknown cause reported in the United States (Khetsuriani, 2007). It is interesting to note that 1 of the 334 cases of encephalitis (0.3%) investigated by the California encephalitis project was diagnosed with rabies (Glaser, 2003). Rabies was not previously suspected in this patient and would almost certainly have remained unrecognized without the extensive testing performed as part of the study. Applying this rate of unrecognized rabies cases to the annual number of reported deaths due to encephalitis of unknown cause suggests there could be over 3 cases of human rabies that go unrecognized each year in the United States alone. This review provides a comprehensive summary of epidemiologic and clinical data of all of the known cases within the last 5 decades which can be used as an aid in recognizing and identifying rabies among patients with encephalitis.

The epidemiology of human rabies in the United States has undergone striking changes over the last century. Prior to the 1960s, the vast majority of human rabies cases in the United State were due to bites from an infected dog. Worldwide, dogs remain the primary source of human rabies (WHO, 2004; Knobel, 2005). However, a dramatic decline in human rabies cases in the United States occurred during the 1940s and 1950s as illustrated in Figure 2. This decrease in cases paralleled the improvement and application of new rabies vaccines for both humans and animals. Key to this approach was the targeting of domestic animals for vaccination to create a barrier of protection from RABV transmission to humans, a strategy that was ultimately successful in eliminating the canine RABV variant from the United States (Velasco-Villa, 2008). Throughout the 1940s and 1950s the number of human rabies cases attributed to domestic animals (primarily dogs) far exceeded those involving wildlife animals. However, a reversal in this relationship took place in the 1960s when the number of human rabies cases associated with wildlife surpassed those due to domestic animals, a trend that continues to this day. Currently the most frequently reported rabid animals in the United States are raccoons, bats, skunks, and foxes (Blanton, 2010). Clinicians should be aware that these species can therefore be considered high risk though must also be careful not to discount exposures to other known vector species.

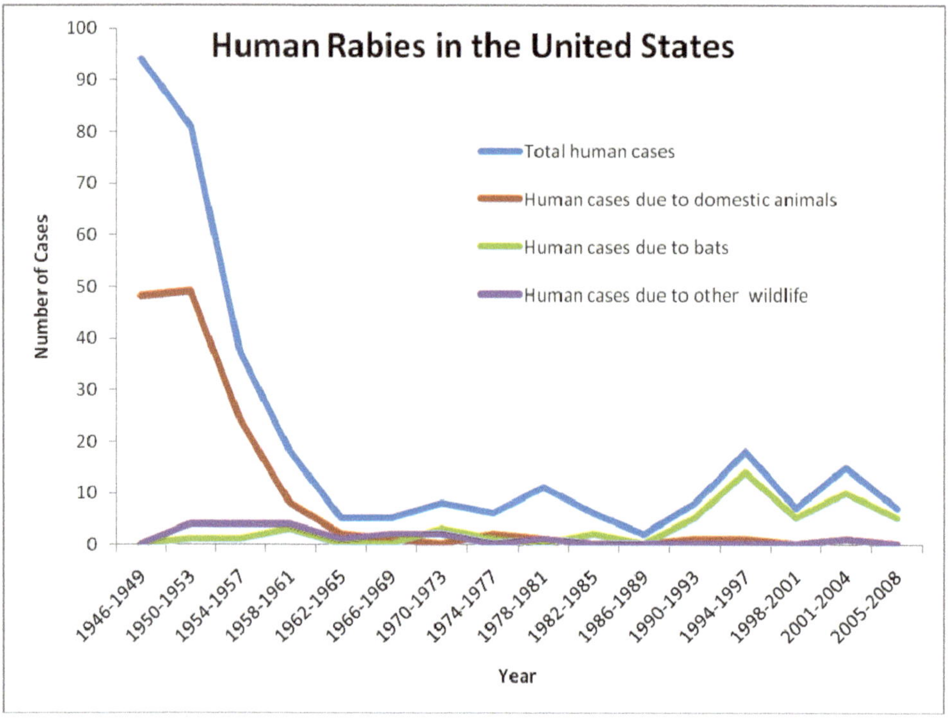

Fig. 2. Human Rabies Cases in the United States, 1946–2008

The increasing number of cases associated with bats illustrates the growing importance of this species in the epidemiology of rabies (Figure 2). The advancement and increased utilization of RABV variant typing methods has led to a greater understanding of rabies epidemiology, particularly with regards to the role of bats (Smith, 1992). Excluding cases acquired through transplantation of infected tissue, a total of 42 RABV variants associated with bats were identified in this series, yet 16 (38%) of these cases had no reported exposure history. Without the availability of antigenic and molecular typing, this epidemiologic link to bats likely would have remained unrecognized in these cases. Many times, possible contact between the patient and a bat was recalled only after a bat RABV variant had been identified. Excluding cases acquired through transplantation, a total of 41/46 (89%) indigenous cases have been associated with bats either through a reported bat exposure or identification of a bat variant. The most common species of bats associated with human cases through variant typing were the silver-haired bat and the tricolored bat (*Lasionycteris noctivagans* and *Perimyotis subflavus*). This is a somewhat curious finding considering that these species of insectivorous bats are considered to be solitary tree-dwelling bats and are infrequently submitted to public health laboratories for rabies diagnostic testing (Krebs, 2000; Messenger, 2002; Blanton, 2010). However, there is some evidence suggesting that the RABV variants in these species have evolved genetic changes that may increase their infectivity (Morimoto, 1996; Dietzschold, 2000). Additional studies of bat RABV will undoubtedly improve understanding of the emergence, perpetuation, and epizootiology of this disease (Streicker, 2010).

Classically, one expects human rabies cases to be preceded by an animal bite exposure. However, a definite history of a recent animal bite was reported in less than half of the cases in this series. The epidemiologic shift in the source of infection of human rabies in the United States provides one possible explanation for this observation. Bites from dogs or other carnivores are more likely to be recognized simply due to the size of the animal. A larger bite wound is also more likely to require medical treatment at which time consideration can be given to the need for rabies PEP. In contrast, North American bats are small and produce bite wounds that are superficial by comparison and less likely to require medical attention. With the advent of modern cell culture vaccines in 1980 and rabies immune globulin, no PEP failures have been reported in the United States. Unless the victim was previously aware of the risk of rabies from a bat bite, the opportunity for lifesaving PEP may be lost. A survey among cavers (spelunkers) in the United States found that 15% indicated a bat bite was not a risk for rabies, suggesting that a significant proportion of the public at large may also be unaware of the risk posed by bats (Gibbons, 2002). Some bat bites go unnoticed entirely because bat teeth are small and sharp (Feder, 1997). If the victim were engaged in an outdoor activity it is not hard to imagine a bat bite being confused for an insect bite or other minor trauma if the bat remained hidden in a tree or crevice (Gibbons, 2002). Furthermore, due to the extended incubation period a patient may not link the symptoms of the disease with an exposure that occurred months before the onset of illness. The median incubation in this series was nearly six weeks with evidence suggesting that long incubation periods on the order of years are possible (Smith, 1991). Thus, it is essential that the public be informed of the risk of rabies from all mammals and to remain vigilant for potential exposures, particularly when engaging in activities that put them at risk for contact with bats and other wildlife animals. Clinicians must also recognize that rabies should not be excluded from the differential diagnosis of a patient with acute progressive encephalitis due to the absence of a recent animal exposure history.

The initial signs and symptoms of human rabies are largely nonspecific and include fever, malaise, headache, nausea, and vomiting. Not surprisingly, almost half of the patients in this series were evaluated for their symptoms at least once prior to being admitted to the hospital without the diagnosis of rabies being considered. Thus, it may be very difficult to diagnose rabies during the prodromal phase in the absence of an animal exposure to alert one to the possibility. However, the progression of illness is rapid with most patients seeking medical care within one day of the appearance of symptoms and requiring hospitalization within 4 days of illness onset. Furthermore, most patients succumbed to their illness within 2 weeks of the onset of symptoms. These data suggest that rabies would be less likely in patients who do not require hospitalization within one week of developing symptoms or in hospitalized patients surviving longer than 2 weeks. Prioritization of testing for other etiologies over rabies would be prudent in these situations. However, several signs and symptoms were found to occur more frequently in patients with rabies when compared to patients with encephalopathy who tested negative for rabies. Aerophobia and hydrophobia were the most specific findings associated with rabies cases despite the fact that these symptoms were found in relatively few cases. Intubation and sedation have become common components of modern medical management of critically ill patients, a practice that may mask these symptoms unless specifically noted by patients early in their course. The neurologic findings of paresthesias or localized pain, dysphagia, and focal weakness were also positively linked to rabies cases. In contrast, headache, malaise or fatigue, seizures, and confusion or delirium were observed more frequently in non-rabies cases than in rabies cases.

The clinical presentation of human rabies is often classified as either encephalitic (furious) or paralytic (dumb) rabies. The encephalitic form of the disease is characterized by overall hyperexcitability with episodes of confusion, agitation or aggressive behavior, and hallucinations. In the paralytic form, localized weakness and/or paralysis are the most prominent feature and are commonly accompanied by paresthesias, pruritis, or localized pain at the site of the bite and a normal mental status. The signs and symptoms associated with rabies cases in this series are those classically used to describe the paralytic rather than the encephalitic form. In general, 80% of human rabies patients are thought to manifest the encephalitic form while 20% have a paralytic form (Jackson, 2002)(Jackson, 2007). As such, clinicians may be more likely to submit cases for testing that resemble their preconceived notion of the more common furious form of human rabies and less likely to consider rabies with the more rare paralytic form. A connection between the paralytic form of rabies and transmission by vampire bats has been noted in several human rabies outbreaks (Nehaul, 1955; Hurst, 1959; Hurst, 1959; Pawan, 1959; Verlinde, 1975; da Rosa, 2006). However, vampire bats do not cause exclusively paralytic disease as the encephalitic form has been described with a vampire bat human rabies outbreak in Peru (Lopez, 1992). Host factors most certainly play a role also as two individuals bitten by the same dog were seen to develop encephalitic rabies in one and paralytic rabies in the other (Hemachudha, 1988). Nevertheless, it is unclear whether the overall preponderance of cases linked to bats may have affected the clinical syndrome observed in this series. Regardless of the source of infection, clinicians should be aware that the clinical presentation of human rabies is a spectrum that can include features of either the encephalitic or paralytic forms. Positive indicators such as hydrophobia, aerophobia, paresthesias or localized pain, focal weakness, and dysphagia in a patient with acute progressive encephalitis should alert the clinician to the possibility of rabies.

The age and sex of a patient in addition to the month of illness onset may also provide clues to the diagnosis of rabies in patients with encephalitis. Globally, human rabies is most likely to be seen in children less than 15 years old (WHO, 2004). However, patients in this series were more likely to be older with a median age of 29 years. The disproportionate number of cases linked with bats and other wildlife species as opposed to dogs is likely responsible for this discrepancy. Children are more likely to unintentionally incite a dog attack through provoking behaviors and inexperience or because their size and movements may be similar to prey. With respect to wildlife, one might expect older age groups to be more likely to engage in outdoor activities or other behaviors that would put them at higher risk of exposure to bats and wildlife animals. Similarly, the predominance of males in this case series may also be due in part to males engaging in these activities more frequently than females. Limited data on the administration of PEP suggests that males may have higher rates of PEP (Helmick, 1983) though this trend was not confirmed in other studies of state level data (Blanton, 2005; O'Bell, 2006). Furthermore, males may be less likely to seek PEP after an exposure occurs. In support of this claim is evidence suggesting that the perception and awareness of health-related risks may be lower in males compared to females (Naslund, 1997; Gustafson, 1998). The observation that most cases occurred during fall months corresponds well with the observation that most contact with wildlife, particularly bats, occurs during the late summer months (Messenger, 2002). Assuming an incubation period of 1-3 months, exposures occurring during summer would then be expected to become ill during the fall. This pattern was particularly significant when analyzing cases associated with bats. Most bat exposures occurred during the early fall months and is consistent with previous research demonstrating that the incidence of rabies-infected bats peaks in August (Constantine, 1979; Pape, 1999). Furthermore, the illness onset month in cases associated with bats was most common during the late fall months. Both exposures and onset of illness were more likely to occur in fall months in cases associated with bats compared with those not associated with bats. Based on these findings, a typical human rabies case in the United States would be a young adult male presenting with signs and symptoms of encephalitis in the fall.

When human rabies is suspected it is important to initiate diagnostic testing as early as possible. Current guidelines for antemortem testing of human patients recommend the collection of samples of skin, serum, saliva, and CSF. In this series, the earliest positive results were found with detection of viral RNA in saliva and viral antigen in skin after a median of 7 days following onset of illness. The earliest diagnosis occurred in patient 98 with both saliva and skin collected 2 days after illness onset reported positive by PCR and DFA respectively on the sixth day of illness. Virus isolation from saliva was also fairly rapid with positive results obtained as early as 3 days after illness onset (median 8 days). The development of a humoral immune response lags behind the secretion of virus in saliva and antibodies were detected in serum and CSF a median of 10 and 14 days respectively following the appearance of symptoms. The earliest detection of rabies specific antibodies after illness onset was 4 days in serum and 5 days in CSF. With respect to sensitivity, identification of viral RNA in saliva was the most sensitive testing modality with 84% of rabies cases tested giving positive results. Detection of antibodies in serum and viral antigens in brain and cutaneous nerves were also relatively sensitive with positive results in 69%, 67%, and 59% of cases tested respectively. Though isolation of RABV from saliva was successful in fewer than half of cases, the utility of virus isolates for variant typing, comparative analyses, investigations of pathogenesis, and other studies is invaluable. Similarly, while antibodies in CSF were found relatively infrequently, their detection is significant as this finding alone is considered diagnostic for rabies regardless of history of rabies vaccination (Moore, 2010). Examination of corneal impressions was positive in only 47% of cases tested and is no longer routinely used for antemortem diagnostic testing given the risk of damage to the eyes when performed by inexperienced practitioners and the relatively poor sensitivity. While the sensitivity of viral antigen detection in antemortem brain samples is high, routine testing of these samples is not recommended due to the invasiveness of the collection procedure. The best approach for maximizing the sensitivity and accuracy of antemortem diagnostic rabies testing is through submission of skin, saliva, serum, and CSF for evaluation with multiple modalities including detection of viral antigen, viral nucleic acid, and rabies specific antibodies, especially because some test results become available in less than 24 hours.

The diagnosis of human rabies can be essential in preventing further cases. Identifying human cases allows for a public health response to investigate the source of infection and provide risk assessments of contacts with potential exposures. If a suspected animal source infestation is discovered, these animals can be removed to avert any further exposures and tested to confirm whether additional animals are rabid. Any individuals with contact with potentially rabid animals can then be assessed for exposures and given PEP when indicated. Public education can also be targeted to increase awareness of the risk of rabies transmission from reservoir species and the importance of seeking medical attention promptly if an exposure does occur. Contacts of rabies patients should also be identified and evaluated for exposures. Although human-to-human transmission of rabies has only been well documented in cases of organ or tissue transplantation, transmission following exposure to human saliva or nervous tissue remains a theoretical possibility (Helmick, 1987). Rare anecdotal reports of direct human to human transmission of rabies through bites, kissing, lactation, intercourse, transplacental transmission, and delivery of healthcare have been reported though possible animal exposures were difficult to exclude and none of these cases were laboratory confirmed (Helmick, 1987; Gibbons, 2002). Healthcare providers can be reassured by the fact that no case of rabies has ever been confirmed in a caregiver of any of the estimated 55,000 cases occurring each year. Moreover, early recognition and contact isolation of suspected cases are effective means of limiting exposures in healthcare settings (Helmick, 1987). Given these facts, the median of 39 individuals receiving PEP per case found in this series may seem excessive. Though the higher rate of PEP of contacts among cases diagnosed postmortem compared to antemortem was not statistically significant, it is still likely that early diagnosis of human rabies will lead to fewer exposures and decrease unnecessary PEP. Lastly, identification of human rabies can avoid transmitting the virus through organ and tissue transplantation. Even if the diagnosis is made after transplantation has already taken place, removal of the transplanted tissue and administration of PEP has been successful in preventing infection in two recipients of corneas from an infected donor (Vetter, 2011).

The early diagnosis of rabies also provides the best opportunity for experimental therapy of victims. The 4 survivors reported in this series demonstrate that survival is rare but does occur. In addition, patient 95 was the first report of a patient recovering from rabies without receiving any vaccination against rabies through the use of the Milwaukee Protocol. Two subsequent survivors attributed to the application of this protocol have been reported among 24 attempts to give an estimated 9% survival by intention-to-treat analysis (Willoughby, 2009). As knowledge is gained from both treatment failures and successes, further refinement of this approach may increase the rate of success. The recovery of patient 104 without application of the Milwaukee Protocol or even need for intensive care is the only well documented case of a presumed human abortive rabies infection. This case hints at the possibility that there may be a much larger spectrum of disease in rabies cases that has not been previously appreciated. It may be only recently recognized due to improved laboratory diagnostic techniques, greater availability of laboratory testing, or increased awareness of the possibility of rabies after several high profile cases in the United States including the survival of patient 95 and the cases transmitted through transplantation (patients 90-93). The association of both of these survivors with exposures to bats has also led to the hypothesis that canine RABV variants may be more virulent than bat variants (Lafon, 2005). However, one case of documented human rabies of canine origin in Equatorial Guinea purportedly survived infection with application of the Milwaukee Protocol, but later succumbed (Rubin, 2009). The patient's death on hospital day 22 was thought to be due to complications of malnutrition. Irrespective of the source of infection, the limited success of treatment attempts emphasizes the importance of prevention. Current treatment protocols require considerable expense and advanced medical facilities making practical application unrealistic in many countries. In contrast, rabies prevention strategies implementing safe, efficacious, and affordable human and animal vaccines have proven to be highly effective, particularly in combination with community outreach and education programs (Rupprecht, 2008; Cleaveland, 2010).

The results of this study are subject to several limitations. Given the relative rarity of human rabies in the United States despite the abundance of the disease in nature, this case series represents a relatively small sample size and several cases had only limited data available. In addition, all of the data from cases were collected retrospectively and are therefore subject to recall bias. Histories of potential animal exposures may be particularly sensitive to poor memory given the lengthy incubation period seen with rabies; this may be exacerbated in cases where rabies was not initially considered or the diagnosis was delayed. In all cases there is a short window of opportunity to communicate directly with patients due to the rapid progression of disease and nearly universal fatal outcome. In the confirmed rabies cases additional clinical and laboratory data were gained through public health investigations. In contrast, data from non-rabies cases relied primarily on patient information forms completed at the time of submission for diagnostic testing. As such, those data represent only a snapshot of the clinical picture making comparisons of temporal patterns in rabies and non-rabies cases unfeasible. Moreover, no follow-up of clinical outcomes (i.e. survival or death) was available for non-rabies cases. Though statistically significant results were obtained, it is possible that other significant findings may have been missed due to the small sample size.

This review complements previous reports of smaller series of human rabies cases in the United States (Held, 1967; Anderson, 1984; Noah, 1998; CDC, 2006). Significant changes in the epidemiology of rabies include the increasing role of bats in human rabies and the concomitant rise in cases with no clear history of animal exposure. These findings underscore the need to increase public awareness of the risk of rabies from wildlife, particularly bats, and the importance of prompt medical evaluation if contact with such animals occurs. Advances in the treatment of human rabies have led to the first reported cases of recovery without immunization with rabies vaccine. These survivors raise hope for continued advancements in the efforts to develop a treatment for rabies. Identification of the first presumptive abortive human rabies case suggests an expanded view of the continuum of disease caused by lyssaviruses is necessary. Our knowledge of human rabies will continue to grow as more cases are identified. As such, increasing the recognition and diagnosis of human rabies will not only enhance our understanding of the disease but ultimately will save human lives as well. Early diagnosis allows the institution of proper biosafety and isolation precautions of rabies patients as well as the initiation of public health action to identify potential exposures to evaluate their need for PEP. Insights gained from human rabies may also prove to be applicable to other zoonoses. As one of the earliest known zoonotic diseases, rabies can be used as a prototype in investigating the interplay between animals and their impact on human health. This relationship is becoming increasingly important as the majority of emerging infectious diseases are now recognized to be zoonotic in nature. Lyssavirus infections and human rabies due to bats should be considered emerging infectious threats themselves. Research into bats and human disease is particularly relevant given the identification of bats as the reservoir of numerous other human pathogens including Ebola virus, Marburg virus, nipah virus, hendra virus, and SARS-like coronaviruses among others (Calisher, 2006). Clearly, the health of humans, animals, and the environment are interconnected and lessons learned from rabies are extremely valuable in relation to this concept of "One Health."

5. Acknowledgements

The authors thank all of the clinicians and public health professionals who provided clinical, epidemiologic, and laboratory data on these cases. The authors also recognize the contributions of Jesse Blanton, Lizette Durand, Richard Franka, Felix Jackson, Ivan Kuzmin, Lillian Orciari, Dustyn Palmer, Sergio Recuenco, Andres Velasco-Villa, and Pam Yager.

6. References

Anderson, L. J., K. G. Nicholson, et al. (1984). "Human rabies in the United States, 1960 to 1979: epidemiology, diagnosis, and prevention." Ann Intern Med 100(5): 728-735.

Blanton, J. D., N. Y. Bowden, et al. (2005). "Rabies postexposure prophylaxis, New York, 1995-2000." Emerg Infect Dis 11(12): 1921-1927.

Blanton, J. D., D. Palmer, et al. (2010). "Rabies surveillance in the United States during 2009." J Am Vet Med Assoc 237(6): 646-657.

Calisher, C. H., J. E. Childs, et al. (2006). "Bats: important reservoir hosts of emerging viruses." Clin Microbiol Rev 19(3): 531-545.

CDC (2006).

CDC (2006). Protocol for Postmortem Diagnosis of Rabies in Animals by Direct Fluorescent Antibody Testing.

Christian, K. A., J. D. Blanton, et al. (2009). "Epidemiology of rabies post-exposure prophylaxis--United States of America, 2006-2008." Vaccine 27(51): 7156-7161.

Cleaveland, S., P. Costa, et al. (2010). "Catalysing action against rabies." Vet Rec 167(11): 422-423.

Constantine, D. G. (1979). "An updated list of rabies-infected bats in North America." J Wildl Dis 15(2): 347-349.

da Rosa, E. S., I. Kotait, et al. (2006). "Bat-transmitted human rabies outbreaks, Brazilian Amazon." Emerg Infect Dis 12(8): 1197-1202.

Dietzschold, B., K. Morimoto, et al. (2000). "Genotypic and phenotypic diversity of rabies virus variants involved in human rabies: implications for postexposure prophylaxis." J Hum Virol 3(1): 50-57.

Feder, H. M., Jr., R. Nelson, et al. (1997). "Bat bite?" Lancet 350(9087): 1300.

Gibbons, R. V. (2002). "Cryptogenic rabies, bats, and the question of aerosol transmission." Ann Emerg Med 39(5): 528-536.

Gibbons, R. V., R. C. Holman, et al. (2002). "Knowledge of bat rabies and human exposure among United States cavers." Emerg Infect Dis 8(5): 532-534.

Glaser, C. A., S. Gilliam, et al. (2003). "In search of encephalitis etiologies: diagnostic challenges in the California Encephalitis Project, 1998-2000." Clin Infect Dis 36(6): 731-742.

Gustafson, P. E. (1998). "Gender differences in risk perception: theoretical and methodological perspectives." Risk Anal 18(6): 805-811.

Held, J. R., E. S. Tierkel, et al. (1967). "Rabies in man and animals in the United States, 1946-65." Public Health Rep 82(11): 1009-1018.

Hellenbrand, W., C. Meyer, et al. (2005). "Cases of rabies in Germany following organ transplantation." Euro Surveill 10(2): E050224 050226.

Helmick, C. G. (1983). "The epidemiology of human rabies postexposure prophylaxis, 1980-1981." Jama 250(15): 1990-1996.

Helmick, C. G., R. V. Tauxe, et al. (1987). "Is there a risk to contacts of patients with rabies?" Rev Infect Dis 9(3): 511-518.

Hemachudha, T., P. Phanuphak, et al. (1988). "Immunologic study of human encephalitic and paralytic rabies. Preliminary report of 16 patients." Am J Med 84(4): 673-677.

Houff, S. A., R. C. Burton, et al. (1979). "Human-to-human transmission of rabies virus by corneal transplant." N Engl J Med 300(11): 603-604.

Hu, W. T., R. E. Willoughby, Jr., et al. (2007). "Long-term follow-up after treatment of rabies by induction of coma." N Engl J Med 357(9): 945-946.

Hurst, E. W. and J. L. Pawan (1959). "A further account of the Trinidad outbreak of acute rabic myelitis: histology of the experimental disease." Caribb Med J 21: 25-45.

Hurst, E. W. and J. L. Pawan (1959). "An outbreak of rabies in Trinidad without history of bites, and with the symptoms of acute ascending myelitis." Caribb Med J 21: 11-24.

Jackson, A. C., M. J. Warrell, et al. (2003). "Management of rabies in humans." Clin Infect Dis 36(1): 60-63.

Jackson, A. C. and W. H. Wunner (2002). Rabies. Amsterdam ; Boston, Academic Press.

Javadi, M. A., A. Fayaz, et al. (1996). "Transmission of rabies by corneal graft." Cornea 15(4): 431-433.

Khetsuriani, N., R. C. Holman, et al. (2007). "Trends in encephalitis-associated deaths in the United States." Epidemiol Infect 135(4): 583-591.

Knobel, D. L., S. Cleaveland, et al. (2005). "Re-evaluating the burden of rabies in Africa and Asia." Bull World Health Organ 83(5): 360-368.

Krebs, J. W., J. S. Smith, et al. (2000). "Mammalian reservoirs and epidemiology of rabies diagnosed in human beings in the United States, 1981-1998." Ann N Y Acad Sci 916: 345-353.

Kusne, S. and J. Smilack (2005). "Transmission of rabies virus from an organ donor to four transplant recipients." Liver Transpl 11(10): 1295-1297.

Kuzmin, I. V., I. S. Novella, et al. (2009). "The rhabdoviruses: biodiversity, phylogenetics, and evolution." Infect Genet Evol 9(4): 541-553.

Lafon, M. (2005). "Bat rabies--the Achilles heel of a viral killer?" Lancet 366(9489): 876-877.

Lopez, A., P. Miranda, et al. (1992). "Outbreak of human rabies in the Peruvian jungle." Lancet 339(8790): 408-411.

Messenger, S. L., J. S. Smith, et al. (2002). "Emerging epidemiology of bat-associated cryptic cases of rabies in humans in the United States." Clin Infect Dis 35(6): 738-747.

Moore, S. M. and C. A. Hanlon (2010). "Rabies-specific antibodies: measuring surrogates of protection against a fatal disease." PLoS Negl Trop Dis 4(3): e595.

Morimoto, K., M. Patel, et al. (1996). "Characterization of a unique variant of bat rabies virus responsible for newly emerging human cases in North America." Proc Natl Acad Sci U S A 93(11): 5653-5658.

Naslund, G. K. (1997). "Relationships between health behavior, knowledge, and beliefs among Swedish blue-collar workers." Scand J Soc Med 25(2): 100-110.

Nehaul, B. B. (1955). "Rabies transmitted by bats in British Guiana." Am J Trop Med Hyg 4(3): 550-553.

Noah, D. L., C. L. Drenzek, et al. (1998). "Epidemiology of human rabies in the United States, 1980 to 1996." Ann Intern Med 128(11): 922-930.

O'Bell, S. A., J. McQuiston, et al. (2006). "Human rabies exposures and postexposure prophylaxis in South Carolina, 1993-2002." Public Health Rep 121(2): 197-202.

Pape, W. J., T. D. Fitzsimmons, et al. (1999). "Risk for rabies transmission from encounters with bats, Colorado, 1977-1996." Emerg Infect Dis 5(3): 433-437.

Pawan, J. L. (1959). "Rabies in the vampire bat of Trinidad, with special reference to the clinical course and the latency of infection." Caribb Med J 21: 137-156.

Rubin, J., D. David, et al. (2009). "Applying the Milwaukee protocol to treat canine rabies in Equatorial Guinea." Scand J Infect Dis 41(5): 372-375.

Rupprecht, C. E., J. Barrett, et al. (2008). "Can rabies be eradicated?" Dev Biol (Basel) 131: 95-121.

Smith, J. S., D. B. Fishbein, et al. (1991). "Unexplained rabies in three immigrants in the United States. A virologic investigation." N Engl J Med 324(4): 205-211.

Smith, J. S., L. A. Orciari, et al. (1992). "Epidemiologic and historical relationships among 87 rabies virus isolates as determined by limited sequence analysis." J Infect Dis 166(2): 296-307.

Srinivasan, A., E. C. Burton, et al. (2005). "Transmission of rabies virus from an organ donor to four transplant recipients." N Engl J Med 352(11): 1103-1111.

Streicker, D. G., A. S. Turmelle, et al. (2010). "Host phylogeny constrains cross-species emergence and establishment of rabies virus in bats." Science 329(5992): 676-679.

Velasco-Villa, A., S. A. Reeder, et al. (2008). "Enzootic rabies elimination from dogs and reemergence in wild terrestrial carnivores, United States." Emerg Infect Dis 14(12): 1849-1854.

Verlinde, J. D., E. Li-Fo-Sjoe, et al. (1975). "A local outbreak of paralytic rabies in Surinam children." Trop Geogr Med 27(2): 137-142.

Vetter, J. M., L. Frisch, et al. (2011). "Survival after transplantation of corneas from a rabies-infected donor." Cornea 30(2): 241-244.

WHO (2004). WHO Expert Consultation on Rabies. First Report. WHO technical report series No 931. Geneva, WHO. 2005: 121.

Willoughby, R. E., Jr. (2009). ""Early death" and the contraindication of vaccine during treatment of rabies." Vaccine 27(51): 7173-7177.

7. Case references

[1] CDC (1960). Human rabies. Morbidity and Mortality Weekly Report, Vol.9, No.31, p.2

[2] Ross, E.; Armentrout, S. (1962). Myocarditis Associated with Rabies: Report of a Case. New England Journal of Medicine, Vol.266, No.21, pp.1087-1089

[3] CDC (1961). Human Rabies – Kentucky. Morbidity and Mortality Weekly Report, Vol.10, No.2, p.2

[4] CDC (1961). Human Rabies – California. Morbidity and Mortality Weekly Report, Vol.10, No.3, p.2

[5] CDC (1961). Human Rabies – Kentucky. Morbidity and Mortality Weekly Report, Vol.10, No.26, p.8

[6] CDC (1962). Rabies in Man – Texas. Morbidity and Mortality Weekly Report, Vol.11, p.258

[7] CDC (1962). Human Rabies – Idaho. Morbidity and Mortality Weekly Report, Vol.11, pp.395,400

[8] CDC (1963). Human Rabies Death – Alabama. Morbidity and Mortality Weekly Report, Vol.12, p.300

[9] Gomez M.; Siekert R. & Hermann E. (1965). A Human Case of Skunk Rabies. Journal of the America Medical Association, Vol.194, , pp.333-335

[10] CDC (1965). Human Rabies Death – West Virginia. Morbidity and Mortality Weekly Report, Vol.14, p.195

[11] Bell, G. (1967). Death from Rabies in a Ten-Year-Old Boy (One of Two Cases in United States in 1966). South Dakota Journal of Medicine, Vol.20, pp.28-30

[12] CDC (1967). Case of Imported Rabies – New York. Morbidity and Mortality Weekly Report, Vol.16, p.258

[13] Cereghino, J.; Mason, L. & Sheehan, T. (1968). A Case of Rabies Encephalitis. Northwest Medcine, Vol.67, pp.857-860

[14] Rubin, R.; Sullivan, L.; Summers, R.; Gregg, M. & Sikes, K. (1970). A Case of Human Rabies in Kansas: Epidemiologic, Clinical, and Laboratory Considerations. Journal of Infectious Diseases, Vol.122, pp.318-322

[15] Emmons, R.; Leonard, L.; Degenaro, F.; Protas, E.; Bazeley, P.; Giamonna, S. & Sturckow, K. (1973). A Case of Human Rabies with Prolonged Survival. Intervirology, Vol.1, pp.60-72

[16] Hattwick, M.; Hochberg, F.; Landrigan, P. & Gregg, M. (1972). Skunk-Associated Human Rabies. Journal of the American Medical Association, Vol.122, No.1, pp.44-47

[17] Hattwick, M.; Weis, T.; Stechschulte, C.; Baer, G. & Gregg, M. (1972). Recovery from Rabies: A Case Reprt. Annals of Internal Medicine, Vol.76, pp.931-942

[18] Bhatt, D.; Hattwick, M.; Gerdsen, R.; Emmons, R. & Johnson, H. (1977). Human Rabies: Diagnosis, Complications, and Management. American Journal of Diseases of Children, Vol.127, pp.862-869

[19] CDC (1971). Human Rabies – New Jersey. Morbidity and Mortality Weekly Report, Vol.20, No.51, pp.459-460

[20] CDC (1972). Human Rabies – California. Morbidity and Mortality Weekly Report, Vol.21, No.9, pp.73-74

[21] Winkler, H.; Fashinell, T.; Leffingwell, L.; Howard, P. & Conomy, J. (1973). Airborne Rabies Transmission in a Laboratory Worker. Journal of the American Medical Association, Vol.126, No.10, pp.1219-1221

[22] CDC (1973). Human Rabies – Kentucky. Morbidity and Mortality Weekly Report, Vol.22, No.39, pp.325-326

[23] Sung, J.; Hayano, M.; Mastri, A. & Okagaki, T. (1976). A Case of Human Rabies and Ultrastructure of the Negri Body. Journal of Neuropathology and Experimental Neurology, Vol.35, pp.541-559

[24] CDC (1976). Human Rabies – Puerto Rico. Morbidity and Mortality Weekly Report, Vol.24, pp.94,99

[25] Baraff, L.; Hafkin, B.; Wehrle, P.; Emmons, R.;Gunn, R.; Overturf, G. & Steinberg, E. (1978). Human Rabies. The Western Journal of Medicine, Vol.128, pp.159-164

[26] CDC (1976). Human Rabies – Maryland. Morbidity and Mortality Weekly Report, Vol.25, pp.235-236

[27] CDC (1977). Human Rabies – Texas. Morbidity and Mortality Weekly Report, Vol.26, pp.31-32

[28] CDC (1977). Rabies in a Laboratory Worker – New York. Morbidity and Mortality Weekly Report, Vol.26, pp.183-184

[29] Houff, S.; Burton, R.; Wilson, R.; Henson, T.;London, W.; Baer, G.;Anderson, L.; Winkler, W.; Madden, D. & Sever, J. (1979). Human-To-Human Transmission of RABV by Corneal Transplant. The New England Journal of Medicine, Vol.300, No.11, pp.603-604

[30] CDC (1978). Human Rabies – Texas. Morbidity and Mortality Weekly Report, Vol.27, p.267

[31] CDC (1979). Human Rabies – Pennsylvania. Morbidity and Mortality Weekly Report, Vol.28, pp.75-76,81

[32] CDC (1979). Two Suspected Cases of Human Rabies – Texas, Washington. Morbidity and Mortality Weekly Report, Vol.28, p.292,297-298

[33] CDC (1979). Human Rabies – United States. Morbidity and Mortality Weekly Report, Vol.28, pp.315-316,321

[34] CDC (1979). Human Rabies – California. Morbidity and Mortality Weekly Report, Vol.28, pp.435-436

[35] CDC (1979). Human Rabies – Oklahoma. Morbidity and Mortality Weekly Report, Vol.28, pp.476-481
[36] CDC (1979). Human Rabies – Kentucky. Morbidity and Mortality Weekly Report, Vol.28, pp.590-591
[37] CDC (1981). Human Rabies – Oklahoma. Morbidity and Mortality Weekly Report, Vol.30, pp.343-344,349
[38] CDC (1981). Human Rabies Acquired Oustide the United States from a Dog Bite. Morbidity and Mortality Weekly Report, Vol.30, No.43, pp.537-540
[39] CDC (1983). Imported Human Rabies. Morbidity and Mortality Weekly Report, Vol.32, No.6, pp.78-80,85-86
[40] CDC (1983). Human Rabies – Michigan. Morbidity and Mortality Weekly Report, Vol.32, No.12, pp.159-160
[41] CDC (1984). Human Rabies – Texas. Morbidity and Mortality Weekly Report, Vol.33, No.33, pp.469-470
[42] Smith, J.; Fishbein, D.; Rupprecht, C. & Clark, K. (1991). Unexplained Rabies in Three Immigrants in the United States. The New England Journal of Medicine, Vol.324, pp.205-211
[43] CDC (1984). Human Rabies – Pennsylvania. Morbidity and Mortality Weekly Report, Vol.33, No.45, pp.633-635
[44] CDC (1985). Human Rabies Acquired Outside the United States. Morbidity and Mortality Weekly Report, Vol.34, No.17, pp.235-236
[45] CDC (1985). Human Rabies Diagnosed 2 Months Postmortem – Texas. Morbidity and Mortality Weekly Report, Vol.34, No.46, pp.700,705-707
[46] CDC (1988). Human Rabies – California, 1987. Morbidity and Mortality Weekly Report, Vol.37, No.19, pp.305-308
[47] Dempsey, D. (1990). The Case of the Missing Animal. The Pediatric Infectious Diseases Journal. Vol.9, No.1, pp.49-50
[48] CDC (1989). Human Rabies – Oregon, 1989. Morbidity and Mortality Weekly Report, Vol.38, No.19, pp.335-337
[49] CDC (1991). Human Rabies – Texas, 1990. Morbidity and Mortality Weekly Report, Vol.40, No.8, pp.132-133
[50] CDC (1991). Human Rabies – Texas, Arkansas, and Georgia, 1991. Morbidity and Mortality Weekly Report, Vol.40, No.44, pp.765-769
[51] CDC (1992). Human Rabies – California, 1992. Morbidity and Mortality Weekly Report, Vol.41, No.26, pp.461-463
[52] CDC (1993). Human Rabies – New York, 1993. Morbidity and Mortality Weekly Report, Vol.42, No.41, pp.799,805-806
[53] CDC (1994). Human Rabies – Texas and California, 1993. Morbidity and Mortality Weekly Report, Vol.43, No.6, pp.93-96
[54] CDC (1994). Human Rabies – California, 1994. Morbidity and Mortality Weekly Report, Vol.43, No.25, pp.455-457
[55] CDC (1994). Human Rabies – Miami, 1994. Morbidity and Mortality Weekly Report, Vol.43, No.42, pp.773-775

[56] CDC (1995). Human Rabies – Alabama, Tennessee, and Texas, 1994. Morbidity and Mortality Weekly Report, Vol.44, No.14, pp.269-272

[57] CDC (1995). Human Rabies – West Virginia, 1994. Morbidity and Mortality Weekly Report, Vol.44, No.5, pp.86-87,93

[58] CDC (1995). Human Rabies – Washington, 1995. Morbidity and Mortality Weekly Report, Vol.44, No.34, pp.625-627

[59] CDC (1996). Human Rabies – California, 1995. Morbidity and Mortality Weekly Report, Vol.45, No.17, pp.353-356

[60] CDC (1996). Human Rabies – Connecticut, 1995. Morbidity and Mortality Weekly Report, Vol.45, No.10, pp.207-209

[61] CDC (1996). Human Rabies – Florida, 1996. Morbidity and Mortality Weekly Report, Vol.45, No.33, pp.719-720,727

[62] CDC (1997). Human Rabies – New Hampshire, 1996. Morbidity and Mortality Weekly Report, Vol.46, No.12, pp.267-270

[63] Scully, R.; Mark, E.; Mcneely, W.; Ebeling, S. & Phillips, L. (1998). Case 21-1998 – A 32-Year-Old Woman with Pharyngeal Spasms and Paresthesias after a Dog Bite. The New England Journal of Medicine, Vol.339, No.2, pp.105-112

[64] CDC (1997). Human Rabies – Kentucky and Montana, 1996. Morbidity and Mortality Weekly Report, Vol.46, No.18, pp.397-400

[65] CDC (1997). Human Rabies – Montana and Washington, 1997. Morbidity and Mortality Weekly Report, Vol.46, No.33, pp.770-774

[66] CDC (1998). Human Rabies – Texas and New Jersey, 1997. Morbidity and Mortality Weekly Report, Vol.47, No.1, pp.1-5

[67] CDC (1999). Human Rabies – Virginia, 1998. Morbidity and Mortality Weekly Report, Vol.48, No.5, pp.95-97

[68] CDC (2000). Human Rabies – California, Georgia, Minnesota, New York, and Wisconsin, 2000. Morbidity and Mortality Weekly Report, Vol.49, No.49, pp.1111-1115

[69] Soun, V.; Eidson, M.; Trimarchi, C.; Drabkin, P; Leach, R.; Wallace, B.; Jones, G.; Cantiello, K.; Qian, J. (2006). Antemortem Diagnosis of New York Human Rabies Case and Review of U.S. Cases. *International Journal of Biomedical Science*. Vol. 2, No. 4, (December 2006), pp.433-444

[70] Krebs, J.; Noll, H.; Rupprecht, C.; Childs, J. (2002). Rabies surveillance in the United States during 2001. *Journal of the American Veterinary Medical Association*. Vol. 221, No. 12, (December 2002), pp.1690-1701

[71] CDC (2002). Human Rabies - California, 2002. Morbidity and Mortality Weekly Report, Vol.51, No.31, pp.686-688

[72] CDC (2002). Human Rabies – Tenessee, 2002. Morbidity and Mortality Weekly Report, Vol.51, No.37, pp.828-829

[73] CDC (2003). Human Rabies – Iowa, 2002. Morbidity and Mortality Weekly Report, Vol.52, No.3, pp.47-48

[74] CDC (2003). First Human Death Associated with Raccoon Rabies – Virginia, 2003. Morbidity and Mortality Weekly Report, Vol.52, No.45, pp.1102-1103

[75] Krebs, J.; Mandel, E.; Swerdlow, D.; Rupprecht, C. (2004). Rabies surveillance in the United States during 2003. *Journal of the American Veterinary Medical Association*. Vol. 225, No. 12, (December 2004), pp.1837-1849
[76] CDC (2004). Human Rabies Death Associated with Bat Rabies – California, 2003. Morbidity and Mortality Weekly Report, Vol.53, No.2, pp.33-35
[77] CDC (2005). Human Rabies – Florida, 2004. Morbidity and Mortality Weekly Report, Vol.54, No.31, pp.767-769
[78] CDC (2004). Investigations of Rabies Infections in Organ Donor and Transplant Recipients – Alabama, Arkansas, Oklahoma, and Texas, 2004. Morbidity and Mortality Weekly Report, Vol.53, pp.1-3
[79] Srinivasan, A.; Burton, E.; Kuehnert, M.; et al (2005). Transmission of RABV from an organ donor to four transplant recipients. The New England Journal of Medicine, Vol.352, No.11, pp.1103-1111
[80] Willoughby, R.; Tieves, K.; Hoffman, G.; Ghanayem, N.; Amlie-Lefond, C.; Schwabe, M.; Chusid, M. & Rupprecht, C. (2005). Survival After Treatment of Rabies with Induction of Coma. The New England Journal of Medicine, Vol.352, No.24, pp.2508-2514
[81] CDC (2004). Recovery of a Patient from Clinical Rabies – Wisconsin, 2004. Morbidity and Mortality Weekly Report, Vol.53, No.50, pp.1171-1173
[82] Krebs, J.; Mandel, E.; Swerdlow, D.; Rupprecht, C. (2005). Rabies surveillance in the United States during 2004. *Journal of the American Veterinary Medical Association*. Vol. 227, No. 12, (December 2005), pp.1912-1925
[83] CDC (2006). Human Rabies – Mississippi, 2005. Morbidity and Mortality Weekly Report, Vol.55, No.8, pp.207-208
[84] Blanton, J.; Hanlon, C.; Rupprecht, C. (2006). Rabies surveillance in the United States during 2006. *Journal of the American Veterinary Medical Association*. Vol. 231, No. 4, (August 2007), pp.540-556
[85] Shah, U. (2007). Rabies Investigation & Response: A Multi-Disciplinary Approach, Proceedings of the 135th APHA Annual Meeting & Exposition, Washington, DC, USA, November 3-7, 2007
[86] CDC (2007). Human Rabies – Indiana and California, 2006. Morbidity and Mortality Weekly Report, Vol.56, No.15, pp.361-365
[87] CDC (2008). Human Rabies – Minnesota, 2007. Morbidity and Mortality Weekly Report, Vol.57, No.17, pp.460-462
[88] CDC (2009). Imported Human Rabies – California, 2008. Morbidity and Mortality Weekly Report, Vol.5, No.26, pp.713-716
[89] CDC (2009). Human Rabies – Missouri, 2008. Morbidity and Mortality Weekly Report, Vol.58, No.43, pp.1207-1209
[90] CDC (2010). Presumptive Abortive Human Rabies – Texas, 2009. Morbidity and Mortality Weekly Report, Vol.59, No.7, pp.185-190
[91] CDC (2010). Human Rabies – Kentucky/Indiana, 2009. Morbidity and Mortality Weekly Report, Vol.59, No.13, pp.393-396
[92] CDC (2011). Human Rabies – Michigan, 2009. Morbidity and Mortality Weekly Report, Vol.60, No.14, pp.437-440

[93] CDC (2010). Human Rabies – Virginia, 2009. Morbidity and Mortality Weekly Report, Vol.59, No.38, pp.1236-1238

[94] CDC (2011). Human Rabies from Exposure to a Vampire Bat – Louisiana, 2010. Morbidity and Mortality Weekly Report, Vol.60, No.31, pp.1050-1052

[95] CDC (2011). Human Rabies – Wisconsin, 2010. Morbidity and Mortality Weekly Report, Vol.60, No.34, pp.1164-1166

Part 3

Protozoan Pathogens

12

Toxoplasmic Encephalitis

Yaowalark Sukthana
Department of Protozoology, Faculty of Tropical Medicine, Mahidol University
Thailand

1. Introduction

Toxoplasmic encephalitis (TE), a life-threatening disease in HIV/AIDS infected individuals, is an inflammation of the brain caused by the reactivation of latent infection of the protozoa *Toxoplasma gondii*. Immunocompetent host when infected with *T. gondii* is almost always unnoticeable or develops mild and non-specific signs and symptoms, then tissue cysts are the consequence harbored in those infected persons life-long, quietly without any problem. However, when host immunity is suppressed by any cause but mostly by HIV/AIDS, the previously quiescent protozoa become active and the aggressive stage, tachyzoite, causes severe clinical manifestations in the Central Nervous System (CNS) such as encephalitis or abscess.

In the early 1980s, at the beginning of AIDS pandemic, there were many alarming case-reports threatening the world medical community with increasing numbers of unknown causes and severe diseases presented in homosexual men, hemophiliacs and Haitian. TE was one of the most common opportunistic infections of this immunocompromised host. Huge efforts have been put on to combat with TE including budget, manpower and research on diagnostic methods, prophylaxis, treatment and prevention. The incidence of TE is now decreasing due to primary and secondary prophylaxis as well as immune restoration because of the HAART (Highly active antiretroviral therapy), but some old problems still exist and new ones have surfaced.

This chapter will focus on all aspects of TE including the etiologic organism, epidemiology, clinical manifestations, diagnostic methods, management and outcome as well as prophylaxis and prevention. Evidences from our research on *T. gondii* and literature review will be used as an input. With those frameworks, an extensive perspective on this fascinating disease will be forthcoming.

2. Etiologic organism: *Toxoplasma gondii*

T. gondii was discovered since 1908 simultaneously by 2 groups of researchers. Firstly, Charles J. H. Nicolle (1866-1936) and Louis H. Manceaux (1865-1943) from the Pasteur Institute in Tunisia isolated a new parasite from the African rodent, *Ctenodactylus gundi*, and differentiated it from *Leishmania*. Secondly, the Italian researcher namely Alfonso Splendore (1871-1953) who worked at Sao Paulo, Brazil identified this protozoan from the liver of rabbit (Dubey et al., 1970; Sukthana, 2006). *T. gondii* was named a year later by Nicolle and Manceaux according to its bow-like shape (Toxoplasma is from a Greek word: toxos means bow or arc; plasma means life) and gondii may result from a misspelling of the scientific name of its original host, the gundii (Ferguson, 2009a). The first congenital case of toxoplasmosis was described in 1923 and the first adult case was diagnosed in 1940 (Frenkel & Fishback, 2000). It was not until 1969 when its life cycle was completely known with cats and other felids as the only definitive host in which sexual reproduction takes place to produce infective oocysts. Human, warm-blooded domestic animals, birds, and rodents including wild and marine mammals are intermediate hosts that harbor tissue cysts in their bodies (Hutchison et al., 1969; Dubey et al., 1970; Dubey, 2007; Ferguson, 2009b). *T. gondii* was classified as coccidian belonging to the phylum Apicomplexa which is an intracellular organism (Dubey et al., 1970).

2.1 Life cycle and mode of transmission of *T. gondii*

There are 3 infective stages of *T. gondii* i.e. 1) oocysts produced and shed by cat and felid animals, 2) an active, rapidly dividing tachyzoite form and 3) an inactive dormant bradyzoite harbored in tissue cysts. Tachyzoite and bradyzoite, sized 2 x 9 µm, cannot be differentiated by light microscope, while the mature oocyst is an oval shape, sized 9 x 13 µm containing 2 sporocysts with 4 sporozoites in each.

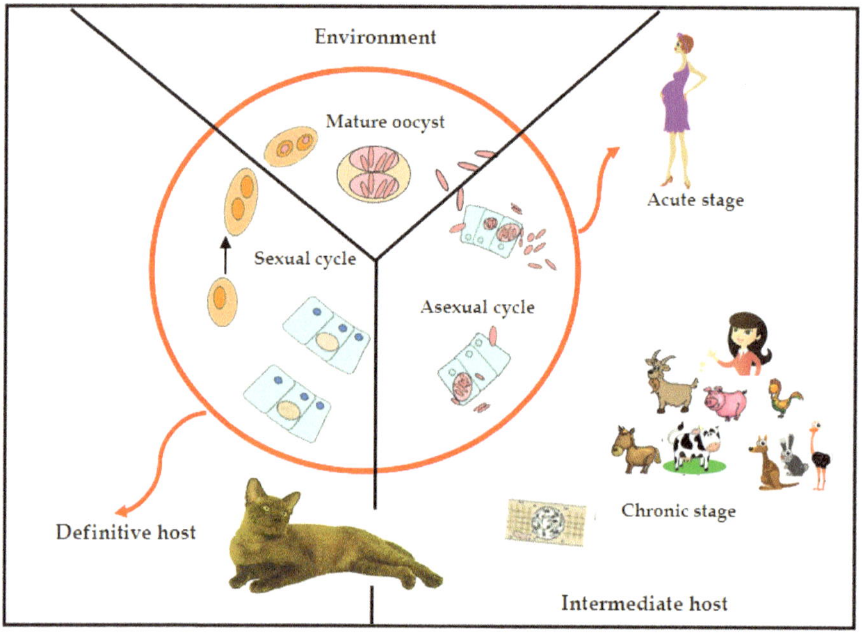

Fig. 1. Life cycle of *Toxoplasma gondii*: Cat and felids are only definitive host where *T. gondii* completes its life cycle. Intermediate hosts are human, warm-blooded domestic animals, bird and rodent including wild and marine mammals. Immature oocysts develop in the environment before becoming infected mature oocysts. Acute stage of infection occurs in both definitive and intermediate hosts, but turns to be chronic and develops as a tissue cyst in the intermediate host. Sexual reproduction occurs in cat producing immature oocysts.

When mature oocysts are ingested by hosts, sporozoites are released after exposure to gastric enzymes and invade enterocytes, whereas in asexual multiplication, multiple

fissions, occurs resulting in many tachyzoites causing cell rupture and subsequently they invade other enterocytes producing the active stage of infection (Figure 1). In intermediate host tachyzoites will shortly transform to be inactive bradyzoites and reside silently in tissue cyst for the whole life of the infected host. Thus the chronic stage of infection occurs. On the contrary, tachyzoites in definitive host modify to be macrogametocyte and microgametocyte and sexual reproduction occurs producing immature oocysts which when shed with cat's fecaes, need about 2-5 days to develop in the environment until mature as infective stage.
Toxoplasma is transmitted to human by 3 routes. The most common two are ingesting contaminated food or water with mature oocysts and consuming undercooked, infected meat where bradyzoites harbor in tissue cysts. The least frequent route is transplacental transmission which occurs only when the mother acquires primary infection during pregnancy. A European multicenter study including cities in Western Europe identified the consumption of undercooked meat as the strong risk factor for acquiring a *T. gondii* infection, whereas in Central and South America it is related with large numbers of stray cats that have access to the outdoor environment of which the climate favours and prolongs the survival of oocysts (Sukthana, 2006). Toxoplasmosis transmitted by cat excreta is not straight forward in Southeast Asia. Due to the religious belief, Malaysian and Indonesian Muslims prefer cats to dog as pet, while lots of stray cats are left in Buddhist temples in Thailand. Those settings should promote cat's excreta as a strong risk factor in that region. Noteworthy, human *Toxoplasma* seroprevalence in Thailand is much lower than in those two countries (21.9% vs. 44.8% and 58%) and correlated with cat seroprevalence (Konishi et al., 2000; Nissapatorn et al, 2004a; Sukthana, 2006). This might be due to high humidity and more rainfall in the latter countries suggesting that ground temperature is an important determinant of oocyst survival.

3. Epidemiology and risk factor

About 20% to 40% of individuals with AIDS develop TE from the reactivation of a latent *T. gondii* infection when the CD4 cell count falls below 100/mm^3 (Luft & Remington, 1992; Sukthana, 2000; Ajzenberg, 2009). The incidence of TE is thus directly proportional to the prevalence of antibodies to *Toxoplasma* in any given population. Before the advent of HIV/AIDS epidemic in 1981, toxoplasmosis was occasionally reported in immunocompromised patients, mostly in those with malignancies of the reticuloendothelial system and cardiac transplant recipients with lesions mostly outside the CNS. But, TE has become one of the commonest causes of focal brain lesions in Western Europe and North America due to AIDS pandemic (Luft & Remington, 1988). Since then, more and more TE cases in HIV/AIDS individuals were diagnosed worldwide. Nearly three decades from that point, nowadays to get a clearer picture of its epidemiology and clinical course, herein, three periods could be divided as: 1) TE during the beginning of AIDS pandemic period (1980s), 2) TE during prophylaxis period (1990s) and 3) TE during HAART period (1997-present).

3.1 TE during the beginning of AIDS pandemic period (1980s)

At the beginning of the 1980s, more and more of the mysterious cases with severe manifestations and fatal outcomes presented in homosexual men, hemophiliacs and Haitian. HIV was subsequently identified as the cause that impaired host immunity causing acquired immunodeficiency syndrome (AIDS) and opportunistic infections. In November 1982, the Centers for Disease Control (CDC) reported 19,744 AIDS cases from the United States, with

287 deaths and 54 cases have been reported from foreign countries (Gapen, 1982). Neurological involvement was seen in three out of four AIDS patients and TE was one of the most common neurological complications. Luft and colleagues (1983) reported acute encephalitis caused by *Toxoplasma* in 10 patients from Belgium, USA and Canada who had no underlying history associated with toxoplasmosis. All patients had a prodrome which varied from one week to 18 months. Three patients had disseminated toxoplasmosis with several organs affected (Table 1). Half of them had concomitant infections including tuberculosis, pneumocystosis, cytomegalovirus infection (CMV) and candidiasis. Other studies revealed similar pictures which reported neurological complications ranging from 20% to 41% with TE as the most or the second most common neurological disorders in HIV/AIDS patients (Luff, et al, 1983; Levy, et al, 1985; Berger, et al, 1987).

A 10-year observational studies from USA (Luft, & Castro, 1991; Richards et al, 1995) revealed at the end of 1989, there were 5,614 cases of toxoplasmosis reported to the CDC as the AIDS indicator disease and it increased to 14,059 (5.1%) of 274,150 adults and adolescents in the United States. The risk factors were observed as black male, intravenous drug users (IVDU), homosexual men, immigrants, Haitian and different geographic location. Richards and colleagues demonstrated that TE was more common among black males than white (5.2% vs. 4.2%, $P < .0001$) and was also more common among IVDU than among men with male sex partners (5.9% vs. 4.6%, $P < .0001$). Immigrants to the USA from Africa, Latin America and Haiti were three to four times more likely to develop TE than American-born (Luft, & Castro, 1991). The rate of TE was higher in the northeastern and southern states of America (5.6% vs. 5.5%) than in the north-central and western states (4.4% vs. 4.1%, $P < .0001$) this was related to the *Toxoplasma* IgG seroprevalence which was observed twice higher in the northern and northeastern regions than those in the western and southwestern regions (Richards et al, 1995).

In Africa, Europe, and South America, where the prevalences of chronic *T. gondii* infection were as high as 60%-75%, patients with AIDS who developed TE were three to four times greater than that in the United States whereas HIV-infected adults with latent *T. gondii* infection was less than 40%, only one-third of those patients developed TE (Luft & Remington, 1992). In France, 11% of AIDS-defining illness was due to TE in 1987, and rose to 23% in 1992 (Oksenhendler et al, 1994). Studies from France and Brazil in 1985 to 1990 reported the prevalence of TE in AIDS patients at 17% and 13% by presumptive diagnosis compared with 22% by definite diagnosis, respectively (Ragnaud et al, 1993; Wainstein et al, 1993). In Asia, the seroprevalence of toxoplasmosis was low, from 4% to 42.5% in Japan, Korea, Taiwan and Thailand, but was higher in India, Malaysia and Indonesia as 22.4% to 67.8% (Nissapatorn, 2009). The first documented case of TE reported in an international journal was from Thailand in 1992 (Sukthana, 2000), but a report in a local textbook showed 9.7% of cerebral toxoplasmosis as AIDS-defining illnesses from 1987 to 1994 and increased to 10.5% in 2001 and to 14.8% in 2002 (Chankrachang, 2004).

3.2 TE during prophylaxis regimen period (1990s)

In the 1990s, numerous TE cases as one of the common opportunistic infections in HIV/AIDS individuals were being diagnosed; medical researchers thus developed a clearer picture of its epidemiology and clinical features. For example, the incidence of TE was found to be 20.5 per 100 patient-years in France (Bossi et al., 1998), 15.9 per 100 patient-years in Swiss HIV Cohort study group (Furrer et al, 1999) and 4.0 per 100 patient-years in nine US cities (Jones et al, 1996). Khetsuriani and colleagues (Khetsuriani et al, 2002) studied the

Study period [References]	Study Location	Patients	Risk factors	TE Prevalence	Clinical features	Diagnostic procedures
1981-1982 [Luft et al, 1983]	Research Institute, Palo Alto Medical Foundation, USA	10 patients with acute encephalitis from Belgium, USA and Canada	Host immune deficiency by unknown cause in homosexual men, IVDU and Haitians.	All developed TE with disseminated toxoplasmosis	1wk-18 mo prodromic period Brain involvement with other organs affected such as lung, retina and heart	Serology (IgG and all negative IgM) Mice inoculation
1980-1984 [Berger et al, 1987]	Jackson Memorial Hospital, Miami, Florida, USA	132 AIDS patients with symptomatic AIDS (including : 55%Haitian, 27%homo-sexual men and 11%IVDU)	Haitian	39%	Fever Headache Alteration of semsorium Hemiparesis Ataxia	Histological diagnosis by Biopsy or Autopsy Immuno-peroxidase staining CT showing multiple enhanced ring-shaped lesions
1985-1990 [Ragnaud et al, 1993]	Bordeaux Regional Hospital, France	428 AIDS patients with initial CD4= 72 cell/mm^3	M:F= 2.8:1 Mean age 36.2 yrs 43% homo-sexual men 30% IVDU	17%	62% focal neurological deficit 58% fever 47%headache 45% altered consciousness 18% seizures	CT findings: focal mass 60% with and 40% without ring enhancement 59% multiple lesions 58% with brain edema
1985-1999 [Wainstein et al, 1993]	Hospital de Clinicas de Porto Alegre, Brasil	516 AIDS patients	-	13% by presumptive diagnosis and 22% by definite diagnosis	Fever with 92% sen and 56% spec Neurological focal signs with 59% sen and 82% spec Headache with 41% sen and 69% spec	65% by blood serology with 95% sen and 30% spec 49% by CSF serology with 77% sen and 56% spec By CT with 65% sen and 82% spec 125 patients by Autopsy

Study period [References]	Study Location	Patients	Risk factors	TE Prevalence	Clinical features	Diagnostic procedures
1981-1990 [Richards et al,1995]	San Francisco, USA	Homosexual men, with AIDS	IVDU, Homo-sexual men, Black male, geographic difference	0.05 cases/person-year of observation	-	-

Table 1. Summary of the data from studies on epidemiology and clinical course of toxoplasmic encephalitis (TE) during the beginning of AIDS pandemic period (1980s). IVDU = Intravenous drug user, mo = month(s), sen = sensitivity, spec = specificity, wk = week(s).

burden of encephalitis in USA from 1988 to 1997 and revealed TE accounted for the majority of 34.1% known causes of hospitalization due to encephalitis (21,504 hospitalizations; SE, ± 2,583). More than 97% of TE had been reactivated from the chronic quiescent *Toxoplasma* infection, nevertheless, few TE cases developed as acute infection (Richards et al, 1995). Only 30%-50% of HIV-positive patients with chronic *T. gondii* infection developed TE when their immune system became severely compromised. These were because host factors or virulence among different strains of *Toxoplasma* played a role in predisposing those patients to recrudescence of active clinical symptoms and signs (Luft & Remington, 1992). The research questions in that period was focused on when and what caused the reactivation to occur and how patients could be taken care of.

There were various retro- and prospective studies on the prevalence of TE, risk factors and prophylaxis worldwide (Table 2). To combat aggressive opportunistic infections (OIs) in HIV/AIDS patients including PCP, CMV infection and toxoplasmosis, medical researchers have unanimously agreed in giving primary prophylaxis to the population at risk of those OIs in suitable time. Primary prophylaxis should be given to prevent OIs when immune deficiency occurs and secondary prophylaxis would be continuously prescribed after acute opportunistic infections subsided. In general, HIV/AIDS individuals were mostly prescribed penthamedine, cotrimoxazole and dapsone as the prophylaxis of PCP and CMV infection which were more aggressive and occurred earlier than toxoplasmosis, when their CD4 were < 200 cell/mm^3. The matters had arisen whether those medications were also preventing TE and were good candidate regimens of appropriate dosage with acceptable adverse effect and adherence or compliance of the patients. In the case of TE, there were two things to be considered for primary prophylaxis which were HIV/AIDS infected person who was also seropositive of *T. gondii* antibody and CD4 was lower than 100 cell/mm^3 (Oksenhendler et al, 1994; Richards et al, 1995; Leport et al, 1996).

Table 2 summarized the data from studies which were carried out in the 1990s concerning TE epidemiology, prophylaxis regimens and outcomes. Cotrimoxazole or trimethoprim-sulfamethoxazole (TMP-SMZ) was the most popular regimen for TE primary prophylaxis, while Fansidar (pyrimethamine-sulfadiazine) was prescribed at the beginning of 1990 when CD4 was lower than 200 cell/mm^3 (Carr et al, 1992; Köppen et al, 1992). However, it was not recommended for the primary prophylaxis of TE because of its side-effects especially rash and allergy. Thus patients discontinued the prophylaxis and had higher TE reactivation. Pyrimethamine had bone marrow toxicity. When patients received without leucovorin supplement the survival rate reduced (Jacobson et al, 1994). Even though pyrimethamine was not recommended as a first-line regimen for primary prophylaxis of TE, some medical researchers considered pyrimethamine for patients who were intolerant to TMP-SMZ, especially in high risk patients with CD4 <100 cell/mm^3 (Leport et al, 1996).

TMP-SMZ was the drug of choice for prophylaxis for both PCP and toxoplasmosis (Carr et al, 1992; Richards et al, 1995). Therefore, there were various regimens ranging from 1 double-strength[1] (DS) tablet twice daily to 1 DS tablet 3 times weekly (14 DS tablets to 3 DS tablets per week) have been used. Ribera and colleagues (1999) found that since 1992, patients received either one of the following 5 regimens of TMP-SMZ for TE prophylaxis i.e.1 DS tablet daily (7DS tab/wk), 2 DS tablets daily 3 times weekly (6 DS tab/wk), 1 DS tablet 5 times weekly (5 DS tab/wk), 1 DS tablet 3 times weekly (3 DS tab/wk), and 1 single-strength (SS) tablet daily (3.5 DS tab/wk), they noticed the more frequent doctors began prescribing low doses of TMP-SMZ the higher number of patients receiving TMP-SMZ prophylaxis developed TE. Therefore, they studied to assess the efficacy of the various doses of TMP-SMZ as primary prophylaxis for TE and concluded that patients receiving low dose TMP-SMZ (<4 DS tab/wk) had a higher risk of developing TE than those who received high dose TMP-SMZ indicating 89% protective efficacy for high doses. An insufficient concentration of the low dose TMP-SMZ within the CNS may be an additional problem in the prevention of toxoplasmosis. Moreover, they also studied the potential interactions between rifampin and TMP-SMZ and hypothesized that rifampin may reduce the efficacy of TMP-SMZ.

Dapsone combined with pyrimethamine (200/75 mg once weekly) was more effective in the primary prophylaxis of TE than aerosolized pentamidine (300 mg every 4 weeks) and had the advantage of a lower cost and easier administration (Torres et al, 1993; Opravil et al, 1995). Girard and colleagues (1993) revealed dapsone plus pyrimethamine prevented first episodes of TE better, but they were more toxic than aerosolized pentamidine (42 patients discontinued dapsone plus pyrimethamine while only 3 patients stopped aerosolized pyrimethamine, $p<0.001$)

In conclusion, primary prophylaxis was the important strategy to prevent TE occurrence in the 1990s period. TMP-SMZ was the drug of first choice which was prescribed when HIV/AIDS seropositive to *T. gondii* antibody had low CD4 <200 cell/mm^3. By this practice, the prevalence of TE was reduced from 19% in 1988 to 6% in 1994 (Katlama, 1995). The incidence of TE was 3.9 cases/100 person-years (95% CI, 3.7-4.1 cases/100 person-years), patients who discontinued TMP-SMZ increased the risk of TE (Abgrall et al, 2001).

3.3 TE during HAART period (1997-present)

Since 1997, protease inhibitor, an antiretroviral drug, had been widely available, HIV-infected persons have lived longer and healthier lives. Since then, in the period of 15 years, that development was considered one of the great success stories of modern medicine. The death rate from HIV disease was reduced by 50 to 80% and changed from a fatal and hopeless illness to what is now a manageable chronic disease. The simultaneous combination of three or more different antiretroviral drugs was known as Highly Active Antiretroviral Therapy or HAART (Cooper 1996). It significantly delayed the onset of AIDS in HIV-infected individuals as well as reduced almost all opportunistic infections. The

---

[1] double-strength (DS) tablet contains 160 mg of trimethoprim and 800 mg of sulfamethoxazole, while single-strength (SS) contains 80 mg of trimethoprim and 400 mg of sulfamethoxazole.

incidence of TE was, with no exception, decreased from 3.9 cases per 100 person-years in the period before the availability of HAART to 1.0 case per 100 person-years in the HAART era (Sacktor et al, 1990; Abgrall et al, 2001). However, TE remained the most prevalent CNS disorder, accounting for one-fourth of all documented cases in both antiretroviral-treated

Study Design [References]	Drug Regimens	Outcomes	Significance
Cohort study in 83 AIDS patients comparing primary and secondary prophylaxis to prevent TE with follow up duration of 3-41 mo (median = 8 mo) [Köppen et al, 1992]	Aerosolized Pentamidine (AP) IAP: Primary prophylaxis IIAP: Secondary prophylaxis Fansidar (pyrimethamine/sulfadiazine PY/S) Ib: Primary prophylaxis IIb: Secondary prophylaxis	TE occurrence • 73% in IAP • 30.9% in IIAP • 5% in IPY/S • 2.3% in IIPY/S	Fansidar (PY/S) was recommended for use as prophylaxis when AIDS patients with ≤ 100 cell/mm³, if CD_4 100-200 /mm³ AP was recommended
Retrospective study in 155 AIDS patients who were referred to tertiary referral teaching hospital after PCP for following up of the TE complication within 3 year periods [Carr et al, 1992]	TMP-SMZ: 60 patients received trimethoprim 160 mg + sulfamethoxazole800 mg Low-dose i.e. 2 tab twice a week AP or P: Pentamidine (AP) and 17 patients received intravenous Pentamidine (P)	No TE occurred in patient who received TMP-SMZ with 1,153 days follow up 33% TE occurred in patients who received AP or P (95% CI, 19% - 51%, P=0.008) and TE occurred even patients have already received prophylaxis for 460 days	Low-dose TMP-SMZ was more effective (P<.008) than AP in preventing TE in HIV-infected patients with previous PCP
Randomized trial in AIDS patients who had CD_4 < 200 cell/mm³ with the 539 days follow up period [Girard et al, 1993]	D/PY: 173 patients received Dapsone 50 mg(D) plus Pyrimethamine 50 mg (PY) AP: 176 patients received aerosolized Pentamidine 300 mg (AP)	TE occurred 10.9% in D/PY gr. (19 out of 173) and 18.2% in AP gr. (32 out of 176) Patients receiving AP had 1.81 times higher risk of TE than those receiving D/PY (95%, CI; 1.12 - 2.94, p= 0.02) Patients infected by *T. gondii*, TE risk was 2.37 times (95% CI, 1.3 -4.4, P =0.006)	D/PY prevents first episodes of TE better, but more toxicity than AP (42 patients discontinued D/PY while only 3 patients stopped AP, p<0.001)
Prospective study in 278 AIDS patients who had CD_4 <250 cell/mm³ and follow up TE occurrence for 42-44 wks [Torres et al, 1994]	D: patients received Dapsone 100 mg, twice per wk AP: 176 patients received aerosolized Pentamidine 100 mg every 2 wk	6 TE events occurring among those receiving AP, compared to none among those taking D (p = 0.01).	D was more effective in the primary prophylaxis of TE and has the advantage of a lower cost and easier administration.
Multicenter, double-blind randomized clinical trial in 378 AIDS patients who had CD_4<200 cell/mm³ with 2.5 yrs follow up period [Jacobson et al, 1994]	PY: 264 patients received Pyrimethamine 25 mg (PY) trice per wk Placebo: 132 patients received placebo	Patients received PY had higher death rate (RR, 2.5; 95% CI, 1.3-4.8; p=.006) No difference between two groups of TE occurrence, this may be due to concomitant PCP prophylaxis with TMP-SMZ in both groups	PY had bone marrow toxicity when patients received without leucovorin supplement will reduce the survival rate, thus primary prophylaxis for TE with PY was not recommended.

Study Design [References]	Drug Regimens	Outcomes	Significance
The placebo-controlled study, randomized, double-blind trial. 554 HIV-infected patients who had CD4 < 200 cell/mm³ were recruited in France, USA and Spain. [Leport et al, 1995]	PY: 50 mg three time a week after a 100-mg loading dose on the first day plus folinic acid 15 mg three time a week Placebo: the similar in appearance and taste to PY plus folinic acid 15 mg three time a week	TE occurrence • 12% in PY gr. • 13%in placebo (RR 0.9; 95% CI, 0.6-1.4), The survival rate was similar, 85% and 80% (RR, 0.9; 95% CI, 0.7-1.2).	PY was not recommended as a primary prophylaxis of TE, but it should be considered for patients who are intolerant to TMP-SMZ, especially in high-risk patients with < 100 CD4 cells/mm3.
Randomized, open label, prospective trial in 197AIDS patients who had CD_4<200 cell/mm³ and no history of previous PCP or TE [Antinori et al, 1995]	AP: aerosolized Pentamidine 300 mg/mo TMP-SMZ: trimethoprim 160 mg and sulfamethoxazole 800 mg every alternative day D/PY: dapsone-pyrimethamine 100 mg/ wk and pyrimethamine 25 mg every 2wk	TE occurred • 25.6/100 person-year in AP gr. • 8.9/100 person-year inTMP-SMZ gr. • 9.4/100 person-year in D/PY gr.	Intermittent TMP-SMZ was more effective preventing TE than low-dose D/PY and AP D/PY was associated with a shorter survival.
Case-control study in 521 HIV-infection cohort study from 1993 - 97 by selecting 32 TE cases compared with 64 non-TE cases who were matched by CD4 and *Toxoplasma gondii* serostatus. [Ribera et al, 1999]	Low doses TMP-SMZ:< 4 DS (8SS) tab/wk (i.e. 3 DS tablets per week and 7 SS tablets per week) H igh doses TMP-SMZ: 14 DS/wk (7, 6, and 5 DS tablets per week).	Patients receiving low dose TMP-SMZ had a higher risk of developing TE than those patients receiving high dose TMP-SMZ (estimated protective efficacy for high doses, 89%).	High doses of TMP-SMZ were more effective than low doses for lowering the risk of TE in HIV-infected patients. Patients receiving concomitant rifampin treatment, rifampin may reduce the efficacy of TMP-SMZ.

Table 2. (cont.) Data from the studies on toxoplasmic encephalitis during prophylaxis regimen period (1990-1997). AP = aerosol pentamidine, D = dapsone, DS = double-strength, gr. = group, mo. = month(s), P= pentamidine, PY/S = pyrimethamine/sulfadiazine, PCP = *Peumocystis carinii* pneumonia, RR = relative risk, SS = single-strength, Tab = tablet, TMP-SMZ = trimethoprim + sulfamethoxazole, TE= Toxoplasmic Encephalitis, wk. = week(s)

and untreated HIV-infected persons, especially among severe immunodeficients and in the absence of prophylaxis (Antinori et al, 2004). The significant risk factors for TE occurrence were identified as decreased CD4 count and lack of prophylaxis against infection with *Toxoplasma* species. As demonstrated by Abgrall and colleagues (2001), patients who discontinued TMP-SMZ prophylaxis, received before and after HAART period, had 4.8 and 4.2 times increased risk of TE respectively. During HAART, patients whose CD4 cell counts increased to >200 cells/mm³, the incidence of TE was only 0.1 case/100 person-years (95% CI, 0.0–0.2) and TE was not increased even with the discontinuation of TMP-SMZ. On other hand, in HIV-infected individuals whose CD4 was lower than 50 cell/mm³, TE occurred in 12.6/100 person-years, the most common opportunistic infection followed by PCP at 11.4/100 person-years (Yazdanpanah et al, 2001). Other problems affecting TE occurrence even with the widespread use of HAART were patients unaware of their HIV serostatus and those who lacked exposure to HAART or prophylaxis. Thus they presented more with TE as AIDS defining illness than the pre HAART era. In cases who were accessible to HAART, the issues of patients' adherence, drug resistance, failure and cross-resistance were major risks for the development of TE (Yazdanpanah et al, 2001; Antinori et al, 2004).

The decreased incidence of TE and other OIs in HIV-infected patients from HAART raised the issue of discontinuation of primary prophylaxis preventing those OIs and secondary prophylaxis against opportunistic diseases. Furrer et al (1999) demonstrated no case of *P. carinii* pneumonia (PCP) and TE in patients receiving a combined antiretroviral therapy and their primary prophylaxis were discontinued after CD4 increased to >200 cells/mm^3 for at least 12 weeks, plus 14% of the total lymphocyte count. They also calculated the upper 99% confidence limits for the incidence of PCP at 1.93/100 patient-years, while it was 4.20/100 patient-years for TE. They thus recommended stopping primary prophylaxis against PCP, but not TE, in HIV-infected patients who received HAART and had a sustained increase (longer than 12 weeks) in their CD4 counts to >200 cells/mm^3 and to at least 14% of total lymphocytes. Because the number of TE patients who had been assessed were insufficient to recommend stopping prophylaxis, the same researcher group thus extended their study by accommodating more patients who were seropositive to *T gondii* with longer follow-up (up to 272 person-years) period. They reassured that stopping primary prophylaxis was safe in HIV- and *T gondii*-infected patients who responded to potent antiretroviral treatment with a sustained elevation in immunological markers (14% of peripheral lymphocyte count and the CD4 count remaining higher than 200 cell/mm^3 for at least 12 weeks), especially in the regions where the prevalence of *Toxoplasma* infection was high as in central and western Europe (Furrer et al, 2000).

Because of high toxicity, the discontinuation of secondary or maintenance prophylaxis of CMV infection and PCP were evaluated first and revealed safety discontinuing for patients receiving HAART whose their CD4 count was increased to >200 cells/mm^3 (Zeller et al, 2002). It was known that the risk of relapse after a TE episode was as high as 50% - 80% among patients who did not receive secondary/maintenance prophylaxis and survived more than 6-12 months (Miro et al, 2006). Studies were later undertaken to evaluate the safety of TE secondary/maintenance prophylaxis discontinuation. Concomitant results supported the recommendations of the US Public Health Service (USPHS) guidelines which suggested that secondary prophylaxis for TE can be discontinued for patients receiving HAART in whom either their CD4 counts remained >200 cells/mm^3 for 3–6 months or CD4 counts were >100 cells/mm^3 with their plasma HIV RNA loads were <500 copies/mL (Soriano et al, 2000; Zeller et al, 2002). However, those studies were primarily aimed at evaluating PCP prophylaxis discontinuation in the patients' CD4 threshold of <200 cells/mm^3. Miro and the GESIDA study group conducted a randomized, multicenter clinical trial by stratified HIV-infected patients according to the high risk of TE reactivation as CD4 count of <100 cell/mm^3. They found no episode of TE during a median follow-up of 25 months (409 person-years). Thus, they recommended discontinuation of primary prophylaxis in patients with sustained increase in the CD4 count of >200 cell/mm^3 for at least 3 months and advised to resume primary prophylaxis when the CD4 count was decreased to <100 cells/mm^3 (Miro et al, 2006). This group also followed 20 patients who developed acute TE and received HAART. It revealed the majority of their T cell responded to *T. gondii* antigen, interferon (IFN)-γ production and CD4 count of >200 cell/mm^3 were restored after at least 1 year of HAART. They concluded that the criteria for safely stopping TE secondary/maintenance prophylaxis should be when patients were on HAART for at least 1 year with an increase in CD4 count to >200 cell/mm^3 and with totally (<5,000 copies/mL) or partially (<10,000 copies/mL) suppressed viral replication for at least 3-6 months. Similar to primary prophylaxis, reintroducing secondary/maintenance prophylaxis whenever the CD4 count was decreased to <200 cell/mm^3 was a prudent practice.

It has been nearly 15 years since HAART was widely administered in advanced AIDS. Many benefits were well recognised and appreciated. However, there were reports of TE relapse after discontinuation of maintenance prophylaxis despite high CD4 count (Tsambiras et al,

2001; Ghosn et al, 2003). TE patients, from two large HIV centres in Germany, receiving HAART was studied regarding the restoration of *T. gondii*-specific immune response and IFN-γ as well as the longitudinal clinical characteristics/outcomes of TE (Hoffmann et al, 2007). Patients were grouped according to the date of TE diagnoses i.e. period 1, 1990-1993; period 2, 1994-1996; period 3, 1997-1999 considered as early HAART period and period 4, 2000-2004 as late HAART period (figure 2). The data from that study indicated several characteristics of TE that have changed since the availability of HAART such as a marked increase in 5-year survival rate as 7% in period 1 compared to 78% in period 3 ($p < 0.0001$). However, accumulative survival in the late HAART era was significantly lower than in the early HAART era (Figure 2). TE was found to be the first AIDS-defining illness more frequently than in earlier periods, therefore, patients who were co-infected with HIV and TE in HAART era did not receive antiretroviral therapy or any prophylaxis. More interestingly, persistent neurological deficits caused by TE such as hemiparesis, seizures, cognitive or other deficits were present in TE patients who survived during HAART higher than in pre HAART era (45% and 37%).

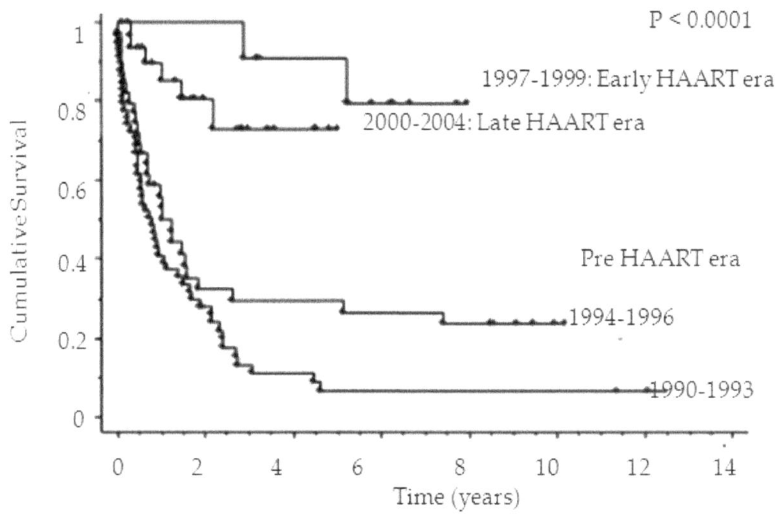

Fig. 2. Comparing cumulative survival of toxoplasmic encephalitis (TE) patients during pre-, early- and late-HAART eras (Hoffmann et al, 2007)

Hoffmann and colleagues found significant decrease in the *T. gondii*-specific immune response and IFN-γ (IL-12 and IL-15) in patients with acute episodes or relapses of TE more than in those who did not relapse even when maintenance therapy was discontinued. The latter was an adequate restoration group, while the former was a poor one in whom TE developed even on HAART and plasma HIV RNA level was below the detection limit for >6 months and their CD4 count were >200 cell/mm^3. There were evidences showing that functional immune restoration during HAART in advanced AIDS patients may be incomplete because quantitative increased CD4 count may not always reflect the quality of antigen-specific responses (Hoffmann et al, 2007; Furco et al, 2008). A multicentre study conducted by Spanish *Toxoplasma gondii* Study Group proposed whether *in vitro* lymphocyte proliferative response (LPR) and IFN-γ production in response to *T. gondii* soluble antigen extract (SATg) could be used as a useful biomarker indicating immune restoration in AIDS patients receiving HAART. They found that severe immunosuppressed patients whose CD4 count <200 cells/mm^3 with experience in current or previous TE did not develop immune restoration indicated by almost absent of SATg-specific LPR and IFN-γ production. Those biomarkers were found in patients receiving successful HAART and in immnunocompetent asymptomatic patients who did not receive TE prophylaxis, however, they may be absent in HIV-1-uninfected and *T. gondii*-positive healthy subjects. Therefore, they cannot be used as biomarkers to detect the status of immune protection against *T. gondii* reactivation. Nevertheless, the discontinuation of TE prophylaxis, especially secondary prophylaxis, can be safely withdrawn after successful HAART as shown by CD4 count >200 cells/mm^3 and a sustained reduction in viral load (Lejeune et al, 2011).

3.3.1 Immune reconstitution inflammatory syndrome (IRIS)

The administration of HAART in HIV-infected patients restores protective immune responses against a wide variety of pathogens and dramatically decreases mortality. An immune restoration process occurs by the suppression of HIV-1 viral replication followed by an increasing CD4 count. In some patients, however, during the initial institution of HAART, the restoration process may be complicated by immune reconstitution inflammatory syndrome or IRIS leading to worsening of clinical, laboratory and/or radiological features. Its histology showed an intense inflammatory reaction against intact subclinical pathogens or residual antigens of opportunistic infections and non-infectious agents. It occurs either by disclosure of occult subclinical infection or enhanced inflammatory response to a treated infection. The former is named "unmasking IRIS" while the latter is called "paradoxical IRIS". About 10-25% of patients on HAART may develop IRIS, particularly in those patients with profound immune suppression, which may occur days to months after starting HAART, but normally within the first 2 months (Howard & Manji, 2009).

The common neurological IRIS had been reported in cryptococcosis, tuberculosis, and mycobacteriosis (Murdoch et al, 2007). Despite TE being the most common opportunistic neurologic disease in HIV-infected patients, neurological IRIS associated with cerebral toxoplasmosis was rarely reported and has been doubted regarding insufficient clinical details challenging the diagnosis of IRIS. In contrast, Subsai and colleagues showed that TE and other abnormalities such as stroke, progressive multifocal leukoencephalopathy (PML), and cytomegalovirus (CMV) retinitis were among the commonest kinds of neurological IRIS in northern Thai AIDS patients (Subsai et al, 2006). Their findings were TE-IRIS accounting for 0.29 and 0.59 per 100 person-years in the first and second year follow-up, respectively. Moreover, they found the incidence rate of TE-IRIS lower than the previous incidence during pre-HAART era.

Sungkanuparpha and colleagues from 4 medical centres in Thailand reported one fatal case of toxoplasmosis after initial HAART institution in HIV-infected patient with very low median (range) CD4 count as 9 (0–147) cells/mm^3. In their study, 20% developed unmasking OIs and tuberculosis was the most common followed by cryptococcal meningitis. They thus proposed that immune reconstitution response to occult pathogens may explain those phenomena (Sungkanuparpha et al, 2002). Researchers from Toulouse University, France reported 9 unmasking TE-IRIS cases; 3 out of 65 TE cases from their institution with a study period of 9 years and the 6 remaining cases from published documents (Martin-Blondel et al, 2010). Their findings with other suggestion (Shelburbe et al, 2006) were proposed as a definition of unmasking TE-IRIS as 1) absence of neurological features related to TE in patients before starting HAART but presented afterwards; 2) at the onset of TE-IRIS, patients' CD4 counts were higher than when starting HAART and their viral load were decreased > 1 log_{10}; 3) histological features showed a profound inflammatory response with predominantly CD8 lymphocytes and 4) symptoms and signs were not due to other newly acquired infections, the expected TE course or drug toxicity.

Paradoxical TE-IRIS cases, in which an exacerbation of a past known and usually treated TE occurred, were also reported (Pfeffer et al, 2009; Tremont-Lukats et al, 2009; Cabral et al, 2010). Two HIV-infected known cases, without antiretroviral treatment, developed TE when their CD4 count was low. They thus received specific TE treatment and HAART and their immune status was restored as indicated by lowering of viral load and increased CD4 count. One and 3 months later, they presented with deterioration of clinical signs and symptoms related to TE. Imaging studies showed significant increase in size and stronger enhancement of the lesions as well as appearance of new nodular areas. Pathological study found an intense perivascular inflammatory infiltration, predominated by CD8 lymphocytes. One case (Pfeffer et al, 2009) showed both stages of cysts containing *Toxoplasma* bradyzoites and few tachyzoites, but negative in another (Cabral et al, 2010). Tremont-Lukats and colleagues (2009) reported a case of paradoxical TE, but was argued by another group (Martin-Blondel et al, 2009) because of finding abundant tachyzoites on brain biopsy, which is an active viable form of *T. gondii*, but not bradyzoite. Also, there was no evidence of an immune response of the affected tissues, so they suggested that the case might be due to an unfavourable course of a previously diagnosed toxoplasmosis than a TE-IRIS.

Despite toxoplasmosis-associated IRIS being a very rare phenomenon, nevertheless, it occurs. Low metabolism of intracellular *Toxoplasma* bradyzoites with less expression of immunogenic surface proteins hides it from the host's immunity, immune reconstitution during HAART is thus attenuated. The patients at highest risk are those with low CD4 count, HAART-naïve, of young age and starting HAART close to a recent diagnosis of opportunistic infections (Shelburne et al, 2006). If TE-IRIS is suspected, close observation is recommended within 2 weeks. The use of magnetic resonance imaging in association with clinical and laboratory data can reduce the number of unnecessary cerebral biopsies (Cabral et al, 2010). A high steroid dose to control IRIS (Venkataramana et al, 2006), uninterrupted HAART, and ongoing treatment for toxoplasmosis could resolve the problem.

4. Clinical features

Toxoplasmic encephalitis (TE) is the most common cause of focal brain lesion (FBL) in HIV/AIDS individuals with profound immune deficiency. Clinical presentations of TE depended on the location, number and size of the lesions. It may present with generalized cerebral dysfunction or focal signs and symptoms of the central nervous system (CNS) or with psychiatric abnormalities (Table 3). The majority of patients present with a combination of generalized and focal CNS abnormalities (Table 1) such as headache, fever, alteration of consciousness, confusion, cognitive impairment, hemiparesis, facial nerve palsy and convulsion (Berger et al, 1987; Ragnaud et al, 1993; Wainstein et al, 1993, Sukthana et al, 2000; Anrinori et al, 2004; Nissapatorn et al, 2004b; Chankrachang, 2004; Miro et al; 2006; Hoffmann et al, 2007; Ho et al, 2008). Headache was a more frequent symptom than fever ranging from 47% to 100%, while fever was found 45.6% to 64.5%. However, Ragnaud and

colleagues (1993) demonstrated that fever was more sensitive than headache when used as diagnostic criteria (92% v. s. 41%sensitivity).
TE has an insidious onset presenting initially by non-focal features such as headache, lethargy, cognitive impairment or confusion followed by focal neurological deficits which develop over a period of days to weeks (up to 4-6 weeks). The common focal neurological deficits are hemiparesis, ataxia and cranial nerve palsies (Mariuz & Steigbigel, 2001; Chankrachang, 2004). Convulsion was found to be the initial manifestations in 14%-39% of TE cases (Nissapatorn et al, 2004b; Chankrachang, 2004).

Neurological manifestations	**Clinical presentations**
Generalized CNS dysfunction	Alteration of consciousness
	Confusion
	Coma
	Cognitive impairment
	Stiffness of neck
	Headache
	Fever
Focal neurological deficits	Hemiparesis, hemiplegia
	Convulsion
	Cranial nerves deficit
	Dysphasia, Aphasia, Dysarthria
	Hemisensory deficit
	Papilledema
Psychiatric abnormalities	Dementia
	Anxiety
	Psychosis
	Personality changes

Table 3. Neurological manifestations and clinical presentations of toxoplasmic encephalitis

Neuropsychiatric abnormalities occasionally dominate the clinical picture (Mariuz & Steigbigel, 2001). Thus the diagnosis will be missed if those were not borne in mind. Meningeal involvement is rare, so that meningeal irritation is unusual on physical examination. However, nearly half of Thai TE patients had positive neck stiffness (Chankrachang, 2004; Mootsikapun et al, 2004). Diffuse form, without focal deficit, of TE showed rapidly progressive generalized cerebral dysfunction which was usually fatal. In such cases, histological study revealed numerous diffuse microglial nodules with *T. gondii* tachyzoites and cysts, hence brain CT scans were negative (Mariuz & Steigbigel, 2001).

Toxoplasmosis of the spinal cord is a rare manifestation and is usually associated with multiple lesions in the brain. Sites of involvement include the cervical, thoracic and lumbar spine. Few cases did not have brain lesions showing myelitis and myelopathic symptoms including a sensory level deficit, paraparesis, incontinence and changes in the deep tendon reflexes (Vyas, & Ebright, 1996; Kung et al, 2011). Kung and colleagues (2011) reported the first case of toxoplasmosis with myelitis in the absence of encephalitis and the diagnosis can be made pre-mortem by muscle biopsy showing multiple *Toxoplasma* bradyzoites and tachyzoites. Ajzenberg et al (2009) found a significantly higher TE occurrence in patients with AIDS than in patients whose immunosuppression was due to other causes than HIV infection (75% v.s. 27,8%). Patients with TE had a better outcome than those whose infection was non-cerebral, whereas pulmonary involvement was more frequently associated with death.

5. Diagnosis

There are no obvious or non-specific clinical manifestations of toxoplasmosis in competent hosts which are unique to the disease. Most of the time, infections are overlooked. Thus, it is not straightforward to diagnose. Serological testing in such patient is the main identifying evidence of specific antibody. In TE reactivation, clinical features are more helpful than serological testing in term of diagnostic criteria.

Centre for Disease Control and Prevention (CDC), the National Institutes of Health, and the HIV Medicine Association of the Infectious Diseases Society of America recommend that making a definitive diagnosis of TE requires 1) compatible clinical features; 2) single or multiple mass lesions by computerized tomography (CT), magnetic resonance imaging (MRI), or other radiographic testing; and 3) the most important is detection of the organism in a clinical sample. This requires a brain biopsy performed by a stereotactic CT-guided needle biopsy. Organisms are demonstrable with hematoxylin and eosin stains and immunohistochemistry staining by experienced laboratories might increase sensitivity (CDC 2009). However, these are always impracticable due to patients' conditions. For clinically suspected TE cases, CDC criteria should be applied for a presumptive diagnosis i.e. 1) the recent onset of a focal neurological abnormality that is consistent with intracranial disease or reduced consciousness; 2) evidence from brain imaging of a lesion with mass effect and ring enhanced appearance after injection of a contrast medium; and 3) positive serum antibody to *T. gondii* or successful response to anti-toxoplasmic treatment (Sukthana, 2006). By using these presumptive diagnostic criteria, the positive predictive value is achievable in approximately 80% (Cohn et al, 1989; Katlama, 1992; Luft et al, 1993).

On brain imaging, most of TE lesions occur in the basal ganglia, thalamus and corticomedullary junction (Lee et al, 2009). MRI is more sensitive than CT, Weenink and colleagues reported a TE patient who showed a normal contrast-enhanced CT scan, but MRI revealed clear abnormalities in the basal ganglia (Weenink et al, 2009). TE usually appears as multiple nodular or ring enhanced lesions with edema and mass effect. However, 14% of cases showing a solitary lesion which need to be differentiated from CNS lymphoma that more commonly presented as a single mass than toxoplasmosis (Legrand et al, 2010). Several techniques such as a diffusion weighted imaging; single-photon emission CT (SPECT) and positron-emission tomography (PET) could provide a more precise diagnosis (Sukthana, 2006; Legrand et al, 2010). Weighted MRI shows a peripheral hyperintensity of

TE mass lesion that is a feature helping to distinguish it from lymphoma. In comparison with TE and other infections, lymphoma displays high thallium uptake on SPET image. The rate of detection will be as high as 100% sensitivity and 89% specificity when the lesion is larger than 2 cm; otherwise it drops significantly if the lesion is smaller than 2 cm. PET imaging need more studies to determine its effectiveness (Lee et al, 2009). Among those techniques, none has high specificity and they are only useful when used in combination (Legrand et al, 2010). Moreover, they are costly and not widely available especially in resource-poor settings (Sukthana, 2006).

Routine laboratory tests of the cerebrospinal fluid (CSF) are not helpful for TE diagnosis because they are usually normal or non-specifically altered. Increased protein level could be seen in about 65% of patients, low glucose level in 8-52% and pleocytosis, predominantly mononuclear cells, in 27-40% (Collazos, 2003). Intrathecal level of *T. gondii* antibody is always low and of limited value for diagnosis because its sensitivity and specificity is about 60-70% (Collazos, 2003; Sukthana, 2006). Parasitic isolation from CSF is very rarely successful. Tachyzoites were seen in only 2 out of 6,090 examined ventricular CSF specimens and only 5 cases existed in the literature where a direct identification of *T. gondii* was possible by cytologic examination (Palm et al, 2008), however, those researchers reported a tachyzoites and bradyzoites of *T. gondii* directly seen in lumbar CSF cytology.

Most patients with TE have an evidence of past infection showing a low titre of *T. gondii* antibody, but it helps the diagnosis. The absence of the antibody thus argues against TE diagnosis (Collazos, 2003; Sukthana, 2006). Nevertheless, it is not impossible since 3-5% of patients with TE have negative serological finding (Collazos, 2003). DNA-amplification-based techniques greatly contribute to the diagnostic improvement. Blood PCR as a single test is not sensitive. CSF PCR produced disappointing results with low sensitivity (50%), although specificity is high (96%-100%) and the results usually are negative once specific anti-toxoplasmic therapy has been started (Collazos, 2003; Sukthana, 2006; CDC, 2009). Repeated testing and combining both CSF and blood PCR enhance sensitivity. Tachyzoite-bradyzoite stage-specific primers could provide a more precise diagnosis of reactivated toxoplasmic encephalitis, especially in recurrent cases (Contini et al, 2002; Cultrera et al, 2002; Mahittikorn et al, 2010). Sukthana used duplex reverse transcriptase PCR (RT-PCR) technique containing tachyzoite (SAG1) and bradyzoite (BAG1) specific genes developed by our colleagues (Mahittikorn et al, 2010) to diagnose Thai TE cases. It was found that RT-PCR technique is simple, easy to perform, and provides 85% positive predictive value when compared with CDC diagnostic criteria (to be published).

6. Treatment

The standard treatment of toxoplasmic encephalitis is a combination of pyrimethamine and sulfadiazine (PY+S). They provide synergistic action, pyrimethamine being an inhibitor of dihydrofolate reductase while sulfadiazine inhibiting dihydrofolic acid synthetase, an enzyme involved in folic acid metabolism. Dose-related bone marrow suppression, thrombocytopaenia and anemia by this combination could occur. Hence, oral folinic acid (leucovorin) is routinely given to prevent those effects without inhibiting the action of pyrimethamine (Petersen & Liesenfeld, 2007). Dose, duration and adverse effects of those drugs are shown in table 4. Serum levels of pyrimethamine on a dose of 25-75 mg/day ranging from 1 to 4.5 mg/l and its CSF level is 10-25% of the serum level. Sulfadiazine is well absorbed with good penetration into CSF (Petersen & Liesenfeld, 2007).

Treatment with PY+S has some limitations including 1) poor compliance due to side effects, particularly sulfadiazine; 2) the large number of pills needed; 3) unavailability in some countries; 4) high cost and 5) lack of an intravenous form. Nearly half of treated patients develop adverse effects such as gastrointestinal upset or rashes (Table 4) and require a change of therapy. Clindamycin is an alternative drug in the case of intolerance to sulfa-compounds. A 600 mg every 6 hours for 3-6 weeks by oral or intravenous route is recommended (Mariuz & Steigbigel, 2001; Sukthana, 2006; Dedicoat & Livesley, 2008). The efficacy and adverse effects of the combination between pyrimethamine and clindamycin (PY+C) seem to be comparable with pyrimethamine and sulfadiazine (PY+S) combination (Table 5). However, when using PY+C as a maintenance regimen, the relapse rate was twice higher (P = .02) than those who received PY+S (Katlama et al, 1996). Diarrheoa was more frequent on PY+C, while skin rash and fever were more commonly encountered in the PY+S group. More drug discontinuation occurred in the PY+S than in PY+C group (11 vs. 30%, p=.001). Therefore, Katlama et al (1996) suggested that a combination of pyrimethamine and clindamycin is a good alternative for acute treatment but is less effective for long-term prevention of the relapses.

Drug	Dosing/duration of treatment	Adverse effects
Pyrimethamine	100 mg orally twice for 1 day, (loading dose) then 50-75 mg orally daily for 3-6 weeks	Gastro-intestinal (GI) upset Rash Cytopaenias
Sulfadiazine	100 mg/kg (4-8 gm in four divided doses) orally daily for 3-6 weeks	GI upset Rash (including Stevens-Johnson syndrome) Cytopaenias Interstitial nephritis Crystalluria Encephalopathy
Or Clindamycin	600 mg every 6 hours for 3-6 weeks, orally or IV use	GI upset Rash Diarrheoa Pseudomembranous colitis
Folinic acid	10-20 mg orally daily for 3-6 weeks	

Table 4. Recommended dose, duration and adverse effects of the standard and alternative drug regimens for toxoplasmic encephalitis (Modified from Mariuz & Steigbigel, 2001).

Cotrimoxazole or trimethoprim-sulfamethoxazole (TMP-SMZ) is another regimen that has been studied and recommended as an alternative treatment in particular areas that pyrimethamine and sulfadiazine are not available especially in developing world (Torr et al, 1998; Béraud et al, 2009). Its efficacy was as high as 70-85.5%, while the mortality rate was low (Table 5). TE relapse occurrence was around one-third of the patients and successfully re-treated by TMP-SMZ. Rash and neutropaenia were the most common side effects which occurred in 12-13.8% of patients but only half required treatment discontinuation. With its low cost, availability in parenteral form with excellent diffusion into the CNS and wide availability in developing countries, TMP-SMZ thus could be the first-line drug regimen for curative treatment and prophylaxis of TE, especially in resource-poor settings (Torr et al, 1998; Dedicoat & Livesley, 2008; Béraud et al, 2009).

Atovaquone was studied as salvage therapy in AIDS patients with TE who were intolerant or failed PY+S or PY+C therapy (Torres et al, 1997). With a dose of 750 mg four times daily, 52% and 37% of patients were clinically and radiologically improved during the acute-therapy phase (the first 6 weeks), respectively, while 26% and 15% remained clinically or radiologically improved by week 18. Few patients' adverse effects that were associated with and resulted in discontinuation of atovaquone were severe rash, fever, hepatomegaly, and toxic epidermal necrolysis. Commonly reported adverse events that did not result in discontinuation of therapy were fever, headache, diarrhea, nausea, and rash.

Outcome		**Drug Regimen [Reference]**			
		PY+C [Mariuz & Steigbigel, 2001]	PY+C vs. PY+ S [Dedicoat & Livesley, 2008]	TMP-SMZ vs. PY+ S [Dedicoat & Livesley, 2008]	TMP-SMZ [Bérau et al, 2009]
Mortality rate		6-20% during the first 3 wk	19% vs. 6% (RR 3.17,95% CI 0.67-15.06)	0% vs. 0%	3.2%
Complete response	clinical response	18-55%	46.2%vs. 48.5% (RR 0.95,95% CI 0.55-1.64)*	70% vs. 70% (RR 1.0, 95% CI 0.74-1.33)*	85.5%
	neurological response	71% by day 7 and 91% by day 14			ND
	radiological response	25%	72-73% vs. 61 - 80%	68% vs. 62%	ND
Partial response		68-95%	-	-	TE relapsed in 30% of patients
Not response		5-12%	ND	ND	7.4%
Adverse effect		40%	60-62% vs. 58-60%	12% vs. 22%	13.8% (only 7.4% required treatment interruption)

Table 5. Outcome of TE cases after receiving different drug regimens therapy. *including complete or partial response defined as a resolution of TE or a greater than 50% improvement in the graded neurological examination. C = clindamycin; ND = no data; PY = pyrimethamine; S = sulfadiazine; TMP-SMZ = trimethoprim-sulfamethoxazole; vs. = versus; wk = week(s).

6.1 Clinical response and outcome

A complete response to standard therapy includes absence of neurological sequelae expected within 10-14 days. Luft and colleagues found that 50%, 86% and over 90% of patients had a clinical response after 5, 7 and 14 days of treatment (Luft et al, 1993). Seizures and headache could not be used to assess the clinical response to therapy. Complete radiological response was defined as disappearance of all initial lesions and the absence of any new lesion. Those who showed clinical response, neuroradiographic abnormalities were also improved within 2-6 weeks in 91% (Mariuz & Steigbigel, 2001). Since patients may have more than one complication, follow-up brain imaging was recommended 10-14 days after starting therapy in each case (Chang et al, 1995). Brain biopsy should be considered in patients who clinically deteriorated after 3 days of treatment or showed no clinical improvement after 10-14 days of therapy. Treatment failure occurs if there is progression of either relevant symptoms and signs or new abnormalities developed within the first 10 days. Many patients died or still had neurological dysfunctions despite receiving standard or alternative therapy as well as developing adverse effects (Table 5).

6.2 Maintenance (secondary) and primary prophylaxis

Life-long maintenance/secondary prophylaxis, after acute-therapeutic phase, using half the dose of therapeutic drugs to prevent TE recurrence is necessary because the available drugs are ineffective against the tissue cyst that could later be reactivated (Sukthana, 2006). The use of highly active antiretroviral therapy (HAART) suppresses the HIV viral load and improves the CD4 count, followed by a strong reduction of opportunistic infections, including TE. It has been confirmed in randomized, controlled clinical trials that maintenance/secondary prophylaxis could be safely discontinued after HAART administration and immune restoration successfully occurred. Table 2 and sections 3.3 entitled 'TE during HAART period' provide more details.

HIV-infected patients with CD4 count <200 cell/mm^3 and positive *T. gondii* antibody is indicated to receive primary prophylaxis preventing toxoplasmosis reactivation. Drug regimens, outcomes and recommendation provided in Table 2 and section 3.2 entitled 'TE during prophylaxis regimen period'. Serological study identifying the past infection is prudent in HIV-infected individual, appropriate primary prophylaxis should thus be administered.

7. Preventive measures

Prevention of *Toxoplasma* infection comprise two important measures i.e. infected-meats and contamination by oocyst from cat excreta. HIV-infected persons with negative *T. gondii* antibody should be recommended to consume only well-cooked meats or those frozen for at least 24 hours. Properly cooked until the internal temperature is over 60°C, correctly smoked or cured in the brine are safe, but microwave cooking is not (Mariuz & Steigbigel, 2001). Noteworthy, increasing animal-friendly production systems might increase *T. gondii* prevalence if cooking practice is not proper. Chumpolbanchorn et al (2009) demonstrated 64.03% *T. gondii* antibody in Thai free-range chickens, while low prevalence (2.3%) was found in animal-friendly pig production systems in the Netherlands (Kijlstra et al, 2004).

Limiting exposure to cats, their litter and soil contamination with cat fecaes are things to be practised as well as avoiding infective oocysts by daily disposal cat litter and thorough hand washing, keeping cats indoor and feeding with canned or well-cooked food.

8. Conclusion

Toxoplasmic encephalitis is the most common cause of focal CNS infections in people with AIDS. Its incidence has been reduced after prophylaxis was widely advocated, but the dramatic reduction occurred since HAART introduction. Although HAART restores immune status and improves the quality of life, some patients were complicated by immune reconstitution inflammatory syndrome (IRIS) with clinical and radiological deterioration. However, TE-IRIS rarely occurs. Clinical features of TE comprise focal and generalized CNS dysfunctions or with psychiatric abnormalities. Its insidious onset and clinical presentations depend on the location, size and number of focal lesions, which is usually multiple. The majority of cases were diagnosed presumptively including clinical relevance to CNS abnormalities, suggestive brain imaging and serological showing past *T. gondii* infection or response to anti-toxoplasmic therapy. Standard treatment is a combination of pyrimethamine and sulfadiazine for 3-6 weeks followed by either life-long maintenance prophylaxis or HAART to prevent TE relapse. Despite the efficacy of currently available drug regimens, the mortality and adverse effects continue to be problems for the responsible physician. Primary prophylaxis should be given to HIV-infected persons whose CD4 count is <200 cell/mm^3 to prevent TE reactivation. HIV-infected individuals with negative *T. gondii* antibody should be instructed on preventing *Toxoplasma* transmission by avoiding either consuming infected meat or ingesting contaminated food and water by oocysts from cat excreta.

9. References

Abgrall, S., Rabaud, C., Costagliola, D. (2001). Incidence and risk factors for toxoplasmic encephalitis in human immunodeficiency virus-infected patients before and during the highly active antiretroviral therapy era. *Clin Infect Dis* Vol. 33, pp.1747-1755.

Ajzenberg, D., Yera, H., Marty, P., et al (2009). Genotype of 88 *Toxoplasma gondii* Isolates Associated with Toxoplasmosis in Immunocompromised Patients and Correlation with Clinical Findings. *The Journal of Infectious Diseases*, Vol. 199,pp.1155–1167.

Antinori, A., Larussa, D., Cingolani, A. et al. (2004). Prevalence, associated factors, and prognostic determinants of AIDS-related toxoplasmic encephalitis in the era of advanced highly active antiretroviral therapy. *Clin Infect Dis*. Vol. 39, pp.1681-1691.

Antinori, A., Murri, R., Ammassari, A., et al. (1995). Aerosolized pentamidine, cotrimoxazole and dapsone-pyrimethamine for primary prophylaxis of Pneumocystis carinii pneumonia and toxoplasmic encephalitis. *AIDS*. Vol.;9, pp.1343-1350.

Béraud, G., Pierre-François, S., Foltzer, A., et al. (2009). Cotrimoxazole for Treatment of Cerebral Toxoplasmosis: An Observational Cohort Study during 1994–2006.*Am J Trop Med Hyg*. Vol. 80, pp. 583–587.

Berger, J.R., Moskowitz, L., Fischl, M., Kelley, R.E. (1987). Neurologic disease as the presenting manifestation of acquired immunodeficiency syndrome. *South Med J*. Vol. 80, pp.683-686.

Bossi, P., Caumes, E., & Astagneau, P. (1998). Epidemiologic characteristics of cerebral toxoplasmosis in 399 HIV-infected patients followed between 1983 and 1994. *Rev Med Interne*.Vol. 19, pp.313-317.

Cabral, R.F., Valle Bahia, P.R., Gasparetto, E.L., et al. (2010). Immune reconstitution inflammatory syndrome and cerebral toxoplasmosis. *Am J Neuroradiol.* Vol.31, pp.E65-66.

Carr, A., Tindall, B., Brew, B.J. et al. (1992). Low-dose trimethoprim-sulfamethoxazole prophylaxis for toxoplasmic encephalitis in patients with AIDS. *Ann Intern Med.* Vol. 15;117, pp.106-111.

Cavalcante, G.T., Aguilar, D.M., & Camargo, .LM. (2006). Seroprevalence of Toxoplasma *gondii* antibodies in humans from rural Western Amazon, Brazil. *J Parasitol.* Vol. 92, pp.:647-649.

CDC Recommendations and Reports. (2009). Guidelines for Prevention and Treatment of Opportunistic Infections in HIV-Infected Adults and Adolescents, Recommendations from CDC, the National Institutes of Health, and the HIV Medicine Association of the Infectious Diseases Society of America, April 10, 2009/58(RR04);1-198

Chang, L., Cornford, M.E., Chiang, F.L., et al. (1995). Radiologic-pathologic correlation. Cerebral toxoplasmosis and lymphoma in AIDS. *AJNR Am J Neuroradiol.* Vol.16, pp.1653-1663.

Chankrachang, S. (2004). CNS Infection in HIV-Infected Patients, In: *Infection: Molecular, Cellular and Clinical Basis,* Wattanasirichaikul, S., Aussadamongkol, K., Rigunti, M., Santiwattanakul, S. eds., pp.1703-13, Medsai Printing, ISBN: 974-92320-7-0, Bangkok, Thailand.

Chumpolbanchorn, K., Anankeatikul, P., Ratanasak, W., et al. (2004). Prevalence of *Toxoplasma gondii* indirect fluorescent antibodies in naturally- and experimentally-infected chickens (*Gallus domesticus*) in Thailand. *Acta Parasitol.*Vol.54, pp.194-196.

Cohn, J.A., McMeeking, A., Cohen, W., et al. (1989). Evaluation of the policy of empiric treatment of suspected Toxoplasma encephalitis in patients with the acquired immunodeficiency syndrome. *Am J Med.* Vol.86, pp.521-527.

Collazos, J. (2003). Opportunistic infections of the CNS in patients with AIDS: diagnosis and management. *CNS Drugs.* Vol.17, pp.869-887.

Contini, C., Cultrera, R., Seraceni, S., et al. (2002). The role of stage-specific oligonucleotide primers in providing effective laboratory support for the molecular diagnosis of reactivated Toxoplasma gondii encephalitis in patients with AIDS. *J Med Microbiol.* Vol.51,pp.879-890.

Cooper, D.A. et al. (1996). Clinical treatment. *AIDS.* Vol. 10, (suppl A), pp. S133-4.

Cultrera, R., Seraceni, S., Contini, C. Efficacy of a novel reverse transcriptase-polymerase chain reaction (RT-PCR) for detecting Toxoplasma gondii bradyzoite gene expression in human clinical specimens. *Mol Cell Probes.* Vol. 16, pp.31-39.

Dedicoat, M. & Livesley, N. (2008). Management of toxoplasmic encephalitis in HIV-infected adults-a review. *S Afr Med J.* Vol. 98, pp.31-32.

Dubey, J. P. (2007). The history and life cycle of *Toxoplasma gondii.* In: *Toxoplasma gondii. The Model Apicomplexan: Perspectives and Methods.* L. M. Weiss, & K. Kim, (Eds.), 1–17, Academic Press, New York.

Dubey, J.P.; Miller, N.L.; Frenkel J.K. (1970). The *Toxoplasma gondii* oocyst from cat fecaes. *J Exp Med,* Vol. 132 pp. 636-662.

Ferguson, D.J. (2009a). *Toxoplasma gondii*: 1908-2008, homage to Nicolle, Manceaux and Splendore. *Mem Inst Oswaldo Cruz.* Vol. 104, No. 2, pp.133-148.

Ferguson, D.J. (2009b). Identification of faecal transmission of *Toxoplasma gondii*: Small science, large characters. *Int J Parasitol.* Vol.39, No.8, pp. 871-875.

Frenkel, J.K. & Fishback J.L. (2000) Toxoplasmosis. In: *Hunter's Tropical Medicine and Emerging Infectious Diseases*, G.T. Strickland, (Ed.), 691-701, W.B. Saunders, London

Furco, A., Carmagnat, M., Chevret, S., et al. (2008). Restoration of *Toxoplasma gondii*-specific immune responses in patients with AIDS starting HAART. *AIDS*. Vol. 18,pp.2087-2096.

Furrer, H., Egger, M., & Opravil, M. (1999). Discontinuation of primary prophylaxis against *Pneumocystis carinii* pneumonia in HIV-1-infected adults treated with combination antiretroviral therapy. Swiss HIV Cohort Study. *N Engl J Med.* Vol. 29, pp.1301-1306.

Furrer, H., Opravil, M., Bernasconi, E., et al. (2000). Stopping primary prophylaxis in HIV-1-infected patients at high risk of toxoplasma encephalitis. Swiss HIV Cohort Study. *Lancet*. Vol. 24;355, pp.2217-2218.

Gapen, P. (1982). Neurological complications now characterizing many AIDS victims. *JAMA*. Vol.248, pp.2941-2942.

Ghosn, J., Paris, L., Ajzenberg, D., et al. (2003). Atypical toxoplasmic manifestation after discontinuation of maintenance therapy in a human immunodeficiency virus type 1-infected patient with immune recovery. *Clin Infect Dis.* Vol.37, pp.112-114.

Girard, P.M., Landman, R., Gaudebout, C. et al. (1993). Dapsone-pyrimethamine compared with aerosolized pentamidine as primary prophylaxis against *Pneumocystis carinii* pneumonia and toxoplasmosis in HIV infection. *N Engl J Med.* Vol.27;328, pp.1514-1520.

Ho, Y.C., Sun, H.Y., Chen, M.Y., et al. (2008). Clinical presentation and outcome of toxoplasmic encephalitis in patients with human immunodeficiency virus type 1 infection. *J Microbiol Immunol Infect.* Vol. 41, pp.386-932.

Hoffmann, C., Ernst, M., Meyer, P., et al. (2007). Evolving characteristics of toxoplasmosis in patients infected with human immunodeficiency virus-1: clinical course and *Toxoplasma gondii*-specific immune responses. *Clin Microbiol Infect.* Vol.13, pp.510-515.

Howard, R. & Manji, H. (2009). Infection in the nervous system, In: *Neurology: A Queen Square Textbook,* Charles Clarke, Robin Howard, Martin Rossor, Simon Sharvon eds, pp. 289-335, Willy Blackwell, ISBN 978-1-4051-3443-3449, Oxford, UK

Hutchison, W.M.; Dunachie J.F.; Siim J. C.; Work, K. (1969). The life cycle of *Toxoplasma gondii*. *Brit Med J,* Vol. 4, pp. 806.

Jacobson, M.A., Besch, C.L., Child, C., et al. (1995). Primary prophylaxis with pyrimethamine for toxoplasmic encephalitis in patients with advanced human immunodeficiency virus disease: results of a randomized trial. *J Infect Dis.* Vol. 169,pp.384-394.

Jones, J.L., Hanson, D.L., Chu, S.Y.et al. (1996). Toxoplasmic encephalitis in HIV-infected persons: risk factors and trends. *AIDS*. Vol.10, pp.1393-13939.

Katlama C. (1992), New perspectives on the treatment and prophylaxis of *Toxoplasma gondii* infection. *Cur Opinion Infect Dis.* Vol. 5,pp. 833-839.

Katlama, C. (1995). The impact of the prevention of cerebral toxoplasmosis. *J Neuroradiol.* Vol. 22, pp.193-195.

Katlama, C., Mouthon, B., Gourdon, D., et al. (1996). Atovaquone as long-term suppressive therapy for toxoplasmic encephalitis in patients with AIDS and multiple drug intolerance. *AIDS*. Vol.10, pp.1107-1112.

Khetsuriani, N., Holman, R.C., & Anderson, L.J. (2002). Burden of Encephalitis-Associated Hospitalizations in the United States, 1988–1997.*CID*. Vol.35, pp. 175-182.

Kijlstra, A., Eissen, O.A., Cornelissen, J., et al. (2004). *Toxoplasma gondii* infection in animal-friendly pig production systems. *Invest Ophthalmol Vis Sci*. Vol. 45, pp.3165-3169.

Konishi, H.Y. *et al.* (2000). High prevalence of antibody to *Toxoplasma gondii* among humans in Surabaya. *J Infect Dis*. Vol. 53, pp.238-241.

Köppen, S., Grünewald, T., Jautzke, G. et al. (1992). Prevention of *Pneumocystis carinii* pneumonia and toxoplasmic encephalitis in human immunodeficiency virus infected patients: a clinical approach comparing aerosolized pentamidine and pyrimethamine/sulfadoxine. *Clin Investig*. Vol. 70, pp.508-512.

Kung, D.H., Hubenthal, E.A., Kwan, J.Y., et al. (2011). Toxoplasmosis myelopathy and myopathy in an AIDS patient: a case of immune reconstitution inflammatory syndrome? *Neurologist*. Vol. 17, pp.49-51.

Lee, G.T., Antelo, F. & Mlikotic, A.A. (2009). Best cases from the AFIP: cerebral toxoplasmosis. *Radiographics*. Vol.29, pp.1200-1205.

Lejeune, M., Miró, J.M., De Lazzari, E., et al. (2011). Restoration of T cell responses to toxoplasma gondii after successful combined antiretroviral therapy in patients with AIDS with previous Toxoplasmic encephalitis. *Clin Infect Dis*. Vol. 52, pp. 662-670.

Legrand, L., Catherine, L., Brivet, F. et al. (2010). Solitary Hypothalamopituitary Toxoplasmosis Abscess in a Patient with AIDS. *AJNR Am J Neuroradiol*. Vol. 24,[Epub ahead of print]

Leport, C., Chêne, G., Morlat, P. et al. (1996) Pyrimethamine for primary prophylaxis of toxoplasmic encephalitis in patients with human immunodeficiency virus infection: a double-blind, randomized trial. *J Infect Dis*. Vol. 173, pp.91-97.

Levy, R.M., Bredesen, D.E., Rosenblum, M.L.(1985). Neurological manifestations of the acquired immunodeficiency syndrome (AIDS): experience at UCSF and review of the literature. *J Neurosurg*. Vol.62, pp.475-495.

López, R., Contreras, R., & Font, L. (1992). Presence of antibodies against *Toxoplasma gondii* in adolescents from the African continent. *Rev Latinoam Microbiol*. Vol. 34, pp. 49-52.

Luft, B.J. & Castro, K.G.(1991) An overview of the problem of toxoplasmosis and pneumocystosis in AIDS in the USA: implication for future therapeutic trials. *Eur J Clin Microbiol Infect Dis*. Vol.10, pp.178-181.

Luft, B.J. & Remington, J.S. (1988). AIDS commentary. Toxoplasmic encephalitis. *J Infect Dis*. Vol. 157, pp.1-6.

Luft, B.J. & Remington, J.S. (1992). Toxoplasmic Encephalitis in AIDS. *Clin Infect Dis*. Vol.15,pp.211-222.

Luft, B.J., Conley, F. & Remington, J.S. (1983). Outbreak of Central Nervous System Toxoplasmosis in Western Europe and North America. *Lancet*. Vol. 9, pp. 781-784.

Luft, B.J., Hafner, R., Korzun, A,H., et al. (1993). Toxoplasmic encephalitis in patients with the acquired immunodeficiency syndrome. *N Engl J Med*. Vol. 329, pp.995-1000.

Mahittikorn, A., Wickert, H. & Sukthana, Y.(2010). *Toxoplasma gondii*: Simple duplex RT-PCR assay for detecting SAG1 and BAG1 genes during stage conversion in immunosuppressed mice. *Exp Parasitol*. Vol.124,pp. 225-231.

Mariuz, P. & Steigbigel, R.T. (2001). *Toxoplasma* infection in HIV-infected patients, In:*Toxoplasmosis A comprehensive clinical guide,* Joynson, D.H.M. & Wreghitt, T.G. eds., pp.147-177,Cambridge University Press, ISBN,0521 44328 8, UK.

Martin-Blondel, G., Alvarez, M., Delobel, P., et al,. (2010). Toxoplasmic encephalitis IRIS in HIV-infected patients: a case series and review of the literature. *J Neurol Neurosurg Psychiatry*. Vol.26, doi: 10.1136/jnnp.2009.199919

Miro, J,M,, Lopez, J.C., Podzamczer, D., et al. (2006). Discontinuation of primary and secondary *Toxoplasma gondii* prophylaxis is safe in HIV-infected patients after immunological restoration with highly active antiretroviral therapy: results of an open, randomized, multicenter clinical trial. *Clin Infect Dis*. Vol.1;43,pp.79-89.

Mootsikapun, P., Chetchotisakd, P.,& Anunnatsiri, S. (2004). Toxoplasmic encephalitis in 110 adult Thai AIDS patients: a retrospective review, *15th International Conference on AIDS*, Bangkok, Thailand, June 2004.

Murdoch, D.M., Venter, W.D., Van Rie, A., et al. (2007). Immune reconstitution inflammatory syndrome (IRIS): review of common infectious manifestations and treatment options. *AIDS Res Ther* Vol. 4, pp.9.

Nissapatorn, V. & Abdullah, K.A. *et al.* (2004). Review on human toxoplasmosis in Malaysia: the past, present and prospective future. *Southeast Asian J Trop Med Public Health.* Vol. 35, pp.24-30.

Nissapatorn, V. (2009). Toxoplasmosis in HIV/AIDS: a living legacy. *Southeast Asian J Trop Med Public Health.* Vol. 40, pp.1158-1178.

Nissapatorn, V., Lee, C., Quek, K.F., et al. (2004). Toxoplasmosis in HIV/AIDS patients: a current situation. *Jpn J Infect Dis.* Vol.57, pp,160-165.

Oksenhendler, E, et al. (1994). *Toxoplasma gondii* infection in advanced HIV infection. *AIDS.* Vol. 8, pp.483-487.

Opravil, M., Hirschel, B., Lazzarin, A. et al. (1995). Once-weekly administration of dapsone/pyrimethamine vs. aerosolized pentamidine as combined prophylaxis for Pneumocystis carinii pneumonia and toxoplasmic encephalitis in human immunodeficiency virus-infected patients. *Clin Infect Dis.* Vol. 20, pp.531-541.

Palm, C., Tumani, H., Pietzcker, T., et al. (2008). Diagnosis of cerebral toxoplasmosis by detection of Toxoplasma gondii tachyzoites in cerebrospinal fluid. *J Neurol.* Vol.255, pp. 939-941.

Petersen, E. & Liesenfeld, O. (2007). Clinical Disease and Diagnostics, In: *Toxoplasma gondii: the Model Apicomplexan: Perspective and Methods,* Wiss, L.M. & Kim, K. eds, pp.81-100, Elsevier, ISBN,13:978-0-12-369542-0, London

Pfeffer, G., Prout, A., Hooge, J., et al. (2009). Biopsy-proven immune reconstitution syndrome in a patient with AIDS and cerebral toxoplasmosis. *Neurology.* Vol. 73,pp.321–322.

Ragnaud, J.M., Morlat, P., Dupon, M., et al. (1993). Cerebral toxoplasmosis in AIDS. 73 cases. Clinical Epidemiology Group on AIDS in Aquitania. *Presse Med.* Vol.22, pp.903-908.

Ribera, E., Fernandez-Sola, A., Juste, C.et al. (1999). Comparison of high and low doses of trimethoprim-sulfamethoxazole for primary prevention of toxoplasmic encephalitis in human immunodeficiency virus-infected patients. *Clin Infect Dis.* Vol. 29, pp.1461-1466.

Richards, F.O. Jr, Kovacs, J.A, & Luft, B.J. (1995). Preventing toxoplasmic encephalitis in persons infected with human immunodeficiency virus. *Clin Infect Dis.* Vol. 21 Suppl 1, pp.S49-56.

Sacktor, N., Lyles, R.H., Skolasky R, et al. (1990). HIV-associated neurologic disease incidence changes: Multicenter AIDS Cohort Study, 1990–1998. *Neurology* Vol. 56, pp.257-260.

Shelburne, S.A., Montes, M., & Hamill, R.J. (2006). Immune reconstitution inflammatory syndrome: more answers, more questions. *J Antimicrob Chemother.* Vol. 57, pp. 167-170.

Soriano, V., Dona, C., Rodríguez-Rosado, R., et al. (2000). Discontinuation of secondary prophylaxis for opportunistic infections in HIV-infected patients receiving highly active antiretroviral therapy. *AIDS.* Vol. 10, pp.383-386.

Subsai, K., Kanoksri, S., Siwaporn, C., et al. (2006). Neurological complications in AIDS patients receiving HAART: a 2-year retrospective study. *Eur J Neurol.* Vol. 13, pp.233-239.

Sukthana, Y. (2006). Toxoplasmosis: beyond animals to humans. *Trends Parasitol,* Vol. 22, pp. 137-142.

Sukthana, Y., Chintana, T., Lekkla, A. (2000). *Toxoplasma gondii* antibody in HIV-infected persons. *J Med Assoc Thai.* Vol. 83, pp. 681-684.

Sungkanuparpha, S., Vibhagoola, A., Mootsikapunb, P., et al, (2002). Opportunistic infections after the initiation of highly active antiretroviral therapy in advanced AIDS patients in an area with a high prevalence of tuberculosis. *The 42nd Interscience Conference on Antimicrobial Agents and Chemotherapy,* San Diego, 2002.

Torre, D., Casari, S., Speranza, F., et al. (1998). Randomized trial of trimethoprim-sulfamethoxazole versus pyrimethamine-sulfadiazine for therapy of Toxoplasmic encephalitis in patients with AIDS. *Antimicrob Agents Chemother* Vol. 42, pp.1346–1349.

Torres, R.A., Barr, M., Thorn, M., et al. (1993). Randomized trial of dapsone and aerosolized pentamidine for the prophylaxis of *Pneumocystis carinii* pneumonia and toxoplasmic encephalitis. *Am J Med.* Vol.95, pp. 573-583.

Torres, R.A., Weinberg, W., Stansell, J., et al. (1997). Atovaquone for Salvage Treatment and Suppression of Toxoplasmic Encephalitis in Patients with AIDS. *CID.* Vol. 24, pp.422-429.

Tremont-Lukats, I.W., Garciarena, P., Juarbe, R., et al. (2009). The immune inflammatory reconstitution syndrome and central nervous system toxoplasmosis. *Ann Intern Med.* Vol. 150, pp. 656–657.

Tsambiras, P.E., Larkin, J.A., Houston, S.H. (2001). Case report. Toxoplasma encephalitis after initiation of HAART. *AIDS Read.* Vol.11, pp. 608-610.

Venkataramana, A., Pardo, C.A., McArthur, J.C., et al. (2006). Immune reconstitution inflammatory syndrome in the CNS of HIV-infected patients. *Neurology.*Vol.67, pp. 383-388.

Vyas, R. & Ebright, J.R. (1996). Toxoplasmosis of the spinal cord in a patient with AIDS: case report and review. *Clin Inf Dis.* Vol.23, pp.1061–1065.

Wainstein, M.V., *et al.* (1993). The sensitivity and specificity of the clinical, serological and tomographic diagnosis of *Toxoplasma gondii* encephalitis in the acquired immunodeficiency syndrome (AIDS). *Rev Soc Bras Med Trop.* Vol.26, pp. 71-75.

Weenink, J.J., Weenink, A.G., Geerlings, S.E., et al. (2009). Severe cerebral toxoplasma infection cannot be excluded by a normal CT scan. *Neth J Med*. Vol.67, pp. 150-152.

Yazdanpanah, Y., Chêne, G., Losina, E. et al. (2001). Incidence of primary opportunistic infections in two human immunodeficiency virus-infected French clinical cohorts. *Int J Epidemiol*. Vol.30, pp. 864-871.

Zeller, V., Truffot, C., Agher, R., et al. (2002). Discontinuation of secondary prophylaxis against disseminated Mycobacterium avium complex infection and toxoplasmic encephalitis. *Clin Infect Dis*. Vol. 34, pp. 662-667.

13

Encephalitis Due to Free Living Amoebae: An Emerging Issue in Human Health

Jacob Lorenzo-Morales, Carmen Mª Martín-Navarro, Enrique Martínez-Carretero, José E. Piñero and Basilio Valladares
University Institute of Tropical Diseases and Public Health of the Canary Islands, University of La Laguna, Tenerife, Canary Islands Spain

1. Introduction

Free-living amoebae (FLA) belonging to *Acanthamoeba* and *Sappinia* genera as well as *Balamuthia mandrillaris* and *Naegleria fowleri* species are aerobic, mitochondriate, eukaryotic protists that occur worldwide and can potentially cause infections in humans and other animals (Visvesvara and Maguire, 2006; Visvesvara et al., 2007). Due to the fact that these amoebae have the ability to exist as free-living organisms in nature and only occasionally invade a host and live as parasites within host tissue, they have also been called amphizoic amoebae (Page, 1988).

All four amoebae are known so far to cause infections of the central nervous system (CNS). Several species of *Acanthamoeba* (i.e. *A. castellanii*, *A. culbertsoni*, *A. hatchetti*, *A. polyphaga*, *A. rhysodes*), the only known species of *Balamuthia*, *B. mandrillaris*, two species of *Sappinia* genus, *S. diploidea* and *S.pedata*, and only one species of *Naegleria*, *N. fowleri*, are known to cause disease in humans and other animals (Khan, 2006; Visvesvara et al., 2007).

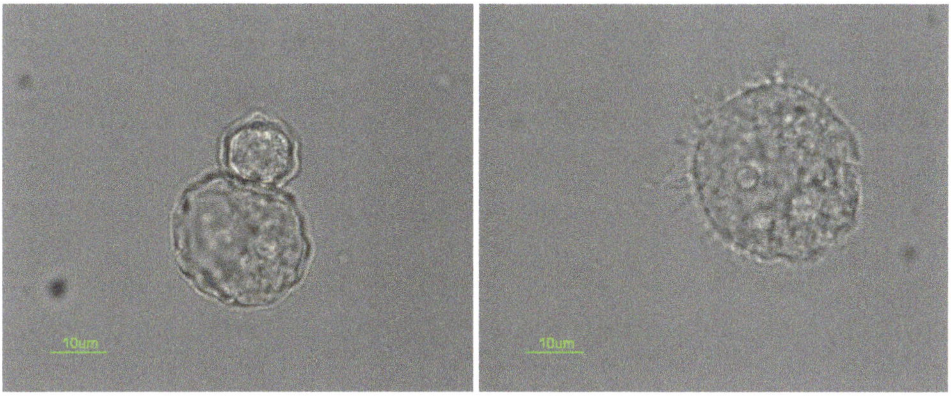

Fig. 1. Trophozoite (right) and Cyst stages (left) in *Acanthamoeba* sp.

2. Central nervous systems infections due to free living amoebae

The waterborne disease Primary Amoebic Meningoencephalitis (PAM) was discovered in Australia in the 1960s. Since then, it has been reported from about 15 other countries in Africa, Asia, Europe and North and South America. PAM is caused by *Naegleria fowleri*, and follows intranasal infection during swimming in warm, contaminated freshwater. Most victims have been children or young adults and the disease is almost invariably fatal. Infections have been linked with warm waters such as above-ground pipelines, tropical lakes, geothermal water, heated swimming pools or discharges of industrial cooling water. Until recent cases in the USA were identified, Australia was the only country where *Naegleria fowleri* has been associated with public water supplies (Visvesvara et al., 2007; Heggie, 2010). Recently, the causal agent of a PAM case in the US was diagnosed as *Paravahlkampfia francinae* n. sp., a new species of the free-living amoeba genus *Paravahlkampfia* that was isolated from the cerebrospinal fluid of a patient with headache, sore throat, and vomiting, presenting typical symptoms of PAM caused by *Naegleria fowleri*. Thus awareness of novel emerging amoebae as causative agents of PAM should also be considered (Visvesvara et al., 2009).

PAM should be suspected in young adults and children with acute neurological symptoms as described below and recent exposure to fresh water. The time from initial contact (swimming, diving, water skiing, or simply immersing head in water) to onset of illness is usually 5–7 days, and may even be as short at 24 h. Because there are no distinctive clinical features that differentiate PAM from acute pyogenic or bacterial meningoencephalitis it is imperative that the attending physician obtains information regarding the patient's contact with fresh water, including hot springs, during the past week. The earliest symptoms are sudden appeareance of headaches, high temperature, nuchal rigidity, followed by nausea, vomiting, irritability and restlessness. Nuchal rigidity usually occurs with positive Kernig and Brudzinski signs. Photophobia may occur late in the clinical course, followed by neurological abnormalities, including lethargy, seizures, confusion, coma, diplopia or bizarre behaviour, leading to death within a week. Cranial nerve palsies (third, fourth, and sixth cranial nerves) may indicate brain edema and herniation. Intracranial pressure is usually raised to 600 mm H_2O or higher. Cardiac rhythm abnormalities and myocardial necrosis have been found in some cases (Martinez, 1980; Visvesvara et al., 2007).

CSF may vary in colour from greyish to yellowish-white, and may be tinged red with a few red cells (250 mm^{-3}) in the early stages of disease. However, as the disease progresses the red blood cell number increases to as high as 24.600 mm^{-3}. The white blood cell count, predominantly polymorphonuclear leukocytes (PMN), also may vary from 300 cells mm^{-3} to as high as 26000 mm^{-3}. No bacteria are seen. The CSF pressure is usually elevated (300–600 mm H_2O). The protein concentration may range from 100 mg per 100 ml to 1000 mg per 100 ml, and glucose may be 10 mg/100 mL or lower (Martinez, 1980; Visvesvara & Maguire, 2006; Visvesvara et al., 2007). The cause of death is usually increased intracranial pressure with brain herniation, leading to cardiopulmonary arrest and pulmonary edema (Martinez, 1980; Visvesvara & Maguire, 2006; Visvesvara et al., 2007).

Many species of *Acanthamoeba* can cause Granulomatous Amoebic Encephalitis (GAE) also known as *Acanthamoeba* Granulomatous Encephalitis (AGE) (Khan, 2006; da Rocha-Azevedo et al., 2009), is a rare, chronic, progressive infection of the CNS that may involve the lungs (da Rocha-Azevedo et al., 2009). AGE is usually associated with an underlying debilitating disease or immune suppressed individuals including HIV-AIDS patients, diabetics, individuals undergoing organ transplants or cancer chemotherapy, and drug abusers (Khan, 2006; Visvesvara et al., 2007; da Rocha-Azevedo et al., 2009).

Therefore, the onset of AGE is slow and subtle and develops as a chronic disease from several weeks to months (Visvesvara & Maguire, 2006, Visvesvara et al. 2007). The usual features of AGE consist of headache, stiff neck, and mental-state abnormalities, as well as nausea, vomiting, low-grade fever, lethargy, cerebellar ataxia, visual disturbances, hemiparesis, seizures and coma. Facial palsy with numbness resulting in facial asymmetry is often seen. Cerebral hemispheres are usually the most heavily affected CNS tissue. They are often edematous, with extensive hemorrhagic necrosis involving the temporal, parietal, and occipital lobes. Computerized tomography (CT) scans of the brain show large, low-density abnormalities mimicking a single or multiple space-occupying mass. Magnetic resonance imaging (MRI) with enhancements shows multiple, ring-enhancing lesions in the brain (Seijo-Martínez et al., 2000; Shirwadkar et al. 2006; Visvesvara et al., 2007).

Acanthamoebae infecting the CNS are not readily found in the cerebrospinal fluid (CSF), although they have been isolated from the CSF in a few cases. *Acanthamoeba* that had apparently entered from the nasopharynx through a fistula have been detected in the CSF of a patient without CNS disease (Petry et al., 2006). CSF examination in general reveals lymphocytic pleocytosis with mild elevation of protein and normal or slightly depressed glucose. Examination of the autopsied brain reveals cerebral edema, areas of cortical and basal ganglia softening, and multiple necrotic and hemorrhagic areas of CNS tissues. The brainstem, cerebral hemispheres and cerebellum may show areas of hemorrhagic infarcts. Histological examination reveals the presence of multinucleated giant cells in the cerebral hemispheres, brain stem, mid-brain, cerebellum, and basal ganglion. Necrotic tissue with lipid-containing macrophages and neovascularization suggesting a tumour is often seen. Trophozoites and cysts of acanthamoebae are usually spread all over the infected tissue. Many blood vessels are thrombotic with fibrinoid necrosis and cuffed by polymorphonuclear leukocytes, amoebic trophozoites, and cysts. Multinucleated giant cells forming granulomas may be seen in immunocompetent patients but less often in immunocompromised patients.

Some infected individuals, mostly with HIV/AIDS, develop chronic ulcerative skin lesions, abscesses, or erythematous nodules (Seijo-Martínez et al., 2000; Visvesvara & Maguire, 2006, Visvesvara et al., 2007), especially of the chest and limbs. These nodules are usually solid but sometimes they become ulcerated and purulent. The prodromal period is unknown and several weeks or months may elapse following infection before the disease becomes apparent. Because of the time delay, the precise portal of entry is not clearly known, but the wide dissemination of these amoebae in the environment allows for many possible contacts and modes of infection. Trophic amoebae and/or cysts of *Acanthamoeba* have been isolated from the nasal mucosa of healthy individuals, suggesting a nasopharyngeal route as one means of invasion. Amoebae may also enter the body through ulcers in the skin, resulting in hematogenous dissemination to the lungs and brain, or by inhalation of amoebic cysts (Visvesvara & Maguire, 2006; Visvesvara et al 2007).

In addition to causing CNS infections, *Acanthamoeba* also causes a vision-threatening disease, ***Acanthamoeba* keratitis** (AK) which mostly affects contact lens wearers although many cases have been reported worldwide in non contact lens users mostly related to a previous corneal trauma [6, 7, 8]. The number of affected individuals is increasing worldwide. Morever, recent outbreaks of *Acanthamoeba* keratitis have been recently reported in the United States and Australia (Verani et al., 2009; Tu and Joslin, 2010; Patel et al., 2010;

Joslin et al., 2010). AK is an acute, painful infection that can occur in immunocompetent individuals. When AK is not treated promptly, loss of visual acuity and blindness can occur [6, 7, 8]. Initial symptoms of AK are not specific and include disproportional eye pain, photophobia, eye redness, and tearing, usually affecting one eye. Using a slit-lamp, corneal inflammation leading to formation of a ring-like stromal infiltrate can be observed. Furthermore, corneal epithelial erosion, irregularities, and edema are present. The radial perineural distribution of the infiltrate (radial keratoneuritis) is characteristic for AK, similar to the type of infiltration observed in *Pseudomonas aeruginosa* keratitis. Later stages of infection can result in epithelial denudation and stromal necrosis. Contact lens usage and/or incidents of corneal trauma are strong indicators for AK. Despite the clinical picture, AK is often misdiagnosed as herpes or bacterial keratitides which present similar clinical symptomatology (Khan, 2006; Visvesvara et al., 2007; Martín-Navarro et al., 2008; da Rocha-Azevedo et al., 2009).

Both *Acanthamoeba* and *Balamuthia* cause infections of the lungs and skin (Khan, 2006; Maciver, 2007; Visvesvara et al., 2007; da Rocha-Azevedo et al., 2009). More recently, *Balamuthia mandrillaris*, has been discovered to cause a fatal encephalitis in humans (Maciver, 2007; Visvesvara et al., 2007; Matin et al., 2008). This encephalitis is known as *Balamuthia* amoebic encephalitis (BAE). There are worrying features of BAE that are emerging, even compared to AGE and PAM. PAM is restricted to bodies of warm freshwater, such as swimming pools and lakes, and so can be avoided after its presence has been identified.

AGE is mostly a disease of the immunocompromised, and so affects a small subpopulation of individuals who could conceivably be monitored for early signs of AGE; for example, by inspection of cerebrospinal fluid (CSF) (Deetz et al., 2003; Maciver, 2007). Present data indicate that BAE is more difficult to detect, as it is sporadic, affecting both immunocompromised and immunocompetent, otherwise healthy, individuals with little evidence of predisposing factors (i.e. working in farms or soil related environments. The unpredictable nature of the disease may mean that BAE is even less likely to be diagnosed in time for medical intervention and, like AGE and PAM, it is essential for BAE to be diagnosed early if it is to be treated successfully (Deetz et al., 2003; Petry et al., 2006; Maciver, 2007]. Worryingly, BAE may be relatively a common type of amoebic encephalitis and some cases reported to be due to *Acanthamoeba* have subsequently been shown to be due to *B. mandrillaris* (Deetz et al., 2003; Maciver, 2007).

Recently, *Sappinia diploidea* and *Sappinia pedata* species, also belonging to the free-living amoeba group, that normally live in soil contaminated with faeces of elk, bison, and cattle, have been identified as causing encephalitis in an otherwise healthy individuals (Gelman et al., 2001; Qvarstrom et al., 2009; Walochnik et al., 2010), indicating that there are probably other amoebae that are capable of causing encephalitis in humans.

A study looking at causes of encephalitis found at least 13. 939 cases of acute encephalitis diagnosed between 1990 and 1999 in California [13, 26]. Amongst these cases, 0.1% was attributed to *Naegleria*, 0.63% to other protozoans, and 34.7% were from unspecified causes. The California Encephalitis Project (CEP) (reviewed in Maciver et al., 2007), identified three fatal cases caused by *Balamuthia* from the 334 patients who met the criteria for CEP. No cases of encephalitis caused by either *Acanthamoeba* or *Naegleria* were seen but immunocompromised patients were excluded from the study [30]. Thus, these data would suggest that in California in the 1990s *Balamuthia* and *Naegleria* each accounted for approximately 0.1% of total encephalitis cases in these studies (reviewed in Maciver et al., 2007).

3. Therapy and prognosis of *FLA* infections

3.1 *Acanthamoeba* spp.

Treatment of AGE is problematic because of the lack of clear-cut symptoms, the lack of a good reliable diagnostic test, and the fact that diagnosis is often made postmortem. However, several patients with GAE caused by *Acanthamoeba* spp., as well as some with *Acanthamoeba* cutaneous infection without CNS involvement, have been successfully treated with a combination of pentamidine isethionate, sulfadiazine, flucytosine, and fluconazole or itraconazole. For *Acanthamoeba* cutaneous infection without CNS involvement, topical applications of chlorhexidine gluconate and ketoconazole cream in addition to the above-noted antimicrobials have resulted in therapeutic success. In many cases, however, therapy had to be discontinued because of undesirable side effects of the medications Visvesvara et al., 2007. A combination of factors -late diagnosis, suboptimal efficacy of antimicrobial therapy, and problems inherent to the immunocompromised host -make for a poor prognosis for GAE patients.
Treatment of *Acanthamoeba* keratitis has been fairly successful. A variety of drugs have been used, including chlorhexidine, polyhexamethylene biguanide, propamidine isethionate, dibromopropamidine isethionate, neomycin, paromomycin, polymyxin B, clotrimazole, ketoconazole, miconazole, and itraconazole (Visvesvara et al., 2007; da Rocha-Azevedo, 2009). Brolene, a commercially available eye medication (in the UK, and other EU countries) containing propamidine isethionate and dibromopropamidine isethionate, was found to be effective in the treatment of *Acanthamoeba* infections but may be accompanied by drug toxicity and development of resistance.
A number of compounds, including a variety of diamidine compounds, synthetic maganins combined with silver nitrate, imidazole and triazole compounds, azithromycin, phenothiazines and povidone-iodine have been screened *in vitro* for efficacy against *Acanthamoeba* spp. Another drug, miltefosine, an alkylphospholipid, has also been shown to have amoebicidal potential. Significantly, medical cure has been achieved with the application of either polyhexamethylene biguanide (PHMB) or chlorhexidine gluconate with or without Brolene. When medical treatment failed, a combination of debridement and penetrating keratoplasty has been used with good results in some cases. Currently, the drugs of for AK are chlorhexidine gluconate, PHMB and Brolene, and they have greatly improved the prognosis for AK sufferers (reviewed in Visvesvara et al., 2007). However, it was recently demonstrated that clinical strains of *Acanthamoeba* are resistant to the concentrations of chlorhexidine gluconate or PHMB present in contact lens maintenance/disinfection solutions (Martín-Navarro et al., 2008). Thus, the latter together with the demonstrated toxicity of these molecules is supporting the need for novel therapies to treat AK worldwide.

3.2 *Balamuthia mandrillaris*

Balamuthia amoebic encephalitis (BAE) is a rare, subacute to chronic disease that is characterized by hemorrhagic necrotizing lesions or brain abscess (normally detected by neuroimaging scans) with severe meningeal irritation and encephalitis. The lesions are mainly detected in the basal ganglia, midbrain, brainstem and cerebral hemiparesis with characteristic lesions in the CNS parenchyma. Typically, encephalitis is of the granulomatous type composed of the amoebae, CD4 and CD8 T cells, B lymphocytes, few plasma cells, macrophages and multinucleate giant cells (Martinez and Visvesvara, 1997;

2001; Matin et al., 2008). However, in immunocompromised patients with an impaired cellular immune response, granuloma formation may be minimal or absent (Martinez and Visvesvara, 1997; 2001).

Post mortem examination often shows severe edema and hemorrhagic necrosis. The amoebae colonize the brain tissue and produce subacute necrotising hemorrhagic encephalitis leading to brain dysfunction. *Balamuthia mandrillaris* trophozoites and cysts are present within the perivascular spaces and within the necrotic CNS parenchyma (Martinez and Visvesvara, 1997). The disease is likely to take a cutaneous route before secondarily attacking the CNS. The time period of transition from the cutaneous form to the CNS ranges from 30 days to 2 years, with an average of 5 –8 months (Bravo and Sanchez, 2003). The skin lesions may appear at the site of an abrasion of the skin surface of the patient, or lesions can appear as single or multiple plaques or nodules (Deetz et al., 2003). These plaques may appear on the face, the trunk or the limbs, with a rubbery to hard consistency (Bravo and Sanchez, 2003). Skin lesions indicate a site of entry and are frequently observed in BAE patients.

Because most of the cases of BAE have presented with no clear-cut clinical profile, they have been treated empirically with steroids as well as with antibacterial, antifungal and antiviral agents with almost no effect upon the course of the infection. Anti-inflammatory steroids that were administered may have actually facilitated spread of the infection by suppressing the inflammatory response. Two patients from California, a 60-year-old man, and a 6-year old girl, in addition to a 70-year-old woman from New York survived balamuthiasis after treatment with a combination of pentamidine isethionate, sulfadiazine, clarithromycin, fluconazole, and flucytosine (5-fluorocytosine) (Deetz et al., 2003).

In the case of the Peruvian balamuthiasis patients with cutaneous lesions (Martínez et al., 2010; Bravo et al., 2011), one recovered without any treatment and two others became well after prolonged therapy with albendazole and itraconazole. The use of multiple antimicrobials in treatment makes it difficult to single out one or more of the drugs that might be the basis for optimal therapy. Furthermore, drugs may show synergistic activities in vivo that are not seen in in vitro testing. In vitro studies have shown that pentamidine and propamidine isethionates were amoebastatic but not amoebicidal. Among other drugs tested with little or no activity were macrolide antibiotics, azole compounds, gramicidin, polymyxin B, trimethoprim, sulfamethoxazole, and a combination of trimethoprim-sulfamethoxazole as well as amphotericin B (Maciver, 2007; Visvesvara et al., 2007).

Recent information based on in vitro data has shown that miltefosine was able to lysed the amoebae. Voriconazole, however, had virtually no effect on *Balamuthia* (Maciver, 2007; Visvesvara et al., 2007). Given the problems with the diagnosis of infection and the lack of effective antimicrobial agents, the prognosis for patients is poor.

3.3 *Naegleria fowleri*

Few patients have survived PAM. One of these survivors, a Californian girl, was aggressively treated with intravenous and intrathecal amphotericin B, intravenous and intrathecal miconazole, and oral rifampin [2, 28]. Over a 4- year follow-up, she remained completely healthy and free of any neurological deficits. It was believed that amphotericin B and miconazole had a synergistic effect but that rifampin was without effect on the amoebae. Based on *in vitro* testing and *in vivo* mouse studies, amphotericin B was reported to be more effective against *Naegleria* than amphotericin B methyl ester, a water-soluble form of the drug. *In vitro* studies of phenothiazine compounds (chlorpromazine and trifluoperazine), which can accumulate in the CNS, were found to have inhibitory effects on

N. fowleri (Visvesvara et al., 2007; da Rocha-Azevedo et al., 2009). Azithromycin, a macrolide antimicrobial, has been shown to be effective against *Naegleria* both in vitro and in vivo (mouse model of disease). However, other macrolides (erythromycin, clarithromycin) are less effective. *Naegleria fowleri* is also sensitive to voriconazole (Marciano-Cabral and Cabral, 2003; Visvesvara et al., 2007; da Rocha-Azevedo et al., 2009).

3.4 *Sappinia* spp.

As it has been recently reported as pathogenic to humans and other animals, no studies have been carried out so far regarding therapy and prognosis of this amoeba.

	Naegleria fowleri (PAM)	*Acanthamoeba (AGE)*	*Balamuthia mandrillaris (BAE)*	*Sappinia spp.*
Life cycle	Three stages: amoeba, cyst and flagellate	Two stages: amoeba and cyst	Two stages: amoeba and cyst	Two stages: amoeba and cyst
Distinctive morphological features	Vesicular nucleus; limacine movement of amoebae; flagellate stage; cyst with pores flush at the surface	Vesicular nucleus; finger-like pseudopodia projecting from surface; cyst wall with two layers and with pores	Vesicular nucleus with single or multiple nucleoli; amoeboid and 'spider-like' movements in culture; cyst wall with three layers	Presence of two abutting nuclei in amoeba and cyst stages
Prodromal period	Days	Weeks to months	Weeks to months	Insufficient data
Epidemiology	Humans typically infected while recreating in warm fresh waters	Infection from soil, water, and air; present in hospital environment (water taps, hydrotherapy pools, air conditioning cooling towers)	Infection from soil, water, and air	Present in soil, water and in air; originally identified from herbivore faeces.
Groups at risk	Children and young adults in good health	Typically, immunocompromised individuals	Immunocompetent (children and elderly) or immunocompromised individuals; Hispanic Americans	Insufficient data
Disease at presentation	Headache, stiff neck, seizures, coma	Headache, stiff neck, behavioural changes, coma	Headache, nausea, seizures, stiff neck, hydrocephalus; sinus infection; nodule formation in cutaneous infections	Headache, vomiting, photophobia, loss of consciousness; preceded by sinus infection
Clinical course	Fulminant disease; death within 1-2 weeks without treatment	Indolent subacute course; acute stage fatal in weeks	Indolent subacute course; once in acute stage, fatal in weeks	Insufficient data

	Naegleria fowleri (PAM)	*Acanthamoeba* (AGE)	*Balamuthia mandrillaris* (BAE)	*Sappinia spp.*
Prevention	Public health monitoring of warm, fresh-water recreational sites	Widespread in soil and water; in hospital setting, monitoring of water supply, ventilators, air conditioning units	Found in soil and water; preventive measures not feasible	Insufficient data; organism found in soil; preventive measures not feasible
Current therapy	Intrathecal amphotericin B, miconazole	Pentamidine, azole compounds, flucytosine, sulfadiazine	Pentamidine, azithromycin, fluconazole, flucytosine	Azithromycin, pentamidine, itraconazole, flucytosine
Prognosis	Fair if diagnosed early (within days); otherwise poor–a few patients have survived	Poor; diagnosis is often postmortem–only a few patients have survived	Poor; diagnosis is often postmortem–three patients have survived	Insufficient data

Table 1. Characteristics of FLA as causal agents of encephalitis (adapted from Visvesvara et al., 2007).

3.5 Novel therapeutic approaches

Recently, the application of siRNA in *Acanthamoeba* species (Lorenzo-Morales et al., 2005; 2008; 2010) has opened a novel approach for the progress of future therapies based on siRNAs alone or in combination with chemical compounds. Also the use of RNAi moleculaes could be very powerful for the identification of novel drug targets and metabolic pathways in these pathogens that could be exploited for the development of new therapeutic agents. Recently, RNAi methodology has been successfully use in *Naegleria fowleri* (Jung et al., 2008) resulting in a reduced pathogenicity of the RNAi-treated amoebae. Therefore, RNAi molecules are currently presenting as very powerful tools that are waiting to be fully exploited in the development of new therapies against pathogenic FLA.

4. Conclusions

Regarding encephalitis caused by FLA, it is important to mention that because most of them are ultimately fatal, diagnosis of these infections is often made at autopsy, even in developed countries where sophisticated diagnostic facilities are readily available. However, in Sub-Saharan Africa and Southeast Asia, where HIV/AIDS rates are increasing, it is quite possible that a large number of cases have gone undetected. A similar case occurs in South America, where skin infections due to *B. mandrillaris* are a common episode in countries like Peru but the lack of diagnostic and treatment facilities in most areas have caused that most of these cases have been unnoticed as well.

This due to a number of reasons: (1) lack of expertise to identify these pathogenic amoebae; (2) cultural methods and expense that prevent autopsies; and (3) an abundance of more prominent diseases such as HIV/AIDS, tuberculosis and malaria that consume national and international resources. Therefore, the actual incidence of the encephalitis caused by FLA is not really known although it seems that these pathogenic amoebae are emerging as causative agents of encephalitis worldwide.

5. References

Bravo F, Sanchez MR. (2003) New and re-emerging cutaneous infectious diseases in Latin America and other geographic areas. Dermatologic Clinics. 2003 Oct;21(4):655-68, VIII. Review

Bravo FG, Alvarez PJ, Gotuzzo E. (2011). Balamuthia mandrillaris infection of the skin and central nervous system: an emerging disease of concern to many specialties in medicine. Current Opinion Infectious Diseases. 2011 Apr;24(2):112-7. Review.

da Rocha-Azevedo B, Tanowitz HB, Marciano-Cabral F. (2009).Diagnosis of infections caused by pathogenic free-living amoebae. Interdisciplinary Perspectives Infectious Diseases. 2009: 251406. Epub 2009 Aug 2.

Deetz TR, Sawyer MH, Billman G, Schuster FL, Visvesvara GS. (2003).Successful treatment of Balamuthia amoebic encephalitis: presentation of 2 cases. Clinical Infectious Diseases. 15;37(10):1304-12.

Gelman BB, Rauf SJ, Nader R, et al. (2001) Amoebic encephalitis due to Sappinia diploidea. JAMA. 16;285(19):2450-

Heggie TW (2010) Swimming with death: Naegleria fowleri infections in recreational waters. Travel Medicine and Infectious Diseases. 2010 8(4):201-6

Joslin CE, Tu EY, Shoff ME, Anderson RJ, Davis FG (2010). Shifting distribution of Chicago-area Acanthamoeba keratitis cases. Arch Ophthalmol. 2010 Jan;128(1):137-9.

Jung SY, Kim JH, Song KJ, Lee YJ, Kwon MH, Kim K, Park S, Im KI, Shin HJ. (2009). Gene silencing of nfa1 affects the in vitro cytotoxicity of Naegleria fowleri in murine macrophages. Molecular and Biochemical Parasitology. 2009 May;165(1):87-93.

Khan NA (2006), Acanthamoeba: biology and increasing importance in human health. FEMS Microbiology Reviews, 30:564–595.

Lorenzo-Morales J, Ortega-Rivas A, Foronda P, Abreu-Acosta N, Ballart D, Martínez E, Valladares B. (2005). RNA interference (RNAi) for the silencing of extracellular serine proteases genes in Acanthamoeba: molecular analysis and effect on pathogenecity. *Molecular and Biochemical Parasitology*. 2005 Nov;144(1):10-5.

Lorenzo-Morales J, Kliescikova J, Martinez-Carretero E, De Pablos LM, Profotova B, Nohynkova E, Osuna A, Valladares B. (2008) Glycogen phosphorylase in Acanthamoeba spp.: determining the role of the enzyme during the encystment process using RNA interference. *Eukaryotic Cell*. 2008 Mar; 7(3):509-17.

Lorenzo-Morales J, Martín-Navarro CM, López-Arencibia A, Santana-Morales MA, Afonso-Lehmann RN, Maciver SK, Valladares B, Martínez-Carretero E. (2010). Therapeutic potential of a combination of two gene-specific small interfering RNAs against clinical strains of Acanthamoeba. *Antimicrobial Agents and Chemotheraty*. 2010 Dec;54(12):5151-5.

Maciver SK.(2007). The threat from Balamuthia mandrillaris. Journal of Medical Microbiology. 56(Pt 1):1-3

Marciano-Cabral F, Cabral G. (2003) Acanthamoeba spp. as agents of disease in humans. *Clinical Microbiology Reviews*. 2003 Apr;16(2):273-307. Review.

Martínez AJ. (1980). Is Acanthamoeba encephalitis an opportunistic infection? Neurology. 1980 Jun;30(6):567-74.

Martinez AJ, Visvesvara GS. (1997). Free-living, amphizoic and opportunistic amebas. Brain Pathology. 1997 Jan;7(1):583-98. Review.

Martínez AJ, Visvesvara GS. (2001) Balamuthia mandrillaris infection. Journal of Medical Microbiology. 2001 Mar;50(3):205-7.

Martínez DY, Seas C, Bravo F, Legua P, Ramos C, Cabello AM, Gotuzzo E. (2010). Successful treatment of Balamuthia mandrillaris amoebic infection with extensive neurological and cutaneous involvement. Clinical Infectious Diseases. 2010 Jul 15;51(2):e7-11.

Martín-Navarro CM, Lorenzo-Morales J, Cabrera-Serra MG, Rancel F, Coronado-Alvarez NM, Piñero JE, Valladares B. (2008). The potential pathogenicity of chlorhexidine-sensitive Acanthamoeba strains isolated from contact lens cases from asymptomatic individuals in Tenerife, Canary Islands, Spain. Journal of Medical Microbiology. 57(Pt 11):1399-404.

Matin A, Siddiqui R, Jayasekera S, Khan NA. (2008).Increasing importance of Balamuthia mandrillaris. Clinical Microbiology Reviews. 2008 Jul;21(3):435-48. Review.

Page, F.C. (1988) A new key to freshwater and soil gymnamoebae. FBA NERC. P26.

Patel DV, Rayner S, McGhee CN (2010).Resurgence of Acanthamoeba keratitis in Auckland, New Zealand: a 7-year review of presentation and outcomes. Clinical Experimental Ophthalmology 38(1):15-20.

Petry F, Torzewski M, Bohl J, et al. (2006). Early diagnosis of Acanthamoeba infection during routine cytological examination of cerebrospinal fluid. Journal of Clinical Microbiology. 44(5):1903-4.

Qvarnstrom Y, da Silva AJ, Schuster FL, Gelman BB, Visvesvara GS. (2009). Molecular confirmation of Sappinia pedata as a causative agent of amoebic encephalitis. Journal of Infectious Diseases. Apr 15;199(8):1139-42.

Seijo Martinez M, Gonzalez-Mediero G, Santiago P, Rodriguez De Lope A, Diz J, Conde C, Visvesvara GS.(2000).Granulomatous amebic encephalitis in a patient with AIDS: isolation of acanthamoeba sp. Group II from brain tissue and successful treatment with sulfadiazine and fluconazole. Journal of Clinical Microbiology. Oct; 38(10):3892-5.

Shirwadkar CG, Samant R, Sankhe M, Deshpande R, Yagi S, Schuster FL, Sriram R, Visvesvara GS. (2006). Acanthamoeba encephalitis in patient with systemic lupus, India. Emerging Infectious Diseases. 2006 Jun;12(6):984-6.

Tu EY and Joslin CE (2010). Recent outbreaks of atypical contact lens-related keratitis: what have we learned?. American Journal of Ophthalmology. 2010 Nov;150(5):602-608.e2.

Verani JR, Lorick SA, Yoder JS, Beach MJ, et al. (2009). National outbreak of Acanthamoeba keratitis associated with use of a contact lens solution, United States. Emerging Infectious Diseases. 15(8):1236-42.

Visvesvara GS and Maguire JH (2006) Pathogenic and opportunistic free-living amebas. Acanthamoeba spp., Balamuthia mandrillaris, Naegleria fowleri, and Sappinia diploidea. Tropical Infectious Diseases, Vol. 2 (GuerrantRL, WalkerDH & WellerPF, eds), pp. 1114–1125. Churchill Livingstone.

Visvesvara GS, Moura H and Schuster F L (2007), Pathogenic and opportunistic free-living amoebae: Acanthamoeba spp., Balamuthia mandrillaris, Naegleria fowleri, and Sappinia diploidea. FEMS Immunology and Medical Microbiology, 50:1–26.

Visvesvara GS, Sriram R, Qvarnstrom Y, Bandyopadhyay K, Da Silva AJ, Pieniazek NJ, Cabral GA. (2009). Paravahlkampfia francinae n. sp. masquerading as an agent of primary amoebic meningoencephalitis. Journal of Eukaryotic Microbiology. Jul-Aug;56(4):357-66.

Walochnik J, Wylezich C, Michel R. (2010)The genus Sappinia: history, phylogeny and medical relevance. Experimental Parasitology. 126(1):4-13.

14

Autoimmunity in the Mediation of Granulomatous Amoebic Encephalitis: Implications for Therapy

Chandirasegaran Massilamany and Jay Reddy
University of Nebraska-Lincoln
School of Veterinary Medicine and Biomedical Sciences
USA

1. Introduction

Acanthamoeba spp. are free-living amoebae that are ubiquitous in the environment. Most healthy individuals carry *Acanthamoeba*-reactive antibodies, suggesting constant exposure to amoebae. In spite of the high prevalence of the amoebae, the incidence of diseases caused by *Acanthamoeba* is very low. Non-opportunistically, Acanthamoebae can induce keratitis in healthy humans, but as an opportunistic pathogen, the amoebae can cause fatal encephalitis especially in immunocompromised individuals and treatments are often ineffective.

Amoebic encephalitis is a life-threatening disease of the central nervous system (CNS) caused by free-living amoebae belonging to the genera *Acanthamoeba, Balamuthia* and *Naegleria*. Because they lack host-specificity, the ubiquitous amoebae can infect a wide range of species (Marciano-Cabral & Cabral, 2003, Schuster & Visvesvara, 2004). The diseases caused by *Acanthamoeba* spp. and *Balamuthia* spp. are generally termed "granulomatous amoebic encephalitis" (GAE), whereas those caused by *Naegleria* spp. are called 'primary amoebic meningioencephalitis (PAM)'(Marciano-Cabral & Cabral, 2003, Schuster & Visvesvara, 2004, Khan, 2006, da Rocha-Azevedo, *et al.*, 2009). While Acanthamoebae induce illness mostly in immunocompromised individuals, *Balamuthia* spp. and *Naegleria* spp. can cause diseases in both immune-sufficient and immune-deficient individuals (Martinez & Visvesvara, 2001, Marciano-Cabral & Cabral, 2003, Schuster & Visvesvara, 2004, Khan, 2006, da Rocha-Azevedo, *et al.*, 2009). Nevertheless, all of them can induce keratitis in healthy individuals, often in contact lens-wearers (Jones, *et al.*, 1975, Martinez & Visvesvara, 1997, Marciano-Cabral & Cabral, 2003, da Rocha-Azevedo, *et al.*, 2009). We recently discovered that *A. castellanii* contains mimicry sequence for immunodominant epitope of CNS myelin proteolipid protein (PLP), suggesting that exposure to *A. castellanii* can lead to the generation of autoimmune responses by antigenic mimicry. In this review, we discuss our understanding of the pathophysiology of *Acanthamoeba*-induced encephalitis, with a special emphasis on autoimmunity in mediation of the disease, and implications for therapy.

2. Characteristics of *Acanthamoeba* infections

Based on morphological characteristics, such as shape and size of amoebic cysts, and growth conditions, the genus *Acanthamoeba* was initially classified into groups I, II, and III, containing 4, 11, and 5 species, respectively (De Jonckheere, 1987). Recently, reclassification was made to group various species into 15 genotypes (T1 to T15) based on 18S rRNA gene sequences, which can distinguish different genotypes showing a variation of as low as 5% (Gast, *et al.*, 1996, Schuster & Visvesvara, 2004). The genotypes T1, T4, T10, and T12 generally cause encephalitis, and *A. castellanii* and *A. polyphaga* that belong to T4 genotype are most frequently implicated as causes of GAE (Garate, *et al.*, 2006). The current trend is to classify Acanthamoebae based on genotype rather than morphology.

2.1 Geographical distribution

Epidemiologically, no clear disease associations have been found with respect to race, gender, and geographical location, except that the disease has not been reported in Africa, an observation attributed mostly to lack of familiarity and diagnostic tools (Tan, *et al.*, 1993, Barker, *et al.*, 1995, Marciano-Cabral & Cabral, 2003). However, serological evidence suggests that Hispanics are 14.5 times less likely to carry *Acanthamoeba*-reactive antibodies than individuals of other ethnicities (Chappell, *et al.*, 2001, Khan, 2006). A study undertaken to measure the seroprevalence of *Acanthamoeba* in different ethnic groups indicated that up to 90 % of healthy humans can carry *Acanthamoeba* antibodies. Seropositivity occurred in the order of Caucasians, followed by Hispanics and African Americans (Chappell, *et al.*, 2001). But it is unknown whether the occurrence of amoebic encephalitis follows a similar pattern in the general population.

2.2 Host distribution and susceptibility

The amoeba has a two-stage life-cycle: trophozoites (infective and invasive) and cysts (dormant). The life cycle can be completed in either the environment or infected hosts (Chagla & Griffiths, 1974, Marciano-Cabral & Cabral, 2003). Under unfavorable conditions, such as extremes of pH and temperature, trophozoites become cysts that are highly resistant to commonly used disinfectants containing chlorine and the cysts can survive environmental temperatures even upto 80° C (De Jonckheere & van de Voorde, 1976, Khunkitti, *et al.*, 1998, Storey, *et al.*, 2004). *Balamuthia* spp. (e.g., *B. mandrillaris*) can cause GAE in a wide range of species such as horses, baboons, sheeps, dogs, and humans (Martinez & Visvesvara, 2001), but development of clinical disease takes months to years. Likewise, *Acanthamoeba* infections are also reported in humans including domestic and non-domestic species such as dogs, monkeys, kangaroos and buffaloes (Schuster & Visvesvara, 2004). Found ubiquitously, Acanthamoebae have been isolated from a variety of sources such as soil; drinking, natural and sea water; hospitals, eye wash stations, and dental irrigation systems; swimming pools; and heating and cooling ducts (Jahnes & Fullmer, 1957, Kingston & Warhurst, 1969, Casemore, 1977, De Jonckheere, 1991, Barbeau & Buhler, 2001, Marciano-Cabral & Cabral, 2003, da Rocha-Azevedo, *et al.*, 2009) and the amoebae generally feed on bacteria, algae, and yeast (Bowers, 1977, Bowers & Olszewski, 1983, Marciano-Cabral & Cabral, 2003, da Rocha-Azevedo, *et al.*, 2009).

Generally, GAE is regarded as a disease of immunocompromised individuals. HIV patients, individuals undergoing immunosuppressive and steroid therapies, and those who have received organ or stem cell transplants are at great risk of developing the disease (Marciano-Cabral, *et al.*, 2000, Seijo Martinez, *et al.*, 2000, Marciano-Cabral & Cabral, 2003, Schuster & Visvesvara, 2004, Khan, 2006, da Rocha-Azevedo, *et al.*, 2009). Other predisposing factors include malignancies and debilitated conditions such as diabetes, chronic alcoholism and malnutrition (Martinez & Janitschke, 1985, Sell, *et al.*, 1997, Marciano-Cabral & Cabral, 2003, Khan, 2006). Exacerbation of GAE lesions was reported in one patient undergoing treatment for cryoglobulinemia with a monoclonal antibody directed against CD20 which selectively depletes mature B cells (Meersseman, *et al.*, 2007). Likewise, GAE can occur in patients with systemic lupus erythematosus, further emphasizing the importance of a compromised immune system for disease-predisposition (Koide, *et al.*, 1998, Uschuplich, *et al.*, 2004, Cha, *et al.*, 2006). Since amoebic encephalitis is not a reportable disease, and diagnosis is often made postmortem, the number of cases documented in the literature does not reflect actual disease-incidence. One study has reported to have documented upto 500 cases of amoebic encephalitis worldwide (Sarica, *et al.*, 2009). However, the recent availability of PCR-based detection of *Acanthamoeba* is greatly facilitating diagnosis (Schroeder, *et al.*, 2001, Khan, 2006, da Rocha-Azevedo, *et al.*, 2009, Maritschnegg, *et al.*, 2011) and as a result, the number of cases reported in recent years show an increasing trend.

2.3 Importance of *Acanthamoeba* in nosocomial infections

Recently, it is proposed that Acanthamoebae might play a role in the increased incidence of nosocomial infections (Michel, *et al.*, 1995, Marciano-Cabral & Cabral, 2003). It is well documented that Acanthamoebae act as natural vectors or reservoirs for a variety of microbes, such as *Escherichia coli, Klebsiella, Bacillus spp., Mycoplasma, Legionella pneumophila, Mycobacterium avium, Mycobacterium leprae, Clostridium frigidicarnis, Porphyromonas gingivalis, Prevotella intermedia, Burkholderia pseudomallei, Afipia felis, Vibrio cholerae, Mobiluncus curtissi, Campylobacter spp., Helicobacter pylori, Cryptococcus neoformans, Candida spp., Coxiella burnetti, Chlamydia, Rickettsia,* and Coxsackievirus among others (Marciano-Cabral & Cabral, 2003, Waldner, *et al.*, 2004, Khan, 2006, Mattana, *et al.*, 2006, Thomas, *et al.*, 2009). Bacteria grown in *Acanthamoeba* show resistance to bactericides and biocides; their survival and virulence are enhanced; and they mechanically transport disease-producing agents to various target organs, thus increasing the risk of multiple infections in the affected patients (King, *et al.*, 1988, Barker, *et al.*, 1995, Turner, *et al.*, 2000, Lloyd, *et al.*, 2001, Marciano-Cabral & Cabral, 2003). The amoebae shed waste through vesicles of 2.1 to 6.4 μm diameter, and they can potentially contain pathogenic microbes. For example, *A. polyphaga* can release up to 20 to 200 bacteria per vesicle and the vesicles can become aerosolized leading to their dispersal to wide-range of geographical locations (Rowbotham, 1980, Berk, *et al.*, 1998).

3. Pathogenesis

The amoebae can gain entry into the CNS through two routes: migration via the olfactory neuroepithelium and/or blood (Fig. 1). *Naegleria* spp. tend to follow the former route. After penetrating the nasal mucosa, the amoebae pass through the cribriform plate and travel along the nerve fibers to the olfactory bulb in the cerebrum (Khan, 2007, Elsheikha & Khan). Alternatively, the amoebae that enter through nasal exposure go to the lungs, enter the blood stream, and reach the CNS possibly by disrupting the blood brain barrier (BBB). The hematogenous route also is a choice for amoeba that enter through the skin (Khan, 2007). However, the mechanism by which amoebae actually enter the CNS is not clearly elucidated. Although it is postulated that they enter through the cerebral capillary endothelium or choroid plexus, the former being the more widely accepted mechanism (Khan, 2003, Marciano-Cabral & Cabral, 2003, Khan, 2005b, Khan, 2006, da Rocha-Azevedo, *et al.*, 2009). These two modes of entry lead to the localization of amoebae in the cerebrum and cerebrospinal fluid (CSF) respectively (Elsheikha & Khan, 2010).

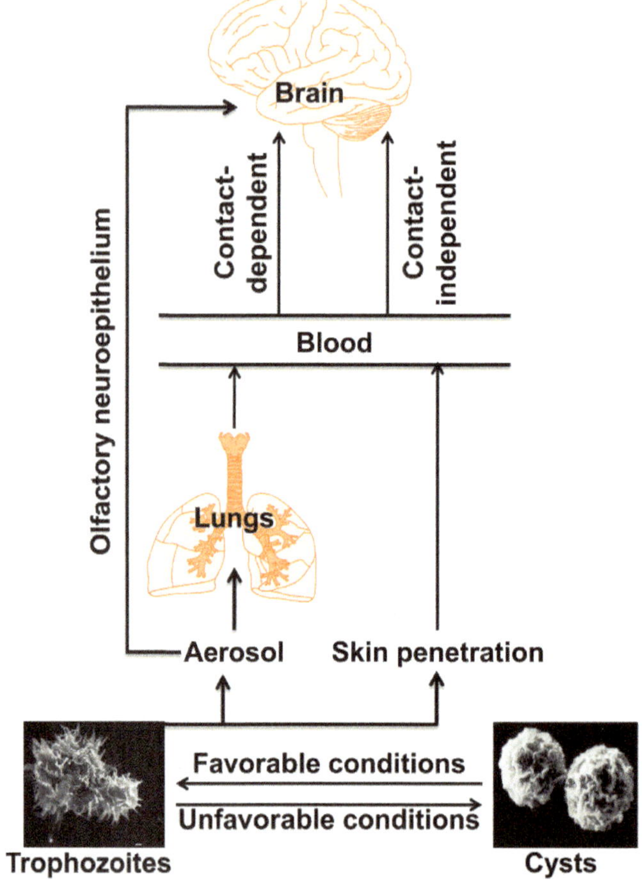

Fig. 1. Proposed routes of entry of *Acanthamoeba* into the CNS. Under favorable conditions, cysts become trophozoites which are the infective stages of *Acanthamoeba*. Upon nasal exposure, trophozoites can reach CNS hematogenously via lungs or through olfactory neuroepithelium. The amoeba that gains entry through the skin can also reach CNS hematogenously. However, actual entry into the brain tissue involves crossing the BBB which appears to be mediated through either contact-dependant mechanisms by inducing apoptosis of the endothelial cells or contact-independent mechanisms via destruction of extracellular matrix by amoebic proteases. The micrographs of *Acanthamoeba* trophozoites and cysts were kindly provided by Dr. Francine Marciano-Cabral, Virginia Commonwealth University, VA, USA

Regardless of route of entry, the amoebae have to cross the BBB, either paracellularly by damaging the tight junctions, or transcellularly, in which the integrity of the BBB is maintained (Khan, 2003, Khan, 2006, Khan, 2007). Disruption of the BBB is thought to be mediated by contact-dependent or contact-independent mechanisms (Khan, 2003, Khan, 2006, Khan, 2007). Contact-dependent mechanisms require attachment of the amoeba to the brain's microvascular endothelial cells through amoebic mannose-binding protein (mannose-BP) causing apoptosis of the endothelial cells, a phenomenon that depends on the phosphatidylinositol 3-kinase signaling pathway (Sissons, *et al.*, 2005, Khan, 2006, Khan, 2007). In contrast, contact-independent mechanisms involve extracellular proteases secreted by *Acanthamoeba*, particularly serine proteases, and these enzymes destroy extracellular matrix proteins comprised of collagen (type I, III, and IV), elastin, and fibronectin (Khan, *et al.*, 2000, Sissons, *et al.*, 2005, Khan, 2007). Alternatively, infected immune cells, most importantly macrophages, may simply act as Trojan horses to carry the amoebae to the CNS (Khan, 2007).

The pathogenicity of *Acanthamoebae* varies by species, depending on their inherent potential to tolerate temperatures, attachment to cellular surfaces, and induction of cytolysis (Marciano-Cabral & Cabral, 2003, Khan, 2006). The principal virulent factors are mannose-BP, Nicotinamide adenine dinucleotide (NADH)-dehydrogenase, GDP-mannose pyrophosphorylase and proteasomal ATPase (Marciano-Cabral & Cabral, 2003, Han, *et al.*, 2006) and of these, the role of mannose-BP has been well-studied. As noted above, the amoebae use mannose-BP for cellular attachment, and the fact that only the infective stage-trophozoites but not cysts upregulates mannose-BP expression suggests that, this protein is critical for amoebic invasion (Garate, *et al.*, 2006). However, once the infection is established, microglial cells produce inflammatory cytokines, such as tumor necrosis factor (TNF)-α, interleukin (IL)-6, IL-1β and IL-1α and they can contribute to tissue damage (Benedetto & Auriault, 2002, Benedetto, *et al.*, 2003, Marciano-Cabral & Cabral, 2003).

4. Immune responses to *Acanthamoeba*

The role of the immune system and immune defense mechanisms in protecting against *Acanthamoeba* has not been well characterized, but protection against amoebae appears to involve both innate and adaptive immune responses. Amoebae are extracellular organisms that lack a sialic acid coat or capsule, making them vulnerable to complement-mediated destruction (Bowers & Korn, 1968, Korn & Olivecrona, 1971, Khan, 2005a). Conversely, amoebae can evade immune mechanisms by binding to a C1q component, as shown in the case of *A. culbertsoni*, and the parasite-derived serine proteases can degrade IgG and IgA (Toney & Marciano-Cabral, 1998, Kong, *et al.*, 2000, Na, *et al.*, 2002, Marciano-Cabral & Cabral, 2003). Neutrophils, macrophages, and microglia can destroy amoebae, and their amoebicidal effects are mediated in part by respiratory burst and nitric oxide under the influence of IL-1β, IL-1α, TNF-α and/or IFN-γ (Ferrante, 1991a, Ferrante, 1991b, Marciano-Cabral & Toney, 1998, Marciano-Cabral, *et al.*, 2000, Benedetto & Auriault, 2002a, Benedetto & Auriault, 2002b, Dudley, *et al.*, 2007, Khan, 2008).

Affected patients, including healthy individuals upto 90%, carry the *Acanthamoeba*-reactive antibodies of IgM, IgG, and IgA isotypes with no significant differences between males (86.2%) and females (89.2%), indicating that humans are regularly exposed to *Acanthamoeba* and become sensitized with the amoebic antigens (Chappell, *et al.*, 2001, McClellan, *et al.*, 2002, Schuster, 2002, Khan, 2005a, Brindley, *et al.*, 2009, da Rocha-Azevedo, *et al.*, 2009). It has been reported that T cells from healthy individuals can react to *Acanthamoeba* antigens obtained from CSF and antigen-specific T cell clones capable of producing IFN-γ also have been derived (Tanaka, *et al.*, 1994). Likewise, peripheral blood mononuclear cells from rheumatoid arthritis patients shows proliferative responses to *A. polyphaga* (Shadidi, *et al.*, 2001). But the significance of these observations is not known. The fact that the individuals exposed to *Acanthamoeba* become seropositive and also carry antigen-specific IFN-γ-secreting cells suggests that the host defenses might involve both antibody- and cell-mediated immune responses but, this aspect requires additional investigations.

4.1 Autoimmunity in the mediation of amoebic encephalitis

In our efforts to identify the disease-inducing microbial mimics for CNS myelin antigens, we recently identified a novel epitope from *A. castellanii* (Fig. 2; Massilamany, *et al.*, 2010, Massilamany, *et al.*, 2011). The epitope termed, ACA 83-95 is derived from rhodanese-related sulfur transferase of *Acanthamoeba*. We tested the disease-inducing ability of ACA 83-95 in the mouse model of experimental autoimmune encephalomyelitis (EAE), which has been traditionally used to study the pathophysiology of multiple sclerosis (MS) in humans (Massilamany, *et al.*, 2010, Massilamany, *et al.*, 2011).

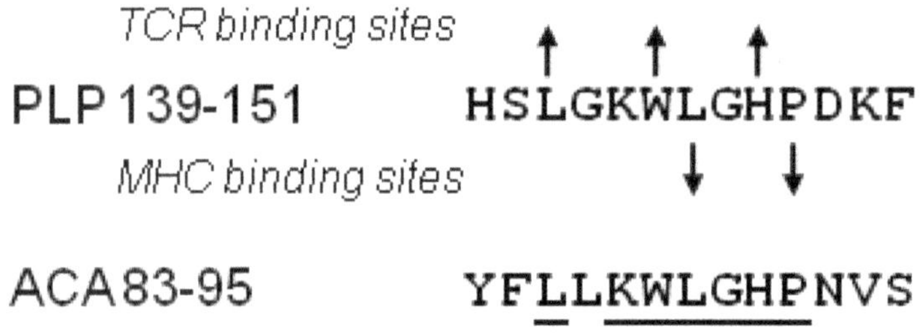

Fig. 2. Comparison of peptide sequences. Peptide sequences of PLP 139-151 and ACA 83-95 are compared. Identical residues are underlined. Top arrows, TCR- contact residues; bottom arrows, MHC-anchor residues (Massilamany, *et al.*, 2010, Massilamany, *et al.*, 2011)

We verified the encephalitogenicity of mimicry epitope in both active immunization and adoptive transfer (AT) EAE protocols in autoimmune-prone SJL mice bearing the H-2^s haplotype. While EAE induction by active immunization requires administration of peptides emulsified in complete Freund's adjuvant (CFA), AT-EAE involves infusion of antigen-sensitized cells into naïve recipients (Miller & Karpus, 2007). The disease induction by active immunization essentially involves two phases: antigen-sensitization and effector T cell-expansion. On the contrary, the pathogenic potential of effector T cells is directly tested in AT-EAE protocol by transferring antigen-stimulated lymph node or spleen cells generated from previously immunized mice, thus eliminating the need to immunize naive recipients prior to disease induction. Figure 3a shows that SJL mice immunized with ACA 83-95 developed clinical signs of EAE reminiscent of disease induced by the cognate peptide PLP 139-151 (Tuohy, *et al.*, 1989, Massilamany, *et al.*, 2010, Massilamany, *et al.*, 2011). Verification of these results in AT-EAE protocol clearly indicated that the disease-induction by ACA 83-95 requires the mediation of antigen-sensitized T cells (Fig. 3b, Fig. 4; Massilamany, *et al.*, 2010, Massilamany, *et al.*, 2011).

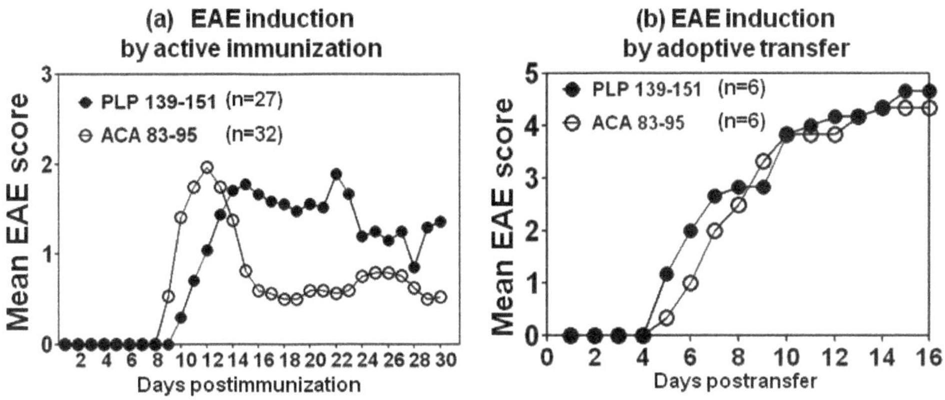

Fig. 3. ACA 83-95 induces autoimmune encephalomyelitis similar to that induced by PLP 139-151. (a) EAE induction by active immunization. SJL mice were immunized with peptides emulsified in CFA, and pertussis toxin was administered on day 0 and 2 postimmunization and the mice were monitored for clinical signs of EAE and scored. (b) EAE induction by adoptive transfer. Short-term T cell lines were derived from mice immunized with the indicated peptides and viable lymphoblasts were injected into naive SJL mice intraperitoneally, and the mice were monitored for signs of EAE and scored (Massilamany, *et al.*, 2010, Massilamany, *et al.*, 2011). Scoring scale: 0, healthy; 1, limp tail or hind limb weakness, but not both; 2, limp tail and hind limb weakness; 3, partial paralysis of hind limbs; 4, complete paralysis of hind limbs; 5, moribund or dead (Tuohy, et al., 1989, Massilamany, et al., 2010, Massilamany, et al., 2011).

4.1.1 ACA 83-95 induces the generation of cross-reactive T cells

We adopted two approaches to prove that EAE induced with ACA 83-95 involves the generation of cross-reactive T cells for PLP 139-151: 1) T cell proliferation assay based on tritiated ^{3}[H] thymidine incorporation and 2) major histocompatibility complex (MHC) class II tetramer staining. The latter assay involves creation of fluorescent dye-labeled MHC class II tetramers for the class II allele of SJL mice, called IA^{s}, into which peptide sequences for ACA 83-95 and PLP 139-151 are covalently tethered. The use of tetramers permitted detection of antigen-specific cells by flow cytometry at a single cell level.

As expected, PLP 139-151 induced dose-dependent proliferative T cell response to PLP, but a fraction of these cells also responded to unimmunized mimicry peptide, ACA 83-95 and vice versa (Fig. 5; Massilamany, *et al.*, 2010, Massilamany, *et al.*, 2011). Consistent with the proliferative responses, PLP 139-151 tetramer^{+} CD4^{+} T cells were evident in mice immunized with either PLP 139-151 or ACA 83-95 as predicted (Fig. 6; Massilamany, *et al.*, 2010, Massilamany, *et al.*, 2011). We verified the specificity of tetramer staining using Theiler's murine encephalomyelitis virus (TMEV) 70-86 tetramers, which stained negligibly. Taken together, the data demonstrate that ACA 83-95 induces T cell response that can cross-react with PLP 139-151.

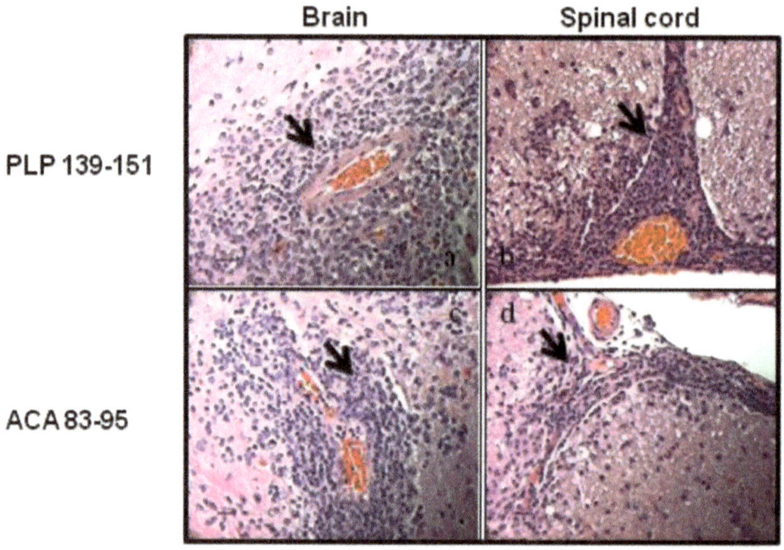

Fig. 4. Histological evaluation of AT-EAE induced by ACA 83-95-sensitized T lymphocytes. Hematoxylin and Eosin-stained sections show perivascular cuffing (arrows) in the brains and spinal cords of mice that received PLP 139-151 (a and b)-, ACA 83-95 (c and d)-sensitized T lymphocytes. Original magnification, x 400 (bar = 20 μm) (Massilamany, *et al.*, 2010, Massilamany, *et al.*, 2011).

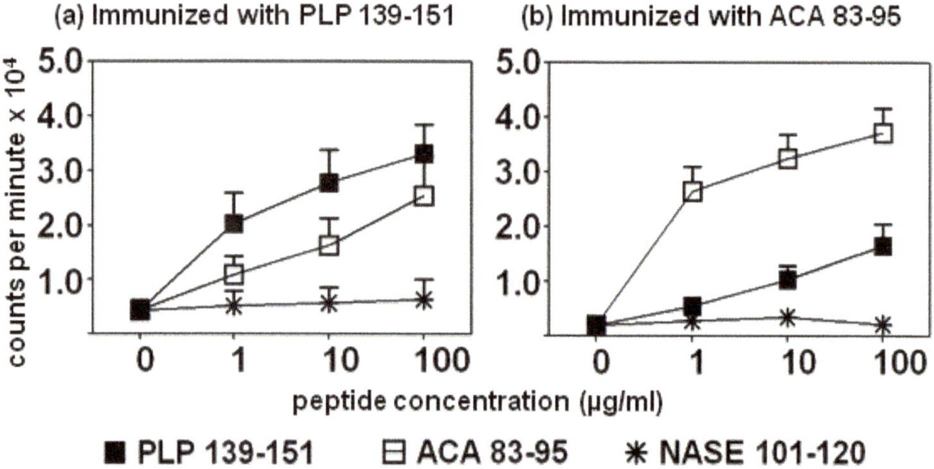

Fig. 5. Cross-reactive T cell responses induced by PLP 139-151 and ACA 83-95. Lymph node cells from PLP 139-151- and ACA 83-95-immunized mice were stimulated with PLP 139-151, ACA 83-95 and NASE 101-120 (control) for two days. After pulsing with tritiated ^{3}[H] thymidine, proliferative responses were measured as counts per minute 16 hours later (Massilamany, *et al.*, 2010, Massilamany, *et al.*, 2011).

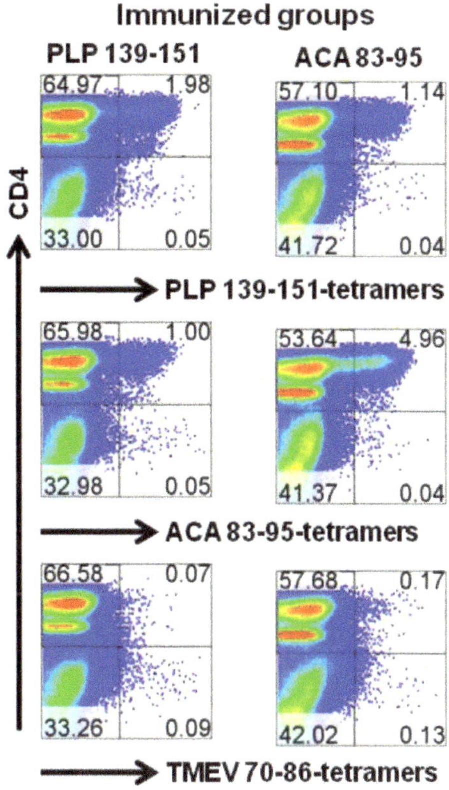

Fig. 6. Cross-reactive T cell responses induced by PLP 139-151 and ACA 83-95 are antigen-specific. Lymph node cells obtained from mice immunized with PLP 139-151 or ACA 83-95 were restimulated with the corresponding peptides, and tetramer staining was performed using PLP 139-151, ACA 83-95 and TMEV 70-86 (control) tetramers, anti-CD4 and 7-amino-actinomycin D (7-AAD). After acquiring the cells by flow cytometry, percentages of tetramer$^+$CD4$^+$ T cells were enumerated in the live (7-AAD$^-$) populations (see upper right quadrant in each plot; (Massilamany, *et al.*, 2010, Massilamany, *et al.*, 2011).

4.1.2 ACA 83-95 induces cytokine responses that favor CNS autoimmunity

One of the hallmarks of CNS autoimmunity is the production of T helper (Th)1 and Th17 cytokines. Although both Th1 and Th17 cells could contribute to EAE pathogenicity, it appears that the ratio between the two subsets of T cells determines the severity of EAE. Predominance of Th17 over Th1 cells exacerbates inflammation and infiltration into the CNS (Bettelli, *et al.*, 2007, Stromnes, *et al.*, 2008). Furthermore, it has been proposed that Th1 cells enter non-inflamed CNS tissues and initiate inflammation, then facilitate the entry of Th17 cells (O'Connor, *et al.*, 2008). Flow cytometrically, we verified Th1 (IL-2, and IFN-γ) and Th17 (IL-17A, IL-17F and IL-22) and Th2 (IL-4 and IL-10) cells, which mediate pro- and anti-inflammatory effects respectively by intracellular staining. As expected, ACA 83-95 induces predominantly Th1 and Th17 cytokines similar to that induced with the cognate peptide,

PLP 139-151 (Fig. 7; Massilamany, *et al.*, 2010, Massilamany, *et al.*, 2011). Based on these data, we expect that animals infected with *A. castellanii* will show the generation of pathogenic PLP-reactive T cells.

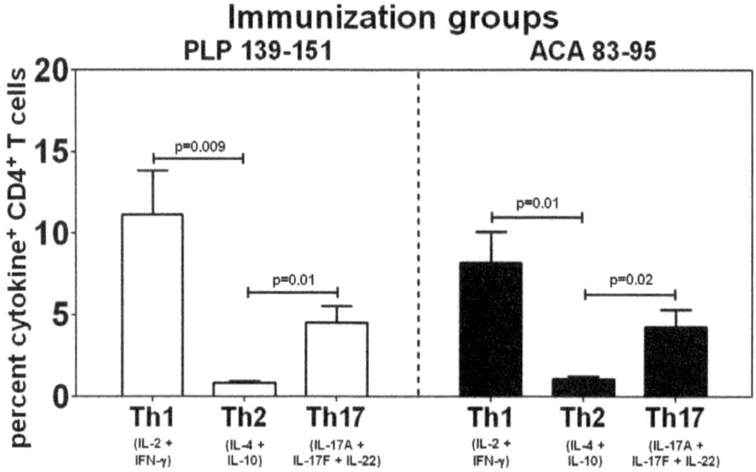

Fig. 7. ACA 83-95 from *A. castellanii* induces cytokines similar to that of PLP 139-151. Lymph node cells obtained from mice immunized with PLP 139-151, or ACA 83-95 were stimulated with the corresponding peptides for two days and then maintained in IL-2 medium. Viable lymphoblasts were harvested on day 4 and stimulated briefly with phorbol 12-myristate 13-acetate and Ionomycin. After staining with anti-CD4 and 7-AAD, intracellular staining was performed using cytokine antibodies and frequencies of cytokine-secreting cells were then determined by flow cytometry in the live (7-AAD-) CD4 subset. Shown are the frequencies of cytokine-secreting cells corresponding to Th1 (IL-2 and IFN-γ), Th2 (IL-4 and IL-10) and Th17 (IL-17A, IL-17F and IL-22) subsets (Massilamany, *et al.*, 2010, Massilamany, *et al.*, 2011).

4.1.3 Murine *Acanthamoeba* granulomatous encephalitis as a disease model of MS

Acanthamoeba spp. can cause choriomeningitis and destructive encephalomyelitis in mice and monkeys (Culbertson, *et al.*, 1958, Culbertson, *et al.*, 1959). The mouse model is widely used to study the pathogenesis of GAE (Kim, *et al.*, 1990, Janitschke, *et al.*, 1996, Marciano-Cabral, *et al.*, 2001, Gornik & Kuzna-Grygiel, 2005, Khan, 2009). Intranasal inoculations of mice with *A. castellanii* produce subacute to chronic granulomatous encephalitis accompanied by rhinitis and pneumonitis (Martinez, *et al.*, 1975, Kim, *et al.*, 1990, Janitschke, *et al.*, 1996, Gornik & Kuzna-Grygiel, 2005). Clinically, GAE in mice is manifested by respiratory distress, pneumonia, head tilt, circling, twirling, seizures, and limb paresis (Culbertson, *et al.*, 1959, Culbertson, 1961, Culbertson, *et al.*, 1966, Martinez, *et al.*, 1975, Kim, *et al.*, 1990, Janitschke, *et al.*, 1996, Gornik & Kuzna-Grygiel, 2005). Histologically, infiltrations consist of microglia, histiocytes and lymphocytes around capillaries, suggestive of formation of foreign body granuloma (Martinez, *et al.*, 1975, Janitschke, *et al.*, 1996, Gornik & Kuzna-Grygiel, 2005). Electron microscopic studies reveal swelling and disintegration of dendrites, astrocytes, oligodendrocyte disruption, and disassociation of the myelin sheath along swollen axon cylinders (Martinez, *et al.*, 1975). In our studies with ACA 83-95-induced autoimmune encephalomyelitis, in spite of the presence of mononuclear cells (MNC), the dominance of plasma cells and giant cells was absent. Instead, the histologic disease resembled typical PLP 139-151-induced EAE (Sobel, *et al.*, 1990, Massilamany, *et al.*, 2010, Massilamany, *et al.*, 2011), suggesting that naturally occurring GAE may involve the mediation of multiple factors and different cell types, which may reflect the host's response to living organisms *in situ*. To date, there are no reports to indicate that autoimmune response is a component of disease pathogenesis in GAE, and our data with ACA 83-95-induced autoimmune encephalomyelitis provide compelling evidence to test this possibility. This notion is further supported by the fact that humans affected with *A. castellanii* infection can never be treated successfully (Marciano-Cabral & Cabral, 2003).

Pathogens that primarily infect the CNS can induce autoimmune responses secondarily. As previously discussed, *A. castellanii* is a pathogen of the CNS that causes granulomatous inflammation of the brain and spinal cord. We propose that *A. castellanii* can induce myelin-reactive T cells by two mechanisms in infected mice (Fig. 8). **(a) Molecular mimicry.** Upon exposure to the parasites, the immune system recognizes parasite-derived mimic of PLP, generating T cells in the periphery, which then migrate into the CNS and cause inflammation. In support of this theory, we have demonstrated that the mimicry epitope from *A. castellanii*,

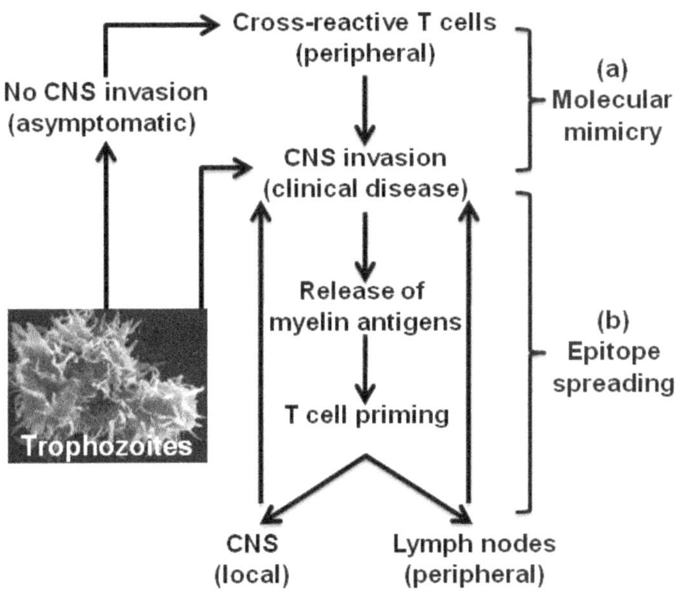

Fig. 8. Proposed mechanisms for the induction of CNS autoimmunity in mice infected with *A. castellanii*. (a) Molecular mimicry. Peripherally, the immune system can recognize mimicry epitope of PLP, and generates cross-reactive T cells, which then migrate into the CNS and cause inflammation. (b) Epitope spreading. Granulomatous CNS inflammation induced by *Acanthamoeba* can lead to the release of myelin antigens and prime T cells locally or peripherally and the *de novo* generated myelin-reactive T cells can further aggravate CNS inflammation. Conversely, mice can remain infected and clinically normal but, cross-reactive cells can still be generated by mimicry.

ACA 83-95, can induce clinical signs of autoimmune encephalomyelitis in the adjuvant protocol of inducing CNS autoimmunity in SJL mice (Massilamany, *et al.*, 2010, Massilamany, *et al.*, 2011). **(b) Epitope spreading.** *A. castellanii* causes granulomatous inflammation in the brain and spinal cord, which can lead to the local release of myelin antigens and prime T cells. Alternatively, the newly released myelin antigens are carried by antigen-presenting cells to the draining lymph nodes and prime T cells, which, in turn, migrate back into the CNS and further aggravate inflammation. Similar events have been earlier demonstrated in the case of murine pathogen, TMEV (Miller, *et al.*, 2001, Olson, *et al.*, 2004, McMahon, *et al.*, 2005).
MS is a disease of the CNS characterized by inflammation and infiltration of MNC and the loss of myelin sheath encapsulating the axons (Noseworthy, *et al.*, 2000, Sospedra & Martin, 2005). Autoimmune responses to myelin antigens have been implicated in MS pathogenesis and this requires the mediation of autoreactive T cells and B cells, but the mechanisms by which the disease is initiated are unknown (Kerlero de Rosbo, *et al.*, 1993, Sospedra & Martin, 2005). Although genetic susceptibility is a major predisposing factor, exposure to environmental microbes such as viruses and bacteria have been suspected in the initiation of autoimmune diseases. In support of the latter, exacerbations of MS attacks or temporal alterations in the disease course have been linked primarily to exposure to virus infections such as Epstein Barr virus and Human Herpes virus-6, but the clinical evidence remains elusive (Cirone, *et al.*, 2002, Pohl, 2009, Salvetti, *et al.*, 2009). The current dogma is that MS does not appear to follow Koch's postulates in that no single organism appears to trigger it; rather, exposure to multiple organisms might be critical for MS predisposition (Sospedra & Martin, 2005). The fact that ACA contains mimicry epitope for PLP, one of the candidate autoantigens implicated in MS pathogenesis, suggests that ACA infection can potentially lead to the generation of PLP reactive T cells and predispose to MS.

5. Clinical signs and histology

Acanthamoeba-induced encephalitis is often overlooked (Schuster & Visvesvara, 2004, da Rocha-Azevedo, *et al.*, 2009), partly due to the rarity of *Acanthamoeba* infections and a lack of familiarity and diagnostic tools. However, when diagnosed, it is difficult to differentiate PAM from GAE because symptoms overlap between each other (da Rocha-Azevedo, *et al.*, 2009). PAM is initially manifested by severe headache, rhinitis, nausea, and fever followed by anosmia, seizures, stiff neck, diplopia, and coma, finally leading to death (Marciano-Cabral & Cabral, 2003, da Rocha-Azevedo, *et al.*, 2009). Histologically, brains contain inflammatory infiltrates comprised of neutrophils, eosinophils, and macrophages (Martinez & Janitschke, 1985, Marciano-Cabral & Cabral, 2003, da Rocha-Azevedo, *et al.*, 2009). In contrast, symptoms of GAE are diverse in that a wide range of clinical manifestations can be expected. These include headache, rise in intracranial pressure, abnormal gait or ataxia, diplopia, stiff neck, confusion, behavioral changes, hemiparesis, cranial nerve palsies, seizures, photophobia, and anorexia; more than 90% of individuals affected with GAE tend to die (Marciano-Cabral & Cabral, 2003, Khan, 2006). The histologic disease is characterized by hemorrhagic or necrotic encephalitis, edema of the brain accompanied by the presence of focal lesions around the cerebrum, cerebellum, and corpus callosum. Cellular infiltrations in histological sections include multinucleated giant cells, plasma cells, polymorphonuclear cells and mononuclear cells (Martinez & Visvesvara, 1997, da Rocha-Azevedo, *et al.*, 2009) and HIV patients can develop granulomas within the CNS possibly due to low CD4 T cell count (Marciano-Cabral & Cabral, 2003, Cha, *et al.*, 2006, Khan, 2006). In some patients, organs other than brain such as skin, liver, lungs, kidneys, prostate glands, lymph nodes, pancreas, and adrenals can also be affected.

6. Diagnosis

Acanthamoeba-induced encephalitis is not routinely suspected, the disease can be misdiagnosed as neurocysticercosis; viral, rickettsial, fungal, and bacterial meningitis; toxoplasmosis; and brain tumors (Schuster & Visvesvara, 2004, khan, 2005b). Serologically, detection of *Acanthamoeba*-reactive antibodies gives an indication of amoebic exposure at a population level (Cursons, *et al.*, 1980, Cerva, 1989, Khan, 2006). However, definitive diagnosis requires the demonstration of amoebic trophozoites or cysts in biological samples. Examination of wet-mount smears prepared from CSF or methanol-fixed smears stained with Giemsa-Wright permit identification of amoebic trophozoites. While evaluating wet-mount smears, careful consideration should be given to differentiate trophozoites from macrophages because of their close morphological resemblance to each other (Cleland, *et al.*, 1982, Lalitha, *et al.*, 1985, Singhal, *et al.*, 2001). In addition to CSF, trophozoites can also be detected in bronchoalveolar lavage fluid from patients with respiratory distress (Newsome, *et al.*, 1992). Detection of trophozoites in fixed tissue sections prepared from brains is usually performed using hematoxylin and eosin and trichrome stainings (Newsome, *et al.*, 1992). In contrast, amoebic cysts in brain tissues are detected using calcofluor white staining (Silvany, *et al.*, 1987). Alternatively, periodic acid-Schiff's stain and Gomori-methenamine silver stain can be used to stain tissue sections in which, cysts appear red whereas tissues appear black in color (Marciano-Cabral & Cabral, 2003).

Other specialized techniques employed to demonstrate the presence of amoeba are transmission electron microscopy and immunofluorescent or immunoperoxidase staining (Willaert & Stevens, 1976, Stevens, *et al.*, 1977, McKellar, *et al.*, 2006, Guarner, *et al.*, 2007). However, because most *Acanthamoeba* spp. are antigenically related, the use of immunohistochemical techniques does not permit identification by species. To identify structural brain lesions, computed tomography and magnetic resonance imaging are widely used (Sell, *et al.*, 1997, Kidney & Kim, 1998). These evaluations can reveal changes such as multifocal areas of signal intensities or ring-like lesions or low-density areas indicating occupying mass of tumor or abscess (Martinez, *et al.*, 1977, Martinez, *et al.*, 1980, Ofori-Kwakye, *et al.*, 1986, Matson, *et al.*, 1988, khan, 2005b, Khan, 2008, da Rocha-Azevedo, *et al.*, 2009). The regions of the brain that are usually affected are midbrain, basal areas of the temporal and occipital lobes, and the posterior fossa (Seijo Martinez, *et al.*, 2000, Marciano-Cabral & Cabral, 2003, Khan, 2006). Molecularly, PCR amplification of the 18S rDNA using sequence-specific primers is currently used as a quick and reliable method of diagnosis (Schroeder, *et al.*, 2001, Khan, 2006, da Rocha-Azevedo, *et al.*, 2009, Maritschnegg, *et al.*, 2011). Hematologically, pleocytosis accompanied by lymphocytosis, neutrophilia, hypoglycemia and hyperprotenemia may be seen in patients with GAE (Marciano-Cabral & Cabral, 2003). In addition, *Acanthamoeba* can be isolated from clinical specimens by plating the samples on non-nutrient agar plates coated with *E. coli* or *Enterobacter aerogenes* (Schuster, 2002, Khan, 2006, da Rocha-Azevedo, *et al.*, 2009).

7. Treatment

The low degree of therapeutic success in treating amoebic encephalitis is due in part to the fact that immunocompromised individuals are most often affected, and the disease outcome thus depends on successful treatment of underlying causes. Furthermore, *Acanthamoeba* infections tend to escape early diagnosis due to the lack of both awareness and diagnostic tools. Nonetheless, if diagnosed early, the disease can be treated successfully (Marciano-Cabral & Cabral, 2003, Schuster & Visvesvara, 2004, Khan, 2006, Khan, 2008, Matin, *et al.*, 2008, Elsheikha & Khan, 2010, Akpek, *et al.*, 2011). Various treatment regimens have been reported in the literature, but there are no reports to indicate that *Acanthamoeba* infections can be treated with a single drug; rather, a combination of multiple drugs is used (Table 1). These include ketoconazole, fluconazole, flucytosine, sulfa-trimethoprim, amphotericin B, pentamidine isothionate, azithromycin, itraconazole and rifampicin. Currently, to enhance BBB-permeability, soluble analogs of the most effective drugs are being tested (Khan, 2006). Likewise, experimental attempts also are being made to use non-viral plasmid DNAs encoding anti-sense RNA sequences for virulence factors of amoebae which can block their entry into the CNS (Elsheikha & Khan, 2010). Based on our data (Massilamany, *et al.*, 2010, Massilamany, *et al.*, 2011), we propose that amoebic encephalitis might involve mediation of autoimmunity, but this hypothesis needs to be tested experimentally in animal models and clinically in GAE patients. Proving that autoimmunity is a component of GAE provides a basis for exploring treatment modalities directed toward autoimmunity in patient subjects.

Species	Disease	Drugs	Outcome	Reference
Acanthamoeba spp.	GAE	Pyrimethamine and fluconazole	Died	Gardner, *et al.*, 1991
Acanthamoeba spp.	GAE	Pyrimethamine and sulfadiazine	Died	Gordon, *et al.*, 1992
Acanthamoeba spp.	Cutaneous amoebiasis and GAE	Fluorocytosine and pentamidine	Died	Murakawa, *et al.*, 1995
Acanthamoeba spp.	GAE	Sulfadiazine, pyrimethamine, fluconazole and sulfadiazine	Survived	Seijo Martinez, *et al.*, 2000
Acanthamoeba T4	GAE	Fluconazole, rifampicin, Metronidazole and sulfadiazine	Survived	Petry, *et al.*, 2006
Acanthamoeba T1	GAE	Fluoxetine, pantoprazole and prednisolone.	Died	Cha, *et al.*, 2006
Acanthamoeba spp.	GAE	Ketoconazole, trimethoprim, sulfamethoxazole, rifampicin and cotrimoxazole	Survived	Gupta, *et al.*, 2008
Acanthamoeba T2	GAE	Miltefosine and amikacin.	Survived	Walochnik, *et al.*, 2008
Acanthamoeba spp.	GAE	Miltefosine and amikacin	Survived	Aichelburg, *et al.*, 2008
Acanthamoeba spp.	GAE	Rifampicin and co-trimoxazole	Survived	Fung, *et al.*, 2008
Acanthamoeba lenticulata T3	GAE	Meropenem, linezolid, moxifloxacin and fluconazole	Survived	Lackner, *et al.*, 2010
Acanthamoeba group II T4	GAE	Trimethoprim-sulfamethoxazole, fluconazole, pentamidine and miltefosine	Survived	Maritschnegg, *et al.*, 2011

Table 1. Drugs used in the treatment of *Acanthamoeba* infections

8. Conclusion

In spite of high prevalence, the diseases induced by Acanthamoebae are extremely low. Although amoebic encephalitis is more commonly seen in immunocompromised individuals, the disease can occur in immunocompetent healthy individuals (Marciano-Cabral & Cabral, 2003, Schuster & Visvesvara, 2004). Our discovery that *A. castellanii* contains mimicry epitope for PLP indicates that exposure to *Acanthamoeba* can accompany autoimmunity through the generation of self-reactive T cells. Acanthamoebae are free-living organisms that are ubiquitous in the environment, leading to constant exposure. It is possible that such coexistence can help microbes acquire some of the genetic elements of their hosts as an evasive mechanism for survival. Alternatively, exposure to such organisms could lead to a break in self-tolerance as a result of antigenic mimicry in genetically susceptible individuals who potentially carry pathogenic autoreactive T cell and B cell repertoires. Further research is required to address these hypotheses, proving which creates opportunities to also target therapy toward autoimmunity in patients affected with GAE.

9. References

Aichelburg AC, Walochnik J, Assadian O, et al. (2008) Successful treatment of disseminated Acanthamoeba sp. infection with miltefosine. Emerg Infect Dis 14: 1743-1746.

Akpek G, Uslu A, Huebner T, *et al.* (2011) Granulomatous amebic encephalitis: an under-recognized cause of infectious mortality after hematopoietic stem cell transplantation. *Transpl Infect Dis.*

Barbeau J & Buhler T (2001) Biofilms augment the number of free-living amoebae in dental unit waterlines. *Res Microbiol* 152: 753-760.

Barker J, Scaife H & Brown MR (1995) Intraphagocytic growth induces an antibiotic-resistant phenotype of Legionella pneumophila. *Antimicrob Agents Chemother* 39: 2684-2688.

Benedetto N & Auriault C (2002a) Complex network of cytokines activating murine microglial cell activity against Acanthamoeba castellani. *Eur Cytokine Netw* 13: 351-357.

Benedetto N & Auriault C (2002b) Prolactin-cytokine network in the defence against Acanthamoeba castellanii in murine microglia [corrected]. *Eur Cytokine Netw* 13: 447-455.

Benedetto N, Rossano F, Gorga F, Folgore A, Rao M & Romano Carratelli C (2003) Defense mechanisms of IFN-gamma and LPS-primed murine microglia against Acanthamoeba castellanii infection. *Int Immunopharmacol* 3: 825-834.

Berk SG, Ting RS, Turner GW & Ashburn RJ (1998) Production of respirable vesicles containing live Legionella pneumophila cells by two Acanthamoeba spp. *Appl Environ Microbiol* 64: 279-286.

Bettelli E, Oukka M & Kuchroo VK (2007) T(H)-17 cells in the circle of immunity and autoimmunity. *Nat Immunol* 8: 345-350.

Bowers B (1977) Comparison of pinocytosis and phagocytosis in Acanthamoeba castellanii. *Exp Cell Res* 110: 409-417.

Bowers B & Korn ED (1968) The fine structure of Acanthamoeba castellanii. I. The trophozoite. *J Cell Biol* 39: 95-111.

Bowers B & Olszewski TE (1983) Acanthamoeba discriminates internally between digestible and indigestible particles. *J Cell Biol* 97: 317-322.

Brindley N, Matin A & Khan NA (2009) Acanthamoeba castellanii: high antibody prevalence in racially and ethnically diverse populations. *Exp Parasitol* 121: 254-256.

Casemore DP (1977) Free-living amoebae in home dialysis unit. *Lancet* 2: 1078.

Cerva L (1989) Acanthamoeba culbertsoni and Naegleria fowleri: occurrence of antibodies in man. *J Hyg Epidemiol Microbiol Immunol* 33: 99-103.

Cha JH, Furie K, Kay J, Walensky RP, Mullins ME & Hedley-Whyte ET (2006) Case records of the Massachusetts General Hospital. Case 39-2006. A 24-year-old woman with systemic lupus erythematosus, seizures, and right arm weakness. *N Engl J Med* 355: 2678-2689.

Chagla AH & Griffiths AJ (1974) Growth and encystation of Acanthamoeba castellanii. *J Gen Microbiol* 85: 139-145.

Chappell CL, Wright JA, Coletta M & Newsome AL (2001) Standardized method of measuring acanthamoeba antibodies in sera from healthy human subjects. *Clin Diagn Lab Immunol* 8: 724-730.

Cirone M, Cuomo L, Zompetta C, Ruggieri S, Frati L, Faggioni A & Ragona G (2002) Human herpesvirus 6 and multiple sclerosis: a study of T cell cross-reactivity to viral and myelin basic protein antigens. *J Med Virol* 68: 268-272.

Cleland PG, Lawande RV, Onyemelukwe G & Whittle HC (1982) Chronic amebic meningoencephalitis. *Arch Neurol* 39: 56-57.

Culbertson CG (1961) Pathogenic Acanthamoeba (Hartmanella). *Am J Clin Pathol* 35: 195-202.

Culbertson CG, Smith JW & Minner JR (1958) Acanthamoeba: observations on animal pathogenicity. *Science* 127: 1506.

Culbertson CG, Ensminger PW & Overton WM (1966) Hartmannella (acanthamoeba). Experimental chronic, granulomatous brain infections produced by new isolates of low virulence. *Am J Clin Pathol* 46: 305-314.

Culbertson CG, Smith JW, Cohen HK & Minner JR (1959) Experimental infection of mice and monkeys by Acanthamoeba. *Am J Pathol* 35: 185-197.

Cursons RT, Brown TJ, Keys EA, Moriarty KM & Till D (1980) Immunity to pathogenic free-living amoebae: role of cell-mediated immunity. *Infect Immun* 29: 408-410.

da Rocha-Azevedo B, Tanowitz HB & Marciano-Cabral F (2009) Diagnosis of infections caused by pathogenic free-living amoebae. *Interdiscip Perspect Infect Dis* 2009: 251406.

De Jonckheere J & van de Voorde H (1976) Differences in destruction of cysts of pathogenic and nonpathogenic Naegleria and Acanthamoeba by chlorine. *Appl Environ Microbiol* 31: 294-297.

De Jonckheere JF (1987) Taxonomy, Amphizoic amoebae human pathology (Rondanelli EG, ed.^eds.), p.^pp. pp 25-48. Piccin Nuova Libraria, Padua, Italy, Padua, Italy.

De Jonckheere JF (1991) Ecology of Acanthamoeba. *Rev Infect Dis* 13 Suppl 5: S385-387.

Dudley R, Alsam S & Khan NA (2007) Cellulose biosynthesis pathway is a potential target in the improved treatment of Acanthamoeba keratitis. *Appl Microbiol Biotechnol* 75: 133-140.

Elsheikha HM & Khan NA (2010) Protozoa traversal of the blood-brain barrier to invade the central nervous system. *FEMS Microbiol Rev* 34: 532-553.

Ferrante A (1991a) Free-living amoebae: pathogenicity and immunity. *Parasite Immunol* 13: 31-47.

Ferrante A (1991b) Immunity to Acanthamoeba. *Rev Infect Dis* 13 Suppl 5: S403-409.

Fung KT, Dhillon AP, McLaughlin JE, et al. (2008) Cure of Acanthamoeba cerebral abscess in a liver transplant patient. Liver Transpl 14: 308-312.

Gardner HA, Martinez AJ, Visvesvara GS & Sotrel A (1991) Granulomatous amebic encephalitis in an AIDS patient. Neurology 41: 1993-1995.

Garate M, Marchant J, Cubillos I, Cao Z, Khan NA & Panjwani N (2006) In vitro pathogenicity of Acanthamoeba is associated with the expression of the mannose-binding protein. *Invest Ophthalmol Vis Sci* 47: 1056-1062.

Gast RJ, Ledee DR, Fuerst PA & Byers TJ (1996) Subgenus systematics of Acanthamoeba: four nuclear 18S rDNA sequence types. *J Eukaryot Microbiol* 43: 498-504.

Gordon SM, Steinberg JP, DuPuis MH, Kozarsky PE, Nickerson JF & Visvesvara GS (1992) Culture isolation of Acanthamoeba species and leptomyxid amebas from patients with amebic meningoencephalitis, including two patients with AIDS. Clin Infect Dis 15: 1024-1030.

Gornik K & Kuzna-Grygiel W (2005) Histological studies of selected organs of mice experimentally infected with Acanthamoeba spp. *Folia Morphol (Warsz)* 64: 161-167.

Guarner J, Bartlett J, Shieh WJ, Paddock CD, Visvesvara GS & Zaki SR (2007) Histopathologic spectrum and immunohistochemical diagnosis of amebic meningoencephalitis. *Mod Pathol* 20: 1230-1237.

Gupta D, Panda GS & Bakhshi S (2008) Successful treatment of acanthamoeba meningoencephalitis during induction therapy of childhood acute lymphoblastic leukemia. Pediatr Blood Cancer 50: 1292-1293.

Han KL, Lee J, Kim DS, Park SJ, Im KI & Yong TS (2006) Identification of differentially expressed cDNAs in Acanthamoeba culbertsoni after mouse brain passage. *Korean J Parasitol* 44: 15-20.

Jahnes WG & Fullmer HM (1957) Free living amoebae as contaminants in monkey kidney tissue culture. *Proc Soc Exp Biol Med* 96: 484-488.

Janitschke K, Martinez AJ, Visvesvara GS & Schuster F (1996) Animal model Balamuthia mandrillaris CNS infection: contrast and comparison in immunodeficient and immunocompetent mice: a murine model of "granulomatous" amebic encephalitis. *J Neuropathol Exp Neurol* 55: 815-821.

Jones DB, Visvesvara GS & Robinson NM (1975) Acanthamoeba polyphaga keratitis and Acenthamoeba uveitis associated with fatal meningoencephalitis. *Trans Ophthalmol Soc U K* 95: 221-232.

Kerlero de Rosbo N, Milo R, Lees MB, Burger D, Bernard CC & Ben-Nun A (1993) Reactivity to myelin antigens in multiple sclerosis. Peripheral blood lymphocytes respond predominantly to myelin oligodendrocyte glycoprotein. *J Clin Invest* 92: 2602-2608.

Khan NA (2003) Pathogenesis of Acanthamoeba infections. *Microb Pathog* 34: 277-285.

Khan NA (2005a) The immunological aspects of Acanthamoeba infections. *American journal of immunology* 1: 24-30.

khan NA (2005b) Granulomatous amoebic encephalitis: Clinical diagnosis and management. *American journal of infectious diseases* 1: 79-83.

Khan NA (2006) Acanthamoeba: biology and increasing importance in human health. *FEMS Microbiol Rev* 30: 564-595.

Khan NA (2007) Acanthamoeba invasion of the central nervous system. *Int J Parasitol* 37: 131-138.

Khan NA (2008) Acanthamoeba and the blood-brain barrier: the breakthrough. *J Med Microbiol* 57: 1051-1057.

Khan NA (2009) Novel in vitro and in vivo models to study central nervous system infections due to Acanthamoeba spp. *Exp Parasitol.*

Khan NA, Jarroll EL, Panjwani N, Cao Z & Paget TA (2000) Proteases as markers for differentiation of pathogenic and nonpathogenic species of Acanthamoeba. *J Clin Microbiol* 38: 2858-2861.

Khunkitti W, Lloyd D, Furr JR & Russell AD (1998) Acanthamoeba castellanii: growth, encystment, excystment and biocide susceptibility. *J Infect* 36: 43-48.

Kidney DD & Kim SH (1998) CNS infections with free-living amebas: neuroimaging findings. *AJR Am J Roentgenol* 171: 809-812.

Kim MJ, Shin CO & Im KI (1990) [Cell-mediated immunity in mice infected with Acanthamoeba culbertsoni]. *Kisaengchunghak Chapchi* 28: 143-154.

King CH, Shotts EB, Jr., Wooley RE & Porter KG (1988) Survival of coliforms and bacterial pathogens within protozoa during chlorination. *Appl Environ Microbiol* 54: 3023-3033.

Kingston D & Warhurst DC (1969) Isolation of amoebae from the air. *J Med Microbiol* 2: 27-36.

Koide J, Okusawa E, Ito T, Mori S, Takeuchi T, Itoyama S & Abe T (1998) Granulomatous amoebic encephalitis caused by Acanthamoeba in a patient with systemic lupus erythematosus. *Clin Rheumatol* 17: 329-332.

Kong HH, Kim TH & Chung DI (2000) Purification and characterization of a secretory serine proteinase of Acanthamoeba healyi isolated from GAE. *J Parasitol* 86: 12-17.

Korn ED & Olivecrona T (1971) Composition of an amoeba plasma membrane. *Biochem Biophys Res Commun* 45: 90-97.

Lackner P, Beer R, Broessner G, et al. (2010) Acute granulomatous acanthamoeba encephalitis in an immunocompetent patient. Neurocrit Care 12: 91-94.

Lalitha MK, Anandi V, Srivastava A, Thomas K, Cherian AM & Chandi SM (1985) Isolation of Acanthamoeba culbertsoni from a patient with meningitis. *J Clin Microbiol* 21: 666-667.

Lloyd D, Turner NA, Khunkitti W, Hann AC, Furr JR & Russell AD (2001) Encystation in Acanthamoeba castellanii: development of biocide resistance. *J Eukaryot Microbiol* 48: 11-16.

Marciano-Cabral F & Toney DM (1998) The interaction of Acanthamoeba spp. with activated macrophages and with macrophage cell lines. *J Eukaryot Microbiol* 45: 452-458.

Marciano-Cabral F & Cabral G (2003) Acanthamoeba spp. as agents of disease in humans. *Clin Microbiol Rev* 16: 273-307.

Marciano-Cabral F, Puffenbarger R & Cabral GA (2000) The increasing importance of Acanthamoeba infections. *J Eukaryot Microbiol* 47: 29-36.

Marciano-Cabral F, Ferguson T, Bradley SG & Cabral G (2001) Delta-9-tetrahydrocannabinol (THC), the major psychoactive component of marijuana, exacerbates brain infection by Acanthamoeba. *J Eukaryot Microbiol* Suppl: 4S-5S.

Maritschnegg P, Sovinz P, Lackner H, *et al.* (2011) Granulomatous amebic encephalitis in a child with acute lymphoblastic leukemia successfully treated with multimodal antimicrobial therapy and hyperbaric oxygen. *J Clin Microbiol* 49: 446-448.

Martinez AJ & Janitschke K (1985) Acanthamoeba, an opportunistic microorganism: a review. *Infection* 13: 251-256.

Martinez AJ & Visvesvara GS (1997) Free-living, amphizoic and opportunistic amebas. *Brain Pathol* 7: 583-598.

Martinez AJ & Visvesvara GS (2001) Balamuthia mandrillaris infection. *J Med Microbiol* 50: 205-207.

Martinez AJ, Markowitz SM & Duma RJ (1975) Experimental pneumonitis and encephalitis caused by acanthamoeba in mice: pathogenesis and ultrastructural features. *J Infect Dis* 131: 692-699.

Martinez AJ, Garcia CA, Halks-Miller M & Arce-Vela R (1980) Granulomatous amebic encephalitis presenting as a cerebral mass lesion. *Acta Neuropathol* 51: 85-91.

Martinez AJ, Sotelo-Avila C, Garcia-Tamayo J, Moron JT, Willaert E & Stamm WP (1977) Meningoencephalitis due to Acanthamoeba SP. Pathogenesis and clinico-pathological study. *Acta Neuropathol* 37: 183-191.

Massilamany C, Steffen D & Reddy J (2010) An epitope from Acanthamoeba castellanii that cross-react with proteolipid protein 139-151-reactive T cells induces autoimmune encephalomyelitis in SJL mice. *J Neuroimmunol* 219: 17-24.

Massilamany C, Thulasingam S, Steffen D & Reddy J (2011) Gender differences in CNS autoimmunity induced by mimicry epitope for PLP 139-151 in SJL mice. *J Neuroimmunol* 230: 95-104.

Matin A, Siddiqui R, Jayasekera S & Khan NA (2008) Increasing importance of Balamuthia mandrillaris. *Clin Microbiol Rev* 21: 435-448.

Matson DO, Rouah E, Lee RT, Armstrong D, Parke JT & Baker CJ (1988) Acanthameba meningoencephalitis masquerading as neurocysticercosis. *Pediatr Infect Dis J* 7: 121-124.

Mattana A, Serra C, Mariotti E, Delogu G, Fiori PL & Cappuccinelli P (2006) Acanthamoeba castellanii promotion of in vitro survival and transmission of coxsackie b3 viruses. *Eukaryot Cell* 5: 665-671.

McClellan K, Howard K, Mayhew E, Niederkorn J & Alizadeh H (2002) Adaptive immune responses to Acanthamoeba cysts. *Exp Eye Res* 75: 285-293.

McKellar MS, Mehta LR, Greenlee JE, *et al.* (2006) Fatal granulomatous Acanthamoeba encephalitis mimicking a stroke, diagnosed by correlation of results of sequential magnetic resonance imaging, biopsy, in vitro culture, immunofluorescence analysis, and molecular analysis. *J Clin Microbiol* 44: 4265-4269.

McMahon EJ, Bailey SL, Castenada CV, Waldner H & Miller SD (2005) Epitope spreading initiates in the CNS in two mouse models of multiple sclerosis. *Nat Med* 11: 335-339.

Meersseman W, Lagrou K, Sciot R, *et al.* (2007) Rapidly fatal Acanthamoeba encephalitis and treatment of cryoglobulinemia. *Emerg Infect Dis* 13: 469-471.

Michel R, Burghardt H & Bergmann H (1995) [Acanthamoeba, naturally intracellularly infected with Pseudomonas aeruginosa, after their isolation from a microbiologically contaminated drinking water system in a hospital]. *Zentralbl Hyg Umweltmed* 196: 532-544.

Miller SD & Karpus WJ (2007) Experimental autoimmune encephalomyelitis in the mouse. *Curr Protoc Immunol* Chapter 15: Unit 15 11.

Miller SD, Katz-Levy Y, Neville KL & Vanderlugt CL (2001) Virus-induced autoimmunity: epitope spreading to myelin autoepitopes in Theiler's virus infection of the central nervous system. *Adv Virus Res* 56: 199-217.

Murakawa GJ, McCalmont T, Altman J, Telang GH, Hoffman MD, Kantor GR & Berger TG (1995) Disseminated acanthamebiasis in patients with AIDS. A report of five cases and a review of the literature. Arch Dermatol 131: 1291-1296.

Na BK, Cho JH, Song CY & Kim TS (2002) Degradation of immunoglobulins, protease inhibitors and interleukin-1 by a secretory proteinase of Acanthamoeba castellanii. *Korean J Parasitol* 40: 93-99.

Newsome AL, Curtis FT, Culbertson CG & Allen SD (1992) Identification of Acanthamoeba in bronchoalveolar lavage specimens. *Diagn Cytopathol* 8: 231-234.

Noseworthy JH, Lucchinetti C, Rodriguez M & Weinshenker BG (2000) Multiple sclerosis. *N Engl J Med* 343: 938-952.

O'Connor RA, Prendergast CT, Sabatos CA, Lau CW, Leech MD, Wraith DC & Anderton SM (2008) Cutting edge: Th1 cells facilitate the entry of Th17 cells to the central nervous system during experimental autoimmune encephalomyelitis. *J Immunol* 181: 3750-3754.

Ofori-Kwakye SK, Sidebottom DG, Herbert J, Fischer EG & Visvesvara GS (1986) Granulomatous brain tumor caused by Acanthamoeba. Case report. *J Neurosurg* 64: 505-509.

Olson JK, Ludovic Croxford J & Miller SD (2004) Innate and adaptive immune requirements for induction of autoimmune demyelinating disease by molecular mimicry. *Mol Immunol* 40: 1103-1108.

Petry F, Torzewski M, Bohl J, et al. (2006) Early diagnosis of Acanthamoeba infection during routine cytological examination of cerebrospinal fluid. J Clin Microbiol 44: 1903-1904.

Pohl D (2009) Epstein-Barr virus and multiple sclerosis. *J Neurol Sci* 286: 62-64.

Rowbotham TJ (1980) Preliminary report on the pathogenicity of Legionella pneumophila for freshwater and soil amoebae. *J Clin Pathol* 33: 1179-1183.

Sakai K, Zamvil SS, Mitchell DJ, Lim M, Rothbard JB & Steinman L (1988) Characterization of a major encephalitogenic T cell epitope in SJL/J mice with synthetic oligopeptides of myelin basic protein. *J Neuroimmunol* 19: 21-32.

Salvetti M, Giovannoni G & Aloisi F (2009) Epstein-Barr virus and multiple sclerosis. *Curr Opin Neurol* 22: 201-206.

Sarica FB, Tufan K, Cekinmez M, Erdogan B & Altinors MN (2009) A Rare But Fatal Case of Granulomatous Amebic Encephalitis with BrainAbscess: The First Case Reported from Turkey. *Turkish Neurosurgery* Vol: 19: 256-259.

Schroeder JM, Booton GC, Hay J, *et al.* (2001) Use of subgenic 18S ribosomal DNA PCR and sequencing for genus and genotype identification of acanthamoebae from humans with keratitis and from sewage sludge. *J Clin Microbiol* 39: 1903-1911.

Schuster FL (2002) Cultivation of pathogenic and opportunistic free-living amebas. *Clin Microbiol Rev* 15: 342-354.

Schuster FL & Visvesvara GS (2004) Free-living amoebae as opportunistic and non-opportunistic pathogens of humans and animals. *Int J Parasitol* 34: 1001-1027.

Seijo Martinez M, Gonzalez-Mediero G, Santiago P, Rodriguez De Lope A, Diz J, Conde C & Visvesvara GS (2000) Granulomatous amebic encephalitis in a patient with AIDS:

isolation of acanthamoeba sp. Group II from brain tissue and successful treatment with sulfadiazine and fluconazole. *J Clin Microbiol* 38: 3892-3895.

Sell JJ, Rupp FW & Orrison WW, Jr. (1997) Granulomatous amebic encephalitis caused by acanthamoeba. *Neuroradiology* 39: 434-436.

Shadidi KR, Aarvak T, Jeansson S, Henriksen JE, Natvig JB & Thompson KM (2001) T-cell responses to viral, bacterial and protozoan antigens in rheumatoid inflammation. Selective migration of T cells to synovial tissue. *Rheumatology (Oxford)* 40: 1120-1125.

Silvany RE, Luckenbach MW & Moore MB (1987) The rapid detection of Acanthamoeba in paraffin-embedded sections of corneal tissue with calcofluor white. *Arch Ophthalmol* 105: 1366-1367.

Singhal T, Bajpai A, Kalra V, Kabra SK, Samantaray JC, Satpathy G & Gupta AK (2001) Successful treatment of Acanthamoeba meningitis with combination oral antimicrobials. *Pediatr Infect Dis J* 20: 623-627.

Sissons J, Kim KS, Stins M, Jayasekera S, Alsam S & Khan NA (2005) Acanthamoeba castellanii induces host cell death via a phosphatidylinositol 3-kinase-dependent mechanism. *Infect Immun* 73: 2704-2708.

Sobel RA, Tuohy VK, Lu ZJ, Laursen RA & Lees MB (1990) Acute experimental allergic encephalomyelitis in SJL/J mice induced by a synthetic peptide of myelin proteolipid protein. *J Neuropathol Exp Neurol* 49: 468-479.

Sospedra M & Martin R (2005) Immunology of multiple sclerosis. *Annu Rev Immunol* 23: 683-747.

Stevens AR, Kilpatrick T, Willaert E & Capron A (1977) Serologic analyses of cell-surface antigens of Acanthamoeba spp. with plasma membrane antisera. *J Protozool* 24: 316-324.

Storey MV, Winiecka-Krusnell J, Ashbolt NJ & Stenstrom TA (2004) The efficacy of heat and chlorine treatment against thermotolerant Acanthamoebae and Legionellae. *Scand J Infect Dis* 36: 656-662.

Stromnes IM, Cerretti LM, Liggitt D, Harris RA & Goverman JM (2008) Differential regulation of central nervous system autoimmunity by T(H)1 and T(H)17 cells. *Nat Med* 14: 337-342.

Tan B, Weldon-Linne CM, Rhone DP, Penning CL & Visvesvara GS (1993) Acanthamoeba infection presenting as skin lesions in patients with the acquired immunodeficiency syndrome. *Arch Pathol Lab Med* 117: 1043-1046.

Tanaka Y, Suguri S, Harada M, Hayabara T, Suzumori K & Ohta N (1994) Acanthamoeba-specific human T-cell clones isolated from healthy individuals. *Parasitol Res* 80: 549-553.

Thomas V, McDonnell G, Denyer SP & Maillard JY (2009) Free-living amoebae and their intracellular pathogenic microorganisms: risks for water quality. *FEMS Microbiol Rev*.

Toney DM & Marciano-Cabral F (1998) Resistance of Acanthamoeba species to complement lysis. *J Parasitol* 84: 338-344.

Tuohy VK, Lu Z, Sobel RA, Laursen RA & Lees MB (1989) Identification of an encephalitogenic determinant of myelin proteolipid protein for SJL mice. *J Immunol* 142: 1523-1527.

Turner NA, Harris J, Russell AD & Lloyd D (2000) Microbial differentiation and changes in susceptibility to antimicrobial agents. *J Appl Microbiol* 89: 751-759.

Uschuplich V, Mileusnic D & Johnson M (2004) Pathologic quiz case. Progressive fatal encephalopathy in an immunosuppressed patient with a history of discoid lupus erythematosus. Subacute granulomatous meningoencephalitis (Acanthamoeba culbertsoni). *Arch Pathol Lab Med* 128: e109-111.

Waldner H, Collins M & Kuchroo VK (2004) Activation of antigen-presenting cells by microbial products breaks self tolerance and induces autoimmune disease. *J Clin Invest* 113: 990-997.

Walochnik J, Aichelburg A, Assadian O, Steuer A, Visvesvara G, Vetter N & Aspock H (2008) Granulomatous amoebic encephalitis caused by Acanthamoeba amoebae of genotype T2 in a human immunodeficiency virus-negative patient. J Clin Microbiol 46: 338-340.

Willaert E & Stevens AR (1976) Indirect immunofluorescent identification of Acanthamoeba causing meningoencephalitis. Pathol Biol (Paris) 24

Part 4

Multicellular Pathogens

15

Encephalitis Due to *Loa loa*

Jean Paul Akue
International Center For Medical Research Franceville (CIRMF), Gabon

1. Introduction

Loa loa encephalitis is becoming an important public health problem, as it impedes the use of some important drugs (ivermectin and DEC) for mass control of filarial disease in parts of West Africa where onchocerciasis is endemic. Loa encephalitis may occur either spontaneously or following chemotherapy targeting *Loa loa*. Although *Loa loa* is restricted to the West African rain forest block, imported cases are described throughout the world, due to intense economic, cultural and touristic population exchanges. The most common clinical features of loiaisis are swelling angioedema (calabar oedema) and ocular passage of the adult worm under the conjunctiva (eye worm). *Loa loa* disease may be particularly severe in expatriates (Nutman et al., 1986). *Loa loa* may cause a localized or systemic disease with involvement of deep organs including the kidney and heart. Only one-third of infected individuals have microfilariae in peripheral blood, leading to an underestimation of the prevalence of this infection. Most expatriates with loiasis have the adult worm but are amicrofilaremic (Churchill et al., 1996). The heterogeneous clinical expression of loisais encephalopathy calls for greater awareness among scientist and medical practitioners worldwide.

2. The pathogen: *Loa loa*

Loa loa is a filarial worm restricted to West Africa (Figure 1), from Guinea in the north through Benin to Uganda in the East, Gabon, Cameroun and Nigeria in the west, and Angola in the South. Parts of Cameroun, Gabon, Nigeria, Congo Brazzaville and Congo Kinshasa (DRC) are hyperendemic. Common clinical signs include eye worm and calabar swelling. *Loa loa* adults produce microfilariae that are released into the peripheral blood. They reach their maximal concentration in peripheral blood during daytime (diurnal periodicity). This larval stage of *Loa loa* is the likely etiologic agent of encephalitis during loiasis. The parasite was first described in 1770 (Mongin, 1770) in the eye of a servant in the island of St Domingue. Only few autochtonous case of loaisis has been reported outside of Africa, in India (Barua et al., 2005; Kethan, 2007), although *Loa loa* can develop successfully in *Chrysops atlanticus*, which is widespread in Louisiana and Mississippi (Orihel & Lowrie, 1975). *Loa loa* is thought to infect 13 million individuals living in endemic zones (Fain, 1978), as well as individuals visiting these areas (Varhaug,2005; Carbonez et al.,2002; Hee-Yoon et al., 2008). However, this prevalence is based on the detection of microfilariae in blood and may therefore be an under-estimation, as about one-third of subjects are amicrofilaremic (Dupont et al., 1988). The adult worm can survive for up to 15 years in its human host.

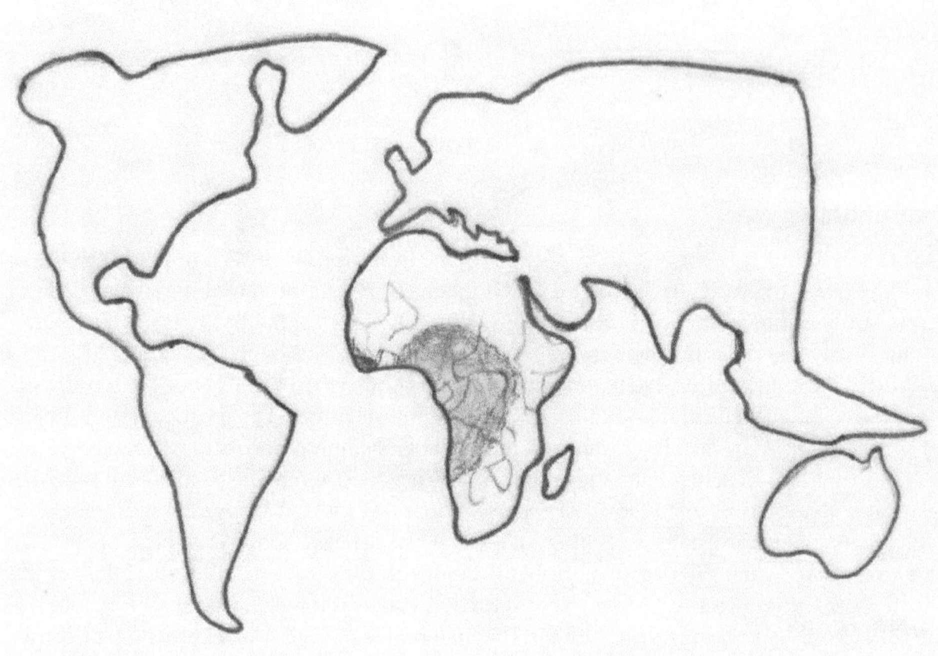

Fig. 1. Distribution of *Loa loa*

The life cycle of *Loa loa* (Figure 2) starts when a female fly of the genus *Chrysops* (*C. silacea*, *dimidiata* or *distinctipennis*) bites an individual harboring *L. loa* microfilariae. The microfilariae reach the stomach of the fly and migrate to the fat body after several mutations to stage L3 (infective larvae). These migrate to the proboscis and are deposited in the host's skin during the next blood meal. Once in the skin, the infective stages moult and reach the adult stage about a year later. The adult remains under the skin but can migrate to different parts of the body, including the ocular conjunctiva (hence the name 'eye worm'). Microfilariae have a diurnal periodicity, being found in peripheral blood from about 5 am to 7 pm, with peak from 9 am to 5 pm (Kershaw, 1950). The existence of an animal reservoir is a possibility (Fain., 1981), as about 10% of blood meals of *C. silacea* and *C. dimidiate* (Gouteux et al., 1989) from hippopotami, rodents, wild ruminants and monitor lizards contain *L. loa* microfilaria, and human L. loa isolates have been successfully maintained in drills (Duke, 1957), baboons, and patas (Orihel & Moore., 1975), rhesus (Grieve et al., 1985), and mandrill monkeys (Pinder et al., 1994).

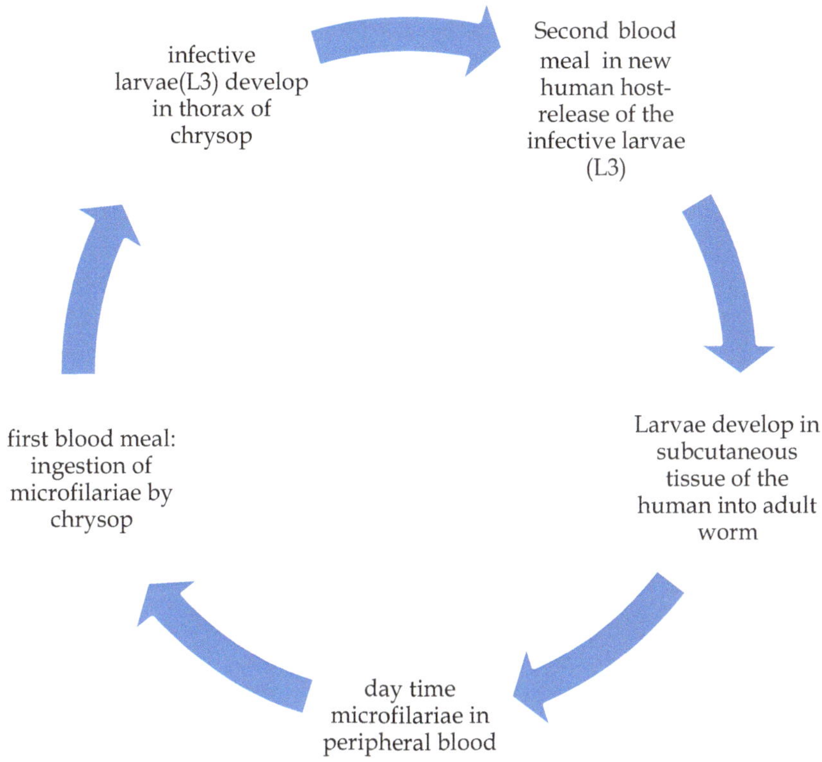

Fig. 2. Life cycle of *Loa loa*

3. The vectors

Chrysops dimidiata and *C. silacea (*Figure 3) (family *Tabanidae*) live in the canopy, and are particularly attracted by smoke and blue tissue. They lay eggs on mud or leaves overhanging water, and the larvae develop in detritus, taking a year before they pupate, with probably seven moults. The pupa is partially buried and the adult emerges after 1-3 weeks. Chrysops is a good intermediate host or vector for *Loa loa*, and it is not unusual to find more than one hundred infective larvae in one fly. For vector control, William (1963) used water emulsions containing various concentrations of DDT, dieldrin, aldrin or gamma-BHC, and found that *Tabanus* larvae were more susceptible than *Chrysops* larvae to all the insecticides tested. Dieldrin emulsion can keep breeding sites free of tabanid larvae for at least eight months (Crewe & Williams, 1964), and has been proposed for the control of chrysops larvae. However, vector control is difficult due to the scale and remote location of breeding sites.

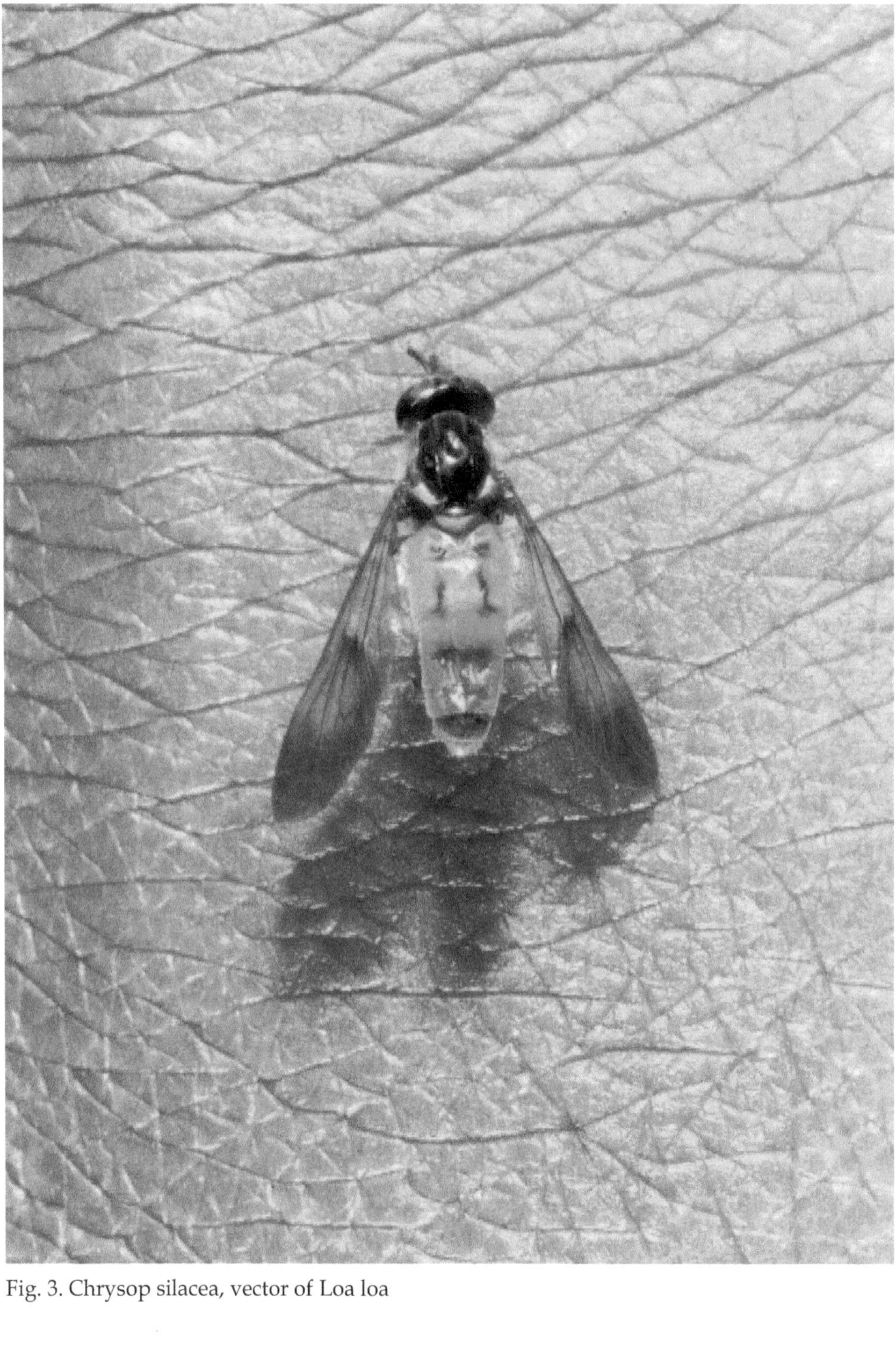

Fig. 3. Chrysop silacea, vector of Loa loa

4. Diagnosis of loaisis

4.1 Clinical diagnosis

Calabar swelling commonly appears on the arm, elbow, face, or chest, and is often accompanied by localized pruritus and discomfort. Another diagnostic sign is ocular passage (Figure 4) of the adult worm (eye worm). These two signs are the most frequent and specific among autochtones and visitors. However, eye worm is more frequent in autochtones than in visitors, while calabar swelling is more common among visitors (82%) (Churchill et al., 1996). Visitors may developed a syndrome of immunological hyper-responsiveness (Nutman et al., 1986) characterized by high titers of antifilarial antibodies, elevated IgE levels (Klion et al., 1991), hypereosinophilia, frequent pruritus around the angiodema, and complications such as endomyocardial fibrosis, renal disease, lymphoma (Gerd et al., 1996), and subcutaneous nodules. Calabar swelling and eye worm may appear alone or simultaneously. Retinal hemorrhage can occur in case of high microfilaremia (Toussaint & Danis 1965), especially after treatment with DEC or ivermectin. Examination of the fundus is therefore necessary, even in the absence of antifilarial treatment. Onset of calabar swelling and eye worm may be followed by cardiac (Andi et al., 1981), renal (Pilay et al., 1973; Bariety et al., 1967) or neurological disorders. Non specific symptoms include pruritus, fever, urticaria, rash, myalgia and arthralgia.

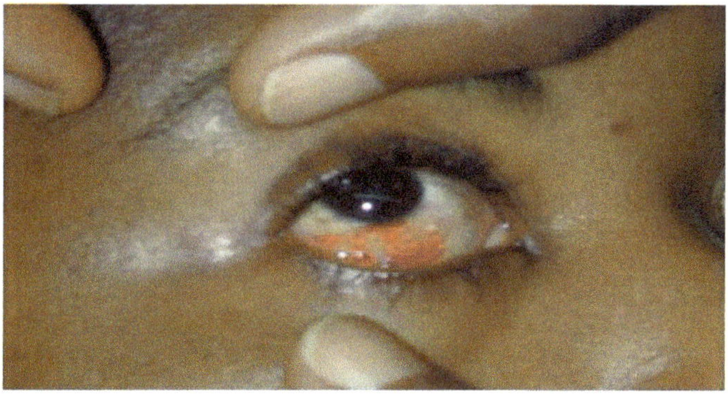

Fig. 4. Ocular passage of *Loa loa* adult worm

4.2 Biological diagnosis

Direct specific diagnosis

Direct specific diagnosis is based on detection of *Loa loa* microfilaria in peripheral blood or of the migrating adult worm. In wet films of blood samples taken around noon, *Loa loa* microfilaria are highly mobile, with a snake-like movement among red blood cells, enveloped in a translucid membrane (sheath). Body size is 231-300 μm by 5-7 μm. A concentration technique on fresh blood can be used: 1 ml of blood is diluted 10X in PBS (Akue et al., 1996), then red cells are lyzed with 2% saponin and the solution is centrifuge at 2000 rpm for 10 minutes. The pellet is smeared on a slide and examined under a microscope. Microfilariae appear as described above. Microfilariae can also be stained with Giemsa in a thick blood film, allowing *Loa loa* to be distinguished from other filariae by their size (253-300 um long), their unstained sheath, and the presence of several nuclei inside the body, reaching the tail but not the cephalic extremity. Direct examination of cerebrospinal fluid (CSF) after centrifugation may be positive for microfilariae in case of neurological signs. The migrating adult worm is most readily detected during its ocular passage. The adult is 2-7 cm long, the female being longer than the male.

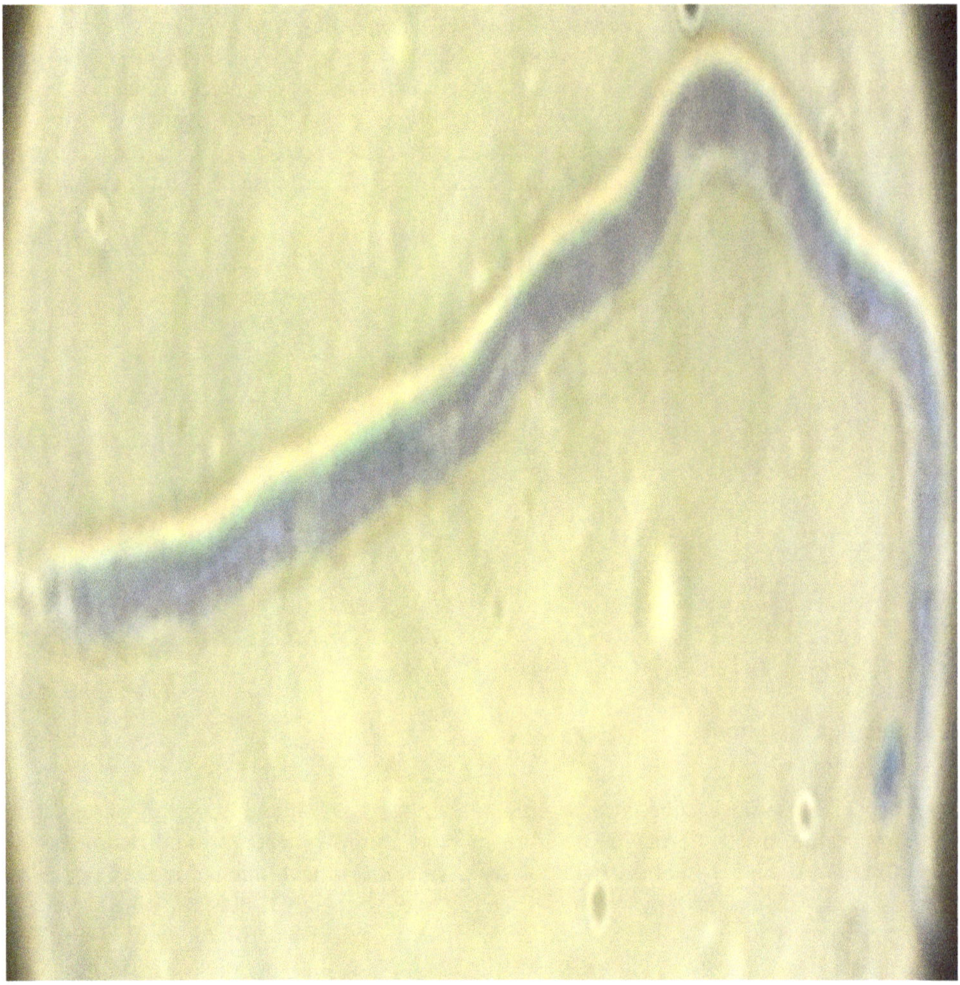

Fig. 5. Stained *Loa loa* microfilaria

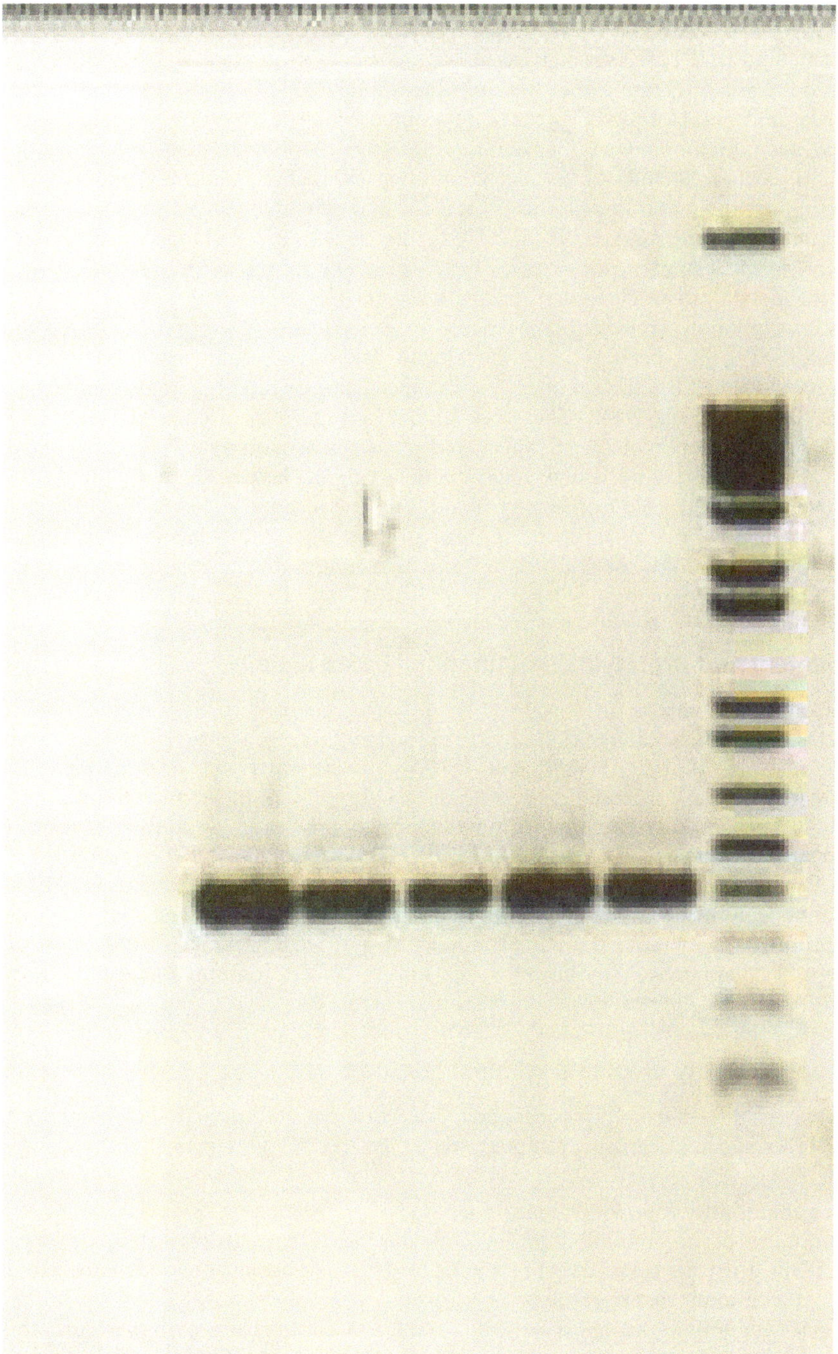

Fig. 6. Amplification of *Loa loa* 15 kDa gene by PCR for diagnosis

Indirect (presumptive) diagnosis

Indirect diagnosis is based on hypereosinophilia (25%) in general among non indigenous population from endemic zone, and elevated total IgE. As most infected people are amicrofilaremic, indirect methods based on antibody or gene detection are valuable. One of the first such methods was the immunofluorescent antibody test (IFAT) using fixed microfilaria. Others include ELISA detection of specific IgG4 against a crude extract of *Loa loa* worm, a method that appears to be specific and sensitive for both microfilaremic and amicrofilaremic forms (Akue et al., 1994). Its sensitivity and specificity (relative to *Mansonnella perstans*) are reported to be better than 90% for parasitologically proven loiasis in a co-endemic area. However, crude extracts are in limited supply. A luciferase immunoprecipitation system (LIPS) based on detection of IgG to *Loa loa* recombinant antigen L1SXP-1 has been recently developed and shows high specificity but limited sensitivity. A rapid LIPS format improves the specificity by limiting cross-reactivity with *O. volvulus* (Burbelo et al., 2008). The same L1XP-1 antigen was used to develop an ELISA method for the detection of specific IgG4 antibodies, but sensitivity was poor (56%) (Klion et al., 2003). Molecular diagnosis may consist of detecting the ladder R3 gene (Ajuh et al., 1995) of *Loa loa* in DNA extracted from whole blood (Touré et al., 1997). However, although highly specific, the test is impractical in rural areas and non specialized laboratories. In general, these methods, although specific, are not sensitive enough to detect all cases of loiasis and are not available at many points of care.

5. Treatment and prophylaxis of uncomplicated loaisis

The treatment of loiasis is based on two major microfilaricides, namely ivermectin (Mectizan® or Stromectol®) and diethylcarbamazine (DEC or Notezine®). With ivermectin, a single dose of 200 µg/kg is sufficient. DEC treatment starts with one-quarter of a tablet (one tablet = 100 mg), then the dose is doubled every day until the maximum dose of 400 mg/day is reached. These treatments must be preceded by precise counting of microfilariae in the patient's blood. If the count is higher than 8000 mf/ml, DEC will be administered at a dose of 8 mg/kg for 21 days under hospital supervision. This treatment is usually combined with antihistamine and corticosteroid therapy during the first week. Proposed chemoprophylaxis includes the use of repellents, and weekly intake of one tablet of DEC (100 mg). Plasmapheresis may be envisaged in case of very high microfilaremia (Muylle et al., 1983; Abel et al., 1986).

6. Encephalopathy in loiasis: clinical features

Loiasis encephalitis is usually a consequence of treatment with dimethyl carbamizine citrate (DEC) or ivermectin (Mectizan), although it may also occur spontaneously.

6.1 Encephalopathy following treatment

The symptoms occur gradually, staring 2 days after ivermectin treatment, or after 24-36 hours of DEC treatment. The patient's condition generally becomes serious after 3 to 5 days. The most common manifestations are vertigo, loss of balance, speaking difficulties, arthralgia, abdominal pain, diarrhea, fever, vomiting, diffuse hypertonia, loss of osteotendinous reflexes, no response to pain, conjunctival or retinal hemorrhage, pruritus, neurological disorders with altered consciousness (obnubilation), renal impairment, coma and death after a few days. Laboratory tests show numerous *Loa loa* microfilaria in peripheral blood, cerebrospinal fluid (CSF) and urine. Loaisis encephalopathy is classified according to the neurological manifestations, their time of onset, and biological findings, in three categories: definite, probable and possible (Scientific working Group on SEA, 2003).

6.1.1 Definite *Loa loa* encephalopathy: microscopic examination of brain tissue obtained by autopsy or needle biopsy is consistent with *Loa loa* encephalopathy (vasculopathy with evidence of *Loa loa* microfilariae), and onset of central nervous system (CNS) disorders within 7 days of treatment with mectizan, progressing to coma without remission.

6.1.2 Probable *Loa loa* encephalopathy: encephalopathy (without seizures, usually febrile) in a previously healthy person with no other cause of encephalopathy, and onset of CNS symptoms and signs within 7 days of treatment with metizan, progressing to coma without remission; and >10 000 mf/ml of peripheral blood pre-treatment, or >1000 mf/ml within 6 months post-treatment, or >2700 mf/ml within 6 months of treatment, and /or L. loa microfilariae in CSF.

6.1.3 Possible L. loa encephalopathy: encephalopathy (without seizures, usually febrile) in a previously healthy person with no other underlying cause of encephalopathy, and onset of CNS symptoms and signs within 7 days of treatment with mectizan, progressing to coma without remission, and semi-quantitatively or qualitatively positive (+, ++ or +++) for L. loa microfilariae in peripheral blood or CSF.

6.2 Spontaneous encephalopathy

Spontaneous cases are rare but may be under-estimated. A number of apparently cases of spontaneous encephalitis have been been reported (Bonet ,1943; Gallais et al., 1954; Carayon et al., 1959; Same Ekobo et al., 1981; Tuna Lukiana et al., 2006). In some case described by Kivit (1952), patients might have taken antifilarial drugs. The symptomatology is variable and may start with calabar swelling accompanied by itching, asthenia, facial edema, abdominal pain, diarrhea, violent headache, renal failure, hemiplegia or double hemiplegia, with mental disorders, functional impairment, altered consciousness including coma, usually terminating in sudden death. The process can last between 1 and 3 months, with hyperthermia in some case. The electroencephalogram may be abnormal (Bogaert et al., 1955). Microfilaria will be present in CSF and usually in peripheral blood, with albuminuria, red blood cells and leukocytes in urine (Lukiana et al., 1996).

7. Treatment of loiasis encephalopathy

Treatment of *L. loa* encephalitis is based on nursing, nutritional support and re-hydration. According to Serious Adverse events (SEA) Experts in *Loa loa* endemic areas (Scientific working Group on SAE, 2003) Corticosteroids and antihistamines should be avoided. The reasons for avoidance of corticosteroids are the lack of evidence of efficacy for this condition and potential harmful effect; while the antihistaminic treatment should be avoid because of the lack of efficacy and they sedate patient with a neurologic condition, interfering with diagnosis and neurologic assessment. The protocol suggested here is based on that described by Gardon et al., 1999. It is based on vital monitoring (pulse, arterial pressure, temperature, consciousness (Glasgow score), hydration, complete neurological and clinical examination every hour then every three hours. When the patient is dehydrated and systolic pressure is below 9 cmHg: perfuse 500 ml of Ringer lactate solution over 30 min; if no improvement, continue to perfuse until systolic pressure reaches 10 cmHg and diuresis 1 ml/kg/hour. Perfuse 2000 ml of 5% glucose (including 6 g of NaCl, 3-4 g of KCl, 2 g of calcium) or mixt sera (with 4 g of KCl and 2 g of calcium) for 24 hours for an adult weighing 60 kg, or 500 ml every 6 hours (28 drops/minute). If dehydration persists, perfuse 1000 ml of these solutions over 8 hours, depending on clinical status. In case of fever, add 1 ml of solution per kilogram for each degree above 37°C. In case of coma, the treatment aim is to avoid bedsores, bronchial accumulation and intercurrent disorders, by mobilizing the patient every three hours and massages to prevent complications of decubitus; urinary probing, mouth care with sodium bicarbonate solution, and eye care with 9% NaCl. Pose of orpharyngeal canicle. If the Glasgow score is less than 10/15, transfer to a specialized intensive care unit. If recovery is slow, use gastric gavage with milk, soja.... Complementary examinations are necessary to rule out any other causes of coma (meningitis, hypo- or hyperglycemia, cerebral malaria, etc.), including thick blood smear (to search for *Loa loa* and malaria); glycemia, glycosuria, proteinuria and lumbar puncture (the liquid should be clear, but *Loa loa* microfilaria should be present between days 3 and 7 in *Loa loa* encephalitis). Removal of eye worm has been reported to cure spontaneous encephalitis (Kenney and Hewitt, 1950).

8. The mechanism of encephalopathy and risk factors in loiasis:

A high density of microfilaria (> 30000 mf/ml) seems to be the most plausible risk factor for *Loa loa* encephalopathy (Figure. 7). In addition, the genetic heterogeneity of this parasite could explain th e higher prevalence of encephalopathy in certain regions. However, parasites isolated in parts of Cameroon with a high prevalence of encephalopathy were not found to differ genetically from those found in other regions of Africa (Gabon and Nigeria) (Higazi et al., 2004). It has also been suggested that hybridization between simian and human strains of *Loa loa* may be a cofactor for encephalopathy, but this remains to be demonstrated. Although it is possible to cross human and simian strains of *Loa loa*, animal strains do not develop in humans, as demonstrated by implantation of simian adult parasites or injection of infective larvae (L3) in human volunteers (Duke, 2004; Nutman et al., 1991). Moreover, vectors of simian strains of *C. langi* and *C. centurionis* do not bite humans and tend to be active after dark. In contrast, human strains of *Loa loa* can be transmitted to non human primates, and hybrids of human and simian strains can be produced experimentally. However, the two sets of strains normally develop in different host-parasite systems (Fain, 1988), and such hybrids are unlikely to occur in natural conditions. A genetic predisposition to developing microfilaremia (Garcia et al., 1999) could also favor the onset of encephalitis in some cases. Coinfection by *Loa loa* and other parasites such as *Plasmodium* (Hartgers et al., 2006; Kamgno et al., 2008) bacteria (Bonnet et al., 1943; Cattan et al., 1960) and viruses (Cauchie et al., 1965), might cause lesions through which microfilaria could enter the nervous system and brain. However, it has been reported that treatment of such coinfections has little impact on the outcome of encephalitis (Kamgno et al., 2008). Finally, alcohol consumption has also been forwarded as a possible risk factor (scientific working group,2003).

The pathophysiologic mechanisms underlying encephalitis in patients with loaisis may involve massive microfilarial death, leading to vascular embolism and inflammation. Interactions with drugs and other substances (alcohol, drugs, dietary components, etc.) may also play a role, through competition for biological carrier molecules. Glycoprotein P, a component of the blood-brain barrier, plays a role in drug entry to the brain. Substance P deficiency could lead to a rise in drug concentrations in the brain, resulting in severe neurotoxicity. This deficiency could be caused by genetic polymorphism, deficient glycoprotein P production, or glycoprotein P inhibition. Indeed, severe neurological adverse effects of ivermectin are observed in CF-I mice, that are deficient in MDRIA glycoprotein P (Kwei et al., 1999). Several drug carrier molecules such as MDR, MRP, OATP and glycoprotein P have been detected on the apical and basolateral membranes of epithelial cells in cerebral capillary membranes (Cordon Cardo et al., 1989; Huai-Yun et al., 1998; Kusuhara et al., 1998; Gao et al., 1999). Glycoprotein P is the most widely studied of these molecules. The risk of encephalitis could also be influenced by genetic factors. Indeed, dogs homozygous for a 4-bp deletion of the *MDR1* gene (resulting in premature termination of glycoprotein P synthesis) are highly sensitive to ivermectin (Mealy et al., 2001). In addition, CFI mice exhibiting low glycoprotein P production are more sensitive to ivermectin neurotoxicity than their wild-type counterparts (Umbenhauer et al., 1997). In addition to the neurotoxicity of ivermectin accumulating in the brain, through a deficiency in glycoprotein P or other carriers, neurotoxicity may result from interactions between drugs competing for the same carrier binding site. Other glycoprotein P substrates may compete with ivermectin, leading to a reduction in ivermectin efflux from the brain. This has been demonstrated in mice treated with both ivermectin and cyclosporine (Marques-Santos et al., 1999). It is important to note that ivermectin and DEC both lead to progressive neurological complications in patients with high microfilaremia and also ocular lesions (retinal or subconjunctival hemorrhage) linked to microemboli created by the parasite. It therefore appears that the etiology of *Loa loa*-associated encephalitis associated with these two drugs is linked to clumping of dead microfilaria in vessels, leading to emboli and local vascular inflammation.

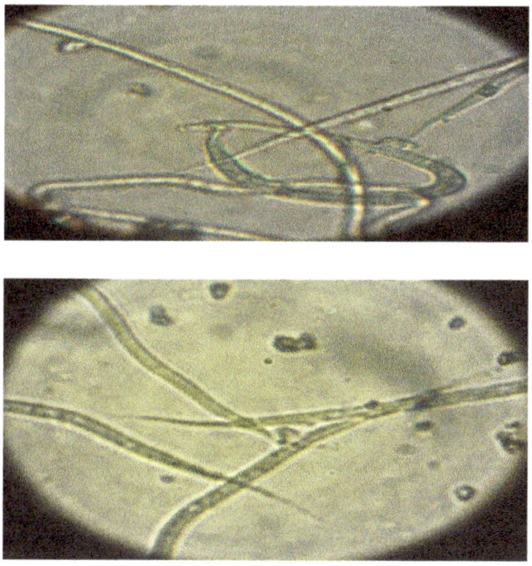

Fig. 7. Two views of *Loa loa* microfilariae in blood of an hypermicrofilaremic individual

It seems that the adult worm and microfilaria are both risk factors for spontaneous encephalitis. Adult worms have been implicated in the neuropsychological complications of loaisis in two European patients (Kenny & Hewitt, 1950). In both cases, extraction of the adult worm led to a clinical improvement and to a decline in eosinophilia from 56-50% to 3%. Location of adult worms in the subarachidonic space at the base of the brain has also been implicated in neuropsychological complications (Bertrand-Fontaine et al., 1948). The abundance of microfilaria is an important risk factor, because of their mobility in small vessels and capillaries and outside the circulatory apparatus. How exactly microfilaria cross the blood-brain barrier remains to be determined. As stated above, coinfection by other pathogens (such as *Plasmodium*) could weaken this barrier, leading to vascular lesions that allow microfilaria to enter the brain. Head trauma could have a similar effect. In well-documented cases of encephalitis (Bogaert et al., 1955), it has been shown that microfilaria cross the vascular barrier and penetrate into deep tissues, where focal necrosis occurs around dead parasites. These foci are surrounded by inflammation and fibrosis, and giant multinucleated cells arise in the spleen, liver and brain. Aggregates of neurological

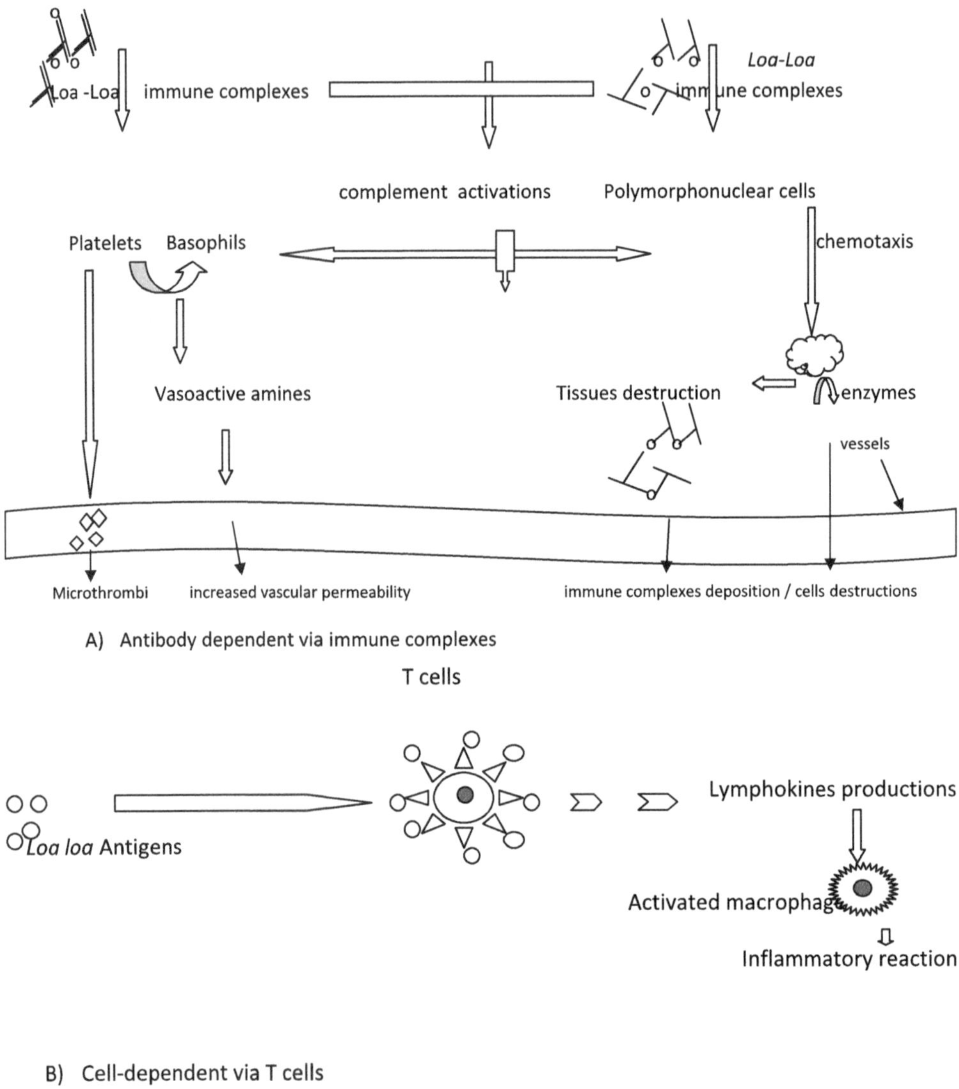

Fig. 8. Potential immunological mechanisms for induction of *Loa loa* encephalitis

lymphocytes and histiocytes may form in cardiac tissue, with a few leukocytes close to microfilaria in extracranial organs. There is no evidence of phagocytosis. Alternatively, complications could be due to obstruction caused by microfilarial and to the toxicity of their metabolic products (Weil et al., 1926).

The immune response could also play a role in encephalitis due to *Loa loa*, for example through the formation of circulating immune complexes that deposit in tissues and vessels. This could result in complement activation and influx of polymorphonuclear cells and basophils, followed by the release of vasoactive amines, causing retraction of endothelial cells and increased vascular permeability. Polymorphonuclear cells that fail to phagocytose deposits of immune complexes may degranulate, causing local tissue damage (Fig. 8A). The large amount of antigens associated with abundant microfilariosis may persistently stimulate an inefficient antibody response resembling type III hypersensitivity. Chronic lesions induced by such phenomena could lead to vessel destruction and encephalitis when they occur in the brain, or nephropathies when the kidneys are affected. Cardiac and renal involvement have both been described in loaisis. Alternatively, T lymphocytes sensitized by *Loa loa* antigens (Fig. 8B) could release cytokines, thus attracting activated macrophages. With the persistence of *Loa loa* antigens, activated macrophages could trigger chronic granulomatous reactions resembling type IV hypersensitivity. Such responses are observed in chronic infections such as schistosomiasis (Brian et al., 1983). Granulomas have been observed in the brain of a person infected by *Loa loa*. These observations suggest that type III and IV hypersensitivity reactions could be involved in the development of *Loa loa* encephalopathy. Finally, it is conceivable that spontaneous encephalitis is the end result of a long process involving deposits of immune complexes in several deep organs, the most sensitive being the brain and kidneys. Cofactors (drugs, coinfection, etc.) could accelerate this process.

9. Ongoing and future directions

Administration of filaricidal drugs in massively infected patients often results in encephalitis, in the absence of any other known cause. The mechanism underlying encephalitis in this setting is unclear. Microfilaria have been found in *parasite*-infected animal brains (Hashimoto, 1939, quoted byJanssens,1952), including those coinfected by trypanosomes (Peruzzi, 1928). Consequently, the presence of *Loa loa* microfilaria in the brain cannot alone explain the onset of encephalitis. The heterogeneous nature of the associated clinical manifestations poses problems for prevention and timely patient management. Studies based on an experimental model, such as non human primates infected by human isolates, could help to identify predictive markers of *Loa loa* encephalitis and specific clinical complications (Orihel & Ebrehard 1985; Duke, 1960). Indeed, clinical expression of this filariosis is similar in humans and non human primates (Pinder et al., 1994), and hypermicrofilaremia can be reproduced in non human primates. Despite the existence of potent microfilaricidal drugs (DEC and ivermectin), new macrofilaricides or compounds capable of inducing a gradual decline in microfilaria without triggering encephalitis are needed. Most cases of encephalitis have been reported in Cameroon during mass treatment with ivermectin, but similar cases may go unreported in other endemic regions, especially if they occur in rural settings without adequate medical facilities. Specific studies are needed to evaluate the prevalence and characteristics of *Loa loa* encephalopathy in endemic areas. Studies of polymorphisms of human drug carrier molecules and proinflammatory cytokine synthesis are also necessary. As all current treatments, including albendazole (Blum et al., 2001), can induce encephalitis in highly microfilaremic patients, the antifilarial activity of African traditional herbal remedies may be of interest. Most of these plants are well accepted and tolerated, and preliminary cytotoxicity results are encouraging (Mengome et al., 2010). There is currently no evidence of the existence of a symbiont in *Loa loa* (McGarry et al., 2003; Buttner et al., 2003), that might warrant concurrent antibiotic therapy for patients with loasis. Because *Loa loa* infection often goes undiagnosed, cases of encephalitis in *Loa loa* endemic areas may be attributed to viruses, bacteria or other parasites. This underdiagnosis is due partly to the lack of a simple, specific and rapid diagnostic test available at points of treatment for use by non specialists. Some candidate antigens have been identified and produced (Azzibrouck et al., 2010). Although spontaneous encephalitis may be caused by the adult worm, life-threatening forms are generally due to massive death of microfilaria. However, in endemic areas, about one-third of infected persons are microfilaremic and only 5% are strongly microfilaremic, the remainder being amicrofilaremic (Van Hoegaerden et al., 1986; Dupont et al., 1988). The fact that these latter persons live permanently in areas of continuous transmission without becoming microfilaremic points to the existence of a natural control mechanism. Further studies of these subjects could help to find ways of clearing microfilaria without triggering encephalitis. Noteworthy immunological differences have been found between microfilaremic and amicrofilaremic subjects. The latter patients exhibit a stronger immune response against *Loa loa* antigens, both qualitatively and quantitatively (Pinder et al., 1988; Pinder et al., 1992; Egwang et al., 1988a; Egwang et al., 1988b;Egwang et al.,1989; Akue et al., 1997; Akue et al., 1998; Baize et al.,1997; Akue & Devaney, 2002). Finally, more work is needed to determine the role of immune complex deposition in the onset of encephalitis in patients with loaisis.

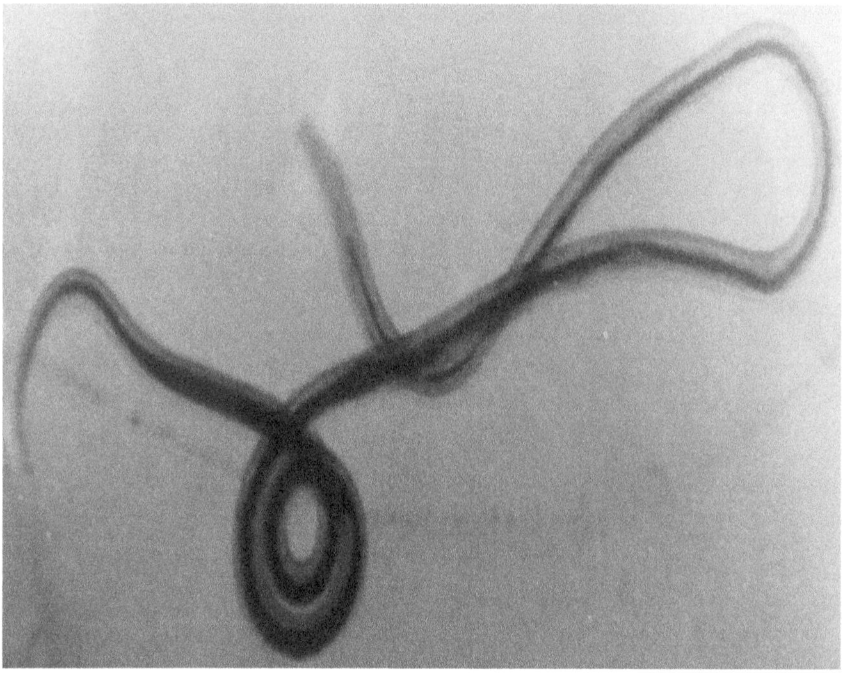

Fig. 9. *Loa loa* adult worm

10. Conclusion

The risk of *Loa loa* encephalitis must be taken in to account when managing patients in and from endemic areas. This severe form can occur spontaneously or be triggered by antifilarial treatment in highly microfilaremic patients. The underlying mechanism appears to include embolism following massive death of microfilaria, genetic polymorphism of biological drug carriers, and immunological processes. More work is needed to develop a diagnostic test, as well as new drugs and possibly a vaccine. Further characterization of *Loa loa* encephalitis in endemic regions and in animal models is needed to understand the mechanisms underlying the onset and outcome of encephalitis in patients with loaisis.

11. Acknowledgement

The work on filariae *Loa loa* is supported by CIRMF. CIRMF is sponsored by total Gabon, Gabonese state and Ministère de la cooperation Française. We thank Ms Line Mengome, Hubert Moukana and Mbou Moutsimbi Roger Antoine for their assistance during the preparation of the manuscript.

12. References

Abel L, Joly v, Yeni P, Carbon C. (1986). Apheresis in the management of loiasis with high microfilariaemia and renal disease. *British Medical Journal* , Vol. 292, No. 4 January 1986) pp 24, ISSN

Andi JJ, FF Bishara, OO Soyinka. (1981). Relation of severe eosinophilia and microfilariasis to chronic African endomyocardial fibrosis. *British Heart Journal*, Vol.45, No. 6, (June 1981), pp. 672-680, ISSN:

Akue Jean Paul, Devaney Eileen. (2002). Transmission Intensity Affects Both Atigen - Specific and Nonspecific T-cell Proliferative Responses in *Loa loa* Infection . *Infection and Immunity*, Vol. 70,pp.1475-1480,ISSN: 0019-9567

Akue JP, Egwang TG, Devaney E. (1994). High level of parasite specific IgG4 in the absence of microfilaremia in Loa loa infection. *Tropical Medicine and Parasitology* ,Vol.45,No. 3, pp. 246-248, ISSN 9177-2392

Akue Jean Paul, Marcel Hommel, Eileen Devaney. (1997). high levels of Parasite-Specific IgG1 correlate with the amicrofilaremic State in *Loa loa* Infection. *Journal of Infectious Diseases*, Vol. 175, pp:158-163 ISSN: 0022-1899

Akue JP Hommel M, Devaney E. (1998). IgG subclass recognition of *Loa loa* antigens and their correlation with clinical status in individuals from Gabon. *Parasite Immunology* , Vol. 20,pp.387-393,ISSN:0141-9838

Akue JP, Hommel M, Devaney E. (1996). Markers of *Loa loa* infection in permanent residents of a loiasis endemic area of Gabon. *Transactions of the Royal Society of Tropical Medicine and Hygiene,* Vol. 90,pp. 115- 118, ISSN:

Ajuh PM, Akue JP, Boutin P, Everaere S Egwang TG. (1995). *Loa loa*: structural diversity of a 15kDa repetitive antigen. *Experimental Parasitology* ,Vol. 81, pp.145-153, ISSN:0014-4894

Baize S, Wahl G, Soboslay P T, Egwang T G, Geaorges AJ. (1997). T helper responsiveness in human *Loa loa* infection: defective specific proliferation and cytokine production by CD4+ T cells from microfilaraemic subjects compared with amicrofilaraemics. *Clinical and Experimental Immunology*, Vol. 108,pp.272-278,ISSN:00099104

Barua P., N Barua, NK Hazarka, S Dia. (2005). *Loa loa* in the anterior chamber of the eye: A case report. *Indian journal of Medical Microbiolog,* Vol. 23, pp 59-60,

Bariety J, Barbier M, Laigre Mc et al. (1967). Proteinurie et loase. Etude histologique, optique et electronique d'une cas. *Bulletin et Memoires de la Societé Médicale des Hopitaux de Paris,* Vol. 118, pp 1015-1025

Bertrand-Fontaine, Schneider, Wolfromm, Cognard. (1948). Un cas de filariose cérébrale (double hémiplégie au cours d'une filariose à F. *loa). Bulletin et Memoires de la Société Medicale des Hopitaux de Paris,* Vol. 32-33, N° 5, pp 1092-1095

Bonnet M.(1943). Réflexions sur un cas de méningite aigue à microfilaria Loa . *Médecine Tropicale,* Vol.3, (Mars, 1943),pp. 273-277, ISSN : 0025-682X

Burbelo P D, Roshan Ramanathan, Klion AD, Iadarola,M J and Nutman TB. (2008). Rapid, novel, specific, high-throughput assay for diagnosis of *Loa loa* infection. *Journal of Clinical Microbiology,* Vol. 46, No 7, (July, 2008), pp.2298-2304, ISSN: 0095-1137, online ISSN: 1098-660X

Buttner DW, Wanji S, Bazzocchi, Bain and Fischer P. (2003). Obligatory symbiotic Wolbachia endobacteria are absent from *Loa loa* . *Filaria Journal,* Vol.2 ,ISSN:1475-2883

Brian R, Ott, N. Peter Libbey, Richard J. Ryter, Wayne M. Trebbin. (1983). Treatment of Schistosome -Induced Glomerulonephritis A cas report and Review of the Literature. *Archives of Internal Medicine.* Vol. 143 No. 7 (July 1983), pp1477-1479

Blampain Azzibrouck G Akue JP, Richard Lenoble D. (2010). Production and immunological characterization of a recombinant subunit of *Loa loa* polyprotein antigen. *Parasitology,* Vol.137, pp.1119-1128, ISSN:0031-1820

Blum M, Wiestner A, Fuhr P and Hatz C. (2001). Encephalopathy following *Loa loa* treatment with albendazole. *Acta Tropica,* Vol.78, pp. 63-65, ISSN: 0001-706X

Cattan R, Frumusan P, Levy C. (1960). Encephalopathie filarienne. *Bulletin et Mémoires de la Société Médicale des Hopitaux de Paris,* Vol. 7,pp. 808-810

Cauchie C, Rutsaert J, Thys O, Bonnyns M, Perrier O. (1965). Encephalite à *Loa loa,* traitée par l'association de cortisone et de carbamazine. *Rev Belg Pathol Med Exp.* ,Vol. 31, pp. 232-244

Carbonez G, Van De Sompel W, Zeyen T. (2002). Subconjunctival *Loa loa* Worm : Case Report. *Bulletin Société Belge Ophtalmologi,e* Vol. 283, pp 45-48

Carayon A, Collomb H, Sankalé M. (1959). Du polymorphisme des complications neuropsychiques des filarioses (A propos de quatre observations personnelles dont deux inédites). *Bulletin Société Médecine Afrique Noire Langue Française,* Vol.4, pp.299-312, ISSN : 0049-1101

Cordon - Cardo C, O'Brien JP, Casals D, Ritman Graver L, Beidler Jl, Melamed MR and Bertino JR. (1989). Multidrug resistance gene P-glycoprotein is expressed by endothelial cells at blood-brain barrier sites. *Proceedings of the National Academic of Science USA* Vol. 86, pp. 695-698

Churchill DR,Morris C,Fakoya A, Wrigt SG, and Davidson RN. (1996). Clinical and laboratory features of patients with loiasis (*Loa loa* filariasis) in The UK. *Journal of infection,* vol.33, No 2, (September, 1996),pp. 103-109, ISSN. 0163-4453

Crew W, and Williams P. (1964). Studies on the control of the vectors of loiasis in west Africa. Effect of low concentrations of dieldrin in the mud of natural tabanid breeding sites in the rain forest of the Cameroons. *Annals of Tropical Medicine Parasitology,*Vol. 58,pp.343-346, ISSN:0003-4983

Duke BOL. (2004). Failed attempts at experimental transplantation and transmission of nocturnally-periodic simian Loa from monkey to man. *Filaria Journal* , Vol. 3, No.5 (29 July 2004), doi: 10.1186/1475-2883-3-5

Duke B O L. (1960). Studies on loiasis in monkeys. II-The population dynamics of the microfilariae of loa in experimentallly infected drills (*Mandrillus leucophaeus*). *Annals of Tropical Medicine and Parasitology*,Vol. 54, pp.15-31, ISSN: 0003-4983

Duke B O L. (1957). Experimental Transmission of *Loa loa* from man to monkey. *Nature*,Vol. 179, pp.1357-1358, ISSN: 0028-0836

Dupont A, Zue-Ndong, J and Pinder M. (1988). Common occurrence of amicrofilaremic *Loa loa* filariasis within the endemic region. *Transactions of the Royal Society of Tropical Medicine and Hygiene*, Vol.8, No. 5, (September, -October 1988),pp.730, ISSN: 0035-9203

Egwang TG, Akue JP, Dupont A, Pinder M. (1988a). The identification and partial characterization of an immunodominant 29-31kilodalton surface antigen expressed by adult worms of the human filarial *Loa loa*. *Molecular and Biochemichal Parasitology*,Vol. 31, pp. 263-272, ISSN: 0166-6851

Egwang TG, Dupont A, Pinder M. (1989). Differential recognition of *Loa loa* antigens by sera of human subjects from a loiasis endemic zone. *American Journal of Tropical Medicine and Hygiene,* Vol. 41, pp. 664-673, ISSN:0002-9637

Egwang TG, Dupont A, Akue JP, Pinder M .(1988b). Biochemical and immunochemical characterization of surface and excretory-secretory antigens of *Loa loa* microfilariae. *Molecular and Biochemical Parasitology*,Vol. 31,pp.251-261, ISSN: 0166-6851

Ekobo Same, Same-Voisin, Eben-Moussi, Ongmagne. (1981). A propos d'un cas de meningo-encephalite filarienne à *Loa loa*. Rappels des critères de diagnostic de certitude. *Afrique Médecine* 20 : 359-361

Fain A. (1978) . Les problèmes actuels de la loase. *Bulletin de l'Organisation Mondiale de la Santé* , vol.56, No. 2,(June ,1978), pp.155-167, ISSN. 0047-96

Fain A.(1981). Epidemiologie et pathologie de la loase. *Annales de la Société Belge de Médecine Tropicale,* vol.61,pp. 277-285, ISSN. 0365-6527

Gao B, steiger B, Noe B, Fritschy JM and Meier PJ. (1999). Localisation of the organic anion transporting polypeptide 2(Oatp2) in capillary endothelium and choroids plexus epithelium of rat brain. *Journal of Histochemistry and Cytochemistry*, Vol. 47,pp. 1255-1263, ISSN: 0022-1554

Garcia A. L Abel, M. Cot, P. Richard, S. Ranque, J. Feingold, F. Demenais, M. Boussinesq and J-P Chippaux. (1999). Genetic epidemiology of host predisposition microfilaremia in human loiasis. *Tropical Medecine and International Health* Vol. 4, No.8, pp.565-574.

Gallais P, Collomb H, Guedel J. (1954).Les manifestations neuropsychique des filarioses. *Médecine Tropicale* Vol.14, pp.663-677, ISSN: 0025-682X

Gardon J, Kamgno J, Fobi G, Essiené, A; Ntep M, Gaxotte P, Boussinesq M, Kollo B. (1999). Depistage , identification et prise en charge des effets secondaires graves imputables à la loase et au traitement par ivermectine au cours des campagnes de lutte contre l' onchocercose. *Bulletin de Liaison Documentation de l' OCEAC* Vol. 32,No.1,pp.37-52, ISSN :0225-5352

Gerd D. Burchard, Ulrike Reimold-Jehle, Volker Burkle, Harald Kretschmer, M Vierbuchen, Paul Racz, and Ying Lu. (1996). Splenectomy for Suspected Malignant Lymphoma in Two Patients with Loiasis. *Clinical Infectious Disease,s* Vol. 23, No. 5 (November 1996), pp 979-982

Grieve, R.B. Eberhard M.L, Jacobson RH, and T C Orihel. (1985). *Loa loa* antibody responses in experimentally infected baboons and rhesus monkeys. *Tropical Medicine and Parasitology*, Vol. 36,pp.225-229

Gouteux JP, Noireau F, Staak C. (1989). The host preference of *Chrysops silacea* and *C. dimidiate* (Diptera:Tabanidae) in an endemic area of *Loa loa* in the Congo. *Annals of Tropical Medicine and Parasitology* Vol.83, pp.167-172, ISSN: 0003-4983

Hartgers Fc and Yazdanbakhsh M. (2006). Co infection of helminthes and malaria: modulation of the immune responses to malaria. *Parasite Immunology*, Vol. 28, No. 10, (October 2006), pp. 497-506

Hee-Yoon Cho, Yoon-Jung Lee, Sun-Young Shin, Hyun-Ouk Song, Myoung-Hee Ahn, Jae-Sook Ryu. (2008). Subconjunctival *Loa loa* with Calabar Swelling. *Journal of Korean Medical Science*, Vol. 23, No. 4, pp 731-733, doi: 10.3346/Kms.2008.23.4.731

Higazi Tarig B, Amy D Klion, Michel Boussinesq, and Thomas R Unnasch. (2003). Genetic heterogeneity in *Loa loa* parasites from southern Cameroon: A preliminary study . *Filaria Journal*, Vol. 3 No. 4 (29 June 2004), doi: 10.1186/1475-2883-3-4

Huai-Yun H,Secrest DT, Mark KS, Carney D, Brandquist C, Elmquist WF and Miller DW. (1998). Expression of multidrug resistance-associated protein (MRP) in brain microvessel endothelial cells. *Biochemical and Biophysical Research Communication*, Vol. 243,pp.816-820, ISSN:0006-291X

Janssens P G.(1952). Remarques au sujet de la possibilité de manifestations nerveuses ou psychiques causes par les filarioses.

Kamgno J, Michel Boussinesq, François Labrousse, Blaise Nkegoum, Bjorn I. Thylefors, and Charles D . Mackenzie (2008). Case Report : Encephalopathy after Ivermectin Treament in a patient Infected with *Loa loa* and *Plasmodium* spp . *American Journal of Tropical Medicine and Hygiene*. Vol. 78, No. 4, pp.546-551

Kenny M and Hewitt R. (1950). Psychoneurotic disturbances in filariasis, and their relief by removal of worms or treatment with hetrazan. *American Journal of Tropical Medicine and Hygien,e* Vol 30, pp 893

Kenney M, and R Hewitt. (1950). Psychoneurotic disturbances in filariasis, and their relief by removed of adult worms or treatment with hetrazan. *American journal of Tropical Medicine and Hygiene*, Vol. 30, No. 6,pp. 895-899

Kershaw, W E. (1950). Studies on the epidemiology of filariasis in West Africa, with special reference to British Camerouns and the Niger delta 1. Methods of survey for infections with *Loa loa* and *Acanthocheilonema perstans*. *Annals of Tropical Medicine and Parasitology* , Vol. 44,pp. 361-378, ISSN: 0003-4983

Kivits M. (1952). Quatre cas d'encéphalite mortelle avec invasion du liquide céphalo-rachidien par Microfilaria Loa. *Annales de la Société Belge de Médecine Tropicale*, Vol. 32, pp.235-242, ISSN : 0365-6527

Kusuhara H, Suzuki H, Naito M, Tsuro T and Sugiyama Y. (1998). Characterization of efflux transport of organic anions in a mouse brain capillary endothelial cell line. *Journal of Pharmacology and Experimental Therapeutic*, Vol. 285, pp.1260-1265, ISSN:0022-3565

Klion AD, Vijaykumar A, Oei T, Martin B and Nutman TB. (2003). Serum immunoglobulin G4 antibodies to the recombinant antigen L1-SXP-1 are highly specific for *Loa loa* infection. *Journal of Infectious Diseases*, Vol.187, pp.128-133, ISSN:0022-1899

Klion AD, Moussougbodji A, Sadeler B C, Ottesen E A, Nutman T B. (1991). Loiasis in endemic and non endemic populations: immunologically mediated differences in clinical presentation. *Journal of Infectious Diseases* Vol.163,pp.1318-1325, ISSN: 0022-1899

Kwei G Y, R F Alvaro, Q Chen, H J Jenkins, C E A C Hop, C A Keohane, V T Ly, J R Strauss, R W Wang, Z Wang, T R Pippert, and D R Umbenhauer. (1999). Disposition of ivermectin and cyclosporin A in CF-I mice deficient in MDR1A p-glycoprotein. *Drug Metabolism and Disposition*, Vol. 27 No. 5, pp. 581-587

Marques-Santos LF, Bernardo RR, de Paula EF and Rumjanek VM. (1999). Cyclosporin A and trifluperazine, two resistance modulating agents, increase ivermectin neurotoxicity in mice. *Pharmacology and Toxicology* Vol. 84, pp. 125-129. ISSN: 0901-9928

Mealey KL, Bentjen SA and Waiting DK. (2001). Frequency of the mutant MDRI allele associated with ivermectin sensitivity in a sample population of collies from the northwestern United States. *American Journal of Veterinary Research* Vol.16, pp.89-94, ISSN: 0002-9645

McGarry HF, Pfarr K, Egerton G, Hoerauf A, Jean Paul Akue , Peter Enyong , Samuel Wanji ,Sabine L. Klager , Albert E Bianco, Nick J.Beeching, and Mark Taylor. (2003). Evidence against *Wolbachia* symbiosis in *Loa loa*. *Filaria Journal*.Vol. 2, ISSN:1475-2883, doi:10.1186/1475-2883-2-9

Mengome Line Edwige, Akue Jean Paul, Souza Alain, Feuya Tchoua Guy Raymond, Nsi Emvo Edouard. (2010). *In vitro* activities of plant extracts on human *Loa loa* isolates and cytotoxicity of eukaryotic cells. *Parasitology Research,* Vol.107,pp.643-650, ISSN: 0031-1820

Mongin.(1770). Observations sur un ver trouvé dans la conjonctive a Maribou, ile Saint Domingue. *Journal de Medicine Chirurgie Pharmacie etc* (Paris), vol.32, pp.338-339

Muylle Ludo, Henri Taelman, Robert Moldenhauer, Roger Van Brabant, Marc E Peetermans. (1983). Usefulness of apheresis to extract microfilarias in management of loiasis. *British Medical Journal,* Vol. 287, N° 20, (August 1983), pp 519-520

Nutman T B. (1991). Experimental Infection of Human with Filariae. *Clinical Infectious Diseases,* Vol. 13, No. 5, pp. 1018-1022, doi: 10.1093/clinids/13.5.1018

Nutman TB, Miller KD, Mulligan M, Ottesen EA. (1986). *Loa loa* infection in temporary residents of endemic regions; recognition of hyperresponsive syndrome with characteristic clinical manifestations. *Journal of Infectious Diseases,* vol.154, No 1, (July, 1986),pp.10-18, ISSN: 0022-1899

Orihel TC and Eberhard ML. (1985). *Loa loa*: the development and course of patency in experimentally-infected primates. *Tropical Medicine and Parasitology* ,Vol.36, pp. 215-224, ISSN 0177-2392

Orihel TC and Lowrie RC. (1975a). *Loa loa*: the development to the infective stage in American deerfly, *Chrysop atlanticus. American Journal of Tropical Medicine and Hygiene*, vol. 24, No. 4 (July,1975) pp.610-615, ISSN : 0002-9637

Orihel TC, and PJ Moore. (1975b). *Loa loa* : Experimental infection in two species of African primates. *American Journal of Tropical Medicine and Hygiene,* Vol. 24, No. 4 (July, 1975), pp. 606-609, ISSN: 0002-9637

Pal Varhaug. (2009). Subconjunctival *Loa loa*: first case report from Norway. *Acta Ophthalmologica*, pp. 929-930, doi:10.1111/j.1755-3768.2009.01600.X

Perruzi, M. (1928). Une filariose cérébrale chez cinq singes atteints de méningo-encephalite à trypanosomes. *Rapport final de la commission Interne de la S.D.N pour l'étude de la trypanosomiase humaine.* Genève, pp322

Pilay VKG, Kirch E, Kurtzman NA. (1973). Glomerulopathy associated with filarial loiasis *JAMA* ,Vol. 225, pp. 179

Pinder M, Leclerc A, Everaere S. (1992). Antibody-dependent cell -mediated immune reactions to *Loa loa* microfilaraemic subjects. *Parasite immunology,* Vol. 14, pp.541-556, ISSN:0141-9838

Pinder M, Dupont A, Egwang TG. (1988). Identification of a surface antigen on *Loa loa* microfilariae the recognition of which correlates with the amicrofilaraemic state in man. *Journal of Immunology,* Vol.141, pp.2480-2486, ISSN:0022-1767

Pinder M, Everaere S, Roelants G E. (1994). *Loa loa*: Immunological responses during experimental infections in mandrills (*Mandrillus sphinx*). *Experimental Parasitology,* Vol. 79, pp. 126-136, ISSN: 0014-4894

Scientific Working Group on serious adverse events in *Loa loa* endemic areas. (2003). Report of a Scientific Working Group on Serious Adverse Events following Mectizan® treatment of onchocerciasis in *Loa loa* endemic areas. *Filaria Journal,* Vol. 2, (October 24, 2003) pp Suppl 1: S2

Toussain D, Danis P. (1965). Retinopathy in generalized *Loa loa* filariasis. A clinicopathological study. *Archive Ophthalmolog,y* Vol.74,pp. 470-476, ISSN: 0003-9950

Touré FS, Egwang TG, wahl G, Millet P, Bain O, and Georges A J. (1997). Species-specific sequence in the repeat 3 region of the gene encoding a putative *Loa loa* allergen: A diagnostic tool for occult loaisis. *American Journal of Tropical Medicine and Hygiene* ,Vol.60, pp.50-57, ISSN: 0002-9637

Tuna Lukiana , Madone Mandina, Nanituma H Situakibanza, Marcel M Mbula, Bompeka F Lepira, Wobin T Odio, Kamgno Joseph and Boussinesq Michel. (2006). A possible case of spontaneous *Loa loa* encephalopathy associated with a glomerulopathy. *Filaria Journal* ,Vol. 5, pp. 1-7, ISSN: 1475-2883

Umbenhauer DR, Lankas GR, Pippers TR, Wise LD, Carwright ME, Hall SJ, and Beare CM. (1997). Identification of the a P-glycoprotein-deficient subpopulation in the CF-I mouse strain using a restriction fragment length polymorphism. *Toxicology and Applied Pharmacology,* Vol. 146, pp. 88-94, ISSN: 0041-008X

Van Bogaert, L, Dubois, A, Janssens P,Radermecker J, Tverdy G and Wanson M. (1955). Encephalitis in *Loa loa* filariasis. *Journal of Neurology, Neurosurgery and Psychiatry,*Vol. 18, No. 2, (May, 1955), pp. 103-119

Van Hoegaerden M, Chabaud B , Akue JP, Ivanoff B. (1987). Filariasi due to *Loa loa* and *Mansonella perstans* : distribution in the region of Okondja, Haut Ogooue Province, Gabon with parasitological and serological follow-up over one year. *Transaction of Royal Society of Tropical Medicine and Hygiene,* Vol. 81,pp. 441-446 ISSN:035-9203

Vijay D Khetan. (2007). Subconjunctival *Loa loa* with calabar swelling. *Indian Journal Ophthalmology,* Vol. 55 No. 2, pp.165-166, doi: 10.4103/0301-4738.30727

Wail S S, Popow P, and Prjadko E. (1926). Uber die pathologisch-anatomischen Veranderungen bei Filariosis *Virchows Archiv,* Vol. 259 ,N° 3, (March 1926), pp 642-646

Williams P (1963) Studies on the control of vectors of loiasis in West Africa. III: comparison of the toxicities of DDT, dieldrin, aldrin and gamma-BHC to late-instan Tabanid larvae. *Annals of Tropical Medicine and Parasitology* Vol. 57,pp.182-190, ISSN:0003-4983

Permissions

The contributors of this book come from diverse backgrounds, making this book a truly international effort. This book will bring forth new frontiers with its revolutionizing research information and detailed analysis of the nascent developments around the world.

We would like to thank Sergey Tkachev, for lending his expertise to make the book truly unique. He has played a crucial role in the development of this book. Without his invaluable contribution this book wouldn't have been possible. He has made vital efforts to compile up to date information on the varied aspects of this subject to make this book a valuable addition to the collection of many professionals and students.

This book was conceptualized with the vision of imparting up-to-date information and advanced data in this field. To ensure the same, a matchless editorial board was set up. Every individual on the board went through rigorous rounds of assessment to prove their worth. After which they invested a large part of their time researching and compiling the most relevant data for our readers. Conferences and sessions were held from time to time between the editorial board and the contributing authors to present the data in the most comprehensible form. The editorial team has worked tirelessly to provide valuable and valid information to help people across the globe.

Every chapter published in this book has been scrutinized by our experts. Their significance has been extensively debated. The topics covered herein carry significant findings which will fuel the growth of the discipline. They may even be implemented as practical applications or may be referred to as a beginning point for another development. Chapters in this book were first published by InTech; hereby published with permission under the Creative Commons Attribution License or equivalent.

The editorial board has been involved in producing this book since its inception. They have spent rigorous hours researching and exploring the diverse topics which have resulted in the successful publishing of this book. They have passed on their knowledge of decades through this book. To expedite this challenging task, the publisher supported the team at every step. A small team of assistant editors was also appointed to further simplify the editing procedure and attain best results for the readers.

Our editorial team has been hand-picked from every corner of the world. Their multi-ethnicity adds dynamic inputs to the discussions which result in innovative outcomes. These outcomes are then further discussed with the researchers and contributors who give their valuable feedback and opinion regarding the same. The feedback is then collaborated with the researches and they are edited in a comprehensive manner to aid the understanding of the subject.

Apart from the editorial board, the designing team has also invested a significant amount of their time in understanding the subject and creating the most relevant covers. They scrutinized every image to scout for the most suitable representation of the subject and create an appropriate cover for the book.

The publishing team has been involved in this book since its early stages. They were actively engaged in every process, be it collecting the data, connecting with the contributors or procuring relevant information. The team has been an ardent support to the editorial, designing and production team. Their endless efforts to recruit the best for this project, has resulted in the accomplishment of this book. They are a veteran in the field of academics and their pool of knowledge is as vast as their experience in printing. Their expertise and guidance has proved useful at every step. Their uncompromising quality standards have made this book an exceptional effort. Their encouragement from time to time has been an inspiration for everyone.

The publisher and the editorial board hope that this book will prove to be a valuable piece of knowledge for researchers, students, practitioners and scholars across the globe.

List of Contributors

Colleen Mikelson and Sean Richards
University of Tennessee Chattanooga, United States of America

Maria Caramelli, Maria Domenica Pintore, Cristiana Maurella, Elena Bozzetta, Cristina Casalone and Barbara Iulini
Istituto Zooprofilattico Sperimentale of Piemonte, Liguria and Valle D'Aosta, Italy

Carlo Cantile
Department of Animal Pathology, University of Pisa, Italy

Gualtiero Gandini
Department of Veterinary Medical Sciences of the University of Bologna, Italy

Maria Teresa Capucchio and Antonio D'angelo
Department of Animal Pathology, University of Turin, Italy

Arianna Calistri
Department of Histology, Microbiology and Medical Biotechnologies University of Padova, Italy

Melanie Denizot, Vincent G. Thon-Hon, Shiril Kumar and Philippe Gasque
GRI/IRG, Immunopathology and Infectious Disease Research Grouping (IRG, GRI), EA4517, University, CHR Felix Guyon and CYROI of La Reunion, France

Jim W. Neal
Neuropathology Laboratory, Dept of Histopathology, Cardiff University Medical School., CF14 4XN, UK

Feyzi Birol Sarica
Başkent University, Faculty of Medicine, Department of Neurosurgery, Turkey

Hideto Fukushi and Tokuma Yanai
Gifu University, Japan

Nicole A. Renner, Andrew A. Lackner and Andrew G. MacLean
Tulane National Primate Research Center, Program in Neuroscience, Covington, USA

Tokuma Yanai, Atsushi Kodama, Hiroki Sakai, Hideto Fukushi, Takeshi Kuraishi, Seisaku Hattori and Chieko Kai
The University of Tokyo, Gifu University, Japan

Pierre J. Talbot, Marc Desforges, Elodie Brison and Hélène Jacomy
Laboratory of Neuroimmunovirology, INRS-Institut Armand-Frappier, Laval (Québec), Canada

Fernandez-Muñoz R., Duque B.M, Serrano-Pardo A., Muñoz-Alia M.A., Porras-Mansilla R., and Celma M.L.

Carabaña J., Caballero M and Liton P.B.
Duke University Medical Center, Durham, NC, USA

Ortego J.
Animal Health Research Center (CISA-INIA), Valdeolmos, Madrid, Spain

Martin-Cortes A.
Complutense University of Madrid, Madrid, Spain

Alvarez-Cermeño J.C.
Neurology Department, Ramón y Cajal University Hospital, Madrid, Spain

Slobodan Paessler and Katherine Taylor
University of Texas Medical Branch, United States of America

Brett W. Petersen and Charles E. Rupprecht
Centers for Disease Control and Prevention, Atlanta, GA, USA

Yaowalark Sukthana
Department of Protozoology, Faculty of Tropical Medicine, Mahidol University, Thailand

Jacob Lorenzo-Morales, Carmen Mª Martín-Navarro, Enrique Martínez-Carretero, José E. Piñero and Basilio Valladares
University Institute of Tropical Diseases and Public Health of the Canary Islands, University of La Laguna, Tenerife, Canary Islands, Spain

Chandirasegaran Massilamany and Jay Reddy
University of Nebraska-Lincoln, School of Veterinary Medicine and Biomedical Sciences, USA

Jean Paul Akue
International Center For Medical Research Franceville (CIRMF), Gabon